Prescription Drugs
and
Medical Terms

BROCKHAMPTON PRESS
LONDON

This edition published 1995 by Brockhampton Press,
a member of Hodder Headline PLC Group

ISBN 1 86019 082 6

2 4 6 8 10 9 7 5 3

Printed and bound in the UK

INTRODUCTION

This listing of prescription medicines provides an insight into the complexity of pharmaceutical preparations and medical diagnosis. It is not, however, intended as a tool for self-diagnosis or self-prescription and can in no way replace the medical practitioner or pharmacist. The book enables the patient to appreciate the vast array of medicines available and understand the likely action and effects of a particular medication.

Each entry provides the name, manufacturer and salient details for each drug. Medical terms used are defined in the dictionary section or, failing that, in the body of the individual entry. The remaining categories in each entry, itemise conditions or goups where care should be exercised (*Special care*), cases where the drug should not be taken (*Avoid use*) and any interactions that may occur with other medications (*Possible interaction*). In *Side effects* are listed the primary possible effects of taking the drug.

No work of this nature can be totally comprehensive, and no one involved with the preparation of publication of this book can be held liable for any omissions, errors or for any consequences resulting from using the book.

Listed below are a number of abbreviations which you may meet and which, in conjunction with the accompanying medical dictionary, will help clarify the information presented.

ACE	angiotensin converting enzyme (ACE inhibitors are used in cardiac failure)
ß-blocker	beta-blocker
BPH	benign prostatic hypertrophy (enlarged prostate gland)
BUN	blood urea nitrogen
CNS	central nervous system
GABA	gamma-aminobutyric acid (an amino acid found in the brain, heart, lungs and kidney that acts as a neurotransmitter)
MAOI	monamine oxidase inhibitor (antidepressant)
NSAID	non-steroidal anti-inflammatory drug
SLE	systemic lupus erythematosus (a chronic inflammatory disease which may be viral or an immune system dysfunction which tends to be commoner in women)
TCAD	tricyclic antidepressant
UTI	urinary tract infection
µg	microgram (10^{-6}g)
CD	signifies a controlled drug, that is one which is subject to the specific restrictions and requirements of the Misuse of Drugs Regulations, 1985.

PRESCRIPTION DRUGS

ACCUPRO

Description: a proprietary preparation of the antihypertensive drug, quinapril; used in conjunction with a diuretic or cardiac glycoside. Available as brown tablets (oval, round or triangular according to strength).

Used for: hypertension and congestive heart failure, especially after other treatments have been tried.

Dosage: in adults only starts at 2.5mg per day usually increasing to 10–20mg per day. The maximum daily dose is 40mg.

Special care: all elderly patients, impairment of kidney function, haemodialysis, severe congestive heart failure, some types of vascular disease and in patients having anaesthesia.

Avoid use: children, pregnant and nursing mothers, some kidney and heart valve diseases.

Possible interaction: potassium-containing supplements, diuretic drugs, NSAIDs, tetracyclines.

Side effects: numerous including hypotension, abdominal, chest and muscle pains, headache, nausea, dizziness, rhinitis, upper respiratory tract infection and allergic reactions.

Manufacturer: Parke-Davis.

ACEPRIL

Description: an ACE inhibitor and preparation of the antihypertensive drug captopril available as white tablets and marked A (12.5mg strength), or ACE and strength (for 25 and 50mg strengths).

Used for: an addition to diuretic drugs and where appropriate digitalis in congestive heart failure. After heart attacks when there is a disorder of the left ventricle.

Dosage: 6.25 or 12.5mg for heart failure, maintenance 25mg two or three times per day. Maximum 150mg per day. treatment to be commenced under close supervision. Diuretics to be reduced or stopped before treatment. Post heart attack-6.25mg, increasing slowly to 150mg per day in divided doses. Start 3 days after attack. For children, contact manufacturer.

Special care: severe congestive heart failure, haemodialysis, kidney disease, anaesthesia, monitor kidney function, white cell count and urinary protein.

Avoid use: pregnancy, lactation, narrowing of the aorta.

Possible interaction: potassium supplements or potassium-sparing diuretics, vasodilators, NSAIDs, lithium, allopurinol, clonidine, probenecid, immunosuppressants.

Side effects: anaemia, loss of taste, hypotension, proteinuria, pancreatitis, rash, angioneurotic oedema, neutropenia, thrombocytopenia.

Manufacturer: Squibb.

ACEZIDE

Description: a combined diuretic/ACE inhibitor anti-hypertensive preparation. Contains captopril (50mg) and hydrochlorothiazide (25mg) in a white, scored tablet, code AZE 50/25.

Used for: mild to moderate hypertension.

Dosage: 1 tablet daily (maximum 2) (in patients who have first become accustomed to the two components given in the same amounts separately).

Special care: patients with renal disorders or undergoing haemodialysis.

Avoid use: in children, pregnant and breast feeding mothers, outflow

obstruction of the heart, aortic stenosis
and renovascular disease.
Possible interaction: NSAIDs,
potassium-containing supplements,
antihypertensives, vasodilatory and
immunosuppressant drugs.
Side effects: protein in urine (proteinuria),
rash, loss of sense of taste, fatigue,
changes in constitution of the blood and,
very unusually, a cough.
Manufacturer: Squibb.

ACHROMYCIN

Description: a preparation of the
antibiotic tetracycline hydrochloride
used to treat a variety of conditions.
Available as orange tablets. Also, as
intramuscular injection and via
intravenous drip. Effective against the
bacterium *Haemophilus influenzae*.
Used for: complications of chronic
bronchitis.
Dosage: 1 or 2 tablets at 6 hourly intervals.
Special care: patients with any liver or
kidney disease. May require avoidance
of use in cases of renal impairment.
Avoid use: in cases of impaired kidney
function. It is absorbed into growing
bone and stains teeth, hence must not be
given to children less than 12 years or to
pregnant women or nursing mothers.
Possible interaction: consumption of milk
which reduces absorption of tetracycline,
contraceptive pill, antacids, iron, magnesium and calcium mineral supplements.
Side effects: digestive upset—diarrhoea
and vomiting, nausea, headache, disturbance of vision, possible allergic response.
Also used for: acne vulgaris.
Description: achromycin topical ointment
containing 3% tetracycline hydrochloride.
Used for: moderate to severe acne and
effective against the bacterium
Propionbacterium acnes.
Dosage: apply to affected skin once a
day or as directed by physician.
Special care: in patients with kidney and
liver disorders or perforated ear drum.
Avoid use: as above.
Possible interaction: as above.

Side effects: possible additional infection,
especially thrush. Occasionally diarrhoea.
Also used for: mild bacterial skin
infections.
Dosage: apply once daily to affected
area or as directed.
Side effects: possible super infection
(infection caused by different micro-
organism, or a strain of the bacterium
causing the original infection which has
become resistant to Achromycin).
Also available as sterile ointment
containing 1% tetracycline hydrochloride.
Used for: bacterial infections of the
outer ear (otitis extrema) which are
sensitive to tetracycline.
Dosage: once or twice daily or as directed.
Special care: patients with perforated ear
drum and for short-term use.
Side effects: localized allergic reactions
and possible superinfection (see above).
Also used for: infections of eyelids, e.g.
styes, surface infections, e.g. conjunctivitis
and chlamydial opthalmia (along with
antibiotic preparations taken orally). Also
following minor abrasions to the surface of
the eye to prevent infections.
Dosage: every 4 hours or as directed by
physician.
Special care: generally as above.
Side effects: possible superinfection.
Manufacturer: Lederle.

ACLACIN

Description: a class II anthracycline,
cytotoxic, antibiotic drug. It contains
aclarubicin hydrochloride in the form of
a powder (20mg) which is reconstituted
as a fluid for rapid infusion.
Used for: non-lymphocytic leukaemia
especially in patients who are resistant to
other forms of chemotherapy or who
have relapsed from these treatments.
Dosage: as infusion, directed by physician.
Special care: elderly, impairment of liver
and kidney functions, heart disorders.
Monitoring of cardiac function is essential
during treatment. High cumulative doses
can lead to cardiac dysfunction.
Side effects: possible tissue damage to

healthy cells adjacent to cancer cells through interference with cell division. Severe nausea and vomiting, loss of hair, suppression of bone marrow so blood cell formation is impaired.
Manufacturer: Lundbeck.

ACTILYSE

Description: a fibrinolytic (disperses blood clots) drug available as a powder for reconstitution and injection. It can only be used under close medical supervision.
Used for: thrombosis, embolisms and particularly myocardial infarction.
Dosage: a total of 100mg, given intravenously over a 2 hour period in adults only.
Special care: in patients with liver or kidney disease, diabetes or hypertension.
Avoid use: in children, pregnant and nursing mothers, those with any form of bleeding (e.g. menstruation), recent surgery including dental treatment, or haemorrhage, any condition likely to bleed, e.g. active peptic ulcer or case of pancreatitis. Should not be administered to those having allergic reactions to streptokinase and anistreplase or who have recently been treated with these.
Possible interaction: with other plasma protein-bound drugs, i.e. anticoagulants.
Side effects: mainly nausea, vomiting and bleeding usually confined to puncture site but can occur elsewhere including intracerebral haemorrhage. Severe bleeding necessitates halting of treatment and possible administration of drugs to counter the fibrinolytic. Hence close monitoring is essential during treatment.
Manufacturer: Boehringer Ingelheim.

ACTINAC

Description: an antibacterial steroid (corticosteroid) preparation with skin softening properties, available as a powder with solvent to be made up as a lotion. Contains the broad spectrum antibiotic chloramphenicol (4%), hydrocortisone acetate (4%) and also sulphur precipitate, allantoin and butoxyethyl nicotinate.
Used for: acne.

Dosage: apply to affected skin morning and night for 4 days then at night only for up to 3 weeks, continuing for 3 days after spots have disappeared.
Special care: pregnant women, avoid contact with jewellery.
Side effects: possible erythema, which may be severe.
Manufacturer: Roussel

ACUPAN

Description: an analgesic non-narcotic drug available in the form of white tablets or as a solution for injection. Contains 30mg nefopam hydrochloride, tablets being marked APN. (Injection contains 20mg nefopam hydrochloride per ml in each ampoule).
Used for: relief of moderate and severe pain, e.g. following surgery, muscle and joint pain, dental cancer.
Dosage: tablets 3 times per day, adults only, total dose in the order of 30–90mg. Injection—one 20mg dose intramuscularly 3 times a day.
Special care: elderly patients (1 tablet, 3 times a day initially), pregnant women, patients with kidney or liver disorders or suffering from urine retention.
Avoid use: children, history of convulsions or heart attack (myocardial infarction) and also glaucoma.
Possible interaction: drugs including sympathomimetics, tricyclics, anticholinergics and MAOIs (antidepressants).
Side effects: nervousness, irritability, dry mouth, dizziness and nausea, headaches. Occasionally insomnia, irregular heartbeat and sweating. Urine may be tinged pink.
Manufacturer: 3M Health Care.

ADALAT

Description: a calcium antagonist and vasodilator, available as liquid-filled orange capsules, containing the active ingredient nifedipine (5mg and 10mg). Also as sustained release tablets and as a preparation for injection.
Used for: angina and Raynaud's phenomenon.

Dosage: 10mg 3 times a day (5mg in elderly patients) in first instance, depending upon response, up to 60mg a day thereafter. Capsules taken with or immediately after food.

Special care: patients with significant left ventricle disorders or congestive heart failure, low blood pressure, kidney and liver disease.

Avoid use: if pain worsens during treatment, pregnant and nursing mothers, children, patients with very low blood pressure.

Possible interaction: antihypertensive drugs; quinidine and cimetidine.

Side effects: dizziness, flushing, nausea, palpitations, sweating, headaches, fluid retention, digestive upset, increased frequency of urination, drowsiness and insomnia. Rarely jaundice and swelling of gums.

Manufacturer: Bayer. Nifedipine capsules also produced by Norton, Evans, APS, Ashbourne (Angiopine), CP, Eastern (Calcilat ®), Kerfoot, Cox.

ADCORTYL

Description: a potent topical steroid preparation (a corticosteroid), containing the active ingredient triamcinolone acetonide 0.1%, as cream or ointment.

Used for: eczema and psoriasis, which has proved unresponsive to less potent preparations of corticosteroids. Can also be used to treat external ear infections and neurodermatitis.

Dosage: apply sparingly to affected area 2–4 times each day and less frequently as condition improves.

Special care: for children and babies, especially face and neck.

Avoid use: acne (including acne rosacea), any skin conditions caused by ringworm, fungi, viruses, tuberculosis, leg ulcers, pregnant women and long term use. Also fungal or bacterial infections which have not been treated.

Side effects: suppression of adrenal gland function, skin thinning and retention of fluid.

Also available: adcortyl witth graneodin (an antimicrobial agent) which includes the antibiotic neomycin. This contains 0.1% triamcinolone acetonide, 0.25% neomycin (as sulphate) and 0.025% gramicidin as cream. It is used as above but where a bacterial infection may additionally be present.

ADCORTYL IN OROBASE is available as an oral paste used to treat mouth ulcers and other oral inflammations. It is applied 2 to 4 times daily and should not be used long term or by pregnant women.

Adcortyl containing 10mg/ml triamcinolone acetonide is available for injection intradermally or into a joint. Used intradermally to treat scaly skin diseases, alopecia areata (patchy hair loss). Used intra-articularly to treat joint pain, stiffness and swelling caused especially by rheumatoid arthritis, bursitis, tenosynovitis and osteoarthrosis (osteoarthritis).

Manufacturer: Squibb

ADIFAX

Description: a preparation containing dexfenfluramine hydrochloride (fenfluramine is chemically related to amphetamine but is not a central nervous system stimulant and is less likely to cause dependence). It is an appetite suppressant which appears to affect the levels of serotonin (a naturally occurring compound in the body) in the brain. It is available in the form of 15mg white capsules marked S5614.

Used for: severe obesity alongside other treatments, mainly control of diet.

Dosage: 1 tablet in the morning and evening, at mealtimes.

Special care: treatment should be limited to three months with gradual withdrawal over 1 or 2 weeks. Elderly patients.

Avoid use: in children, pregnant and nursing mothers, patients with history of psychiatric illness, drug/alcohol abuse, anorexia, glaucoma, epilepsy, liver and kidney disorders.

Possible interaction: anorectic drugs; MAOIs, antidepressants, sedatives,

antihypertensive drugs, antidiabetics.
Side effects: dependence effects possible
on withdrawal including depression,
breathlessness, headache, nervousness
and irritability, sleep disturbance, dry
mouth, dizziness, nausea, diarrhoela,
constipation, more frequent urination.
Manufacturer: Servier

ADIZEM

Description: a calcium antagonist and
vasodilator containing the active ingredient
diltiazem hydrochloride. Available as
tablets in 3 forms:
ADIZEM 60—coded 60/DL, 60mg
white capsules. **ADIZEM-SR**—white
90mg; brown 120mg; white/brown
180mg. Also as 120mg white tablets
(DL/120). All continuous-release capsules.
ADIZEM XL—pink/blue 120mg; pink/
blue 180mg; red/blue 240mg; maroon/
blue 300mg . All continuous-release
capsules marked with strength.
Used for: angina and hypertension.
Dosage: 60mg 3 times a day increasing
if required to a maximum of 480mg.
Elderly, twice a day in first instance.
Special care: patients with heart block,
reduced function in left ventricle of
heart, bradycardia, diabetes.
Avoid use: in children, pregnant and
nursing mothers, severe heart block or
bradycardia, impairment of kidney and
liver function.
Possible interaction: digoxin, ß-blockers,
antihypertensive drugs, cardiac
depressants, diazepam, cyclosporin,
cimetidine, theophylline, cartamazepine.
Side effects: swelling of ankles, nausea,
headache, bradycardia, rash, first degree
heart block.
Manufacturer: Napp

AEROLIN AUTOHALER

Description: a preparation of a selective
Beta$_2$-agonist (beta receptor stimulant)
salbutamol which causes dilation or
expansion of air passages in the lungs.
Salbutamol (as sulphate) is present as
100 µg per dose.

Used for: prevention (prophylaxis) and
treatment of bronchial asthma and
breathing difficulties associated with
bronchitis.
Dosage: Aerolin is administered by
means of a breath-activated aerosol
inhalant which delivers a metered dose.
Dose is 1–2 puffs 3–4 times daily for
prevention. Half dose for children.
Special care: thyroid gland disorders
(hyperthyroidism) hypertension, heart
disorders, e.g. myocardial insufficiency,
during pregnancy and breastfeeding.
May cause thyrotoxicosis with
associated symptoms.
Possible interaction: corticosteroids—
increased risk of hypokalaemia with
high doses.
Side effects: headache, nervousness and
irritability, fine tremor (in hands),
vasodilation in peripheral areas of body.
Manufacturer: 3M Health Care

AKINETON

Description: an anticholinergic preparation
containing the active ingredient biperiden
hydrochloride, used to counter the effects
of Parkinsonism. It is available as white,
scored tablets with Knoll logo, containing
2mg biperiden hydrochloride and as a
preparation containing biperiden lactate
5mg/ml, for slow intravenous or
intramuscular injection.
Used for: Parkinsonism and treatment of
symptoms of drug-induced Parkinsonism.
Dosage: *Tablets*: in adults, 1mg twice
daily in first instance gradually
increasing to 2mg 3 times a day. After
initial period, the usual daily dose is in
the order of 3–12mg 3 times a day.
Injection: 2.5–4mg per ml up to 4 times
per day.
Special care: in patients with liver,
kidney or heart disease. Treatment must
be discontinued gradually.
Avoid use: children, pregnant and
nursing mothers, some types of
glaucoma, patients with untreated urine
retention or gastro-intestinal obstruction.
Possible interaction: CNS depressant

drugs and other anti-Parkinsonism drugs. *Side effects*: dry mouth, drowsiness, blurred vision and gastro-intestinal disorders. More rarely, urine retention and tachycardia and possible allergic reactions. *Manufacturer*: Knoll.

AKNEMIN

Description: an antibiotic drug, containing minocycline hydrochloride, available as 50mg red/fawn coloured capsules and 100mg red capsules.
Used for: acne.
Dosage: adults, twice daily dose of 50mg or 100mg. Tablets required for a minimum period of 6 weeks to 3 months with improvement not expected until after first month.
Special care: liver or kidney disorders.
Avoid use: pregnant and nursing mothers, children, kidney failure, SLE.
Possible interaction: alcohol, antacid stomach preparations, mineral supplements, anticoagulant drugs, penicillin.
Side effects: skin rashes, dizziness, blood abnormalities. Possible intracranial hypertension—drug should be discontinued.
Manufacturer: Stiefel.

ALDACTIDE

Description: a proprietary preparation containing a potassium-sparing diuretic (encourages potassium to be retained and not eliminated in kidney) combined with a thiazide (a drug which inhibits the reabsorption of chloride and sodium in the kidney). The preparation is available in two strengths. **ALDACTIDE 25** contains 25mg spironalactone and 25mg hydroflumethiazide in buff-coloured tablets marked Searle 101. **ALDACTIDE 50** (Gold Cross) contains 50mg of each drug.
Used for: congestive heart failure.
Dosage: *Aldactide 25*: adults, 4 tablets daily with food in first instance with a maximum of eight. *Aldatide 50*: two tablets daily with a maximum of four. In children: 1.5–3mg per kg of body weight

given at intervals through the day.
Special care: elderly, liver and kidney disorders, pregnant mothers, diabetic patients, gout, long-term use in young people. Blood tests and monitoring of electrolyte levels may be required.
Avoid use: nursing mothers, patients with liver or kidney failure, hypercalcaemia, hyperkalaemia, Addison's disease, sensititivity to sulphonamide drugs.
Possible interaction: potassium supplements, other potassium-sparing diuretic drugs, NSAIDs, anti-diabetic drugs, antihypertensive drugs, ACE inhibitors and cardiac glycosides.
Side effects: metabolic disorders, disturbance of electrolyte balance in blood, rash, drowsiness, sensitivity to light, gastro-intestinal upset, menstrual irregularities, deepening of voice.
Manufacturer: Searle.

ALDACTONE

Description: a diuretic, potassium-sparing preparation containing spironolactone. Tablets available: 25mg buff marked Searle 39, 50mg off-white (Searle 916), 100mg buff (Searle 314).
Used for: congestive heart failure, oedema caused by cirrhosis of the liver, malignancy or nephrotic syndrome, primary aldosteronism (over-production of the adrenal hormone, aldosterone).
Dosage: in adults with congestive heart failure, 100mg daily in first instance increasing to 400mg taken with food. Thereafter, 75–200mg per day. Children, 3mg per kg of body weight in first instance in several doses.
Special care: pregnant mothers, long-term use in young people patients with liver or kidney disorders. Blood electrolyte levels may need to be monitored.
Avoid use: nursing mothers, patients with kidney failure, Addison's disease, and hyperkalaemia.
Side effects: gastro-intestinal upset, rash, headache, disturbance of electrolyte levels, metabolic disturbance, breast

enlargement, deepening of voice, menstrual irregularities, confusion, ataxia (unsteadiness).
Manufacturer: Searle.

ALDOMET

Description: a centrally acting (on central nervous system), antihypertensive preparation containing the drug methyldopa. It is available as tablets or in ampoules for injection. May be used in combination with a diuretic drug. Aldomet tablets are available in three strengths all marked Aldomet and coloured yellow: Aldomet 125mg code 135; Aldomet 250mg code 401, Aldomet 500mg code 516.
Used for: hypertension, especially useful for hypertension of pregnancy.
Dosage: in adults, 250mg 2 to 3 times a day in first instance with an eventual maximum of 3 grams at 2-day intervals. In children, 10mg per kg of body weight each day in 2 to 4 separate doses.
Special care: history of liver disease, kidney disorders, haemolytic anaemia, undergoing anaesthesia.
Avoid use: liver disease, a disease of the adrenal glands called phaeochromocytoma, patients with depression.
Possible interaction: sympathomimetics, other hypertensives, MAOIs, tricyclic antidepressants, lithium and phenothiazines.
Side effects: depression, sleepiness, headache, dry mouth, nasal congestion, gastro-intestinal upsets, bradycardia, jaundice, haemolytic anaemia, positive Coombs test.
Manufacturer: MSD.

ALEXAN

Description: a preparation of the antimetabolite, cytotoxic drug, cytarabine. It is available as ampoules for intravenous injection in two strengths, 20mg/ml and 100mg/ml (ALEXAN 100).
Used for: acute kind of leukaemia, especially myeloblastic leukaemia, to induce remission.

Dosage: as directed by cancer specialist.
Special care: careful monitoring of the blood is essential as this drug significantly reduces the ability of the bone marrow to manufacture blood cells.
Side effects: hair loss, nausea, vomiting.
Manufacturer: Pfizer.

ALFA D

Description: a manufactured form of vitamin D containing alfacalcidol (1α-hydroxycholcalciferol), a hydroxylated derivative. Since the conversion of vitamin D to its active form (which can be used by the body) requires hydroxylation by the kidneys, alfacalcidol is especially useful for patients suffering from any form of renal disorder. Alfa D is available in two strengths and contains 0.25 µg of alfacalcidol in a pink capsule or 1 µg in an orange capsule, each marked appropriately.
Used for: rickets and osteomalacia (adult rickets, possibly caused by liver disease or malabsorption of vitamin D), overactivity of the parathyroid glands (and bone disease) (hyperparathyroidism), underactivity of the parathyroid glands (hypoparathyroidism), renal osteodystrophy (bone disease associated with chronic kidney failure).
Dosage: adults: 1 µg each day in first instance, adjusted according to response. Elderly patients: 0.5 µg at first followed by adjustment of dose. Children over 20kg weight, 1 µg daily, then adjusted dose.
Special care: pregnant and breast feeding mothers; vitamin D is passed into breast milk and can cause hypercalcaemia in infants. Patients with kidney failure. Monitoring of blood plasma levels of calcium is essential during treatment.
Avoid use: children under 20kg body weight.
Possible interaction: barbiturate and anticonvulsant drugs, digitalis, danazol, thiazides, mineral supplements, cholestyramine, sucralfate, colestipol.
Side effects: (associated with overdose)

diarrhoea, vomiting, nausea, weight loss,
vertigo, headache, sweating, lethargy,
thirst, elevated levels of calcium and
phosphate in urine.
Manufacturer: Du Pont

ALGITEC

Description: a preparation, containing
the H$_2$-receptor antagonist, cimetidine,
which acts to reduce the production of
gastric acid in the stomach. It is also a
reflux suppressant which is available in
chewable tablets called Chewtab and as
a liquid suspension. Algitec tablets are
off-white in colour and contain 200mg
cimetidine and 500mg alginic acid and
are marked ALGITEC 120. Also,
ALGITEC SUSPENSION containing
100mg cimetidine and 250mg sodium
alginate in each 5ml.
Used for: gastric and duodenal ulcers,
Zollingen-Ellison syndrome, reflux
oesophagitis.
Dosage: adults, one to two tablets
chewed four times a day following
meals, or 10–20mls of suspension, and at
night time, for four to eight weeks.
Special care: the presence of gastric
cancer should first be eliminated.
Patients suffering from kidney disorders
and pregnant and nursing mothers.
Avoid use: not for children.
Possible interaction: oral anticoagulants,
warfarin, phenytoin, theophylline or
aminophylline.
Side effects: generally few but dizziness,
fatigue, rash, diarrhoea may occur, and
rarely, headache, confusion, joint and
muscle pains, reversible liver damage
and gynaecomastia (breast enlargement).
Manufacturer: SK & F.

ALIMIX

Description: a preparation containing the
active ingredient, asapride, which acts to
promote stomach and intestine motility
and emptying. It is thought to work by
promoting the release of acetylcholine in
the wall of gastro-intestinal tract. It is
available as white scored tablets, marked

J/Y and C and containing 10mg of
cisapride (as monohydrate).
Used for: gastro-oesophageal reflux,
delayed gastric emptying accompanying
such conditions as diabetes, systemic
sclerosis and autonomic neuropathy
(nerve supply to gastro-intestinal tract is
disrupted), non-ulcer dyspepsia (short-
term treatment).
Dosage: depending upon condition being
treated but usually 1 tablet 3 or 4 times
daily, a quarter or half an hour before
meals, for 6–12 weeks.
Special care: nursing mothers, elderly
patients, kidney and liver disorders.
Avoid use: children and pregnant
women, gastro-intestinal bleeding,
obstruction or perforation. Any condition
where stimulation of gastro-intestinal
tract might prove to be harmful.
Possible interaction: anticholinergic
drugs, anticoagulants, sedatives, opiod
analgesics, antimuscarines.
Side effects: diarrhoea and abdominal
pains, borborygmi (stomach and
abdominal rumbling caused by fluid and
gas), rarely headaches and convulsions.
Manufacturer: Janssen.

ALKERAN

Description: a preparation of the
alkylating, cytotoxic drug melphalan, for
use by a physician skilled in cancer
chemotherapy. It is available in tablets of
two strengths, a white tablet coded A2A
(2mg), and a white tablet coded B2A
(5mg). Also available as a powder for
reconstitution, containing 50mg melphalan
(as hydrochloride), for injection.
Used for: myeloma (or multiple myeloma,
myelomatosis) a malignant bone marrow
disease, ovarian and breast cancer.
Dosage: 150–300 µg per kg of body
weight each day for four to six days. This
may be repeated after four to eight weeks.
Special care: bone marrow suppression
occurs but not immediately. Hence blood
counts must be checked before each stage
of treatment. Dose must be reduced in
patients with impaired kidney function.

Possible interaction: antibacterial drugs, nalidixic acid cyclosporin.
Side effects: nausea, vomiting, hair loss, bone marrow suppression.
Manufacturer: Wellcome.

ALLEGRON

Description: a TCAD, nortriptyline, available in tablets of two strengths. It has less of a sedative efect than some other TCAD drugs. It is available as white scored tablets marked DISTA, containing 10mg nortriptyline hydrochloride, and orange scored tablets marked DISTA (25mg).
Used for: depressive illnesses and bedwetting in children.
Dosage: adults, 20 to 40mg each day in divided doses, increasing to 100mg if required. Maintenance, 30 to 75mg a day. Elderly persons; 10mg three times daily in first instance. Children (for bedwetting), seven to ten years, 10 to 20mg, 11 to 16 years, 25 to 50mg, given half an hour before bedtime.
Special care: patients with heart disease, elderly people (reduced doses), nursing mothers, those with diabetes, thyroid disease, liver disorders, tumours of the medulla of adrenal glands, epilepsy, glaucoma, urine retention, psychosis, suicidal tendencies. Withdrawal should be gradual. May reduce ability to perform skilled tasks such as driving.
Avoid use: pregnant mothers, heart block, heart attack, serious liver disorders.
Possible interaction: alcohol, MAOIs, barbiturate drugs, anticholinergic drugs, other antidepressant and antihypertensive drugs, adrenaline, noradrenaline, oestrogens, cimetidine.
Side effects: drowsiness, blurred vision, dry mouth, insomnia, urine retention, palpitations and shakiness, low blood pressure, weight changes, skin reactions, jaundice, blood changes, loss of libido.
Manufacturer: Dista.

ALMEVAX

Description: a preparation of vaccine against German measles (Rubella) containing the live, but attenuated, strain Wistar RA 27/3 virus. It is available in one and ten dose vials for injection.
Used for: immunization against Rubella in non-pregnant women and girls aged 10–14 who have not received MMR vaccine.
Dosage: one dose given intramuscularly or subcutaneously,
Special care: contraceptives should be used during the first three months although there is thought to be little risk of harm to the foetus.
Avoid use: pregnancy, cancer, acute fevers, hypogamma globulinaemia (gamma globulin blood deficiency).
Possible interaction: other live vaccines, transfusions, irradiation, cytotoxic drugs, corticosteroids, immunoglobulins.
Side effects: sore throat, rash, malaise, aching joints, possible anaphylaxis.
Manufacturer: Evans.

ALOMIDE

Description: a preparation containing lodoxamide tromethamine with additives benzalkonium chloride and disodium edetate, available as 1% solution.
Used for: allergic conjunctivitis.
Dosage: one to two drops in each eye four times daily.
Special care: pregnant and nursing mothers.
Avoid use: those who wear soft contact lenses, children under four years of age.
Side effects: irritation, stinging, watering of eyes.
Manufacturer: Galen.

ALPHADERM

Description: a moderately strong steroid with a hydrating agent (to moisten the skin). Alphaderm combines 1% hydrocortisone, 10% urea in a slightly oily cream.
Used for: dermatitis and eczema.
Dosage: wash and dry affected skin and apply thinly twice a day.
Special care: short-term use only (especially in children or on face).

Avoid use: acne, scabies, tuberculosis, ringworm, untreated bacterial and fungal infections, viral skin diseases, leg ulcers, pregnant mothers.
Side effects: usually few but skin thinning, adrenal gland suppression, fluid retention possible.
Manufacturer: Procter and Gamble.

ALPHOSYL HC

Description: a preparation of coal tar and hydrocortisone used in the treatment of psoriasis. It contains 5% coal tar extract, 0.5% hydrocortisone and 2% allantoin in a water-based cream.
Used for: psoriasis.
Dosage: adults and children over 5 years, apply to affected skin twice each day.
Special care: use should be limited to 5 days with children or on face. If treatment in adults is prolonged, withdrawal should be gradual.
Avoid use: extensive or prolonged use in pregnant women, acne or untreated fungal and bacterial infections, tuberculosis, viral skin disease, leg ulcers, ringworm. Children under 5 years.
Side effects: thinning of skin, suppression of adrenal glands, fluid retention.
Manufacturer: Stafford-Miller.

ALRHEUMAT

Description: a NSAID preparation available as capsules and suppositories. Alrheumat contains 50mg ketoprofen and propionic acid in off-white cream-coloured capsules or as anal suppositories.
Used for: pain and inflammation caused by musculo-skeletal diseases and rheumatoid and osteoarthritis, acute gout, pain following orthopaedic surgery, ankylosing spondylitis.
Dosage: capsules—adults one 2–4 times each day with food. Suppositories—100mg at bedtime. Combined capsules and suppositories no more than 200mg daily.
Special care: pregnancy and lactation, patients with heart, kidney or liver diseases, elderly people.
Avoid use: children, patients with

asthma, allergy to aspirin or NSAIDs, active peptic ulcer or history of peptic ulcer, gastrointestinal haemorrhage.
Possible interaction: high doses of methotrexate, sulphonamide antibiotic drugs, quinolones, hydantoins and anticoagulant drugs.
Side effects: gastrointestinal upsets, rash, rectal irritation (suppositories).
Manufacturer: Bayer.

ALUPENT

Description: a bronchodilator, containing the partially selective drug orciprenaline sulphate. It is available as off-white scored tablets marked A7 containing 20mg orciprenaline sulphate. Also as alupent sugar-free syrup (10mg/5ml of solution) and alupent aerosol containing 0.75mg per metered puff.
Used for: bronchial spasm due to asthma, chronic bronchitis and emphysema.
Dosage: tablets and syrup: adults, one tablet or 10mls four times a day. Children under 1 year 2.5 to 5mls three times daily; 1–3 years, 2.5 to 5mls four times daily; 3–12 years, 5mls four times daily up to 10mls three times daily depending on age and symptoms.
Aerosol: adults, 1–2 puffs which can be repeated after 30 minutes if required. Maximum dose 12 puffs in 24 hours. Children, 6 years and under, one puff, 6–12 years, one or two puffs. Must not be repeated within 30 minutes and maximum dose is four puffs in 24 hours.
Special care: patients with diabetes or hypertension. Patients should follow instructions carefully.
Avoid use: acute heart disease, hyperthyroidism or cardiac asthma.
Possible interaction: sympathomimetic drugs, tricyclic antidepressants, MAOIs.
Side effects: tachycardia, arrythmia, fine tremor, headache and nervous tension, dilation of blood vessels.
Manufacturer: Boehringer Ingelheim.

AMBAXIN

Description: a broad-spectrum antibiotic

preparation, containing a form of penicillin, available as scored, oblong-shaped tablets marked Upjohn and 130.
Used for: respiratory, ear, nose, throat, soft tissue and skin infections. Also urinary tract infections and venereal diseases such as gonorrhoea. Para-typhoid fever.
Dosage: adults, 1–2 tablets, 2 or 3 times a day. Venereal disease, 4 tablets plus 1g of probenecid as a single dose. Children over 5 years, half a tablet 3 times daily.
Special care: patients suffering from liver and kidney diseases or infectious mononucleosis (glandular fever).
Avoid use: children under five years. Allergy to penicillin.
Side effects: gastro-intestinal upsets, possible allergic responses, e.g. rash (discontinue treatment).
Manufacturer: Upjohn.

AMFIPEN

Description: a broad-spectrum antibiotic penicillin, ampicillin, available as capsules, Amfipen syrup and in vials for injection; Amfipen capsules are grey/red and available in 2 strengths containing 250mg and 500mg, marked with name and strength. AMFIPEN SYRUP is also available in 2 strengths and contains 125mg and 250mg ampicillin per 5ml.
Used for: respiratory and ear, nose and throat infections. Also, soft tissue, urinary tract and veneral infections (gonorrhoea).
Dosage: adults, 250mg–1g 4 times each day. Children, half adult dose.
Special care: patients with kidney disease or glandular fever (infectious mononucleosis).
Avoid use: allergy to penicillin.
Side effects: gastro-intestinal upsets, allergic responses, e.g. rash (discontinue treatment).
Manufacturer: Brocades

AMIKIN

Description: a preparation of the aminoglycoside antibiotic drug,

amikacin, produced in the form of solutions for intramuscular or slow intravenous injection or infusion. Amikin contains 500mg per 2mls.
AMIKIN PAEDIATRIC contains 100mg amikacin (as sulphate) per 2ml.
Used for: serious bacterial infections particularly those caused by Gram-negative bacteria which are resistant to the more usual aminoglycosides, gentamicin and tobramycin.
Dosage: adults, 15mg per kg of body weight intramuscularly or intravenously in two divided doses for up to 10 days. Maximum total dose 15g. For urinary tract infections, 7.5mg per kg of body weight each day in two divided doses. Children, 10mg–15mg per kg of body weight daily in two divided doses.
Special care: patient should receive adequate fluid intake, caution with kidney disease. Monitor for toxicity.
Avoid use: pregnant women.
Possible interaction: anaesthetics, neuromuscular blocking drugs, ethacrynic acid, frusemide.
Side effects: temporary kidney impairment and irreversible deafness can occur with prolonged or too high dosage.
Manufacturer: Bristol-Myers.

AMIL-CO

Description: a potassium-sparing diuretic available in the form of peach-coloured, diamond-shaped tablets with the name and logo. They contain 5mg amiloride hydrochloride and 50mg hydrochlorothiazide (co-amilozide 5/50).
Used for: cirrhosis of the liver (with fluid retention), congestive heart failure, hypertension.
Dosage: adults, 1–2 tablets each day increasing up to 4, if required, in single or divided dose.
Special care: patients with gout, kidney or liver disease, diabetes, acidosis.
Avoid use: children, pregnant and nursing mothers, hyperkalaemia, severe or progressive kidney failure.
Possible interaction: other potassium-

sparing diuretics, potassium supplements, antihypertensive drugs, ACE inhibitors, lithium, digitalis (digoxin). *Side effects*: gout, rash, sensitivity to light, blood dyscrasias.
Manufacturer: Baker-Norton.

AMOXIL

Description: preparations of the broad-spectrum antibiotic, amoxycillin, which is a derivative of ampicillin and available as maroon/gold capsules (250mg or 500mg amoxycillin trihydrate), marked with name and strength; dispersible, sugar-free tablets containing 500mg; **AMOXIL FIZTAB** chewable tablets, sugar-free (125mg). Not suitable for children under 3 years of age; AMOXIL SYRUP SF sugar-free, containing either 125mg or 250mg per 5ml for reconstitution with water; **AMOXIL PAEDIATRIC SUSPENSION**, 125mg amoxycillin (as trihydrate) per 1.25ml; **AMOXIL 3g SACHETS SF**—3g in sucrose-free sorbitol base as a powder in a sachet. **AMOXIL 750mg SACHET SF** containing 750mg in sugar-free, sorbitol base as a powder in a sachet; **AMOXIL INJECTION**—Either 250mg, 500mg or 1g amoxycillin (as sodium salts), in a vial as a powder for reconstitution.
Used for: one or more of the different forms are used for soft tissue infections, urinary tract infections, respiratory, ear, nose, throat, infections, gonorrhoea, dental abscess and to prevent endocarditis during dental treatment. Glandular fever.
Dosage: infants under 6 months, Amoxil Paediatric suspension is appropriate. Adults, 250–500mg three times each day, children half adult dose. Injection, (used for glandular fever), adults, 500mg intramuscularly at 8-hour intervals or 1g intravenously at 6-hourly intervals if infection is severe. Children, 50–100mg per kg of body weight in divided doses.
Special care: patients with allergy to penicillin.
Side effects: gastro-intestinal upsets,

allergic responses, e.g. rash, especially in patients with glandular fever, HIV virus, lymphatic leukaemia.
Manufacturer: Bencard.

AMPICLOX

Description: a broad-spectrum antibiotic ampicillin with cloxacillin available as capsules, black/purple (250mg ampicillin trihydrate) and 250mg cloxacillin (as sodium salt); Also **AMPICLOX SYRUP** containing 125mg/125mg per 5ml, available as powder for reconstitution; **AMPICLOX NEONATAL**, a sugar-free suspension containing 60mg/30mg per 0.6ml when reconstituted; **AMPICLOX NEONATAL INJECTION** containing 50mg/25mg as powder for reconstitution; **AMPICLOX INJECTION** containing 250mg/250mg as powder for reconstitution.
Used for: emergency treatment of serious bacterial infections of urinary tract, ear, nose, throat, upper respiratory tract while bacteriology is being investigated. Also as a preventative against infection when the patient is to undergo major surgery.
Dosage: adults, capsules, 1–2 every four to six hours; syrup, 10–20ml every four to six hours. Children, babies under one month, neonatal suspension, 0.6ml every four to six hours or neonatal injection intravenously or intramuscularly, 1 vial three times a day. Children 1 month to 2 years 2.5ml–5ml Ampiclox syrup both every 4 to 6 hours. Adults, Ampiclox injection, intravenously or intramuscularly, 1 to 2 vials every 4 to 6 hours. Children 1 month to 2 years, one-quarter adult dose, children 2 to 10 years, half adult dose.
Special care: allergic patients, kidney disease, rashes especially in glandular fever, HIV, chronic lymphatic leukaemia.
Avoid use: patients with known penicillin allergy.
Side effects: gastro-intestinal upsets, allergic responses.
Manufacturer: Beecham.

AMSIDINE

Description: a cytotoxic, antibiotic, anti-cancer preparation containing amsacrine. This is available as a preparation for intravenous infusion for use by a physician skilled in cancer therapy. Amsidine concentrate contains 5mg amsacrine (as lactate) per ml when reconstituted.
Used for: acute myeloid leukaemia.
Dosage: as directed by physician. Usually no more than 450mg/m^2 of body surface area as a total cumulative dose.
Special care: patients with cardiac disorders, liver or kidney disease (reduced doses), elderly people, pregnant women. Caution in handling as irritant to tissues and skin; glass apparatus should be used for mixing. Cardiac monitoring and monitoring of electrolyte levels is essential during treatment.
Side effects: suppression of bone marrow function (myelosuppression), hair loss, mucositis. Rarely, tachycardia associated with ventricles of heart. Heart disease and potentially fatal heart failure.
Manufacturer: Parke-Davis

AMYTAL

Description: a barbiturate preparation containing amylobarbitone, available as white tablets containing 50mg amylobarbitone.
Used for: severe intractable insomnia of a persistent nature for use by those patients already taking barbiturates.
Dosage: adults, 100–200mg at bedtime.
Special care: extremely dangerous, addictive drug with narrow margin of safety. Liable to abuse by overdose leading to coma and death or if combined with alcohol. Easily produces dependence and severe withdrawal symptoms. Drowsiness may persist next day affecting driving and performance of skilled tasks.
Avoid use: should be avoided if possible in all patients. Not to be used for children, young adults, pregnant and nursing mothers, elderly pesons, those with drug or alcohol related problems, patients with

liver, kidney or heart disease, porphyria, insomnia where the cause is pain.
Possible interaction: alcohol, central nervous system depressant drugs, Griseofulvin, metronidazone, rifampicin, phenytoin, chloramphenicol. Anticoagulant drugs of the coumarin type, steroid drugs including contraceptive pill.
Side effects: hangover with drowsiness, shakiness, dizziness, headache, anxiety, confusion, excitement, rash and allergic responses, gastro-intestinal upsets, urine retention, loss of sexual desire.
Manufacturer: Kite.

ANAFRANIL

Description: a TCAD containing clomi-pramine hydrochloride, available as capsules, syrup and in ampoules for injection. There are three strengths: yellow/caramel (10mg), orange/caramel (25mg), grey/caramel (50mg) all marked Geigy. Also **ANAFRANIL SR** sustained release pink capsules containing 75mg, marked Geigy on one side and GD on the other. In addition, **ANAFRANIL SYRUP** containing 25mg per 5ml. Also, **ANAFRANIL INJECTION**, containing 25mg per 2ml in ampoules.
Used for: depression, phobic and obsessional states.
Dosage: adults, capsules for depression, 10mg each day gradually increasing to 30–150mg (maximum 250mg) in divided doses or as a single dose at bedtime. Obsession and phobia, 25mg at first increasing to 100–150mg daily. Elderly, 10mg each day at first increasing to a maximum of 75mg. Intramuscular injection, 25mg–50mg each day increasing by 25mg to 100–150mg. Intravenous infusion, 25–50mg then about 100mg for 7–10 days.
Special care: nursing mothers, elderly, psychoses or suicidal tendencies. Persons with heart disease, liver disorders, thyroid disease (hyperthyroidism), epilepsy, diabetes, urine retention, glaucoma, tumour of the adrenal glands. Blood tests are advisable during therapy.

Avoid use: children, pregnant women, patients with heart block, heart attack, serious liver disease.

Possible interaction: MAOIs or within 14 days of their use, other antidepressant drugs, anticholinergic drugs, alcohol, adrenaline, noradrenaline (or anaesthetics containing these), antihypertensive drugs, barbiturates, cimetidine, oestrogens.

Side effects: gastro-intestinal disturbances such as constipation, blurred vision, dry mouth, anxiety, drowsiness, insomnia, urine retention, sweating, tremor, disturbance of heartbeat rate, weight gain or loss. Also low blood pressure, allergic skin reactions, jaundice, loss of libido and impotence may occur. Occasionally, symptoms of schizophrenia and mania may be activated particularly in elderly persons.

Manufacturer: Geigy

ANAPOLON 50

Description: a preparation containing the anabolic steroid drug, oxymethalone. Available as white scored tablets containing 50mg and marked Syntex 50.

Used for: certain types of anaemia (especially aplastic anaemias and hypoplastic anaemias which have not improved after other therapy).

Dosage: children over 2 years, 2–4mg per kg of body weight daily. Adults, 2–5mg per kg of body weight in first instance reducing to half or less as condition improves. All in divided doses.

Special care: patients with diabetes, cardiac failure, enlarged prostate gland in men. Liver tests should be carried out during therapy.

Avoid use: children under 2 years, pregnant and nursing mothers, liver or kidney disease, men with breast or prostate cancer, women with breast cancer and hypercalcaemia.

Possible interaction: anticoagulant and corticosteroid drugs.

Side effects: vomiting, nausea, diarrhoea, sleeplessness, muscle cramps. Toxic effect on liver including jaundice, pruritis

(itching), tumours, hepatic coma. Also oedema, congestive heart failure, masculinization in women and pre-pubertal children, loss of menstruation (amenorrhoea) in women, changes in blood, hypercalcaemia (therapy should be halted).

Manufacturer: Syntex.

ANDROCUR

Description: an anti-androgen hormonal preparation containing cyproterone acetate, for use under hospital supervision. Available as white, scored tablets (50mg), marked BV in a hexagon.

Used for: male sexual deviation and severe hypersexuality. (Also, acne and abnormal hair growth in women, prostate cancer in men).

Dose: adult men only, 1 tablet in morning and evening after food.

Special care: patient consent is vital. Drug inhibits sperm production resulting in reversible infertility. Abnormal sperm are produced and liver tumours have been produced in animals. Ability to drive and perform skilled tasks impaired. Ineffective where hypersexuality is caused by chronic alcoholism. Special care in patients with diabetes mellitus and disorders of adrenal glands. Blood (haemoglobin) and sperm tests and monitoring of liver and adrenal gland function is advisable.

Avoid use: males under 18 years of age or those in whom bones and testes are not fully matured. Patients with thrombosis, embolism, severe liver disease, malignant or wasting diseases. Severe chronic depression.

Side effects: depression, tiredness, weight gain, breast enlargement, changes in hair growth, rarely, osteoporosis.

Manufacturer: Schering H.C.

ANECTINE

Description: a depolarizing muscle relaxant, the effect of which lasts for only 5 minutes and is used during anaesthesia. It is available as ampoules for injection, and contains 50mg

suxamethonium chloride per ml.
Used for: muscle relaxation during anaesthesia to facilitate the insertion, e.g. of a ventilator, into the windpipe.
Dosage: according to body weight, usually 0.3–1.1mg/kg depending on degree of muscle relaxation needed.
Special care: premedication with atropine is desirable. More prolonged muscle paralysis may occur in patients with dual block (after several doses of suxamethonium) and in those with low pseudocholinesterase enzymes in blood plasma, requiring continued artificial ventilation until normal muscle function is resumed
Avoid use: patients with burns and those with serious liver disease.
Manufacturer: Wellcome.

ANEXATE

Description: an antagonist to the effects of benzodiazepines used in anaesthesia, diagnostic procedures and intensive care. It contains 100 µg of flumazenil per ml of solution and is administered by means of intravenous injection or infusion.
Used for: reversal of sedative effects of benzodiazepines in anaesthesia, intensive care and diagnostic investigations.
Dosage: by injection, 200µg given over 15 seconds. Repeated doses of 100µg at one minutes intervals if needed. Usual dose in the order of 300–600µg with a maximum of 1mg (possibly 2mg in intensive care procedures). By infusion (if drowsiness persists after initial injection), 100–400µg per hour according to patient response.
Special care: rapid injection should be avoided especially in patients who have had major surgery, head injury or liver disorders.
Avoid use: epileptic patients who have received sustained doses of benzodi-azepines.
Side effects: vomiting, nausea, flushing. If wakening is too rapid patient may be anxious, agitated and fearful. Intensive care patients may have short-lived

increase in heart rate and blood pressure. Rarely, convulsions may occur especially in epileptic patients.
Manufacturer: Roche.

ANHYDROL FORTE

Description: an anti-perspirant solution containing 20% aluminium chloride hexahydrate in an alcohol base. It is available as a solution in a bottle with a roll-on applicator.
Used for: excessive sweating (hyperhid-rosis) of armpits, hands and feet.
Dosage: apply at night to dry skin and wash off the following morning. Use less as condition improves.
Special care: avoid bathing immediately before use or use of depilatory creams and shaving of armpits within 12 hours of applying. Should only be used on feet in children.
Avoid use: contact with eyes, broken or inflamed skin. Contact with clothing and jewellery.
Manufacturer: Dermal.

ANQUIL

Description: an antipsychotic drug available as white tablets containing 0.25mg (butyrophenone) benperidol marked Janssen, A and 0.25.
Used for: antisocial, deviant sexual behaviour.
Dosage: adults, 0.25mg to 1.5mg per day in divided doses. Elderly or debilitated patients, half adult dose.
Special care: patients with epilepsy, Parkinsonism, heart disease, kidney or liver disorders, glaucoma, acute infections, elderly persons, pregnant or nursing mothers. Also, those with history of jaundice, underactive thyroid gland, myasthenia gravis, enlarged prostate gland. Regular blood counts and tests of liver function should be carried out during extensive therapy.
Avoid use: children, symptoms of central nervous system disturbance (pyramidal or extrapyramidal effects).
Possible interaction: alcohol, antihyper-

tensive, antidepressant and anticonvulsive drugs, analgesic drugs, central nervous system depressants, levodopa and antidiabetic drugs.
Side effects: muscle spasms of eyes, neck, back, face, Parkinson-like symptoms (tremor and rigidity), dry mouth, nasal stiffness, irregular heartbeat, palpitations, blurring of vision, blood changes, jaundice, drowsiness, fatigue, low blood pressure, weight gain, impotence, breast enlargement, hypothermia (in elderly), constipation, rarely, fits.
Manufacturer: Janssen.

ANTABUSE

Description: a preparation containing the drug disulfiram, an enzyme (aldehyde dehydrogenase) inhibitor used in the treatment of alcoholism. It is available as white, scored tablets (200mg) marked ANY 200 and CP.
Used for: adjunct in therapy for alcohol dependence.
Dosage: adults, 800mg as single dose on first day. Afterwards reducing to 200–100mg over period of five days. Should not be used for longer than six months.
Special care: liver or kidney disease, respiratory disease, diabetes mellitus, epilepsy. Careful counselling of patient essential before use as reaction of disulfiram with even a minute quantity of alcohol causes extremely unpleasant and possibly fatal consequences due to accumulation of acetaldehyde in body. With small amounts of alcohol reactions include severe throbbing headache, palpitations, nausea, vomiting, raised heartbeat, flushing of face. The quantity of alcohol in many medicines may be sufficient to precipitate this. Larger quantities of alcohol can cause hypotension, heart arrhythmias and collapse. No alcohol should be consumed until one week after stopping the drug or for 24 hours prior to start of treatment.
Avoid use: patients with heart failure, coronary artery disease or high blood

pressure. Children and pregnant women. Patients with severe mental disorders or suicidal tendencies.
Possible interaction: alcohol, some TCADs, paraldehyde, warfarin, barbiturate drugs, antiepileptic drugs, metronidazole (antibacterial drug).
Side effects: fatigue and drowsiness, vomiting and nausea, bad breath (halitosis), reduced libido, allergic skin reactions, liver damage. Rarely, mental disturbances (mania, paranoia, schizophrenia, depression).
Manufacturer: CP Pharmaceuticals.

ANTEPSIN

Description: a cytoprotectant (cell-surface protectant) preparation available in the form of tablets and suspension. The tablets are scored, white, oblong in shape and contain 1g sucralfate, marked Antepsin on one side and WY39 on reverse. ANTEPSIN SUSPENSION contains 1g/5ml of solution.
Used for: gastric and duodental ulcers, chronic gastritis, prevention of haemorrhage from stress, ulceration in patients who are seriously ill.
Dosage: tablets, adults 2g twice a day in the morning and at bedtime or 1g four times a day one hour before meals. Maximum dose 8g per day. Treatment period usually 4–6 weeks, sometimes up to 12 weeks. Prevention (prophylaxis) of stress ulceration, 1g suspension 6 times a day with a maximum of 8g daily.
Special care: patients with kidney failure, pregnancy and lactation.
Avoid use: children and patients with severe kidney failure.
Possible interaction: antibacterial drugs (ciproflxacin, ofloxacin, norfloxacin and tetracycline), warfarin, antiepileptics (phenytoin).
Side effects: gastro-intestinal upsets—constipation, diarrhoea, indigestion, nausea, dry mouth, rash, back pain, dizziness, sleeplessness, drowsiness, vertigo are possible.
Manufacturer: Wyeth.

ANTHRANOL

Description: an ointment available in three strengths, containing 0.4%, 1% and 2% dithranol, and also 0.5% salicylic acid. Dithranol is the most potent of the preparations used in the treatment of psoriasis and must be applied with caution.

Used for: psoriasis.

Dosage: starting with low concentrations initially once a day, ointment is applied to skin lesions and washed off after ten minutes. The concentration and time period may be gradually increased (the ointment may be left on for half an hour), depending upon the response of the patient's condition.

Special care: may cause severe skin irritation in some people (especially those with fair skin) even at low concentrations hence must be used with caution. Stains clothing and skin.

Avoid use: acute psoriasis, pustular psoriasis.

Side effects: skin irritation which may be severe, burning, allergic reactions.

Manufacturer: Stiefel.

ANTURAN

Description: a preparation containing the active ingredient, sulphinpyrazone, which promotes the excretion of uric acid by preventing its reabsorption in the kidney tubules. Anturan is available in the form of yellow, sugar-coated tablets marked Geigy in 2 strengths, (100mg and 200mg).

Used for: hyperuricaemia (high blood levels of uric acid), chronic gout, recurrent gouty arthritis.

Dosage: adults, 100mg to 200mg with food per day at first increasing over a 2–3 week period to 600mg. After this the amount is reduced (once uric acid level has dropped) to a maintenance dose which may be as low as 200mg daily.

Special care: pregnant and breastfeeding mothers, kidney disease or heart failure. Plenty of fluids should be taken during treatment and blood and kidney function tests may be necessary.

Avoid use: children. Patients with known allergies to anti-inflammatory drugs, severe liver or kidney disease, acute gout, history of peptic ulcers or acute peptic ulcer, blood disorders, porphyria.

Possible interaction: salicylates, aspirin, hypoglycaemic drugs, anticoagulants, sulphonamides, penicillins, phenytoin, theophylline.

Side effects: gastro-intestinal upset and bleeding, ulcers, acute gout, kidney stones, renal colic, liver and kidney disorders, rash, blood changes (treatment should stop).

Manufacturer: Geigy.

ANUGESIC H-C

Description: a preparation containing corticosteroid combined with antiseptic and soothing properties, available in the form of a cream and as suppositories. The cream contains 1.25% benzyl benzoate, 0.875% bismuth oxide, 0.5% hydrocortisone acetate, 1.85% Peru balsam, 1% pramoxine hydrochloride and 12.35% zinc oxide. ANUGESIC H-C SUPPOSITORIES contain 33mg benzyl benzoate, 24mg bismuth oxide, 59mg bismuth subgallate, 5mg hydrocortisone acetate, 49mg Peru balsam, 27mg pramoxine hydrochloride and 296mg zinc oxide.

Used for: haemorrhoids, anal itching and other ano-rectal disorders.

Dosage: adults, 1 suppository or application of cream morning and night and after bowel movement.

Special care: pregnant women. Avoid prolonged use—no more than 7 days.

Avoid use: children. Fungal and viral infections. Tuberculosis.

Side effects: systemic (affecting body as a whole) corticosteroid effects.

Manufacturer: Parke-Davis.

ANUSOL HC

Description: an astringent antiseptic with soothing properties in the form of an ointment and suppositories. The ointment contains 1.25% benzyl

benzoate, 0.875 bismuth oxide, 2.25% bismuth subgallate, 0.25% hydrocortisone acetate, 1.875% Peru balsam, 10.75% zinc oxide. The suppositories contain 33mg benzyl benzoate, 24mg bismuth oxide, 59mg bismuth subgallate, 10mg hydrocortisone acetate, 49mg Peru balsam and 296mg zinc oxide.
Used for: haemorrhoids, ano-rectal inflammation.
Dosage: adults, one application of ointment or one suppository night and morning and after bowel movement.
Special care: pregnant women. Not to be used for longer than 7 days.
Avoid use: children, patients with fungal or viral infections or suffering from tuberculosis.
Side effects: systemic (affecting whole body) corticosteroid effects.
Manufacturer: Parke-Davis.

APISATE[CD]

Description: a preparation which combines an appetite suppressant with vitamin B. It contains the central nervous system stimulant, and sympathomimetic agent, diethylproprion, which should only be taken for a few days as it can cause dependence and psychiatric effects. Apisate is available in the form of two-layer yellow, sustained-release tablets marked Wyeth containing 75mg diethylproprion hydrochloride, 5mg thiamine hydrochloride, 4mg riboflavine, 2mg pyridoxine hydrochloride, 30mg nicotinamide.
Used for: patients suffering from obesity.
Dosage: adults, 1 daily in early morning or mid-afternoon.
Special care: patients with severe liver or kidney disorders, peptic ulcer, angina, heart arrhythmias, high blood pressure, enlargement of prostate gland, depression, first three months of pregnancy. May affect the performance of skilled tasks such as driving. Prolonged use should be avoided.
Avoid use: children and elderly persons, patients with a history of psychiatric

illness, drug or alcohol abuse, arteriosclerosis, glaucoma, severe high blood pressure, hyperthyroidism.
Possble interaction: sympathomimetic drugs, MAOIs, psychotropic drugs, guanethidine, methyldopa, other anoretics.
Side effects: dependence and tolerance, psychiatric disorders, anxiety, insomnia, agitation and nervousness.
Manufacturer: Wyeth.

APRESOLINE

Description: a vasodilator available in the form of tablets of two strengths and as a powder for reconstitution for injection. It contains hydralazine hydrochloride. Yellow tablets (25mg) are sugar-coated and marked CIBA and GF, while the deep pink tablets are marked in the same way and contain 50mg.
APRESOLINE INJECTION contains 20mg hydralazine hydrochloride as a powder in an ampoule for reconstitution.
Used for: moderate and severe chronic heart failure. Also used for moderate to severe hypertension.
Dosage: for hypertension in adults (along with ß-blocker and thiazide diuretic), 25mg twice a day at first increasing to a maximum of 200mg daily. For cardiac failure in adults (with diuretics and cardiac glycosides), 25mg 3–4 times each day increasing to 50–75mg 4 times a day every second day.
Special care: patients with coronary or cerebrovascular disease, liver disorders, severe kidney failure, nursing mothers. Withdrawal should be gradual.
Avoid use: children, first half of pregnancy, patients with certain heart disorders (aortic, mitral stenosis, tachycardia, idiopathic SLE, constructive pericarditis, dissecting aortic aneurysm, cor pulmonale).
Possible interaction: anaesthetics, TCADs, MAOIs, antihypertensive drugs, diazoxide, CNS depressants.
Side effects: hypotension, tachycardia, angina, headache, flushes, especially with daily dose exceeding 100mg.

Protein in urine, blood in urine, kidney failure, urine retention. Possible though rare, liver damage, nerve disorders and blood changes.
Manufacturer: CIBA

APRINOX

Description: a thiazide preparation which has diuretic properties and is available as white tablets of two strengths containing 2.5mg or 5mg of bendrofluazide.
Used for: hypertension, oedema such as occurs in mild to moderate heart failure.
Dosage: adults, for oedema, 5–10mg in morning or on alternate days at first and then 5–10mg once or twice per week for maintenance. For hypertension, 2.5–5mg once each day.
Special care: pregnancy and breastfeeding, elderly persons. Patients with liver or kidney disease, liver cirrhosis, gout, diabetes, SLE. Advisable to monitor fluid, electrolytes and glucose levels.
Avoid use: children. Patients with severe liver or kidney failure, hypercalcaemia, Addisons disease, allergy to sulphonamide drugs.
Possible interaction: alcohol, opioids, barbiturates, antidiabetic drugs, NSAIDs, corticosteroids, tubocurarine, carbenoxolone, cardiac glucosides, lithium.
Side effects: metabolic disturbance and upset of electrolyte balance, gastrointestinal disturbance, blood changes, rash, dizziness, impotence, pancreatitis, anorexia.
Manufacturer: Boots.

ARAMINE

Description: a sympathomimetiuc amine that acts as a vasoconstrictor available as ampoules for injection containing 10mg metraminol tartrate per ml.
Used for: acute hypotension such as may occur in patients in severe shock or during general anaesthesia.
Dosage: 15–100mg according to response.
Special care: possible localized tissue death at injection site.
Avoid use: pregnancy, heart attack.

Side effects: reduced blood flow to kidneys, heart arrhythmias and tachycardia.
Manufacturer: MSD.

AREDIA

Description: a preparation of the disophonate drug disodium pamidronate available as a powder for reconstitution and intravenous infusion. Vials contain 15mg or 30mg.
Used for: hypercalcaemia caused by malignancy.
Dosage: adults, depending upon levels of calcium in blood plasma, maximum dose of 90mg each treatment given by slow infusion at a rate not exceeding 30mg in two hours. Dose may be divided over 2–4 days.
Special care: severe kidney disorders, may cause convulsions due to disturbance of electrolyte balance.
Avoid use: pregnancy and breastfeeding.
Possible interaction: other infusions containing calcium disophonates, drugs for hypocalcaemia, plicamycin.
Side effects: diarrhoea, nausea, short-lived rise in body temperature, hypocalcaemia, lowering of magnesium levels, decrease in number of white blood cells (lymphocytes) in blood.
Manufacturer: CIBA

ARELIX

Description: a powerful diuretic (a *loop diuretic*) which acts on the parts of the kidney tubules known as the loops of Henle. It is available as orange/green sustained release capsules containing 6mg of piretanide.
Used for: mild to moderate hypertension.
Dosage: 1 or 2 capsules taken in the morning with food.
Special care: hypokalaemia may develop and monitoring of electrolyte levels may be necessary especially in patients with impaired kidney or liver function. Also, in patients with enlarged prostate gland or impaired urination. Pregnancy and nursing mothers, persons with diabetes or gout.

Avoid use: patients with severe imbalance of electrolytes, liver cirrhosis, children.
Possible interaction: antihypertensive drugs, NSAIDs, digoxin, lithium, cephalosporin antibiotic drugs, aminoglycosides.
Side effects: electrolyte imbalance, rarely gastro-intestinal upset, muscle pain after high doses.
Manufacturer: Hoechst.

ARFONAD

Description: trimetaphan camsylate, a ganglion blocker, available in ampoules for injection or infusion (50mg per ml).
Used for: controlled lowering of blood pressure (hypotension) during surgery.
Dosage: by intravenous infusion at a rate of 3–4mg per minute in first instance and thereafter adjusted according to the patient's response.
Special care: patients with impaired liver or kidney function, coronary disease, cerebral vascular disease, degenerative conditions of the central nervous system, Addison's disease, reduced adrenal gland function. Also in elderly persons and patients with diabetes mellitus.
Avoid use: pregnant women, serious heart disease, severe arteriosclerosis, pyloric stenosis.
Side effects: depression of breathing (especially in combination with muscle relaxant drugs), tachycardia, dilation of pupils, increased intra-ocular pressure in eyes, constipation.
Manufacturer: Cambridge.

ARPICOLIN

Description: an anticholinergic preparation of the drug procyclidine hydrochloride available in the form of a syrup in two strengths, containing 2.5mg or 5mg per 5ml.
Used for: Parkinsonism, including that which is drug-induced.
Dosage: 2.5mg–5mg 3 times each day at first. This is increased at 2 to 3 day

intervals to a usual maximum of 30mg daily (exceptionally, 60mg).
Special care: patients with obstruction of gastro-intestinal tract, enlarged prostate gland, heart disease, narrow-angle glaucoma. Drug should be withdrawn gradually.
Avoid use: children, patients with a movement disorder called tardive dyskinesia.
Possible interaction: antidepressant and antihistamine drugs. Phenothiazines.
Side effects: anticholinergic effects, with high doses there may be mental confusion.
Manufacturer: R.P. Drugs.

ARTANE

Description: an anticholinergic containing benhexol hydrochloride, an antimuscarine drug used in the treatment of Parkinsonism. White-scored tablets are available in two strengths (2mg and 5mg) coded 4434 and 4436 respectively. Both are marked Lederle.
Used for: Parkinsonism including drug-induced Parkinson's disease.
Dosage: first day, 1mg, second day, 2mg, then increased by 2mg daily every 3 to 5 days. The maintenance dose is usually 5–15mg per day.
Special care: patients with obstruction of gastro-intestinal tract, kidney or liver disease, heart disorders, enlargement of prostate gland, narrow angle glaucoma.
Avoid use: children.
Possible interaction: antihistamine and antidepressant drugs. Phenothiazine drugs.
Side effects: anticholinergic effects. After high doses, agitation and confusion.
Manufacturer: Lederle.

ARTHROTEC

Description: an NSAID containing diclofenac sodium, a phenylacetic acid prostaglandin analogue. Arthrotec tablets contain 50mg diclofenac sodium, 200 μg misoprostol and are marked with a symbol and Searle 1411.
Used for: osteoarthritis, rheumatoid arthritis.

Dosage: adults, one tablet twice a day with food increasing to one three times a day if required.

Special care: women of childbearing age should use effective contraception. Patients with gastric or duodenal ulcer, heart disease, coronary, cerebrovascular, peripheral vascular disease, kidney or liver disorders. Patients taking the drug for a long period should be monitored.

Avoid use: children, pregnant women or those planning pregnancy, breastfeeding. Patients with gastro-intestinal bleeding, those with allergy to aspirin or other anti-inflammatory drugs.

Possible interaction: NSAIDs, anticoagulants, quinolone, methotrexate, digoxin, lithium, steroids, diuretic drugs, oral hypoglycaemics.

Side effects: gastro-intestinal upset, erosion of gastro-intestinal tract, heavy menstrual bleeding and intermenstrual bleeding, dizziness, headache, oedema, nausea, skin reactions.

Manufacturer: Searle.

ARYTHMOL

Description: a class I antiarrhythmic drug used to treat disturbances of heart rhythm. Arythmol contains propafenone hydrochloride and is available in tablets of two strengths (150 and 300mg) which are white, scored and film-coated.

Used for: treatment and prevention of ventricular arrhythmias.

Dosage: adults, 150mg 3 times daily in first instance, gradually increasing at 3-day intervals to 300mg twice a day. Maximum dose is 300mg 3 times a day.

Special care: patients with heart failure or who are fitted with pacemakers, those with liver or kidney disorders, elderly persons.

Avoid use: children, pregnant women, some particular forms of heart rhythm disturbance, patients with uncontrolled congestive heart failure, electrolyte balance disturbances, obstructive lung disease, severe hypotension, myasthenia gravis.

Possible interaction: other class I antiarrhythmic drugs, myocardial (heart muscle) depressant drugs, warfarin, digoxin, cimetidine rifampicin, propranolol, metoprolol.

Side effects: gastro-intestinal upset including constipation, diarrhoea, vomiting, nausea, unpleasant bitter taste, fatigue, headache, allergic skin rashes, disturbances of heart rhythm.

Manufacturer: Knoll.

ASACOL

Description: a preparation of the salicylate drug, mesalazine, available as tablets and suppositories. Tablets (400mg strength) are oblong, red and resin-coated. Suppositories are available in two strengths containing 250mg and 500mg. Also, **ASACOL FOAM ENEMA** is available.

Used for: to induce and maintain remission in ulcerative colitis and to treat acute attacks of this condition.

Dosage: adults, tablets, acute attack, 6 daily in divided doses. For maintenance, 3–6 tablets daily in divided doses. Asacol suppositories, adults 750–1500mg daily in divided doses with last dose at night.

Special care: elderly persons, pregnant and nursing mothers, patients with kidney disease, elevated blood urea levels, proteinuria.

Avoid use: children, patients with severe kidney disease.

Possible interaction: lactulose, substance which increases acidity of motions.

Side effects: gastro-intestinal upset, blood changes, headache, kidney failure.

Manufacturer: S.K. & F.

ASENDIS

Description: a TCAD preparation containing amoxapine, available in tablets of various strength, all seven-sided, scored tablets: 25mg, white, marked LL25; 50mg, orange, marked LL50; 100mg, blue, marked LL100 and 150mg, white, marked LL150.

Used for: depression.

Dosage: 100–150mg per day at first increasing to a maintenance dose in the region of 150–250mg. Maximum daily dose is 300mg. Elderly persons, 25mg twice a day at first increasing, after 5–7 days, to 50mg 3 times daily if required.

Special care: patients with psychoses or suicidal tendencies, elderly persons, pregnant and nursing mothers, people with cardiac disorders, epilepsy, hyperthyroidism, urine retention, closed angle glaucoma, liver disease, tumours of adrenal gland, diabetes.

Avoid use: children, patients with recent heart attack, heart arrhythmias, heart block, porphyria (rare blood disorder).

Possible interaction: alcohol, barbiturate drugs, local anaesthetics (containing adrenaline or noradrenaline), antihypertensive and sympathomimetic drugs, anticholineric drugs, cimetidine, oestrogens.

Side effects: anticholinergic effects including urine retention, dry mouth, constipation, blurred vision, rapid heartbeat, palpitations, nervousness, insomnia, sweating, dizziness, fatigue, weight changes, jaundice, blood changes, allergic skin rashes, changes in libido, breast enlargement and impotence.

Manufacturer: Novex.

ASPAV

Description: a combined salicylate and opiate analgesic containing aspirin and papaveretum available as dissolvable tablets. Aspav white tablets contain 500mg aspirin, 10mg papaveretum.

Used for: relief of post-operative pain and chronic pain caused by inoperable cancers.

Dosage: adults, 1–2 tablets in water every four to six hours. Maximum daily dose, 8 tablets in 24 hours.

Special care: women in labour, pregnant women and nursing mothers, elderly persons. Patients with head injury, liver or kidney disease, gastro-intestinal

ulcers, heart failure, hypothyroidism, history of bronchospasm or allergy to anti-inflammatory drugs.

Avoid use: children, patients in comatose states with depressed breathing, or obstructed airways.

Possible interaction: central nervous system depressants, NSAIDs, anticoagulants, MAOIs, sulphonamide antibiotics, hypoglycaemic drugs, uric acid-lowering drugs, methotrexate.

Side effects: allergic responses, asthma, bleeding of gastro-intestinal tract, confusion, nausea, constipation.

Manufacturer: Roussel.

ATAVAX

Description: an antihistamine preparation containing hydroxyzine hydrochloride available as sugar-coated tablets of two strengths (10 and 25mg) coloured orange and green respectively and in the form of a syrup. **ATARAX SYRUP** contains 10mg hydroxyzine hydrochloride per 5ml.

Used for: anxiety (short-term treatment) and itching caused by allergy (chronic urticaria and dermatitis).

Dosage: anxiety, adults only, 50–100mg 4 times each day. Itching, adults, 25mg taken at night increasing to 25mg 3–4 times a day if required. Children, 6 months to 6 years, 5–15mg daily increasing to 50mg in divided doses if required; 6 years and over, 15–25mg daily increasing to 50–100mg in divided doses if required.

Special care: patients with kidney disease. Patients must be warned that judgement and dexterity is impaired. Children should be given reduced doses for itching only.

Avoid use: pregnant women.

Possible interaction: central nervous system depressants, alcohol.

Side effects: drowsiness, anticholinergic effects, if high doses are taken there may be involuntary muscle movements.

Manufacturer: Pfizer.

ATIVAN

Description: an anxiolytic benzodiazepine, lorazepam. which is for short-term use only as it carries a risk of dependency. It is available as tablets of two strengths and also in the form of ampoules for injection. Blue, oblong, scored tablets, marked A1 contain 1mg and yellow, oblong, scored tablets, marked A2.5 contain 2.5mg. **ATIVAN INJECTION** contains 4mg lorazepam per ml.

Used for: anxiety, status epilepticus (a condition where a person with epilepsy suffers a series of fits in close succession and is deprived of oxygen), a sedative premedication prior to full anaesthesia.

Dosage: tablets, adults, for anxiety, 1–4mg each day in divided doses. Elderly persons, 0.5mg–2mg each day. For status epilepticus, adults, 4mg by intravenous injection, children half the adult dose. For premedication, adults, tablets, 2–4mg 1 or 2 hours prior to operation or 0.05mg per kg of body weight intravenously about 30–45 minutes before operation.

Special care: women in labour, pregnancy, breastfeeding, elderly, liver or kidney disorders, lung disease. Short-term use only, withdraw gradually.

Avoid use: children, acute lung diseases, depression of breathing, those with chronic psychoses, obsessional states and phobias.

Possible interaction: CNS depressant drugs, alcohol, anticonvulsants.

Side effects: light-headedness, drowsiness, vertigo, confusion, unsteadiness in walking, gastro-intestinal upset, disturbance of vision, rash, retention of urine, changes in libido, low blood pressure. Rarely, blood changes and jaundice. Risk of dependence especially with high doses.

Manufacturer: Wyeth.

ATROMID-S

Description: an isobutyric acid derivative which lowers the concentration of cholesterol and other fats (lipids) found in blood plasma. It is available as red, gelatin-coated capsules, marked ICI, containing 500mg of clofibrate.

Used for: elevated plasma lipid levels (hyperlipidaemias) of types IIb, III, IV and V which have not been lowered by dietary changes or other appropriate treatments.

Dosage: adults, 20–30mg per kg of body weight two to three times daily after meals in divided doses.

Special care: patients with low levels of albumin (protein) in blood serum. Regular blood checks may be carried out.

Avoid use: children, pregnant women, patients with diseases of the gall bladder, liver or kidney disorders.

Possible interaction: hypoglycaemics, phenytoin, anticoagulants.

Side effects: gastro-intestinal upset, muscle pains, gallstones.

Manufacturer: Zeneca.

ATROVENT

Description: an anticholinergic containing ipratropium bromide available available in various forms: aerosol inhalation, 20 µg per dose delivered by metered dose inhaler; **ATROVENT AUTOHALER**, 20 µg per dose delivered by breath-actuated metered dose aerosol; **ATROVENT FORTE**, 40 µg per dose delivered by metered dose inhaler; **ATROVENT SOLUTION**, 250 µg per ml, in preservative-free isotonic solution in unit dose vials for use with nebulizer.

Used for: severe obstruction of airways, especially that caused by chronic bronchitis.

Dosage: adults, inhaler, 1–2 puffs three or four times a day. Children under 6 years, one puff, 6–12 years, 1–2 puffs, both three times a day. Adults, Atrovent Forte, 1 or 2 puffs three to four times daily; children 6–12 years, 1 puff three times daily. Adults, Atrovent solution, 0.4–2ml nebulised up to four times each day. Children over 3 years, 0.4–2ml nebulised up to three times each day.

Special care: patients with enlarged prostate gland (prostate hypertrophy), glaucoma.
Side effects: urine retention, constipation, dry mouth.
Manufacturer: Boehringer Ingelheim.

AUDICORT

Description: a combined antibacterial, antifungal and anti-inflammatory (corticosteroid) preparation available in the form of ear drops. Audicort contains 1mg triamcinolone acetate and neomycin undecylenate (antibiotic) (equivalent to 3.5mg neomycin base).
Used for: chronic and acute inflammation and/or bacterial infection of the outer ear.
Dosage: adults, 2–5 drops three of fopur times each day.
Special care: pregnant and nursing mothers avoid prolonged use.
Avoid use: children, patients with perforated ear drum.
Side effects: localized irritation, additional infection.
Manufacturer: Lederle.

AUGMENTIN

Description: a broad-spectrum, penicillin-like antibiotic, amoxycillin as the trihydrate, with clavulanic acid as the potassium salt. The latter makes the antibiotic effective against a wider range of infections by combating certain enzymes produced by some bacteria. Available as white film coated tablets, Augmentin 375mg (250mg/125mg) and 625mg (500mg/125mg). Also, **AUGMENTIN DISPERSABLE** (250mg/125mg), white tablets marked Augmentin. Also **AUGMENTIN SUSPENSION 125/31 SF** (sugar-free) contains 125mg amoxycillin as trihydrate, 31mg clavulanic acid as potassium salt, per 5 ml when reconstituted with water. Similarly, **AUGMENTIN SUSPENSION 250/62 SF** (250/62mg). **AUGMENTIN INTRAVENOUS** is a powder for intravenous injection available in 2 strengths containing amoxycillin as sodium salt and clavulanic acid as potassium salt (500/100mg, and 1g/200mg).
Used for: respiratory tract and ear, nose and throat infections, skin and soft tissue infections, urinary tract infections.
Dosage: adults, tablets, 375mg three times a day (severe infections 625mg) for 14 days. Children, use suspension, under 6 years use lower strength 125/31. Under one year 25mg per kg body weight each day; 1–6 years, 5ml three times a day for 14 days. 6–12 years use 250/62 suspension, 5ml 3 times each day for 14 days.
Intravenous injection: adults, 1.2g or by intermittent infusion 6 to 8-hourly for 14 days. Children, under 3 months, 30mg per kg of body weight every 12 hours in newborns increasing to every 8 hours in older infants. 3 months–12 years, 30mg per kg of body weight every 8 or 6 hours. By intravenous or intermittent infusion for up to 14 days.
Special care: pregnant and breastfeeding mothers, patients with liver and kidney disease, glandular fever. Review after 14 days.
Avoid use: allergy to penicillin.
Side effects: gastro-intestinal upset, allergic responses, rarely cholestatic jaundice, hepatitis, phlebitis at site of injection.
Manufacturer: Beecham.

AUREOCORT

Description: a combined antibacterial and steroid preparation available in the form of cream or ointment, containing 0.1% of the corticosteroid triamcinolone acetonide and 3% of the tetracycline antibiotic, chlortetracycline hydrochloride.
Used for: inflammation and irritation of the skin where infection is present also.
Dosage: apply sparingly to affected skin two or three times daily.
Special care: limit use to a short time

period. In children and on face, treatment should not exceed 5 days.
Avoid use: on extensive areas of skin or for long time periods or for prevention. Acne (including rosacea), urticaria, scabies, leg ulcers, viral skin infections, tuberculosis, ringworm.
Side effects: thinning of skin and skin changes, adrenal gland suppression, fluid retention.
Manufacturer: Lederle.

AUREOMYCIN

Description: a broad-spectrum antibiotic preparation, containing chlortetracycline hydrochloride, available as cream and ointment both of which contain 3% chlortetracycline hydrochloride. Aureomycin is also available as an eye ointment containing 1% tetracycline hydrochloride.
Used for: superficial skin infections with bacterial origin. Eye infections sensitive to tetracycline.
Dosage: skin infections, apply on gauze once or twice daily. Eye infections, apply into eye every two hours then reduce frequency as condition improves. Continue to use for 48 hours after symptoms have disappeared.
Avoid use: Possible interaction:
Side effects: additional infections.
Manufacturer: Lederle.

AVENTYL

Description: a TCAD, nortriptyline hydrochloride, available in capsules of two strengths: white/yellow capsules coded H17 (10mg) and white/yellow capsules coded H19 (25mg). All marked Lilly.
Used for: depression and also bed-wetting in children.
Dosage: depression, adults, 20–40mg each day in divided doses increasing to 100mg daily if necessary. Usual maintenance is in the order of 30–75mg. Elderly persons, 10mg three times daily. Bed-wetting in children over six years, 10–35mg 30 minutes before bedtime.

Special care: patients with heart disease, tumours of adrenal gland, enlarged thyroid gland, liver disease, diabetes, epilepsy, glaucoma, urine retention. Persons with psychoses or suicidal tendencies. Also, in nursing mothers.
Avoid use: children under six years, pregnant women, serious liver disease, heart attack, heart block.
Possible interaction: other antidepressants, MAOIs, alcohol, barbiturates, local anaesthetics containing adrenaline or noradrenaline, anticholinergics, antihypertensives, oestrogens, cimetidine.
Side effects: constipation, urine retention, dry mouth, blurred vision, raised heartbeat, palpitations, insomnia, anxiety, drowsiness, tremor, sweating, dizziness, fatigue, unsteadiness, weight changes, low blood pressure. Allergic skin rashes, blood changes, jaundice, heart arrhythmias, changes in libido, impotence. Mania and schizophrenic symptoms may be activated especially in elderly persons.
Manufacturer: Eli Lilly.

AVLOCLOR

Description: an antimalarial drug containing chloroquine phosphate, available as white, scored tablets containing 250mg chloroquine phosphate.
Used for: prevention and treatment of malaria, rheumatoid arthritis, lupus erythematosus (inflammatory disease of skin and some internal organs), amoebic hepatitis.
Dosage: prevention of malaria; adults, 2 tablets as one dose on the same day each week commmencing 2 weeks before entering affected area and continuing for 4 weeks after leaving. Children should take in the same way at a dose rate of 5mg per kg of body weight. Treatment of hepatitis, adults only, four tablets each day for two days then one tablet twice daily for two to three weeks.
Special care: pregnancy, liver or kidney disease, breastfeeding, patients with

epilepsy and some other neurological
conditions, psoriasis, porphyria, severe
gastro-intestinal disorders. Regular eye
tests may be needed during treatment.
Side effects: gastro-intestinal upset,
headache, hair loss, loss of pigment, skin
rashes, blurred vision, opacity of cornea,
retinal damage.
Manufacturer: Zeneca.

AXID

Description: a preparation containing
nizatidine (an H₂ blocker) available in
the form of capsules: pale, yellow/dark
yellow, coded 3144 (150mg) and yellow/
brown coded 3145 (300mg). AXID
INJECTION contains 25mg nizatidine
per ml.
Used for: duodenal and benign gastric
ulcers and their prevention. Gastro-
oesophageal reflux disease.
Dosage: adults, for duodenal and gastric
ulcers, 300mg taken in the evening or
150mg morning and evening for 4–8
weeks. Prevention, 150mg in evening for
up to one year. Adults, for gastro-
oesophageal reflux disease, 150mg–
300mg twice a day for up to 12 weeks.
Axid injection, adults, dilute before use,
100mg by slow intravenous injection
three times each day or 10mg per hour
by intravenous infusion. Maximum
480mg per day.
Special care: patients with liver or kidney
disease, pregnant or breastfeeding mothers.
Avoid use: children.
Possible interaction: salicylates.
Side effects: sweating, sleepiness,
itchiness, headache, muscle and joint
pain, jaundice, raised levels of liver
enzymes, hepatitis, anaemia.
Manufacturer: Lilly.

AXSAIN

Description: a topical counter-irritant
analgesic preparation available as a
cream containing 0.075% capsaicin.
Used for: post-herpetic neuralgia.
Dosage: adults only, massage in 3 to 4
times daily once lesions have healed.

Avoid use: children, on broken, irritated
skin.
Side effects: local skin irritation.
Manufacturer: Euroderma.

AZACTAM

Description: a powder for injection and
infusion, containing 500mg aztreonam
available as 1g or 2g powder in vials.
Used for: serious infections caused by
Gram-negative bacteria, including those
of the lower respiratory tract and lung
infections in cystic fibrosis sufferers.
Also, soft tissue, skin, joint, bone,
gynaecological and abdominal
infections. Urinary tract infections and
gonorrhoea, meningitis (where H.
influenzae or N. Menigitidis is the causal
organism), septicaemia and bacteraemia
(bacteria in blood indicating infection).
Dosage: adults, 1g by intramuscular or
intravenous injection every eight hours
or 2g intravenously every 12 hours. If
infection is severe, 2g six to eight hourly
intravenously. Maximum daily dose is
8g. For urinary tract infections, 0.5–1g
intramuscularly or intravenously every
eight to twelve hours. For cystitis, 1g
intramuscularly as a single dose.
Children, one week to two years, 30mg
per kg of body weight every six to eight
hours. Severe infections in children over
two years, 50mg per kg of body weight
every six to eight hours. Maximum dose
is 8g each day.
Special care: patients with allergy to
penicillin or cephalospoin. Persons with
kidney or liver disease.
Avoid use: children under one year,
pregnant or breastfeeding mothers.
Side effects: gastro-intestinal upset,
vomiting and diarrhoea, local skin
inflammation at injection site.
Manufacturer: Squibb.

AZAMUNE

Description: an immunosuppressant,
cytotoxic preparation containing
azathioprine available as yellow, scored
tablets marked AZA 50 (50mg).

Used for: to lessen the likelihood of rejection following organ transplants and donor skin grafts. Also, some auto-immune diseases.

Dosage: adults and children, following transplant, 5mg per kg of body weight at first then 1–4mg per kg of body weight each day for 3 months in divided doses. For chronic hepatitis, 1–1.5mg per kg of body weight daily. Auto-immune diseases, 2–2.5mg per kg of body weight daily.

Special care: Azathioprine causes suppression of bone marrow function, hence careful monitoring of blood count for toxic effects is necessary and dosage must be adjusted accordingly. Pregnant women, patients with over-exposure to sun, any infection, kidney disorders.

Avoid use: toxic hepatitis, stoppage of bile flow.

Possible interaction: muscle relaxant drugs, cytostatics, allopurinol.

Side effects: bone marrow suppression, liver toxicity, gastro-intestinal upset, rashes.

Manufacturer: Penn Pharmaceuticals.

BACTRIM

Description: a preparation combining an antibacterial sulphonamide with a folic acid inhibitor. Elongated, orange, film-coated capsules marked Roche contain 80mg trimethoprim and 400mg sulphamethoxazole. Also, **BACTRIM DISPERSIBLE**: yellow tablets, scored, containing 480mg co-trimoxazole. **BACTRIM DOUBLE STRENGTH**: white scored tablets containing 160mg trimethoprim and 800mg sulphmethoxazole and marked Roche 800 and 160. **BACTRIM ADULT SUSPENSION** is a yellow syrup containing 480mg co-trimoxazole per 5ml and **BACTRIM PAEDIATRIC SYRUP** contains 40mg

trimethoprim and 200mg sulphmethoxazole per 5ml (sugar-free and fruit-flavoured).

Used for: urinary tract infections, infections of joints, bones and skin, gastro-intestinal and respiratory tract.

Dosage: adults, ordinary strength tablets, 1–3 tablets twice each day; children 6 to 12 years, 1 twice a day. Children under 6 years use paediatric syrup. Six weeks to 5 months, 2.5ml; 6 months to 5 years, 5ml. Six to 12 years, 10ml, all doses twice each day. Adults, double strength tablets, $1/2$ to $1\,1/2$ tablets twice each day.

Special care: breastfeeding, elderly, kidney disease (reduce dose, increase interval between doses). Regular blood tests should be carried out.

Avoid use: children under 6 weeks, pregnant women, patients with severe kidney or liver disease or blood changes.

Possible interaction: antidiabetics, anticoagulants, antiepileptic drugs, antimalarial drugs, cyclosporin, cytotoxics, folate inhibitors.

Side effects: vomiting, nausea, blood changes, skin rashes, inflammation of the tongue (glossitis), folate (folic acid) deficiency. Rarely, Lyell syndrome, erythema multiformae (circular red patches on skin).

Manufacturer: Roche

BACTROBAN

Description: a broad-spectrum antibiotic preparation containing 2% mupirocin in the form of an ointment. **BACTROBAN NASAL** is an ointment containing 2% mupirocin in a soft white paraffin base.

Used for: bacterial skin infections. Nasal ointment, infections of the nose and nostrils caused by staphlocci bacteria.

Dosage: ointment, apply to skin 3 times a day for up to 10 days. Nasal ointment, apply to the inner surface of nostrils 2 or 3 times daily.

Special care: patients with kidney disorders, avoid eyes.

Side effects: may sting on application.

Manufacturer: Beecham.

BAMBEC

Description: a preparation containing bambuterol hydrochloride which is a selective ß₂-agonist used in the treatment of asthma. Bambec is available as tablets of 2 strengths containing 10mg (marked A/BA) and 20mg (marked A/BM). Tablets are oval, white and scored.

Used for: asthma (bronchospasm) and reversible airways obstruction.

Dosage: 10mg as one dose taken at night increasing to 20mg once a day if necessary. If the patient has been used to treatment with a ß₂-agonist, then 20mg may be taken from the start.

Special care: pregnant women and breastfeeding mothers, diabetics, moderate or severe kidney disorders, heart disorders, thyrotoxicosis. In cases of severe asthma, potassium levels in blood should be monitored.

Avoid use: children.

Possible interaction: Other ß-blockers, suxamethonium.

Side effects: headache, palpitations, cramps, tremor, hypokalaemia.

Manufacturer: Astra.

BARATOL

Description: an antihypertensive, alpha-adrenoreceptor blocking drug, indoramin hydrochloride, available in 2 strengths, blue tablets (25mg, marked MPL020 and 25) and green tablets (50mg, marked MPL 021 and 50). Both are film-coated and scored.

Used for: hypertension (high blood pressure).

Dosage: adults, 25mg twice each day at start increasing by 25mg or 50mg each fortnight. Maximum dose is 200mg per day in 2 or 3 divided doses.

Special care: patients with liver or kidney disorders, Parkinson's disease, epilepsy, history of depression. Patients with incipient heart failure should be treated with digoxin and diuretics. Performance of skilled tasks such as driving may be impaired.

Avoid use: children, cardiac failure.

Possible interaction: alcohol, antihypertensive drugs, MAOIs.

Side effects: drowsiness, dizziness, depression, dry mouth, blocked nose, weight gain, failure to ejaculate.

Manufacturer: Monmouth.

BAXAN

Description: a cephalosporin antibiotic preparatiton available as tablets and as powder for reconstitution with water, in 3 strengths. Baxan white capsules contain 500mg cefadroxil (as monohydrate) and are marked 7244. BAXAN SUSPENSION contains either 125mg, 250mg or 500mg per 5ml when reconstituted with water, available as powder to make 60ml.

Used for: various infections of skin, urinary and respiratory tracts, ear and soft tissues.

Dosage: adults, 500mg–1g twice each day (1 to 2 tablets); children under 1 year, 25mg per kg of body weight in divided doses; 1 to 6 years, 250mg twice each day; 6 years and over, 500mg twice each day.

Special care: patients with penicillin allergy or kidney disease.

Avoid use: cephalosporin allergy, porphyria.

Possible interaction: some diuretics.

Side effects: gastro-intestinal upset, allergic responses.

Manufacturer: Bristol-Myers.

BAYCARON

Description: a thiazide-like diuretic preparation, mefruside, available as white scored tablets marked Bayer and L/1 (strength 25mg).

Used for: oedema and hypertension.

Dosage: 1-2 tablets as a single dose taken in the morning for 10-14 days, then 1 daily or on alternate days for maintenance. Maximum dose for oedema is 4 tablets daily.

Special care: elderly, pregnancy and breastfeeding, liver or kidney disease, gout, diabetes, liver cirrhosis. Fluid, electrolytes and glucose levels should be monitored.

Avoid use: children, patients with liver or kidney failure, Addison's disease, hypercalcaemia, sensitivity to sulphonamide drugs.

Possible interaction: alcohol, opioids, barbiturates, NSAIDs, antidiabetic drugs, tubocurarine, lithium, corticosteroids, cardiac glycosides, carbenoxolone.

Side effects: gastro-intestinal upset, rash, blood changes, disturbance of electrolyte levels and metabolism, dizziness, sensitivity to light, pancreatitis, anorexia, impotence.

Manufacturer: Bayer.

BECLAZONE

Description: a corticosteroid preparation containing either 50 or 100µg beclomethasone dipropionate per dose, delivered by metered dose aerosol. Also **BECLAZONE 250**, containing 250µg per metered dose.

Used for: chronic reversible obstructive airways disease (asthma).

Dosage: adults, 100µg 3 to 4 times each day. If very severe, 600–800µg (maximum 1g) in divided doses each day. Children, 50–100µg 2 to 4 times each day. Beclazone 250, adults only, 500µg twice each day or 250µg 4 times each day. This may be increased to 1500–2000µg each day in divided doses if required.

Special care: pulmonary tuberculosis, pregnant women, patients who have been taking systemic steroid drugs.

Side effects: hoarseness, fungal infections of throat and mouth.

Manufacturer: Baker Norton.

BECLOFORTE

Description: a corticosteroid preparation in a variety of forms for inhalation containing 250µg beclomethasone dipropionate per dose delivered by metered dose aerosol. **BECLOFORTE VM** is available as a pack consisting of 2 Becloforte inhalers and Volumatic.

Also, **BECLOFORTE DISKHALER** consisting of blisters containing 400µg beclomethasone dipropionate per dose delivered by breath-actuated inhaler.

Used for: patients with chronic and severe asthma, emphysema or chronic bronchitis who require high doses of Beclomethasone.

Dosage: adults only, 500µg twice each day or 250µg 4 times a day. May be increased to 500µg 3 or 4 times each day if necessary. Diskhaler, adults, 2 blisters each day.

Special care: pregnancy, patients with active or quiescent pulmonary tuberculosis, those transferring from systemic steroids.

Avoid use: children.

Side effects: hoarseness, fungal infections of throat and mouth.

Manufacturer: A & H.

BECODISKS

Description: a corticosteroid preparation available as a dry powder for inhalation with Diskhaler. Beige disks contain 100µg beclomethasone dipropionate; brown disks contain 200µg; light brown disks contain 400µg.

Used for: bronchial asthma.

Dosage: adults, 400µg twice each day or 200µg 3 to 4 times each day. Children, 100µg 2 to 4 times each day or 200µg twice each day.

Special care: pregnant women, patients with active or quiescent pulmonary tuberculosis, those transferring from systemic steroids.

Side effects: hoarseness, fungal infections of throat and mouth.

Manufacturer: A & H.

BECOTIDE

Description: a corticosteroid preparation, beclomethasone diproprionate, available in the form of an aerosol of different strengths for inhalation. Becotide-50 (50µg per metered inhalation), Becotide-100 (100µg) and Becotide-200 (200µg).

Used for: bronchial asthma.
Dosage: adults, 400µg each day in 2, 3 or 4 divided doses. If asthma is severe, 600–800µg may be required in first instance in daily divided doses. This should be reduced as condition improves. Children, 200µg twice each day using Becotide-50 or 100 only.
Special care: pregnant women, patients with active or quiescent pulmonary tuberculosis, those transferring from systemic steroids.
Side effects: hoarseness, fungal infections of throat and mouth.
Manufacturer: A & H.

BECOTIDE ROTACAPS

Description: a corticosteroid preparation, beclomethasone diproprionate, available as a dry powder in capsules for inhalation: buff/clear (100µg), brown (200µg), dark brown/clear (400µg), all marked with name and strength and each is a single dose for use with a Rotahaler.
Used for: bronchial asthma.
Dosage: adults, 400µg twice each day or 200µg 3 or 4 times each day. Children, 100µg 2 or 4 times each day or 200µg twice each day.
Special care: pregnant women, patients with active or quiescent pulmonary tuberculosis, those transferring from systemic steroids.
Side effects: hoarseness, fungal infections of throat and mouth.
Manufacturer: A & H.

BENEMID

Description: a uricosuric preparation (one which enhances the excretion of uric acid from the kidneys), available as white, scored tablets containing 500mg probenecid, and marked MSD 501.
Used for: gout, hyperuricaemia (elevated uric acid levels in blood). Also, with certain antibiotics (e.g. penicillin) to prolong their effects and maintain high blood levels. This occurs because excretion of the antibiotic is inhibited.
Dosage: for gout and hyperuricaemia,

half a tablet twice a day for 1 week then 1 twice daily. Adults, with certain antibiotics, 4 tablets daily in divided doses. Children over 2 years, with antibiotics, 25mg per kg of body weight, then 40mg per kg each day in divided doses.
Special care: pregnancy, elderly, history of peptic ulcer or kidney disorders. Plenty of fluids should be taken.
Avoid use: children under 2 years, patients during acute attack of gout (the start of treatment should be delayed), uric acid stones in kidneys, blood changes.
Possible interaction: β lactam antibiotics, methotextrate, indomethacin, sulphonamides, salicylates, pyrazinamide, sulphonylureas.
Side effects: gastro-intestinal upset, headache, sore gums, flushes, frequency of urination, hypersensitivity, kidney colic, kidney stones, acute gout.
Manufacturer: M & D.

BEROTEC 100

Description: a proprietary bronchodilator and short-acting β₂-agonist that acts rapidly to relax smooth muscle in the walls of the airways and relieves symptoms for about 3 to 6 hours. Berotec is produced in the form of an aerosol of 2 strengths or as a solution for use with a nebulizer, for inhalation. Berotec 100 contains 0.1mg fenoterol hydrobromide per metered dose inhalation. **BEROTEC 200** contains 0.2mg per metered dose inhalation. **BEROTEC NEBULIZER** solution contains 0.5% fenoterol hydrobromide.
Used for: reversible obstruction of airways as in bronchial asthma, emphysema and bronchitis.
Dosage: adults, aerosol starting with lower strength (100), 1 to 2 puffs up to 3 times each day with a maximum of 2 puffs every 6 hours. Berotec 200, 1 to 2 puffs up to 3 times each day with a maximum of 2 puffs every 6 hours. Nebulized solution, 0.5–1.25mg us to 4 times a day with strength adjusted as necessary by dilution with sterile sodium

chloride solution. Children, lower strength 100 aerosol, over 6 years of age, 1 puff up to 3 times each day with a maximum of 2 puffs every 6 hours. Berotec 200 and nebuliser solution should not be given to children under 16 years of age.

Special care: pregnant women, patients with hypertension, heart arrhythmias, heart disorders, angina, hyperthyroidism.

Avoid use: children under 6 years.

Possible interaction: sympathomimetic drugs.

Side effects: headache, dilation of blood vessels in skin, nervousness.

Manufacturer: Boehringer Ingelheim.

BETA-ADALAT

Description: a cardio-selective ß-blocker/Class II calcium antagonist containing atenolol and nifedipine available as red-brown capsules marked with the Bayer cross and name and containing 50mg atenolol and 20mg nifedipine.

Used for: hypertension, angina (where therapy with a calcium-channel blocker or beta-blocker alone proves to be ineffective).

Dosage: for hypertension, 1 capsule each day increasing to 2 if required. Elderly persons, 1 capsule. Angina, 1 capsule twice each day.

Special care: weak heart, liver or kidney disease, diabetes, anaesthesia.

Avoid use: children, pregnancy, breast-feeding, heart block, heart shock or heart failure.

Possible interaction: cardiac depressant drugs, cimetidine, quinidine.

Side effects: headache, dizziness, flushing, dryness of eyes, skin rashes, oedema, swelling of gums, allergic jaundice.

Manufacturer: Bayer.

BETA CARDONE

Description: a non-cardioselective ß-blocker, sotalol hydrochloride, available as tablets in 3 strengths: green-scored tablets marked Evans/BC4 (40mg) :

pink-scored tablets marked Evans/BC8 (80mg) and white-scored tablets marked Evans/BC20 (200mg).

Used for: heart arrhythmias, angina, hypertension and as an additional therapy for thyrotoxicosis.

Dosage: heart arrhythmias, 40mg 3 times daily for 7 days increasing to 120–240mg each day either all at once or in divided doses. Angina, 80mg twice each day in first instance for 1 week to 10 days, increasing to 200–600mg daily either all at once or in divided doses. Hypertension, 80mg twice each day in first instance for 1 week to 10 days, increasing to 200–600 mg daily, either all at once or in divided doses. Thyrotoxicosis, 120–240 mg each day as a single amount or in divided doses.

Special care: patients with diabetes, liver or kidney disorders, those undergoing general anaesthesia (drug may need to be stopped). Pregnant women and nursing mothers. Patients with weak hearts may need to be treated with digitalis and diuretic drugs.

Avoid use: children, patients with asthma or history of bronchospasm, those with heart block, heart attack, heart shock and some other cardiac disorders. Drug should be stopped gradually.

Possible interaction: verapamil, clonidine withdrawal, hyperglycaemics, class I anti-arrhythmic drugs, some anaesthetics, reserpine, sympathomimetics, antidepressants, ergotamine, indomethacin, cimetidine.

Side effects: slow heartbeat, disruption of sleep, cold hands and feet, fatigue in exercise, gastro-intestinal upset, wheezing, heart failure, skin rash, dry eyes (withdraw drug gradually).

Manufacturer: Evans.

BETAGAN

Description: a ß-blocker in the form of eye drops containing 0.5% levobunolol hydrochloride and 1.4% polyvinyl alcohol, and as single dose units.

Used for: chronic simple open-angle

glaucoma, reduction of intra-ocular pressure.
Dose: adults, 1 drop once or twice each day.
Special care: patients with breathing disorders, breastfeeding mothers, diabetics.
Avoid use: children, patients with asthma, pregnant women, those with various heart disorders including heart block, heart failure, heart shock, slow heartbeat, history of obstructive lung disease.
Possible interaction: ß-blockers, reserpine.
Side effects: local allergic irritation or dry eyes, respiratory difficulties, dizziness, headache, ß-blocker effects.
Manufacturer: Allergan.

BETA-PROGRANE

Description: a non-cardioselective ß-blocker produced in the form of sustained-release capsules which are white and contain 160mg propranolol hydrochloride. Also available, **HALF BETA-PROGRANE** white sustained-release capsules containing 80mg propranolol hydrochloride.
Used for: angina, high blood pressure, as additional therapy for over-active thyroid gland (thyrotoxicosis), prevention of migraine.
Dosage: angina, 80–160mg each day increasing to a maximum of 240mg if needed. Hypertension, 160mg each day increasing to 320mg by 80mg each day if necessary. Thyrotoxicosis, 80mg to 160mg each day increasing to 240mg if necessary. Prevention of migraine, 80mg–160mg each day increasing to 240mg if necessary.
Special care: pregnancy and lactation, diabetes, liver or kidney disease, metabolic acidosis, those undergoing general anaesthesia, patients with weak hearts should be treated with digitalis and diuretics. The drug should be stopped gradually.
Avoid use: children, patients with various heart disorders including heart

shock, heart block, heart failure, asthma.
Possible interaction: some anaesthetics, antidiabetic drugs, antihypertensives, sympathomimetics, sedatives, indomethacin, reserpine, class I antiarrhythmics, verapamil, clonidine withdrawal.
Side effects: disturbance of sleep, cold feet and hands, slow heartbeat rate, fatigue with exercise, wheezing, heart failure, gastro-intestinal disorders; dry eyes or skin rash (gradually withdraw drug).
Manufacturer: Tillomed.

BETALOC

Description: a cardioselective ß-blocker, metoprolol tartrate, available as tablets of 2 strengths, as modified-release tablets and in ampoules for injection. Betaloc tablets are white, scored and contain 50mg (marked A/BB) or 100mg (marked A/ME). Also, **BETALOC-SA** modified-release tablets (Durules®), containing 200mg and marked AMD. Also, **BETALOC INJECTION** containing 1mg per ml in 5ml ampoules.
Used for: heart arrhythmias, angina, maintenance therapy in heart attack, hypertension, additional therapy in thyrotoxicosis, prevention of migraine.
Dosage: heart attack, 200mg each day; heart arrhythmias, 50mg 2 or 3 times each day increasing to maximum daily dose of 300mg. Angina, 50–100mg twice or three times each day. Hypertension, 50mg twice each day at first increasing to 400mg if required. Thyrotoxicosis, 50mg 4 times each day; migraine prevention, 100mg–200mg each day in divided doses.
Special care: pregnancy, breastfeeding, liver or kidney disease, diabetes, metabolic acidosis, those undergoing anaesthesia; patients with weak hearts should be treated with digitalis and diuretics. Drug should be stopped gradually.
Avoid use: children, patients with asthma, various forms of heart disease including heart block, heart shock, slow heartbeat rate, heart failure.

Possible interaction: cardiac depressant, anaesthetics, reserpine, sedatives, antihypertensives, sympathomimetics, cimetidine, indomethacin, ergotamine, class I antiarrhythmic drugs, verapamil, clonidine withdrawal, hypoglycaemics.
Side effects: sleep disturbance, cold feet and hands, slow heartbeat, fatigue on exercise, wheeziness, heart failure, gastro-intestinal disorders; dry eyes or skin rash (stop use gradually).
Manufacturer: Astra.

BETHANIDINE

Description: an antihypertensive drug, bethanidine sulphate, which acts by blocking the release of noradrenaline (a neurotransmitter) from nerve endings. It is available in the form of tablets containing 10mg bethanidine sulphate.
Used for: hypertension, especially that which has failed to respond to other antihypertensive drugs. It is usually used in conjunction with a diuretic (e.g. a thiazide) or beta-blocker.
Dosage: adults, 10mg, 3 times each day after food at first increasing by 5mg once a week to a maximum daily dose of 200mg.
Special care: kidney disease, pregnant women, asthma, peptic ulcer or history of peptic ulcer, cerebral or coronary arteriosclerosis. Low blood pressure when rising from a prone position may cause falls in elderly people.
Avoid use: children, patients with kidney or heart failure, phaeochromocytoma.
Possible interaction: tricyclic antidepressants, sympathomimetics, MAOIs.
Side effects: low blood pressure associated with lying down (postural hypotension), blocked nose, headache, drowsiness, oedema, failure of ejaculation.

BETIM

Description: a non-cardioselective beta-blocker available as white, scored tablets containing 10mg timolol maleate and marked with 102 and symbol.
Used for: prevention of second heart

attack following initial episode, angina, hypertension, prevention of migraine.
Dosage: adults, prevention of secondary heart attack, 5mg twice each day for first 2 days, thereafter 10mg twice each day. Angina, 10mg twice each day at first, adjusted according to response to a maximum of 60mg. Hypertension, 10mg a day at first in single or divided dose increasing by 10mg every 3 to 4 days to a maximum of 60mg. Usual maintenance dose is in the order of 10–30mg. Prevention of migraine, 10–20mg each day in 1 or 2 divded doses.
Special care: pregnancy, breastfeeding, liver or kidney disease, diabetes, those undergoing general anaesthesia, patients with weak hearts should receive digitalis and diuretics. Drug should be stopped gradually.
Avoid use: children, patients with asthma or history of breathing difficulties, those with various forms of heart disease including heart block, heart shock, slow heartbeat, heart failure.
Possible interaction: class I antiarrhythmics, cardiac depressant anaesthetics, ergotamine, sedatives, sympathomimetics, cimetidine, indomethacin, reserpine, hypoglycaemic drugs, clonidine withdrawal, verapamil.
Side effects: sleep disturbance, cold feet and hands, slow heartbeat, fatigue in exercise, wheeziness, heart failure, gastro-intestinal upset, dry eyes or skin rash (stop drug gradually).
Manufacturer: Leo.

BETNELAN

Description: a corticosteroid preparation containing the glucocorticoid betmethasone, in the form of white, scored tablets (0.5mg strength) and marked with the name and Evans.
Used for: allergic conditions, severe asthma, rheumatoid arthritis, collagen diseases.
Dosage: adults, 0.5mg–5mg daily then reduce to effective maintenance dose according to response. Children, 1 to 7

years, quarter to half adult dose, 7 to 12 years, half to three-quarters adult dose. *Special care*: pregnant women, patients who have recently undergone intestinal surgery, some cancers, inflamed veins, peptic ulcer, active infections and those with viral or fungal origin, tuberculosis. High blood pressure, kidney diseases, osteoporosis, diabetes, glaucoma, epilepsy, underactive thyroid, liver cirrhosis, stress, psychoses. Patients should avoid contact with chicken pox or *Herpes zoster* virus while on steroid treatment and for 3 months afterwards. In the event of exposure to chicken pox, patients should be immunized within 3 days (if chicken pox is contracted specialist care is required). Drug should be stopped gradually.
Avoid use: children under 12 months.
Possible interaction: NSAIDs, anticoagulants taken by mouth, diuretics, hypoglycaemics, cardiac glycosides, anticholinesterases, phenobarbitone, phenytoin, rifampicin, ephedrine.
Side effects: mood swings (euphoria and depression), hyperglycaemia, osteoporosis, peptic ulcers, Cushing's syndrome caused especially by high doses.
Manufacturer: Evans.

BETNESOL

Description: a corticosteroid containing the glucocorticoid betmethasone (as sodium phosphate), available as soluble tablets— pink, scored and marked with the name and Evans and containing 0.5mg. Also, **BETNESOL INJECTION** containing 4mg per ml in 1ml ampoules.
Used for: allergic conditions, severe asthma, rheumatoid arthritis, collagen diseases. Injection: adrenal crisis and shock.
Dosage: adults, 0.5mg–5mg in water as daily dose reducing to minimum effective dose for maintenance. Children, 1 to 7 years, one quarter to half adult dose; 7 to 12 years, half to three-quarters adult dose. Injection: adults, 4–20mg intravenously 3 or 4

times a day if needed. Children, 1 year and under, 1mg; 1 to 5 years, 2mg; 6 to 12 years, 4mg by intravenous injection.
Special care: pregnancy, recent intestinal surgery, some cancers, inflamed veins, peptic ulcer, active infections and those with fungal or viral origin, tuberculosis, high blood pressure, kidney diseases, osteoporosis, diabetes, glaucoma, epilepsy, underactive thyroid, liver cirrhosis, stress, psychoses. Patients should avoid contact with chicken pox or *Herpes zoster* while on steroids and for 3 months after treatment has ceased. In the event of exposure to chicken pox, patients should be immunized within 3 days. (If chicken pox is contracted, specialist care is required). Drug should be stopped gradually.
Avoid use: children under 12 months.
Possible interaction: NSAIDs, oral anticoagulants, diuretics, hypoglycaemics, cardiac glycosides, anticholinesterases, phenobarbitone, phenytoin, rifampicin, ephedrine.
Side effects: mood swings (euphoria and depression), hyperglycaemia (elevated blood sugar levels), osteoporosis, peptic ulcers, Cushings syndrome, especially caused by high doses.
Manufacturer: Evans.

BETNOVATE

Description: a group of moderate to potent corticosteroid preparations containing betmethasone and available as ointment, cream or lotion. Betnovate cream and ointment both contain 0.1% betmethasone (as valerate); **BETNO-VATE SCALP APPLICATION**, (0.1%) **BETNOVATE C** cream and ointment contains an antimicrobial drug (antifungal and antibacterial), 3% clinoquinol and 0.1% betmethasone (as valerate); **BETNOVATE N** cream and ointment also contain an antimicrobial (antibacterial) drug, 0.5% neomycin sulphate and 0.1% betmethasone (as valerate). **BETNOVATE RD** cream and ointment are less potent containing

0.025% betmethasone (as valerate).
Used for: eczema, seborrhoeic and contact
dermatitis, psoriasis, other skin disorders
(lichen simplex and planus). For infected
conditions, Betnovate C or N are used
depending upon causal organism.
Dosage: adults, apply sparingly 2 or 3
times each day. More potent preparations
may be used first with Betnovate RD
then used for maintenance treatment.
Children over 1 year same as adult dose.
Special care: should not be used
extensively or for a prolonged period.
Should be used for only 5 days on
children or on face. Stop use gradually.
Avoid use: children under 1 year,
continuous use especially by pregnant
women, any conditions caused by
ringworm, fungi, viruses, tuberculosis,
acne, leg ulcers, scabies.
Side effects: thinning of skin, suppression of adrenal glands, hair growth,
symptoms associated with Cushings
syndrome, e.g. reddening of skin on face
and neck.
Manufacturer: Glaxo.

BETNOVATE RECTAL

Description: a steroid, vasoconstrictor
and local anaesthetic preparation
produced in the form of an ointment
with applicator. The ointment contains
2.5% lignocaine hydrochloride, 0.1%
phenylephrine hydrochloride and 0.05%
betmethasone valerate.
Used for: haemorrhoids and mild
proctitis (inflammation of the rectum).
Dosage: adults, apply 2 or 3 times daily
at first and then once each day.
Special care: avoid use for a long period,
especially pregnant women.
Avoid use: children, patients with tuberculosis, bacterial, viral or fungal infections.
Side effects: systemic corticosteroid
effects.
Manufacturer: Glaxo.

BETOPTIC

Description: a cardio-selective beta-
blocker that reduces pressure within the
eye. Betoptic contains 0.5% betaxolol
hydrochloride in the form of eye drops.
Used for: chronic open angle glaucoma
and hypertension of eyes.
Dosage: 1 drop twice each day into eye.
Special care: patients with diabetes,
thyrotoxicosis, blocked airways disease,
those undergoing general anaesthetic.
Avoid use: children, patients with certain
heart diseases including heart shock,
cardiac failure, slow heart beat, those
using soft contact lenses.
Side effects: passing slight discomfort,
rarely staining or reddening of cornea
and decreased sensitivity of cornea.
Manufacturer: Alcon.

BEZALIP

Description: a preparation used to
reduce high levels of fats (lipids) in the
bloodstream, and available in the form
of white, film-coated tablets marked
BM/G6, containing 200mg bezafibrate.
Bezalip-MONO are white, film-coated,
modified-release tablets marked BM/D9
containing 400mg bezafibrate.
Used for: hyperlipidaemias (high blood
levels of lipids, classified as type IIa,
IIb, III, IV and V) which are resistant to
changes in diet.
Dosage: adults, Bezalip-MONO, 1 tablet
after food at night or in morning. Bezalip,
1 tablet 3 times each day with food.
Special care: patients with kidney disease.
Avoid use: children, patients with serious
kidney or liver disease, nephrotic
disease, pregnant and breastfeeding
women.
Possible interaction: MAOIs,
antidiabetic and anticoagulant drugs.
Side effects: gastro-intestinal upset, rash,
muscle pain.
Manufacturer: Boehringer Mannheim.

BICILLIN

Description: a preparation of 2 types of
penicillin used in the treatment of a
variety of infections. Bicillin is available
as a powder for reconstitution and
injection containing 1.8g procaine

penicillin and 360mg benzylpenicillin (300mg procaine penicillin, 60mg benzylpenicillin per ml).
Used for: gonococcal, streptococcal, pneumococcal, meningococcal infections, gas-gangrene, anthrax, syphilis, tetanus, diphtheria, yaws, Lyme disease in children. Other penicillin-sensitive infections where prolonged effect of antibiotic in tissues is desirable.
Dosage: adults, 1ml given by intramuscular injection once or twice each day. Early syphilis, 3ml by intramuscular injection (or 4ml for patients over 80kg), each day for 10 days. Gonorrhoea, up to 12ml as a single intramuscular injection. Children, under 25kg body weight dose adjusted in proportion to that given to a light adult. Over 25kg, same as adult dose.
Special care: patients with history of allergy or kidney disease.
Avoid use: patients with penicillin allergy.
Side effects: allergic responses including rash, fever, joint pains (anaphylactic shock in patients with penicillin allergy), gastro-intestinal upset.
Manufacturer: Brocades.

BICNU

Description: an alkylating cytotoxic drug used in the treatment of certain cancers and produced in the form of a powder for reconstitution and injection. Bicnu contains 100mg carmustine as a powder in a vial, with 3ml sterile ethanol for reconstitution.
Used for: leukaemia, lymphomas, myelomas, brain tumours.
Dosage: as directed by skilled cancer specialist.
Special care: patients should receive regular checks for blood count.
Side effects: vomiting and nausea, hair loss, bone marrow suppression (onset of which is delayed) necessitating regular blood checks, adverse effects on fertility. Possible kidney and liver damage may occur.
Manufacturer: Bristol-Myers.

BINOVUM

Description: a combined oestrogen/pro-gesterone oral contraceptive preparation produced as a course of 21 tablets: 7 white tablets marked C over 535 contain 0.5mg (500µg) norethisterone and 35µg ethenyloestradiol; 14 peach tablets, marked C over 135, contain 1mg nore-thisterone and 35µg ethinyloestradiol.
Used for: oral contraception.
Dosage: 1 tablet each day starting with white tablets on first day of period. There are 7 tablet-free days before the process is repeated.
Special care: hypertension, asthma, diabetes, varicose veins, multiple sclerosis, Raynaud's disease, kidney dialysis, chronic kidney disease, obesity, severe depression. Family history of heart disease, inflammatory bowel disease, Crohn's disease. Risk of arterial thrombosis especially in older women, those who smoke and those who are obese. Regular checks on blood pressure, breasts and pelvic organs should be carried out at intervals.
Avoid use: pregnancy, history of heart disease or thrombosis, hypertension, sickle cell anaemia, liver disease, cholestatic jaundice of pregnancy, abnormalities of liver function, porphyria, undiagnosed vaginal bleeding, some cancers, (hormone-dependent ones), infectious hepatitis, recent trophoblastic disease.
Possible interaction: barbiturates, tetracycline antibiotics, rifampicin, griseofulvin, carbamezapine, chloral hydrate, primidone, phenytoin, ethosuximide, glutethimide, dichloral-phenazone.
Side effects: oedema and bloatedness, leg cramps, reduction in sexual desire, headaches, depression, weight gain, vaginal discharge, breakthrough bleeding, cervical erosion, nausea, chloasma (brownish patches on skin).
Manufacturer: Ortho.

BIOPLEX

Description: a cytoprotectant produced in the form of granules for reconstitution with water to form a mouthwash. Bioplex contains 1% carbenoxolone sodium (20mg per 2g sachet).
Used for: mouth ulcers.
Dosage: use as mouthwash 3 times each day and at night.
Special care: do not swallow.
Manufacturer: Thames

BIORPHEN

Description: an antimuscarine or anticholinergic preparation used in the treatment of Parkinsonism. It is thought that antimuscarine drugs act to correct the excess of acetylcholine believed to be the result of dopamine deficiency in Parkinsonism. Biorphen is produced as a sugar-free liquid containing 25mg orphenadrine hydrochloride per 5ml.
Used for: Parkinsonism including drug-induced symptoms.
Dosage: adults and children, 150mg each day at first in divided doses, increasing by 25–50mg every 2 or 3 days. Usual maintenance dose is in the order of 150–300mg.
Special care: heart disorders, gastro-intestinal blockage, liver or kidney disease, avoid abrupt withdrawal of treatment.
Avoid use: narrow or closed angle glaucoma, enlarged prostate gland, some disorders of movement (tardive dyskinesia).
Possible interaction: antidepressants, antihistamines, phenothiazines.
Side effects: euphoria, agitation, confusion, anticholinergic effects and rash (high doses).
Manufacturer: Bioglan.

BLOCADREN

Description: a non-cardioselective beta-blocker produced in the form of blue scored tablets, marked MSD 135, containing 10mg timolol maleate.
Used for: prevention of secondary heart attack, angina, prevention of migraine, hypertension.
Dosage: adults, prevention of secondary heart attack, starting 1 to 4 weeks after first heart attack, 5mg twice each day for 2 days, then 10mg. Adults, angina, 5mg 2 or 3 times each day at first, increasing if required to 10–15mg daily every 3 days. Usual maintenance dose is in the order of 35–45mg. Adults, hypertension, 10mg each day at first as single or divided doses, increasing to a maximum of 60mg daily if required. Adults, prevention of migraine, 10–20mg each day, either as a single or as divided doses.
Special care: patients with kidney or liver disease, diabetes, metabolic acidosis, those undergoing general anaesthesia, pregnant women and nursing mothers. Persons with weak hearts should receive diuretics and digitalis. May need to halt drug before planned surgery. Withdraw gradually.
Avoid use: children, patients with asthma, heart block, heart failure, slow heartbeat, heart shock, severe peripheral arterial disease.
Possible interaction: cardiac depressant anaesthetic drugs, antihypertensives, sedatives, class I antiarrhythmic drugs, verapamil, clonidine withdrawal, ergotamine, cimetidine, indomethacine, sympathomimetics.
Side effects: disturbance of sleep, cold hands and feet, fatigue on exercise, slow heartbeat, bronchospasm, heart failure, rash, dry eyes (withdraw gradually).
Manufacturer: MSD

BOLVIDON

Description: a tetracyclic antidepressant available in various strengths, containing 10mg mianserin hydrochloride (coded CT4); 20mg marked CT6, 30mg marked CT7. All tablets are white film-coated and marked ORGANON.
Used for: depressive illnesses, particularly those requiring sedation.
Dosage: adults, 30–40mg each day either as divided doses or a single one

taken at night. May be gradually increased over a period of days to a maintenance dose in the order of 30–90mg each day according to response. Elderly persons, 30mg each day which may be carefully increased over a period of days if required.
Special care: elderly persons, pregnant women, patients with heart block or heart attack, enlarged prostate gland, epilepsy. Regular blood counts may be required.
Avoid use: children, breastfeeding mothers, patients with serious liver disease, those suffering from mania.
Possible interaction: alcohol, MAOIs, anticoagulant drugs.
Side effects: blood changes, drowsiness, if signs of influenza-like infection, convulsions, jaundice, hypomania occur, the drug should be withdrawn gradually.
Manufacturer: Organon.

BONEFOS

Description: a preparation of the drug, sodium clodronate (a diphosphonate) which affects bone metabolism, preventing the increased rate of bone turnover associated with certain malignant conditions. Bonefos is available in the form of capsules and as a solution for intravenous infusion. Yellow capsules contain 400mg and intravenous solution contains 60mg per ml in 5ml ampoules.
Used for: hypercalcaemia of malignancy. Bone pain and lesions associated with secondary bone growths as a result of multiple myeloma (malignant bone marrow disease) or breast cancer.
Dosage: adults, 4 tablets each day as single or divided dose avoiding food for 1 or 2 hours before and after treatment, especially anything containing calcium, mineral supplements or iron. Infusion, adults, 1500mg as single infusion over 4 hours or 300mg given by slow intravenous infusion for up to 7 days. Afterwards, capsules should be taken.
Special care: moderate kidney disorders. Ensure adequate fluid intake, monitor

blood calcium levels and kidney function.
Avoid use: children, pregnancy, breast-feeding, severe kidney failure.
Possible interaction: other diphosphonates, NSAIDs, mineral supplements, antacid preparations.
Side effects: skin rashes, gastro-intestinal upset, disturbance of kidney function, parathyroid hormone, lactic acid dehydrogenase, creatinine, transaminase, alkaline phosphatase (enzymes) levels may be elevated for a time. Rarely, there may be hypocalcaemia which does not cause symptoms. There may be transient proteinurea.
Manufacturer: Boehringer Ingelheim.

BRELOMAX

Description: a broncho-dilator of a type known as a selective β_2-agonist. It is available as white scored tablets, marked with logo, contain 2mg tulobuterol hydrochloride.
Used for: prevention and control of bronchospasm in reversible airways disease (asthma).
Dosage: adults, 1 tablet twice each day at first increasing to 1 tablet 3 times daily if needed. Children over 10 years, $1/2$ to 1 tablet twice daily.
Special care: patients with diabetes, epilepsy, mild kidney failure, hypertension, heart-circulatory disease (cardiovascular disease), hyperthyroidism.
Avoid use: children under 10 years, serious liver disease or liver failure, moderate to severe kidney failure.
Possible interaction: Other ß-blockers, corticosteroids, theophylline (increased risk of hypokalaemia with high doses).
Side effects: hypokalaemia, which may be serious, raised heartbeat rate, palpitations, headache, tremor, nervous tension.
Manufacturer: Abbott.

BRETYLATE

Description: a proprietary class III antiarrhythmic drug used to treat irregularities of heartbeat and available in the form of a solution for injection

containing 50mg bretylium tosylate per ml in 10ml ampoules.
Used for: heartbeat irregularities (ventricular arrhythmias) especially those resistant to other forms of treatment.
Dosage: 5–10mg per kg of body weight at first given intramuscularly or intravenously and repeated after 1–2 hours if necessary. The treatment is continued every 6 to 8 hours for up to 5 days.
Special care: patients with kidney disorders.
Avoid use: children, patients with phaeochromocytoma.
Possible interaction: noradrenaline, other sympathomimetics.
Side effects: passing worsening of arrhythmia, hypotension, vomiting and nausea.
Manufacturer: Wellcome.

BREVIBLOC

Description: a cardio-selective beta-blocker available in the form of a solution for injection. Brevibloc contains either 10mg esmolol hydrochloride per ml in a 10ml vial or 250mg per ml (for dilution before use) in 10ml ampoules.
Used for: cardiac arrhythmias of various types, (sinus tachycardia; atrial flutter, atrial fibrillation), raised heartbeat rate and hypertension.
Dosage: 50–200μg per kg body weight per minute by intravenous infusion.
Special care: women in late pregnancy, breastfeeding, liver disease, kidney disease, angina, diabetes.
Avoid use: asthma, history of obstructive airways disease, heart failure, heart block, heart shock.
Possible interaction: other antiarrhythmic drugs.
Manufacturer: Gensia.

BREVINOR

Description: a combined oestrogen/progestogen contraceptive preparation available as white tablets, marked B and Syntex contain 35μg ethinyloestradiol and 0.5mg norethisterone.

Used for: contraception.
Dosage: 1 each day for 21 days starting on 5th day of period, then 7 tablet-free days.
Special care: women with asthma, hypertension, Raynaud's disease, diabetes, multiple sclerosis, chronic kidney disease, kidney dialysis, varicose veins, depression, smoking, age and obesity increase the risk of thrombosis.
Avoid use: pregnant women, patients with history of thrombosis or who may be at risk of this, heart disease, sickle cell anaemia, liver diseases, infectious hepatitis, history of cholestatic jaundice (caused by a failure of bile to reach the small intestine), porphyria, chorea, ostosclerosis, haemolytic uraemic syndrome, hormone-dependent cancers, recent trophoblastic disease, undiagnosed vaginal bleeding.
Possible interaction: tetracycline antibiotics, barbiturates, chloral hydrate, griseofulvin, rifampicin, carbamazepine, phenytoin, primidone, dichloralphenazone, ethosuximide glutethimide.
Side effects: oedema and bloatedness, leg cramps, enlargement of breasts, loss of libido, headaches, nausea, depression, weight gain, breakthrough bleeding, cervical erosion, vaginal discharge, brownish patches on skin (chloasma).
Manufacturer: Syntex.

BRICANYL

Description: a bronchodilator and a selective B_2-agonist (a selective beta receptor stimulant) and muscle relaxant containing terbutaline sulphate. Bricanyl is available as tablets, a syrup and as a variety of preparations suitable for use with different kinds of inhaler.
Dosage: Bricanyl white scored tablets, marked 5 contain 5mg. Adult dose: 1 tablet twice each day or at 8-hour intervals. Children: 7 to 15 years, half adult dose. Young children under 7 should use syrup.
Also, **BRICANYL SA** (sustained release) tablets, white, marked A/BD, contain 7.5mg. Adult dose: 1 twice each

day. Aerosol inhalation, capsules contain 0.25mg per metered dose aerosol. Adults and children: 1 to 2 puffs as required, maximum dose 8 puffs in 24 hours.
BRICANYL TURBOHALER is a breath-actuated dry powder inhaler containing 0.5mg per metered dose. Adults and children, 1 inhalation as needed with a maximum of 4 in 24 hours. **BRICANYL SPACER INHALER** (with extended mouthpiece which is collapsible) contains 0.25mg per dose. Adults and children, 1 to 2 puffs as required with a maximum of 8 in 24 hours. **BRICANYL RESPULES** (for use with nebuliser) contain 5mg per 2ml solution as single dose units. Adults: 5–10mg 2, 3 or 4 times each day. Children over 25kg body weight: 5mg 2, 3 or 4 times daily. Both with nebuliser.
BRICANYL RESPIRATOR SOLUTION (for use with power-operated nebuliser) contains 10mg per ml (diluted before use with sterile physiological saline). Adults and children 2–10mg diluted and used with nebuliser. **BRICANYL SYRUP** (sugar-free) contains 1.5mg per 5ml. Adults: 10–15ml; children under 3 years: 2.5ml; 3 to 7 years, 2.5–5ml, 7 to 15 years, 5–10ml. All at 8-hour intervals.
BRICANYL INJECTION contains 0.5mg per ml in ampoules. Adults; 0.25–0.5mg by subcutaneous, intramuscular or slow intravenous injection. Children; 2 to 15 years, 10µg per kg of body weight, subcutaneously, intramuscularly or by slow intravenous injection.
Special care: pregnancy, angina, heart disorders and arrhythmias, hypertension, hyperthyroidism. Caution in diabetic persons if given intravenously.
Possible interaction: sympathomimetics.
Side effects: headache, nervous tension, trembling, dilation of blood vessels.
Manufacturer: Astra.

BRITAJECT

Description: a dopamine agonist used in the treatment of Parkinson's disease.

Britaject contains 10mg apomorphine hydrochloride per ml in ampoules for injection.
Used for: treatment of involuntary muscle movements in Parkinson's disease which have not responded to other methods of treatment.
Dosage: as directed by hospital physician.
Special care: patients require 3 or more days of treatment prior to start of therapy.
Manufacturer: Britannia

BRITIAZEM

Description: a vasodilator which is a class III calcium antagonist, available as white tablets, scored on one side contain 60mg diltiazem hydrochloride.
Used for: angina.
Dosage: 1 tablet 3 times daily increasing if required to a maximum of 6 each day in divided doses. Elderly, 1 tablet twice each day.
Special care: monitoring of heartbeat rate may be required during therapy especially in elderly patients, those with a slow heartbeat and those with kidney or liver disorders.
Avoid use: children, pregnant women, those with marked bradycardia, heart block (2nd- and 3rd-degree atrio-ventricular block) sick sinus syndrome.
Possible interaction: beta-blockers, carbamazepine, digoxin, cardiac depressants, other antihypertensive drugs, cyclosporin, diazepam, lithium, cimetidine, dantrolene infusion.
Side effects: bradycardia, 1st degree heart block (atrio-ventricular block), headache, rash, nausea, swelling of ankles caused by oedema.
Manufacturer: Thames

BRITLOFEX

Description: a preparation acting on the central (sympathetic) nervous system available as peach, film-coated tablets with 0.2mg lofexidine hydrochloride.
Used for: control of withdrawal symptoms in patients undergoing detoxification from opioid drug dependency.

Dosage: adults, 1 tablet twice each day in first instance increasing by 1 or 2 daily if necessary. Maximum daily dose is 12 tablets. Therapy usually should be carried out over a period of 7 to 10 days and then is gradually withdrawn over 2 to 4 days.

Special care: pregnancy, breastfeeding, heart and circulatory diseases, recent heart attack or chronic kidney failure, severe bradycardia, depression.

Avoid use: children.

Possible interaction: alcohol, sedatives.

Side effects: dry mouth throat and nose, drowsiness, hypotension, rebound hypertension on withdrawal.

Manufacturer: Britannia.

BROCADOPA

Description: a preparation of the drug, Levodopa, which is a dopamine precursor. Levodopa is converted into dopamine inside the body, and it is a lack of dopamine in the brain which is associated with Parkinson's disease. Brocadopa is produced in capsule strengths 125mg, 250mg and 500mg.

Used for: Parkinsonism but not drug-induced.

Dosage: 250mg each day in divided doses at first, gradually increasing by 250mg every 3 to 4 days until best response is achieved. Usual dose is in the order of 1–8g in divided doses.

Special care: pregnancy, heart, lung, liver, kidney diseases, disorders of the endocrine (hormones) system, wide angle glaucoma or peptic ulcers. Heart, liver and kidney function should be monitored and blood checks carried out.

Avoid use: children, patients with narrow angle glaucoma, history of malignant melanoma, severe psychoses.

Possible interaction: sympathomimetics, MAOIs, drugs affecting amine levels in central nervous system, pyroxidine, ferrous sulphate antihyptertensive drugs.

Side effects: vomiting and nausea, anorexia, low blood pressure on rising from sitting or lying down (postural hypotension), heart and central nervous system disturbance, involuntary movements, discolouration of urine.

Manufacturer: Yamanouchi.

BROFLEX

Description: an antimuscarine or anticholinergic preparation, produced in the form of a pink syrup containing 5mg benzhexol hydrochloride per 5ml.

Used for: Parkinsonism including drug-induced.

Dosage: adults, 1mg each day at first increasing over a period of days by 1 or 2mg to a usual maintenance dose of 5–15mg. Maximum daily dose is 20mg.

Special care: narrow angle glaucoma, enlarged prostate gland, obstruction of gastro-intestinal tract, heart, liver or kidney disease. Withdraw drug slowly.

Avoid use: children, tardive dyskinesia (movement disorder), closed angle glaucoma, severe gastro-intestinal obstruction, untreated urinary retention.

Possible interaction: antidepressants, antihistamines, phenothiazines.

Side effects: gastro-intestinal disturbances, dry mouth, dizziness, blurred vision, sometimes nervousness, hypersensitivity, tachycardia (raised heart beat rate), urinary retention. In susceptible patients and/or with higher doses, psychiatric disturbances, mental confusion, excitability which may require treatment to be discontinued.

Manufacturer: Bioglan.

BRONCHODIL

Description: a bronchodilator and selective beta$_1$-agonist available in the form of an aerosol containing 0.5mg reproterol hydrochloride per metered dose inhalation.

Used for: reversible airways obstruction in bronchitis, bronchial asthma and emphysema.

Dosage: adults, 1 or 2 puffs every 3 to 6 hours. Prevention of symptoms, 1 puff 3 times each day. Children, 6 to 12 years, 1 puff 3- to 6-hourly; prevention of

symptoms, 1 puff 3 times each day.
Special care: pregnant women, patients with weak hearts, heart arrhythmias, hypertension, angina, hyperthyroidism.
Avoid use: children under 6 years.
Possible interaction: sympathomimetics.
Side effects: headache, dilation of blood vessels, fine tremor of hands, nervous tension.
Manufacturer: ASTA Medica.

BRUFEN

Description: an NSAID used as an analgesic to treat a variety of disorders and available as tablets, granules and syrup containing ibuprofen: magenta-coloured, oval, sugar-coated tablets are available in 3 strengths; coded BRUFEN (200mg); coded BRUFEN 400 (400mg) and coded BRUFEN 600 (600mg).
BRUFEN GRANULES are effervescent, orange-flavoured granules in sachet containing 600mg. BRUFEN SYRUP contains 100mg per 5ml and BRUFEN RETARD, contain 800mg as white, oval film-coated sustained release tablets.
Used for: pain and inflammation in such conditions as rheumatic disorders, joint pain, juvenile arthritis, periarticular disorders, rheumatoid arthritis, seronegative arthritis, ankylosing spondylitis, osteoarthrosis, post-operative pain, period pain, soft tissue injuries.
Dosage: adults, 1200–1800mg each day in divided doses (after food) with a maximum daily dose of 2400mg. A maintenance dose in the region of 600–1200mg may be sufficient. Children, over 7kg body weight, use syrup. Age 1 to 2 years, 2.5ml; 3 to 7 years, 5ml; 8 to 12 years, 10ml. All 3 to 4 times each day.
Special care: pregnancy, nursing mothers, elderly, asthma, gastro-intestinal disorders, heart, liver or kidney disease. Patients on long-term therapy should receive monitoring.
Avoid use: patients with known allergy to aspirin or anti-inflammatory drugs, those with peptic ulcer. Children under 7kg body weight.

Possible interaction: quinolones, anticoagulants, thiazide diuretics.
Side effects: gastro-intestinal upset and bleeding, rash, low levels of blood platelets.
Manufacturer: Boots.

BUCCASTEM

Description: an anti-emetic and dopamine antagonist belonging to a group called the phenothiazines, available as pale yellow (buccal) tablets containing 3mg prochlorperazine maleate.
Used for: severe nausea, vomiting, vertigo due to labyrinthine disorders or Ménière's disease.
Dosage: 1 to 2 tablets twice each day, the tablet being placed high up between upper lip and gum and left to dissolve.
Special care: pregnancy, nursing mothers.
Avoid use: children under 14 years of age (may cause dystonia, a movement disorder, and other extra-pyramidal symptoms in children and young people). Patients with Parkinson's disease, blood changes, narrow angle glaucoma, enlarged prostate gland, liver or kidney disease, epilepsy.
Possible interaction: alcohol, alpha-blockers, CNS depressants (sedatives).
Side effects: hypotension (low blood pressure), especially in elderly persons or dehydrated patients, anticholinergic effects, drowsiness, skin reactions, insomnia. Rarely extra-pyramidal symptoms may occur and parkinsonism, especially in elderly patients.
Manufacturer: Reckitt & Colman.

BURINEX

Description: a loop diuretic preparation, (acting on the part of the kidney tubules called loops of Henle), available in the form of tablets, liquid and in ampoules for injection containing bumetanide. White, scored tablets marked 133 and with logo contain 1mg, those marked with strength contain 5mg. BURINEX LIQUID contains 1mg per 5ml. BURINEX INJECTION contains

0.5mg per ml in ampoules.
Used for: oedema caused by congestive
heart failure, liver and kidney disease
including nephrotic syndrome.
Dosage: adults, tablets or liquid, 1mg
daily according to response of patient's
condition. Injection, 1–2mg given
intravenously (for pulmonary oedema),
repeated after 20 minutes if necessary.
Special care: pregnancy, breastfeeding,
diabetes, gout, liver or kidney disease,
enlarged prostate gland, impaired
micturition (urination). Potassium
supplements may be needed.
Avoid use: children, patients in precomatose states as a result of liver cirrhosis.
Possible interaction: digoxin, lithium,
antihypertensives, aminoglycosides.
Side effects: gastro-intestinal upset,
cramps, skin rash, blood changes,
enlarged breasts, thrombocytopenia.
Manufacturer: Leo.

BURINEX A

Description: a combined loop and
potassium-sparing diuretic preparation
available as scored, cream, oval-shaped
tablets, marked with lion and 149,
containing 1mg bumetanide and 5mg
amiloride hydrochloride.
Used for: patients requiring immediate
diuresis, especially those in whom
hypokalaemia may be a problem.
Dosage: adults, 1 to 2 tablets each day.
Special care: pregnancy, breastfeeding,
diabetes, impaired micturition
(urination). Blood electrolyte levels
should be monitored.
Avoid use: children, patients with severe
imbalance of electrolyte levels (salts),
kidney or liver disease, disorders of
adrenal glands, hepatic pre-coma.
Possible interaction: antihypertensive
drugs, digitalis, potassium supplements,
potassium-sparing diuretics, lithium,
ACE inhibitors, cephalosporins,
aminoglycosides.
Side effects: gastro-intestinal upset, skin
rash, cramps, thrombocytopenia.
Manufacturer: Leo.

BURINEX K

Description: a combined loop diuretic,
potassium supplement preparation
available in the form of white, oval
tablets, containing 0.5mg bumetanide,
and 573mg potassium in a slow release
wax core.
Used for: oedema accompanying
congestive heart failure, kidney and liver
disease in which a potassium supplement
is needed.
Dosage: adults, 1 to 4 tablets each day.
Special care: pregnancy, breastfeeding,
gout, diabetes, kidney or liver disorders,
enlarged prostate gland, impaired
micturition (urination).
Avoid use: children, patients with
Addison's disease, hyperkalaemia,
precomatose states in liver cirrhosis.
Possible interaction: aminoglycosides,
digitalis, lithium, antihypertensives,
potassium-sparing diuretics.
Side effects: gastro-intestinal upset,
cramps, skin rash, enlarged breasts,
thrombocytopenia. Drug should be
discontinued if obstruction of ulceration
of small bowel occurs.
Manufacturer: Leo.

BUSPAR

Description: an anxiolytic (anxiety-
relieving) preparation, and an azapirone.
It is thought to be less open to abuse
than the benzodiazepine drugs which are
also used to relieve severe anxiety, and
also to be less sedating in its effect.
Buspar is produced in tablets of 2
strengths, containing 5mg or 10mg
buspirone hydrochloride. The tablets are
white, oval-shaped and marked with
strength.
Used for: short-term relief of severe
anxiety, i.e. that which is causing
extreme distress and inability to function
normally. This may or may not be
accompanied by depression.
Dosage: adults, 5mg 2 or 3 times each
day at first, increasing every 2 or 3 days
to a usual dose in the order of 10mg
twice daily. Maximum dose is 45mg daily.

Special care: if patient has been taking a benzodiazepine this should be slowly withdrawn before starting Buspirone therapy. Special care in patients with liver or kidney disorders.
Avoid use: children, patients with severe kidney or liver disease, epilepsy, pregnant women, breastfeeding mothers.
Possible interaction:
Side effects: headache, nervous tension, dizziness. Rarely, confusion, fatigue, dry mouth, chest pain, tachycardia.
Manufacturer: Bristol-Myers.

CAFERGOT

Description: an analgesic preparation containing ergotamine which is available as white, sugar-coated tablets containing 1mg ergotamine tartrate and 100mg caffeine. **CAFERGOT SUPPOSITORIES** contain 2mg ergotamine tartrate and 200mg caffeine.
Used for: migraine.
Dosage: 1 or 2 tablets at start of attack with no more than 4 in 24 hours; should not be repeated within 4 days. Suppositories, 1 at start of attack with maximum of 2 in 24 hours. Must not repeat within 4 days.
Avoid use: children, pregnancy, breastfeeding, liver or kidney disease, coronary, occlusive or peripheral vascular disease, sepsis, severe hyptertension.
Possible interaction: ß-blocker, erythromycin.
Side effects: vomiting, nausea, abdominal pains, impairment of circulation, weakness in legs. If pleural or retroperitoneal fibrosis occurs drug should be immediately stopped.
Manufacturer: Sandoz.

CALCIPARINE

Description: an anticoagulant available in the form of pre-filled syringes containing 25,000 units heparin calcium per ml for use as subcutaneous injection only.
Used for: deep vein thrombosis, pulmonary embolism and prevention of these before surgery.
Dosage: 5000 units 2 hours before surgery then every 8 to 12 hours for 7 days.
Special care: pregnancy, kidney or liver disease. Blood platelet counts are required and therapy should be halted in patients who develop thrombocytopenia.
Avoid use: patients with allergy to heparin, those with haemophilia, haemorrhagic disorders, severe hypertension, peptic ulcer, cerebral aneurysm, recent eye surgery or concerning central nervous system, serious liver disease.
Side effects: haemorrhage, thrombocytopenia, allergic reactions. After prolonged use, osteoporosis and rarely, baldness may occur.
Manufacturer: Sanofi Winthrop.

CALCITARE

Description: a preparation of thyroid hormone (derived from pig), available as a powder for reconstitution and injection, consisting of 160 units porcine calcitonin in a vial with gelatin diluent.
Used for: Paget's disease of bone, hypercalcaemia.
Dosage: Paget's disease, 80 units 3 times a week to 160 units daily in single or divided doses, but subcutaneous intramuscular injection. Hypercalcaemia, 4 units per kg of body weight daily by subcutaneous or intramuscular injection, adjusted according to response. Children per kg of body weight in similar way but should not receive treatment for periods exceeding a few weeks.
Special care: if history of allergy, scratch skin test should be carried out. Pregnant women, breastfeeding mothers.
Possible interaction: cardiac glycosides.
Side effects: vomiting and nausea, tingling in hands, flushing, unpleasant taste in mouth.
Manufacturer: Theraplix.

CALMURID HC

Description: a topical, moderately potent steroid with keratolytic and hydrating agents which have a softening and moistening effect on the skin. Available as a cream containing 1% hydrocortisone, 10% urea and 5% lactic acid.

Used for: dry eczemas and dermatoses.

Dosage: wash and dry affected skin, apply thinly twice a day at first and reduce frequency as condition improves.

Special care: limit use in children to 5 to 7 days, use extreme care with infants (napkin rash and infantile eczema). Also, use on face should be limited to 5 to 7 days. If stinging occurs, dilute to half-strength with water-based cream for 1 week before reverting to full strength preparation.

Avoid use: long-term use especially in pregnant women, patients with acne or skin conditions caused by tuberculosis, viral, fungal, bacterial infections which are untreated or ringworm, leg ulcers.

Side effects: not usually severe but thinning of skin, lines in skin (striae), blotchy red patches caused by distended blood vessels (capillaries) (telangiectasia), suppression of adrenal glands may occur.

Manufacturer: Novex.

CALSYNAR

Description: a manufactured form of a hormone, calcitonin, which is concerned with the regulation of calcium levels in the body. It is produced in ampoules for injection and contains 100 units salcatonin per ml in saline, (salcatonin is synthetic salmon calcitonin). Calcitonin lowers levels of calcium in blood plasma by inhibiting resorption of bone.

Used for: osteoporosis in post-menopausal women, Paget's disease, hypercalcaemia, in bone cancer, bone pain resulting from cancer.

Dosage: hypercalcaemia, 5–10 units per kg of body weight each day to 400 units 6- to 8-hourly according to response, by subcutaneous or intramuscular injection.

Paget's disease of bone, 50 units 3 times each week to 100 units daily in single or divided doses, by subcutaneous or intramuscular injection. Post-menopausal osteoporosis, 100 units each day by subcutaneous or intramuscular injection along with 600mg calcium and 400 units vitamin D taken by mouth. Bone pain in cancer, 200 units every 6 hours or 400 units every 12 hours, for 48 hours by subcutaneous or intramuscular injection. Children should not receive therapy for more than a few weeks, as directed by physician.

Special care: history of allergy, perform scratch skin test. Pregnant women, breastfeeding mothers.

Possible interaction: cardiac glycosides.

Side effects: vomiting and nausea, tingling sensation in hands, flushing, allergic responses, unpleasant taste in mouth.

Manufacturer: Theraplix.

CAMCOLIT

Description: an antidepressant preparation of lithium salts available as tablets of 2 strengths. Camcolit 250® tablets are white, scored, film-coated and contain 250mg lithium carbonate (equivalent to 6.8mmol Li⁺). CAMCOLIT 400® tablets are white, scored, modified release, film-coated and contain 400mg lithium carbonate (10.8mmol Li⁺), marked S and CAMCOLIT.

Used for: treatment and prevention of mania, recurrent bouts of depression, manic depression, aggressive and self-mutilating behaviour.

Dosage: adults, prevention 0.5–1.2g each day at first (elderly patients 0.5–1g). Maintain serum levels of lithium in range of 0.5 to 1mmol per litre. Treatment: 1.5 to 2g each day at first, (elderly patients, 0.5 to 1g). Maintain serum levels of lithium in range of 0.6 to 1.2 mmol per litre. Camcolit 250 should be given in divided doses; Camcolit 400 in single or divided doses.

Special care: treatment should be started

in hospital with monitoring of plasma lithium concentrations at regular intervals. (Overdosage usually with plasma concentrations in excess of 1.5mmol Li* per litre can be fatal). Adequate fluid and salt intake should be maintained. Monitor thyroid function.
Avoid use: children, pregnancy, breastfeeding, heart or kidney disease, hypothyroidism, Addison's disease, imbalance in sodium levels.
Possible interaction: NSAIDs, diuretics, haloperidol, phenytoin, metoclopramide, carbamazepine, flupenthixol.
Side effects: oedema, hypo and hyperthyroidism, weight gain, gastro-intestinal upset, diarrhoea and nausea, trembling in hands, muscular weakness, heart and central nervous system disturbance, skin reactions, intense thirst, large volumes of dilute urine.
Manufacturer: Norgine.

CANESTEN-HC

Description: a mildly potent steroid with an antifungal and antibacterial drug in the form of a cream containing 1% hydrocortisone and 1% clotrimazole.
Used for: fungal infections accompanied by inflammation.
Dosage: apply to affected skin twice each day.
Special care: limit use on face or in children to 5 to 7 days, especially on infants. Withdraw gradually, short term use only.
Avoid use: prolonged or extensive use on pregnant women, patients with untreated bacterial or fungal infections, acne, leg ulcers, scabies, viral skin infections, tuberculosis, ringworm, peri-oral dermatitis.
Side effects: slight burning or irritation, allergic reactions.
Manufacturer: Bayer.

CANTIL

Description: an anticholinergic preparation which acts as a smooth muscle relaxant, available as tablets which are yellow, scored and contain 25mg mepenzolate bromide.
Used for: spasm and overactivity of smooth muscle of the lower gastro-intestinal tract.
Dosage: adults, 1 to 2 tablets 3 or 4 times daily.
Special care: enlarged prostate gland.
Avoid use: children, pregnancy, breast-feeding, glaucoma, myasthenia gravis, unstable angina, tachycardia, liver and kidney disease, ulcerative colitis, reflux obstructive disease, hiatus hernia.
Possible interaction: antihistamines, tricyclic antidepressants, benzodiazepines.
Side effects: gastro-intestinal upset, nausea, constipation, vomiting, dry mouth, difficulty in swallowing (dysphagia), tachycardia, flushing, blurred vision, insomnia, weakness, retention of urine.
Manufacturer: Boehringer Mannheim.

CAPASTAT

Description: a peptide antituberculous preparation available as a powder for reconstitution and injection. Capastat consists of 1 mega unit (million units) of capreomycin sulphate (equivalent to approximately 1g capreomycin).
Used for: treatment of tuberculosis which has failed to respond to other drugs.
Dosage: usually 1g each day given by deep intramuscular injection for a period of 60–120 days. Thereafter, 1g 2 or 3 times a week by intramuscular injection.
Special care: pregnancy, breastfeeding, kidney and hearing disorders, history of liver disease or allergy. Liver, kidney and vestibular (concerned with balance and controlled by organs in the inner ear) functions should be monitored and hearing tests carried out.
Avoid use: children.
Possible interaction: other antibacterial drugs, streptomycin, viomycin, vancomycin, colistin, aminoglycosides.
Side effects: allergic reactions, e.g. skin rash and urticaria, changes in blood (thrombocytopenia, leucocytosis—an increased number of white blood cells,

leucopenia), nephrotoxicity (toxic effects on the kidney), ototoxicity (damage to the organs of hearing and balance), liver damage, electrolyte level disturbances, loss of hearing accompanied by tinnitus and vertigo.
Manufacturer: Dista.

CAPOTEN

Description: an antihypertensive preparation, captopril, which is an ACE inhibitor, produced in tablets of 3 strengths: white (12.5mg); mottled white square (25mg); mottled white oval (50mg).
Used for: mild to moderate hypertension (with diuretics and digitalis), severe hypertension, where other methods have not been successful, congestive heart failure, heart attack, diabetic nephropathy in insulin-dependent diabetes.
Dosage: adults, mild to moderate hypertension, 12.5mg twice each day at first with usual maintenance dose in the order of 25mg twice daily. Maximum dose is 50mg twice each day. Addition of a thiazide may be needed. Severe hypertension, 12.5mg twice each day at first, increasing to a maximum of 50mg 3 times each day if needed. Diabetic nephropathy, 75–100mg each day in divided doses. Heart failure, 6.25–12.5mg daily at first increasing to usual maintenance in the order of 25mg 2 or 3 times each day. Maximum dose is 150mg each day. N.B. therapy should be initiated in hospital under strict medical supervision with any diuretics being stopped or reduced before treatment begins. Post heart attack, 6.25mg daily at first beginning 3 days after attack increasing to 150mg daily in divided doses.
Special care: severe congestive heart failure, kidney disease, reno-vascular hypertension, undergoing dialysis or anaesthesia. Those with collagen vascular disease. White blood cell counts and checks on protein in urine and kidney function should be carried out before and during therapy. Contact manufacturer before use in children.
Avoid use: pregnancy, breastfeeding, various heart disorders (aortic stenosis, outflow obstruction).
Possible interaction: NSAIDs, potassium supplements, potassium-sparing diuretics, immunosuppressants, vasodilators, allopurinol, probenecid, clonidine, procainamide.
Manufacturer: Squibb.

CAPOZIDE

Description: a combined thiazide diuretic with an ACE inhibitor, produced in the form of white, scored tablets marked SQUIBB containing 25mg hydrochlorothiazide and 50mg captopril. CAPOZIDE LS tablets are white, scored and contain 12.5mg hydrochlorothiazide and 25mg captopril and are marked SQUIBB 536.
Used for: mild to moderate hypertension in patients who are stable when taking the same proportions of captopril and hydrochlorothiazide individually.
Dosage: adults, 1 tablet daily with a possible maximum of 2. Capozide LS, 1 tablet each day.
Special care: patients with kidney disease or receiving dialysis, liver disease, gout, collagen vascular disease, diabetes, undergoing asnaesthesia. Kidney function, urinary protein and white blood cell count shoudl be checked before and during treatment.
Avoid use: pregnant women, breastfeeding mothers, patients with certain heart diseases (aortic stenosis, outflow obstruction), anuria.
Possible interaction: NSAIDs, potassium supplements, potassium-sparing diuretics, immunosuppressants, vasodilators, allopurinol, probenecid, clonidine, procainamide.
Side effects: blood dyscrasias (blood changes), hypotension, rash, proteinuria, loss of sensation of taste, sensitivity to light, pancreatitis, tiredness, rarely, a cough.
Manufacturer: Squibb

CARACE

Description: an ACE inhibitor produced in the form of blue, oval tablets marked NSD15 containing 2.5mg lisinopril; white, oval, scored tablets contain 5mg lisinopril; yellow, oval, scored tablets contain 10mg lisinopril; orange, oval, scored tablets contain 20mg lisinopril. All except 2.5mg tablets are marked with name and strength.

Used for: congestive heart failure (in conjunction with diuretics and possibly digitalis), hypertension.

Dosage: adults, congestive heart failure, (reduce dose of any diuretic being taken before start of treatment) 2.5mg once each day at first increasing gradually to maintenance dose in the order of 5–20mg once daily, after 2 to 4 weeks. Hypertension, (discontinue any diuretic being taken 2 to 3 days before treatment starts); 2.5mg once a day increasing to a maintenance dose in the order of 10–20mg once daily. Maximum daily dose, 40mg.

Special care: breastfeeding, patients with kidney disease, receiving dialysis, renovascular hypertension, severe congestive heart failure, undergoing anaesthesia. Kidney function should be monitored before and during treatment. Treatment should begin under hospital supervision for heart failure patients.

Avoid use: pregnancy, children, patients with various heart disorders (aortic stenosis, outflow obstruction), cor pulmone (a lung disorder), angioneurotic odema as a result of previous ACE inhibitor treatment.

Possible interaction: potassium supplements, potassium-sparing diuretics, antihypertensives, indomethacin, lithium.

Side effects: headache, dizziness, diarrhoea, nausea, tiredness, palpitations, hypotension, rash, angioedema, asthenia (weakness), cough.

Manufacturer: DuPont.

CARACE PLUS

Description: an ACE inhibitor with a thiazide diuretic produced in the form of blue, hexagonal tablets marked 145 containing 10mg lisinopril and 12.5mg hydrochlorothiazide. CARACE 20 PLUS are yellow, hexagonal scored tablets containing 20mg lisinopril and 12.5mg hydrochlorothiazide.

Used for: mild to moderate hypertension in patients who are stable when taking the same proportions of lisinopril and hydrochlorothiazide individually.

Dosage: adults, 1 Carace Plus or Carace 20 Plus each day with a possible maximum of 2 tablets.

Special care: patients with liver or kidney disease receiving dialysis, heart and circulatory diseases, gout, hyperuricaemia (excess uric acid levels in blood), undergoing anaesthesia or surgery, with imbalances in salts (electrolytes) or fluid levels, children.

Avoid use: pregnancy, breastfeeding, anuria, angioneurotic oedema as a result of previous ACE inhibitor treatment.

Possible interaction: potassium supplements, hypoglycaemics, NSAIDs, lithium, tubocurarine.

Side effects: cough, headache, nausea, weariness, hypotension, diarrhoea, angioneurotic oedema, impotence, dizziness.

Manufacturer: Du Pont.

CARBO-CORT

Description: a mildly potent topical steroid combined with a cleansing agent, produced in the form of an antipsoriatic cream. Carbo-Cort contains 0.25% hydrocortisone and 3% coal tar solution.

Used for: eczema, lichen planus (a type of skin disease).

Dosage: apply to affected skin 2 or 3 times each day.

Special care: use in children or on face should be limited to 5 to 7 days. Special care in infants. Extensive or prolonged use should be avoided and the preparation withdrawn gradually.

Avoid use: patients with acne, untreated fungal or bacterial infections, tuberculosis, ringworm, viral skin infections, leg ulcers, scabies, peri-oral dermatitis.

Side effects: adrenal gland suppression, skin thinning, striae (lines on skin), telangiectasia (red blotches on skin).
Manufacturer: Lagap.

CARDENE

Description: a Class II calcium antagonist produced in the form of capsules: blue/white capsules contain 20mg nicardipine hydrochloride and pale blue/blue capsules containing 30mg .
Used for: chronic angina which is stable.
Dosage: adults, angina, 20mg 3 times each day in first instance increasing with 3-day intervals to a maintenance dose in the order of 30mg 3 times daily. Maximum daily dose, 120mg.
Special care: congestive heart failure, liver or kidney disease, weak heart.
Avoid use: children, pregnancy, breast-feeding, advanced aortic stenosis (a heart valve disease).
Possible interaction: cimetidine, digoxin.
Side effects: headache, dizziness, nausea, palpitations, flushing and feeling of warmth; chest pain within half an hour of taking dose or on increasing dose, drug should be withdrawn.
Manufacturer: Syntex.

CARDENE SR

Description: a Class II calcium antagonist produced in the form of sustained-release capsules: white capsules marked SYNTEX 30 contain 30mg nicardipine hydrochloride; blue capsules marked SYNTEX 45 contain 45mg.
Used for: mild to moderate hypertension.
Dosage: adults, 30mg twice each day at first increasing to 60mg twice daily if required.
Special care: congestive heart failure, liver or kidney disease, weak heart.
Avoid use: children, pregnant women, breastfeeding mothers, patients with advanced aortic stenosis (a heart valve disease).
Possible interaction: cimetidine, digoxin.
Side effects: headache, dizziness, nausea, palpitations, flushing and feeling of

warmth; chest pain within half an hour of taking dose or on increasing dose, drug should be withdrawn.
Manufacturer: Syntex

CARDURA

Description: an antihypertensive alpha-blocker, doxazosin mesylate, available as white, pentagonal tablets, marked DXP1 (1mg); white, oval tablets, marked DXP2 (2mg); white, square tablets, marked DXP4 (4mg). All tablets are marked Pfizer.
Used for: hypertension.
Dosage: adults, 1mg once a day at first increasing to 2mg after 1 or 2 weeks and then to 4mg once each day if needed. Maximum daily dose is 16mg.
Special care: pregnant women.
Avoid use: children, breastfeeding.
Side effects: headache, weariness, dizziness, vertigo, postural hypotension, asthenia (weakness), oedema.
Manufacturer: Invicta.

CARISOMA

Description: a carbamate preparation which acts as a muscle relaxant and available as white tablets containing 125mg carisoprodol and white tablets marked with P in a hexagon contain 350mg carisoprodol.
Used for: muscle spasm resulting from bone and muscle disorders.
Dosage: 350mg, elderly, 125mg, both 3 times each day.
Special care: history of drug abuse or alcoholism, liver or kidney disease. Long term treatment should be avoided and the drug withdrawn gradually.
Avoid use: children, pregnancy, breast-feeding, acute intermittent porphyria.
Possible interaction: oral contraceptives, steroids, CNS depressants, tricyclics, griseofulvin, phenothiazines, rifampicin, phenytoin, anticoagulants.
Side effects: nausea, constipation, flushes, rash, weariness, drowsiness, headache.
Manufacturer: Pharmax.

CATAPRES

Description: an antihypertensive preparation, clonidine hydrochloride, produced in the form of tablets of 2 strengths, modified release capsules and in ampoules for injection. White scored tablets, marked with symbol and C over C, contain 0.1mg; white scored tablets marked with symbol and C over 03C, contain 0.3mg . Also, **CATAPRES PERLONGETS** are yellow/red sustained-release capsules marked with name, 11P and symbol and contain 0.25mg. Additionally, **CATAPRES INJECTION** contains 0.15mg per ml in ampoules.

Used for: hypertension.

Dosage: tablets, 0.05–1mg 3 times each day, gradually increasing every second or third day. Perlongets, 1 at night increasing, if required, to 1 tablet night and morning.

Special care: breastfeeding, depression, peripheral vascular disease. Tablets should be stopped gradually especially if beta-blockers are being withdrawn.

Avoid use: children.

Possible interaction: other antihypertensives, tricyclics, CNS depressants, alpha-blockers.

Side effects: dry mouth, oedema, drowsiness, dizziness.

Manufacturer: Boehringer Ingelheim.

CCNU

Description: an alkylating cytotoxic preparation produced in the form of blue/white capsules containing 10mg lomustine, and blue capsules containing 40mg lomustine.

Used for: Hodgkin's disease and some solid tumours.

Dosage: 120–130mg per square metre of body surface every 6 to 8 weeks.

Side effects: nausea, vomiting, bone marrow suppression, the onset of which is delayed.

Manufacturer: Lundbeck.

CEFIZOX

Description: a cephalosporin antibiotic preparation available as powder in vials for reconstitution and injection. Cefizox contains cefizoxime in the form of sodium salts as 500mg, 1g and 2g powder in vials.

Used for: septicaemia, urinary tract infections and gonorrhoea, skin and soft tissue infections and those of the lower respiratory tract.

Dosage: by intravenous infusion, deep intramuscular injection or slow intravenous injection, 1–2g 8- to 12-hourly increased in severe infections to a maximum of 8g daily, in 3 divided doses. Children over 3 months old, 30–60mg per kg of body weight each day in 2 to 4 divided doses. When infection is severe, 100–150mg per kg of body weight may be required.

Special care: patients with known allergy to penicillins and those with kidney disorders.

Avoid use: patients with allergy to cephalosporins, those with porphyria.

Possible interaction: amino glycosides, loop diuretics.

Side effects: allergic reactions, pain at site of injection, gastro-intestinal upset, rise in level of liver enzymes and urea in blood, candidosis eosinophils (increase in blood of number of eosinophils, a variety of white blood cell), thrombocytopenia, neutropenia. Positive Coomb's test.

Manufacturer: Wellcome.

CELANCE

Description: a dopamine agonist, pergolide mesylate, produced in the form of tablets: ivory, marked 4131 contain 0.05mg , green marked 4133, contain 0.25mg, and pink tablets, marked 4135 contain 1mg. All are rectangular, scored and marked LILLY.

Used for: additional therapy (to levodopa) in treatment of Parkinson's disease.

Dosage: 0.05mg each day at first increasing every third day by 0.1–0.15mg for a period of 12 days. Then the dose is increased by 0.25mg every third day until the best response is achieved. Maximum daily dose is 5mg. Levodopa dose should be carefully reduced.

Special care: pregnancy, breastfeeding, heart disease, heart arrhythmias, history of hallucinations. Drug should be gradually withdrawn.

Avoid use: children.

Possible interaction: anticoagulants, antihypertensives, other dopamine antagonists.

Side effects: disturbances of heartbeat, movement disorder (dyskinesia), drowsiness, hypotension, inflammation of the nose, dyspepsia, nausea, dyspnoea (laboured breathing), diplopia.

Manufacturer: Lilly

CELECTOL

Description: an antihypertensive preparation which is a cardioselective beta$_1$-blocker and partial beta$_2$-agonist. It is produced in heart-shaped tablets of 2 strengths, yellow scored tablets contain 200mg celiprolol hydrochloride and white tablets contain 400mg. The tablets are film-coated and marked with logo and strength.

Used for: mild to moderate hypertension.

Dosage: adults, 200mg once each day half an hour before food, maximum dose 400mg.

Special care: pregnancy, nursing mothers, anaestheseia or planned surgery, diabetes, liver or kidney disease, metabolic acidosis. Patients with weak hearts should receive diuretic and digitalis. Patients with history of bronchospasm. Drug should be gradually withdrawn.

Avoid use: children, patients with various forms of heart disease including heart block, heart failure, slow heart beat rate; sick sinus syndrome, peripheral arterial disease. Patients with obstructive airways disease (unless absolutely no alternative).

Possible interaction: sympathomimetics, central nervous system depressants, indomethacin, antihypertensives, ergotamine, reserpine, cimetidine,

cardiac depressant anaesthetics, hypoglycaemics, verapamil, Class I antiarrhythmics, clonidine withdrawal.

Side effects: gastro-intestinal disorders, fatigue with exercise, cold feet and hands, disruption of sleep, slow heartbeat rate. If dry eyes or skin rash occur, drug should be gradually withdrawn.

Manufacturer: Rhône-Poulenc Rorer.

CEPAREX

Description: a cephalosporin antibiotic produced in the form of tablets, capsules and syrup. Pink, film-coated tablets, containing 250mg, 500mg and 1g cephalexin are marked GLAXO and with name and strength. **CEPOREX CAPSULES** coloured grey/caramel contain 250mg and 500mg and are marked GLAXO and with capsule name and strength. **CEPOREX ORANGE SYRUP** (produced as granules for reconstitution), contains 125mg, 250mg and 500mg per 5ml when made up with water. **CEPOREX SUSPENSION** coloured yellow, contains 125mg or 250mg per 5ml. **CEPOREX PAEDIAT-RIC DROPS** coloured orange contain 125mg per 1.25ml solution (produced as granules for reconstitution with 10ml water).

Used for: urinary tract infections, gonorrhoea, middle ear infections, respiratory tract, skin and soft tissue infections.

Dosage: adults, 1–2g daily in 2, 3 or 4 divided doses. Children, under 3 months, 62.5mg–125mg twice each day; 4 months to 2 years, 250–500mg each day; 3 years to 6 years, 1–2g each day, all in 2, 3 or 4 divided doses.

Special care: patients with allergy to penicillins or kidney disease.

Side effects: allergic reactions, gastro-intestinal upset.

Manufacturer: Glaxo.

CESAMET

Description: an anti-emetic preparation, which is a cannabinoid drug thought to have an effect in the central nervous system involving opiate receptors. It is produced as blue/white capsules, for hospital use only, containing 1mg babilone.

Used for: nausea and vomiting caused by cytotoxic drugs.

Dosage: 1mg twice each day increasing to 2mg twice daily if required. First dose is taken the night before and the second, 1 to 3 hours before cytotoxic therapy begins. Maximum dose is 6mg in 3 divided doses. If necessary, it may be continued for 48 hours after cytotoxic therapy has ceased.

Special care: elderly persons, patients with heart disease, severe liver disorders, hypertension, history of psychiatric disorders. Performance of skilled tasks, e.g. driving may be affected.

Possible interaction: alcohol, hypnotics and sedatives (enhances the effect of drowsiness).

Side effects: dry mouth, disturbance of vision, headache, drowsiness, vertigo, inability to concentrate, sleep disturbances, unsteady gait, hypotension, nausea. Mental disturbances including confusion, euphoria, disorientation, hallucinations, psychosis, depression, lack of co-ordination, loss of appetite, increased heartbeat rate, tremor, abdominal pain.

Manufacturer: Lilly.

CHEMOTRIM PAEDIATRIC

Description: an antibiotic preparation produced in the form of a suspension specifically intended for children. It combines a sulphonamide with a folic acid inhibitor, containing 200mg sulphamethoxazole and 40mg trimethoprim per 5ml of suspension.

Used for: urinary tract, skin, respiratory and gastro-intestinal infections.

Dosage: children 6 weeks to 5 months, 2.5ml; 6 months to 5 years, 5ml; 6 years to 12 years, 10ml. All twice each day.

Special care: elderly, breastfeeding, kidney disease (reduce and/or increase

time between doses). During long-term therapy, regular blood counts should be carried out.

Avoid use: neonates (babies from birth to 1 month of age), pregnancy, patients with serious liver or kidney disease or blood changes.

Possible interaction: hypoglycaemics, anticoagulants, anticonvulsants, folate inhibitors.

Side effects: skin rashes, glossitis (inflammation of tongue), nausea, vomiting, blood changes, folate deficiency. Rarely erythema multiforme, Lyell syndrome.

Manufacturer: RP Drugs.

CHENDOL

Description: a bile acid preparation produced in the form of orange/ivory capsules, marked CHENDOL contain 125mg chenodeoxycholic acid.

Used for: to dissolve cholesterol gallstones which are not calcified.

Dosage: adults 10–15mg per kg of body weight as a single nightly dose or divided doses. Continue for 3 months after gallstones have been dissolved.

Special care: liver function should be carefully monitored.

Avoid use: children, women planning a pregnancy, patients with chronic liver disease or inflammatory intestinal disease.

Possible interaction: oral contraceptives.

Side effects: pruritis (itching), diarrhoea.

Manufacturer: CP Pharmaceuticals.

CHENOFALK

Description: a bile acid preparation produced in the form of tablets and available as white capsules containing 250mg chenodeoxycholic acid.

Used for: to dissolve cholesterol gallstones which are not calcified.

Dosage: adults, 15mg per kg of body weight each day in divided doses. Should be continued for 3 to 6 months after stones have been dissolved.

Special care: liver function should be carefully monitored.

Avoid use: women planning pregnancy or who are not using contraception. Patients with non-functioning gall bladder, inflammatory intestinal disease, chronic liver disease.
Possible interaction: oral contraceptives.
Side effects: pruritis (itching), diarrhoea.
Manufacturer: Thames.

CHLORASEPT

Description: a proprietary disinfectant preparation available as a pink solution and containing 0.05% chlorhexidine acetate.
Used for: cleansing of wounds.
Dosage: apply as required.
Manufacturer: Baxter

CHLORDIAZEPOXIDE

Description: an anxiolytic and long-acting benzodiazepine produced in the form of tablets of strengths 5mg, 10mg and 25mg chlordiazepoxide. Also, **CHLORDIAZEPOXIDE HYDRO-CHLORIDE** tablets are available in strengths of 5mg, 10mg and 25mg and **CHLORDIAZEPOXIDE CAPSULES**, available in strengths of 5mg and 10mg.
Used for: relief of anxiety.
Dosage: adults, 30mg each day in divided doses increasing to 40–100mg if symptoms are severe. Elderly persons, 10mg each day at first, carefully increased if needed.
Special care: use for short-term relief of severe and disabling anxiety (for a period of 2–4 weeks). Lowest possible dose and withdraw drug gradually. Special care needed for elderly persons, pregnant women, breastfeeding mothers, women in labour. Patients with lung, liver or kidney disease.
Avoid use: patients with severe lung disease or depressed respiration. Those with psychiatric disorders including obsessional and phobic states and psychosis.
Possible interaction: alcohol, CNS depressants, anticonvulsant drugs.
Side effects: gastro-intestinal upset,

drowsiness, light headedness, unsteadiness, vertigo, confusion, impaired judgment and dexterity. Disturbance of vision, hypotension, skin rashes. Urine retention, changes in libido. Rarely, jaundice and blood changes. Risk of dependency with higher doses or longer period of use.
Manufacturer: non-proprietary.

CHLOROMYCETIN

Description: a broad-spectrum antibiotic, chloramphenicol, produced in the form of capsules, as a suspension and as a powder for reconstitution and injection. White/grey capsules marked PARKE-DAVIS contain 250mg, **CHLOROMYCETIN PALMITATE SUSPENSION** contains 125mg per 5ml. **CHLOROMYCETIN INJECTION** produced as a powder in vials for reconstitution contains cholamphenicol (as sodium succinate).
Used for: severe infections where there are no effective alternatives, typhoid fever, influenzae meningitis.
Dosage: adults, 50mg per kg of body weight each day in divided doses at 6 hourly intervals. Children under 2 weeks of age, half adult dose; over 2 weeks, same as adult.
Special care: regular blood tests are advisable during course of treatment.
Avoid use: for minor infections or for prevention.
Possible interaction: paracetamol, anticonvulsants, anticoagulants.
Side effects: gastro-intestinal upset, allergic reactions, blood changes, neuritis, and optic (eye) neuritis with prolonged use. Newborn babies may develop Grey syndrome.
Manufacturer: Parke-Davis.

CHLOROMYCETIN EYE OINTMENT

Description: a broad-spectrum antibiotic eye ointment containing 1% chloramphenicol and also eye drops, **CHLORO-MYCETIN REDIDROPS**, containing

0.5% chloramphenicol.
Used for: bacterial conjunctivitis.
Dosage: 2 drops or apply ointment every 3 hours or more often if needed. Continue for 2 days after symptoms have gone.
Side effects: rarely, aplastic anaemia (caused by bone marrow failure) a form of anaemia in which there is a lack of all blood elements.
Manufacturer: Parke-Davis.

CHLOROMYCETIN HYDROCORTISONE

Description: a proprietary antibiotic and corticosteroid ointment containing 1% chloramphenicol and 0.5% hydrocortisone acetate.
Used for: eye infections.
Dosage: apply to eye once an hour if infection is severe, or less frequently if infection is less severe.
Special care: infants or prolonged use.
Avoid use: glaucoma, viral, fungal or purulent infections.
Manufacturer: Parke-Davis

CICATRIN

Description: an aminoglycoside, antibacterial preparation available in the form of a cream, dusting powder and aerosol. The cream and powder contain 3300 units neomycin sulphate, 250 units bacitracin zinc, 2mg l-cysteine, 10mg glycine and 1mg threonine per g. The aerosol contains 16,500 units neomycin sulphate, 1250 units bacitracin zinc, 12mg l-cysteine, 60mg glycine/g in the form of a spray powder.
Used for: minor bacterial skin infections.
Dosage: adults and children, cream, aerosol and dusting powder, apply 3 times each day to affected skin for 3 weeks.
Special care: on large areas of affected skin. Do not repeat for 3 months.
Side effects: allergic responses, ototoxicity (damage to organs of hearing and balance).
Manufacturer: Wellcome.

CIDOMYCIN

Description: an aminoglycoside antibiotic preparation containing gentamicin as sulphate and produced in a variety of different forms for injection. Cidomycin injection contains 40mg gentamicin (as sulphate) per ml produced in ampoules and vials. **CIDOMYCIN PAEDIATRIC INJECTION** contains 10mg/ ml in 2ml vials. **CIDOMYCIN INTRATHECAL INJECTION** contains 5mg/ml in ampoules.
Used for: serious infections sensitive to gentamicin; urinary tract infections.
Dosage: adults, 5mg per kg of body weight by intramuscular or intravenous injection each day in 3 or 4 divided doses. Children, up to 2 weeks of age, 3mg per kg of body weight at 12 hour intervals; over 2 weeks, 2mg per kg of body weight at 8-hour intervals. Both intramuscularly or intravenously for a period of 7–10 days.
Special care: patients with kidney disease, myasthenia gravis; regular blood tests are necessary as blood concentrations over 10µg per ml can cause damage to the organs of hearing and balance.
Avoid use: pregnant women.
Possible interaction: anaesthetics, neuromuscular blocking drugs, frusemide, ethacrynic acid.
Manufacturer: Roussel.

CIDOMYCIN CREAM AND OINTMENT

Description: an aminoglycoside antibiotic preparation containing 0.3% gentamicin (as sulphate) in the form of a cream or ointment.
Used for: skin infections (including impetigo), of a primary and secondary nature.
Dosage: apply to affected skin 3 or 4 times each day.
Special care: large areas of affected skin.
Side effects: allergic reactions, ototoxicity.
Manufacturer: Roussel.

CIDOMYCIN EYE AND EAR DROPS

Description: an antibiotic preparation containing 0.3% gentamicin (as sulphate) in the form of ear and eye drops. Also, **CIDOMYCIN EYE OINTMENT** containing 0.3% gentamicin as sulphate.

Used for: bacterial infections of the external ear and eye.

Dosage: ear drops, adults and children, 2 to 4 drops 3 or 4 times each day and at night. Eye drops and ointment, adults and children, 1 to 3 drops or applications of ointment 3 to 4 times each day.

Avoid use: ear infections where drum is perforated.

Side effects: risk of superinfection (another infection occurring during treatment).

Manufacturer: Roussel.

CILEST

Description: a combined oestrogen/progestogen contraceptive preparation containing 35μg ethinyloestradiol and 0.25mg norgestimate in the form of blue tablets marked C250.

Used for: oral contraception.

Dosage: 1 tablet each day for 21 days starting on first day of period, followed by 7 tablet-free days.

Special care: patients with asthma, diabetes, Raynaud's disease, varicose veins, hypertension, serious kidney disease, kidney dialysis, multiple sclerosis, hyperprolactinaemia (an excess of prolactin, a hormone, in the blood), serious depression. The risk of thrombosis increases with age and if woman smokes or is obese. Pelvic organs, breasts and blood pressure should be checked regularly during the time oral contraceptives are being taken.

Avoid use: pregnancy, history of thrombosis or at risk, those with various forms of heart disease, heart valve disease and angina. Patient with sickle cell anaemia, infectious hepatitis, certain liver and kidney disorders, hormone-dependent cancers, undiagnosed vaginal bleeding.

Possible interaction: tetracyclines, barbiturates, carbamazepine, primidone, griseofulvin, phenytoin, chloral hydrate, glutethimide, ethosuximide, dichloralphenazone.

Side effects: nausea, headaches, bloatedness due to fluid retention, enlargement of breasts, cramps and leg pains, reduction in libido, depression, weight gain, bleeding, vaginal discharge, erosion of cervix.

Manufacturer: Ortho.

CINOBAC

Description: a quinolone antibiotic drug produced as green/orange capsules containing 500mg cinoxacin and marked LILLY 3056.

Used for: infections of the urinary tract.

Dosage: 1 tablet twice each day for 7 to 14 days. For prevention of infection, 1 tablet at night.

Special care: patients with kidney disorders or history of liver disease.

Avoid use: children, pregnancy, breast-feeding, severe kidney disorders.

Possible interaction: NSAIDs, anticoagulant drugs taken by mouth, theophylline.

Side effects: gastro-intestinal upset, disturbance of CNS, allergic reactions.

Manufacturer: Lilly.

CIPROXIN

Description: A 4-quinolone antibiotic preparation, ciprofloxacin hydrochloride monohydrate, produced in the form of tablets of 3 different strenths and as a solution for infusion. White, film-coated tablets, marked with BAYER logo and CIP 250 contain 250mg; BAYER logo and CIP 500 (500mg); marked with BAYER logo and CIP 750 (750mg). **CIPROXIN INFUSION** contains 2mg ciprofloxacin (as lactate) per ml.

Used for: ear, nose, throat, respiratory tract infections. Skin, bone, joint, soft tissue and eye infections. Also, pelvic and gastro-intestinal infections, gonorrhoea and pneumonia caused by Gram-negative bacteria. Prevention of infection in endoscopy and surgery on upper gastro-intestinal tract.

Dosage: adults, tablets, 250mg to 750 mg twice each day for 5 to 10 days. For gonorrhoea, one 250mg dose. For prevention of infection, 750mg 1 hour to 1½ hours before operation. Infusion, 100–200mg twice each day by intravenous infusion for 5 to 7 days. For gonorrhoea, 100mg by intravenous infusion.

Special care: severe kidney and liver disorders, epilepsy or disorders of central nervous system, history of convulsions. Plenty of fluids should be drunk.

Avoid use: children and adolescents (except in exceptional circumstances), pregnancy, breastfeeding.

Possible interaction: alcohol, NSAIDs, opiates, theophylline, cyclosporin, glibenclamide, iron, magnesium or aluminium salts.

Side effects: headache, tremor, dizziness, confusion, impaired judgment and dexterity (ability to drive and operate machinery may be affected), disturbance of sleep, convulsions. Sensitivity to light, skin rash, pains in joints, disturbance of vision, tachycardia. There may be changes in liver, kidneys and in blood.

Manufacturer: Bayer.

CITANEST

Description: a local anaesthetic preparation produced as solutions of various strengths, for injection and containing prilocaine hydrochloride. Citanest is available in strengths of 0.5% (5mg prilocaine hydrochloride per ml), 1% (10mg per ml), 2% (20mg per ml) and 4% (40mg per ml). Also, **CITANEST WITH OCTAPRESSIN** containing 3% and 0.03 units per ml of felypressin.

Used for: local anaesthesia.

Dosage: adults, (adjusted according to patient response and nature of operation), maximum 400mg if used alone or 600mg with felypressin or adrenaline. Children according to body weight and nature of operation.

Special care: patients with liver, kidney or respiratory disorders, epilepsy or conduction disturbances.

Avoid use: patients with anaemia, methaemoglobinaemia (presence in the blood of methaemoglobin derived from the blood pigment, haemoglobin, which results in a lack of oxygen being carried in the blood and various symptoms arising from this).

Side effects: allergic reactions, rarely, whole body (systemic) effects.

Manufacturer: Astra.

CLAFORAN

Description: a cephalosporin antibiotic preparation produced in the form of a powder for reconstitution and injection. Claforan contains 500mg, 1g or 2g of cefotaxime (as sodium salt), as powder in vials.

Used for: urinary tract and soft tissue infections, septicaemia, meningitis and respiratory tract infections.

Dosage: adults, 1g by intravenous or intramuscular injection at 8-hourly intervals. For serious infections dose may need to be increased to 6g (maximum 12g) daily in 3 or 4 divided doses. The 2g dose should be given intravenously. Children, newborn babies, 50mg per kg of body weight daily in 2, 3 or 4 divided doses; older infants and children, 200mg per kg of body weight daily in 2, 3 or 4 divided doses.

Special care: pregnancy, breastfeeding, penicillin allergy and serious kidney failure.

Possible interaction: aminoglycosides, loop diuretics.

Side effects: gastro-intestinal upset, pain at injection site, allergic reactions, candidosis, blood changes, haemolytic anaemia, rise in liver enzymes and blood urea.

Manufacturer: Roussel.

CLARITYN

Description: an antihistamine preparation produced in the form of oval, white, scored tablets containing 10mg loratadine, and marked with strength and logo. Also, **CLARITYN SYRUP** containing 5mg per 5ml.

Used for: relief of symptoms of allergic rhinitis, e.g. hay fever, urticaria.

Dosage: adults, 1 tablet each day, or 10ml syrup. Children, syrup only, 2 to 7 years, 5ml; 7 to 12 years, 10ml, both once each day.

Avoid use: children under 2 years of age, pregnancy, breastfeeding.

Side effects: headache, nausea, fatigue.

Manufacturer: Schering-Plough.

CLEXANE

Description: an anticoagulant preparation produced in pre-filled syringes for injection containing either 20mg (low molecular weight heparin) enoxaparin per 0.2ml or 40mg enoxaparin per 0.4ml.

Used for: prevention of deep vein thrombosis especially associated with orthopaedic and general surgery. Prevention of blood clot formation during haemodialysis.

Dosage: adults, low to medium risk of thrombosis (in general surgery), 20mg 2 hours before operation by deep subcutaenous injection and then 20mg once each day for 7 to 10 days. High risk of thrombosis (orthopaedic surgery), 40mg 12 hours before operation by deep subcutaenous injection, and 40mg once a day for 7 to 10 days. Haemodialysis, 1mg per kg of body weight with a further dose of 0.5 to 1mg/kg if process lasts for longer than 4 hours.

Special care: pregnancy, breastfeeding, hypertension, history of liver disorders or ulcers.

Avoid use: children, patients with peptic ulcer, serious bleeding disorders (e.g. haemophilia), those at risk of haemorrhage, thrombocytopenia, cerebral aneurysm, severe liver disease. Patients who have had recent CNS or eye surgery.

Possible interaction: aspirin, NSAIDs, dextran, anticoagulants taken by mouth, antiplatelet drugs.

Side effects: effects on liver, thrombocytopenia, less commonly, bruising and haemorrhage.

Manufacturer: Rhône-Poulenc Rorer.

CLIMAGEST

Description: a combined oestrogen, progestogen hormonal preparation, produced in the form of tablets. Climagest 1mg consists of 16 blue-grey tablets containing 1mg oestradiol valerate, coded E1, and 12 white tablets, containing 1mg oestradiol valerate and 1mg norethisterone, coded N1. Also, **CLIMAGEST 2MG** consists of 16 blue tablets containing 2mg oestradiol valerate, coded E2, and 12 yellow tablets containing 2mg oestradiol valerate and 1mg norethisterone, coded N2.

Used for: relief of menopausal symptoms.

Dosage: 1 tablet daily starting with oestradiol valerate (coded E) on first day of period (if present), and finishing with the 12 tablets (coded N), containing norethisterone.

Special care: patients considered to be at risk of thrombosis, those with diabetes, epilepsy, hypertension, multiple sclerosis, migraine, fibroids in uterus, ostosclerosis, tetany, liver disease, porphyria, gallstones. Regular examination of breasts and pelvic organs should be carried out and blood pressure checked. Drug should be stopped if there are any signs of jaundice, headaches which are severe, migraine, rise in blood pressure before planned surgery.

Avoid use: pregnancy, breastfeeding, hormone-dependent cancers, breast or uterus cancer, endometriosis, undiagnosed vaginal bleeding, sickle cell anaemia. Serious heart, kidney or liver disease, thrombosis. Patients suffering from Dublin-Johnson syndrome or Rotor syndrome.

Possible interaction: drugs which induce liver enzymes.

Side effects: weight gain, enlargement and tenderness of breasts, fluid retention, cramps, gastro-intestinal upset, nausea and vomiting, headaches, breakthrough bleeding, dizziness.
Manufacturer: Sandoz.

CLIMAVAL

Description: a hormonal oestrogen preparation produced in tablets of 2 strengths. Climaval 1mg are grey/blue tablets containing 1mg oestradiol valerate marked E1; Climaval 2mg are blue tablets containing 2mg oestradiol valerate and marked E2.
Used for: treatment of menopausal symptoms in women who have had a hysterectomy.
Dosage: 1 tablet each day either 1mg or 2mg according to response. May be taken continuously for up to 2 years.
Special care: only in elderly women for post-menopausal symptoms, otherwise avoid use; patients considered to be at risk of thrombosis, those with diabetes, epilepsy, hypertension, multiple sclerosis, migraine, fibroids in uterus, ostosclerosis, tetany, liver disease, porphyria, gallstones. Regular examination of breasts and pelvic organs should be carried out and blood pressure checked. Drug should be stopped if there are any signs of jaundice, severe headaches and migraine, a rise in blood pressure and before planned surgery.
Avoid use: pregnancy, breastfeeding, hormone-dependent cancers, breast and uterine cancer, endometriosis, undiagnosed vaginal bleeding, sickle cell anaemia, serious heart, kidney or liver disease, thrombosis. Patients suffering from Dublin-Johnson syndrome or Rotor syndrome.
Possible interaction: drugs which induce liver enzymes.
Side effects: weight gain, enlargement and tenderness of breasts, fluid retention, cramps, gastro-intestinal upset, nausea and vomiting, headaches, dizziness.
Manufacturer: Sandoz.

CLINORIL

Description: a proprietary analgesic NSAID produced in the form of hexagonal yellow scored tablets containing 100mg or 200mg sulindac and marked MSD 943 and MSD 942 respectively.
Used for: inflammation and pain in rheumatic diseases including gout, rheumatoid arthritis and osteoarthritis.
Dosage: adults, 200mg twice each day with food or drink.
Special care: elderly persons with history of lithiasis (gallstones, kidney stones, stones in lower urinary tract), patients with heart failure, liver or kidney disease, history of gastro-intestinal haemorrhage or ulcers. Plenty of fluids should be taken and liver function monitored.
Avoid use: children, pregnancy, breast-feeding, allergy to aspirin or anti-inflammatory drugs, those with gastro-intestinal bleeding or peptic ulcer.
Possible interaction: aspirin, anticoagulants, diflunisal, hypoglycaemic drugs, methotrexate, dimethyl sulphoxide, cyclosporin.
Side effects: allergic responses including liver failure and fever (stop drug immediately). Disturbance of vision, central nervous system effects, heart arrythmias, changes in blood, kidney stones and disturbance of kidney function, pancreatitis, hyperglycaemia, gastro-intestinal bleeding and upset. Also rash, dizziness, glossitis (inflammation of tongue), tinnitus, muscle weakness, effects on urine including discolouration, proteinuria (protein in urine), crystals in urine (crystalluria), oedema.
Manufacturer: MSD.

CLOBAZAM

Description: an anxiolytic long-acting benzodiazepine drug also used as an additional treatment for epilepsy. It is produced in the form of capsules containing 10mg clobazam.

Used for: short-term relief of symptoms of anxiety; additional therapy for epilepsy.

Dosage: anxiety, 20–30mg each day in divided doses or as 1 dose taken at night. In severe cases (under hospital supervision) dose may be increased to 60mg each day in divided doses. Elderly or debilitated persons, reduced daily dose of 10–20mg. Adults, epilepsy, 20–30mg each day (maximum 60mg) in divided doses. Children, for epilepsy only, age 3 to 12 years, half adult dose.

Special care: children under 3 years (epilepsy) and not for children in cases of anxiety, pregnancy, women in labour, breastfeeding, elderly (reduced dose), patients with liver or kidney disease or respiratory disorders. Prolonged use and abrupt withdrawal of drug should be avoided.

Avoid use: severe respiratory or lung disorders.

Possible interaction: CNS depressants, alcohol, anticonvulsant drugs.

Side effects: impaired judgment and dexterity interfering with performance of skilled tasks, lightheadedness, confusion, drowsiness, unsteadiness, vertigo. Also disturbance of vision, gastro-intestinal upset, retention of urine, skin rashes, change in libido, hypotension. Rarely, jaundice and blood changes.

Manufacturer: non-proprietary but available from Hoechst as **Frisium**.

CLOMID

Description: an anti-oestrogen hormonal preparation produced in the form of pale yellow scored tablets, containing 50mg clomiphene citrate, and marked with a circle containing the letter M.

Used for: treatment of sterility in women due to failure of ovulation.

Dosage: 1 tablet each day for 5 days starting on the fifth day of menstruation.

Special care: ensure patient is not pregnant before and during the course of treatment.

Avoid use: women with large ovarian cyst, cancer of the womb, undiagnosed uterine bleeding, liver disease.

Side effects: hot flushes, enlargement of ovaries, abdominal discomfort, blurring of vision (withdraw drug).

Manufacturer: Merrell Dow.

CLOPIXOL

Description: an antipsychotic drug and thioxanthene produced in the form of tablets and as solutions for injection. Tablets are produced in various strengths and all are film-coated; pink tablets contain 2mg zuclopenthixol hydrochloride; light brown tablets contain 10mg; brown tablets contain 25mg.
CLOPIXOL INJECTION contains 200mg per ml (as oily injection) contained in ampoules and vials.
CLOPIXOL CONCENTRATED INJECTION contains 500mg per ml (as oily injection) contained in ampoules.
CLOPIXOL ACUPHASE contains 50mg per ml (as oily injection) contained in ampoules.

Used for: psychoses, particularly schizophrenia and especially when accompanied by aggression and agitated behaviour.

Dosage: tablets, 20–30mg each day in divided doses in first instance. Usual maintenance dose is in the order of 25–50mg each day with a maximum daily dose of 500mg. Clopixol injection, 200–400mg every 2 to 4 weeks by deep intramuscular injection with a maximum weekly dose of 600mg. Clopixol concentrated injection, 250–500mg every 1 to 4 weeks by deep intramuscular injection with a maximum weekly dose of 600mg. Clopixol acuphase (for immediate treatment of acute psychoses), 50–150mg by deep intramuscular injection repeated after 1, 2 or 3 days if required. Maximum total dose is 400mg and maintenance should be by means of tablets or other Clopixol injections.

Special care: pregnancy, breastfeeding, heart and circulatory disorders, liver or kidney disease, Parkinsonism, an intolerance to neuroleptic drugs taken by mouth.

Avoid use: children, coma, states of withdrawal and apathy.

Possible interaction: alcohol, antidiabetic drugs, levodopa, anticonvulsant drugs, analgesics, CNS sedatives, antihypertensive drugs.

Side effects: Parkinsonism-like effects, spasms in muscles and involuntary, repetitive movements, rapid heartbeat rate, vision disturbance, tremor. Also hypotension, changes in weight, difficulty in passing urine, dry mouth and stuffiness in nose, impotence, enlargement of breasts, hypothermia (especially in elderly persons). There may be blood changes, dermatitis, weariness and lethargy, fits and jaundice.

Manufacturer: Lundbeck.

CLOSTET

Description: a preparation of tetanus toxoid vaccine (40iu per 0.5ml) adsorbed onto aluminium hydroxide and contained in pre-filled (0.5ml) syringes.

Used for: immunisation against tetanus and for "booster" injections to reinforce immunity.

Dosage: adults, a course of 0.5ml by subcutaneous or intramuscular injection given a total of 3 times at 4 week intervals. After 10 years, a "booster" reinforcing dose of 0.5ml may be given by subcutaneous or intramuscular injection. If an injury is received which might give rise to tetanus, a booster reinforcing dose should be given to patients previously immunised. Those who have not, should be given a first dose of the primary course and an injection of antitetanus immunoglobin at a different site. Children normally receive a combined triple vaccine consisting of adsorbed tetanus, diphtheria and pertussis (whooping cough) vaccine, and can later receive booster reinforcing doses against tetanus.

Special care: allergic reactions especially in persons receiving vaccine within 1 year of receiving a previous booster dose. Normally, 10 years should have elapsed before a reinforcing dose is given.

Avoid use: patients with serious infections unless there is a wound likely to be prone to tetanus.

Side effects: malaise, fever, slight soreness and local reactions.

Manufacturer: Evans.

CLOZARIL

Description: an antipsychotic drug and dibenzodiazepine, clozapine, produced as yellow scored tablets (25mg strength) and marked CLOZ 25, and 100mg strength, marked CLOZARIL 100.

Used for: schizophrenia which has failed to respond to, or patient is intolerant of other conventional antipsychotic drugs.

Dosage: first day, 12.5mg once or twice. Second day, 25mg once or twice; dose is gradually increased over a period of 2 to 3 weeks by 25–50mg each day until patient is receiving 300mg daily in divided doses. Depending upon response, a further increase may be required by giving an additional 50–100mg every 4 to 7 days to a maximum of 900mg each day in divided doses. Usual maintenance dose is in the order of 150–300mg in divided doses. Elderly persons, 12.5mg each day in first instance slowly increasing by 25mg daily.

Special care: patient, prescribing doctor and pharmacist must be registered with Sandoz Clorazil Patient Monitoring Service (CPMS). Patients should report signs of infection and must take contraceptive precautions. Special care in pregnant women, patients with enlarged prostate gland, liver disease, glaucoma, paralytic ileus. Persons with epilepsy should be monitored. Regular blood counts of leucocytes should be carried out before and during treatment. Drug should be immediately withdrawn if whole blood count falls below 3000/

mm³ or neutrophil (a type of white blood cell) count below 1500/mm³.

Avoid use: children; patients with history of drug induced blood disorders—neutropenia, agranulocytosis (a serious fall in the number of white blood cells called eosinophils, basophils and neutrophils), bone marrow disorders. Also, patients with history of drug intoxication, toxic and alcoholic psychoses, CNS depression or those in comatose states. Avoid use in breastfeeding mothers, persons with serious kidney or liver disease or circulatory collapse and cardiac failure.

Possible interaction: benzodiazepines, alcohol, MAOIs, CNS depressants, other drugs which cause agranulocytosis, anticholinergics, antihistamines, hypotensive drugs, lithium, phenytoin, warfarin, cimetidine.

Side effects: neutropenia leading to agranulocytosis (characterized by fever, collapse, bleeding ulcers of vagina, rectum and mouth) which may be fatal, effects on heart muscle and brain activity, tachycardia, fits, fatigue, dizziness, headache, over-production of saliva in mouth, retention of urine, gastro-intestinal upset, disturbance of body temperature regulation.

Manufacturer: Sandoz

CO-BETALOC

Description: an antihypertensive preparation combined with a cardioselective β-blocker with a thiazide diuretic produced in the form of white scored tablets, marked A/MH, contain 100mg metoprolol tartrate and 12.5mg hydrochlorothiazide. Also **CO-BETALOC SA** are yellow, film-coated tablets, marked A/MC, containing 200mg metoprolol tartrate and 25mg hydrochlorothiazide and having a sustained-release coat.

Used for: mild to moderate hypertension.

Dosage: adults, 1 to 3 tablets each day in single or divided doses, or 1 Co-Betaloc SA tablet daily.

Special care: pregnancy, breastfeeding, diabetes, kidney or liver disorders, metabolic acidosis, undergoing general anaesthesia, (may need to be withdrawn before planned surgery). Monitor electrolyte levels. Patients with weak hearts may need treatment with digitalis and diuretics. Drug should be gradually withdrawn. Potassium supplements may be required.

Avoid use: children, patients with history of obstructive airways disease, bronchospasm, asthma, heart block, heart shock, heart failure, severe peripheral arterial disease, sick sinus syndrome, severe kidney failure, anuria.

Possible interaction: sympathomimetics, cardiac depressant anaesthetics, clonidine withdrawal, hypoglycaemics, class I antiarrhythmic drugs, other antihypertensives, verapamil, ergotamine, reserpine, indomethacin, cimetidine, CNS depressants, lithium, digitalis.

Manufacturer: Astra.

CO-DANTHRAMER

Description: a preparation which combines a stimulant laxative and faecal softener produced in the form of a liquid. It contains 200mg of Poloxamer '188' and 25mg of danthron per 5ml of liquid. Also, **STRONG CO-DANTHRAMER** which contains 1g Poloxamer '188' and 75mg danthron per 5ml of liquid.

Used for: treatment and prevention of constipation in terminally ill persons (which has been caused by analgesic drugs). Also, constipation in elderly persons and patients with coronary thrombosis or cardiac failure.

Dosage: adults, 5–10ml Co-Danthramer or 5ml Strong Co-Danthramer taken at night. Children, 2.5–5ml Co-Danthramer only, taken at night.

Special care: pregnant women, patients suffering from incontinence (avoid prolonged contact with skin as irritation and soreness may occur).

Avoid use: babies in nappies, breastfeed-

ing, severe painful abdominal disorders, any intestinal obstruction.
Side effects: red discolouration of urine and skin with which urine comes into contact.
Manufacturer: non-proprietary, available from Napp as variations of **Codalax**.

CO-DANTHRUSATE

Description: a preparation which combines a stimulant laxative and faecal softener produced in the form of capsules and as a suspension. The capsules contain 50mg danthron and 60mg docusate sodium and **CO-DANTHRUSATE SUSPENSION** contains 50mg danthron and 60mg docusate sodium per 5ml.
Used for: treatment and prevention of constipation in terminally ill patients (which has been caused by analgesic drugs). Also, constipation in elderly persons and patients with coronary thrombosis and cardiac failure.
Dosage: adults, 1 to 3 capsules or 5–15ml suspension taken at night. Children over 6 years of age, 1 capsule or 5ml suspension taken at night.
Special care: pregnancy, breastfeeding.
Avoid use: children under 6 years, patients with intestinal obstruction.
Side effects: red discoloration of urine and skin with which urine may come into contact.
Manufacturer: non-proprietary, available from Evans as **Normax**.

CO-DYDRAMOL

Description: a compound opiate analgesic preparation combining 10mg dihydrocodeine tartrate with 500mg paracetamol in the form of tablets.
Used for: relief of mild to moderate pain.
Dosage: adults, 1 to 2 tablets every 4 to 6 hours with a maximum of 8 daily.
Special care: pregnant women, elderly persons, patients with allergies, underactive thyroid, liver or kidney disease.
Avoid use: children, patients with

obstructive airways disease or respiratory depression.
Possible interaction: CNS sedatives, alcohol.
Side effects: headaches, constipation, nausea.
Manufacturer: Non-proprietary, available from several companies.

CO-PROXAMOL

Description: a compound opiate analgesic preparation combining 32.5mg dextropropoxyphene hydrochloride and 325mg paracetamol in tablet form. .
Used for: relief of mild to moderate pain.
Dosage: adults, 2 tablets 3 or 4 times each day.
Special care: pregnant women, elderly persons, patients with liver or kidney disease.
Avoid use: children.
Possible interaction: CNS sedatives, alcohol, anticonvulsant and anticoagulant drugs.
Side effects: risk of dependence and tolerance, dizziness, rash, nausea, constipation, drowsiness.
Manufacturer: non-proprietary, available from several companies.

COBADEX

Description: a mildly potent topical corticosteroid preparation produced in the form of a cream containing 1% hydrocortisone and 20% dimethicone.
Used for: mild inflammatory skin conditions such as eczema which are responsive to steroids. Also, anal and vulval pruritis (itching).
Dosage: apply thinly 2 or 3 times daily to affected area.
Special care: use in children or on face should be limited to a maximum period of 5 days. Should be gradually withdrawn after prolonged use.
Avoid use: various skin conditions including acne, leg ulcers, scabies, viral skin disease, ringworm, tuberculosis, untreated bacterial or fungal infections. Continuous use or long-term use in pregnancy.

Side effects: thinning of skin, suppression of adrenal glands, hair growth.
Manufacturer: Cox.

COBALIN-H

Description: a preparation of vitamin B$_{12}$ produced in ampoules for injection containing 1000µg hydroxocobalamin per ml.
Used for: B$_{12}$ responsive macrocytic anaemia (a disorder of the blood characterized by reduced production of red blood cells and the presence of large, fragile red blood cells), megaloblastic anaemia, tobacco amblyopia (an eye disorder).
Dosage: for anaemias, 250–1000µg by intramuscular injection on alternate days for 1 to 2 weeks. Afterwards, 250µg once a week until normal blood count is achieved. Maintenance dose is 1000µg every 2 to 3 months.
Special care: should only be given when cause of anaemia (either lack of vitamin B$_{12}$ or of folate) has been established.
Manufacturer: Link.

CODAFEN CONTINUS

Description: a combined opiate analgesic and NSAID produced in the form of pink/white tablets containing 20mg codeine phosphate and 300mg of sustained-release ibuprofen.
Used for: relief of pain including post-operative, dental and period pain.
Dosage: adults, 2 tablets every 12 hours at first increasing to 3 tablets every 12 hours if needed. Maintenance dose is 1 to 3 tablets each 12 hours.
Special care: Pregnancy, elderly, allergy to anti-inflammatory drugs or aspirin. Those with liver or kidney disease, heart failure, hypotension, hypothyroidism, head injury, history of bronchospasm.
Avoid use: children, patients with peptic ulcer or history of peptic ulcer, respiratory depression, breathing disorders.
Possible interaction: CNS sedatives, anticoagulants taken by mouth, thiazides, MAOIs, quinolones.

Side effects: dizziness, blurring of vision, headache, gastro-intestinal upset and bleeding, peptic ulcer, drowsiness. Rarely, disturbance of liver and kidney function, thrombocytopenia, agranulocytosis (abnormal blood disorder in which there is a reduction in the number of certain white blood cells).
Manufacturer: NAPP.

CODALAX

Description: a preparation which combines a stimulant laxative and faecal softener produced in the form of a solution of 2 different strengths. It contains 200mg Poloxamer '188' and 25mg danthron per 5ml. CODALAX FORTE contains 1g Poloxamer '188' and 75mg danthron per 5ml.
Used for: treatment and prevention of constipation in terminally ill persons (which has been caused by analgesic drugs). Also, constipation in elderly persons and patients with coronary thrombosis or cardiac failure.
Dosage: adults, Codalax, 5–10ml taken at night; Codalax Forte, 5ml taken at night. Children, Codalax only, 2.5–5ml taken at night.
Special care: pregnancy, incontinence.
Avoid use: babies in nappies, patients suffering from severe painful conditions of the abdomen or intestinal blockage.
Side effects: red discoloration of urine and skin with which urine comes into contact.
Manufacturer: Napp

CODEINE PHOSPHATE

Description: an opiate analgesic preparation which additionally acts as a cough suppressant, and is available in the form of tablets and as a solution. The tablets are available in 3 strengths of 15mg, 30mg and 60mg codeine phosphate. The solution contains 25mg codeine phosphate per 5ml.
Used for: relief of mild to moderate pain.
Dosage: adults, 10–60mg every 4 hours

with a maximum dose of 200mg each day. Children, 1 to 12 years, 3mg per kg of body weight, in divided doses, each day.

Special care: elderly persons, women in labour, patients with hyperthyroidism or serious liver disease.

Avoid use: children under 1 year of age, patients with obstructive airways disease or respiratory depression.

Possible interaction: central nervous system sedatives, MAOIs.

Side effects: blurred vision, drowsiness, dry mouth, dependence and tolerance, constipation.

Manufacturer: non-proprietary.

COGENTIN

Description: an anticholinergic preparation produced as tablets and in ampoules for injection. White, scored tablets, contain 2mg benztropine mesylate and are coded MSD 60.
COGENTIN INJECTION contains 1mg per ml in 2ml ampoules.

Used for: treatment of Parkinsonism including drug-induced symptoms of tremor and involuntary muscle movements (dyskinesia).

Dosage: tablets 0.5mg each day at first increasing gradually as required by 0.5mg every 5 or 6 days. Maximum dose is 6mg daily. Children over 3 years consult manufacturer. Adults, injection (for emergency treatment), 1–2mg given intramuscularly or intravenously.

Special care: narrow angle glaucoma, tachycardia, enlarged prostate gland, gastro-intestinal blockage. Drug should be withdrawn slowly.

Avoid use: patients with movement disorder (tardive dyskinesia) or children under 3 years.

Possible interaction: antidepressants, phenothiazines, antidopaminergic drugs.

Side effects: agitation and confusion, anticholinergic effects; with higher doses, rash.

Manufacturer: MSD.

COLESTID

Description: a form of a resin which is a bile acid sequestrant acting as a lipid-lowering agent. Colestid is available as 5g yellow granules in sachets containing colestipol hydrochloride. Also,
COLESTID ORANGE granules consisting of 5g orange-flavoured powder containing colestipol hydrochloride with aspartame.

Used for: hyperlipidaemias (high fat levels in blood) particularly type IIa.

Dosage: adults, 5–30g each day in 1 or 2 divided doses taken with liquid. Children, consult manufacturer.

Special care: pregnancy, nursing mothers, additional vitamins A, D and K may be needed.

Avoid use: complete biliary blockage (total obstruction of bile duct).

Possible interaction: diuretics, digitalis, antibiotics. Any drug should be taken 1 hour before or 4 hours after Colestid as there may be intereference with absorption.

Side effects: constipation.

Manufacturer: Upjohn.

COLIFOAM

Description: a corticosteroid produced in the form of an aerosol foam containing 10% hydrocortisone acetate in mucoadherent foam.

Used for: ulcerative colitis and inflammation of the bowel.

Dosage: adults, 1 applicatorful into rectum once or twice each day for 2 or 3 weeks. Afterwards the same dosage every second day.

Special care: pregnant women, patients with severe ulcerative disease. Avoid use for prolonged periods.

Avoid use: children, patients with intestinal obstruction, abscess, perforation, peritonitis. Also, patients with recent anastomoses within the intestine, or extensive fistulas. Patients suffering from fungal or viral infectioins or tuberculosis.

Side effects: systemic corticosteroid

effects including mood changes, thinning of bones, mood swings, elevated blood sugar levels.

Manufacturer: Stafford-Miller.

COLOFAC

Description: an anticholinergic, antispasmodic preparation produced in the form of tablets and as a liquid. White, sugar-coated tablets contain 135mg mebeverine hydrochloride. Yellow banana-flavoured, sugar-free COLOFAC SUSPENSION contains mebeverine pamoate (equivalent to 50mg mebeverine hydrochloride per 5ml).

Used for: bowel spasm and gastro-intestinal spasm in irritable bowel syndrome and gastro-intestinal disorders.

Dosage: adults, 1 tablet or 15ml suspension 20 minutes before a meal 3 times each day. Children over 10 years, same as adult dose.

Avoid use: children under 10 years.

Manufacturer: Duphar.

COLOMYCIN

Description: a polymyxin antibiotic preparation produced in the form of powder in vials for reconstitution with water and injection, syrup, tablets and as powder for topical application. Colomycin powder for injection consists of 500,000 units colistin sulphomethate sodium or 1 million units colistin sulphomethate sodium in vials. COLOMYCIN SYRUP contains 250,000 units colistin sulphate per 5ml. COLOMYCIN TABLETS are quarter-scored and white containing 1.5 million units colistin sulphate and are marked with P inside a hexagon. COLOMYCIN POWDER for topical application contains 1g colistin sulphate in vial.

Used for: burns and wounds, surgery, skin infections, ENT infections, gram-negative infections, aerosol therapy.

Dosage: adults (over 60kg body weight), injection, 2 mega units every 8 hours; children 50,000 units/kg body weight each day 8-hourly. Adults, tablets, 1 to 2

8-hourly; children, syrup, up to 15kg body weight, 5–10ml; 15–30kg, 15–30ml; over 30kg same as adult. All taken 8-hourly.

Special care: patients with kidney disease, porphyria.

Avoid use: pregnancy, breastfeeding, myasthenia gravis.

Possible interaction: muscle relaxant drugs, other antibiotic drugs, anticoagulants, cytotoxics, cholinergics, diuretics, bisophonates, cyclosporin.

Side effects: paruesthesia ("pins and needles"), vertigo, muscle weakness, apnoea (temporary halt in breathing), toxic effects on kidneys. Rarely, confusion, slurred speech, psychosis, bronchospasm (on inhalation).

Manufacturer: Pharmax.

COMBANTRIN

Description: a broad-acting anti-helmintic preparation produced in the form of orange tablets containing 125mg pyrantel embonate.

Used for: to treat infestations of hookworm, roundworm, threadworm and trichostrongyliasis.

Dosage: adults and children over 6 months of age, 10mg per kg of body weight as a single dose.

Special care: patients with liver disorders.

Side effects: central nervous system effects, rash, gastro-intestinal upset.

Manufacturer: Pfizer.

COMBIDOL

Description: a bile acid preparation available in the form of white, film-coated tablets containing 125mg chenodeoxycholic acid marked COMBIDOL 60.

Used for: to dissolve small or medium sized radiolucent gallstones in patients who have slight symptoms and unimpaired gall bladder function.

Dosage: adults, 2 or 3 tablets each day (5mg per kg of body weight) either as single night time dose, or in divided

---

doses after meals with final dose taken before bedtime. If patient is 120% or more above ideal body weight, 6 tablets (7.5mg per kg of body weight) should be taken daily.
Avoid use: children, pregnancy, breast-feeding, women who are not using contraception, patients with non-functioning or impaired gall bladder, those with inflammatory diseases of colon and small intestine, peptic ulcer, chronic liver disease.
Possible interaction: bile acid sequestrants, antacids, oestrogens, oral contraceptives, other drugs which influence cholesterol levels.
Side effects: minor effects on liver and a rise in serum levels of transaminases (enzymes), diarrhoea, pruritis (itching), gallstones may become opaque.
Manufacturer: CP Pharmaceuticals.

CONCORDIN
Description: a TCAD preparation available as pink film-coated tablets containing 5mg protryptyline hydrochloride and marked MSD 26, and white, film-coated tablets contain 10mg and marked MSD 47.
Used for: depression.
Dosage: adults, 15–60mg each day in divided doses. Reduced dose of 5mg 3 times each day in elderly persons.
Special care: breastfeeding, liver or kidney disease, epilepsy, heart and circulatory diseases, diabetes, hyperthyroidism, tumours of adrenal gland, retention of urine, glaucoma. Also, certain psychiatric conditions, suicidal tendencies and psychoses.
Avoid use: pregnant women, children, patients with serious liver disease, heart atack or heart block.
Possible interaction: alcohol, barbiturates, other antidepressant drugs, antihypertensives, cimetidine, oestrogens, local anaesthetics containing adrenaline or noradrenaline, anticholinergic drugs.
Side effects: nervousness, drowsiness,

dizziness, sweating, tremor, weariness, gastro-intestinal upset, insomnia, hypotension. Anticholinergic effects including constipation, urine retention, blurring of vision, dry mouth. Allergic skin rashes, blood changes, jaundice, heart arrhythmias, weight gain or loss, changes in libido, enlargement of breasts, production of milk, blood sugar changes. Mania and schizophrenic symptoms may be activated, especially in elderly persons.
Manufacturer: MSD.

CONDYLINE
Description: a preparation available in the form of a solution with applicators containing 0.5% podophyllotoxin in alcoholic base.
Used for: genital warts.
Dosage: adults, apply solution twice each day for 3 days directly on to warts. Repeat at 4 day intervals if required for maximum of 5 weeks.
Avoid use: children, open wounds.
Side effects: irritation at site of application.
Manufacturer: Yamanouchi.

CONOVA 30
Description: a combined oestrogen/progestogen oral contraceptive produced in the form of white film-coated tablets containing 30μg of ethinyloestradiol and 2mg ethynodiol diacetate, marked with the maker's name and 930.
Used for: oral contraception.
Dosage: 1 daily for 21 days starting on fifth day of period followed by 7 tablet-free days.
Special care: patients with asthma, varicose veins, hypertension, diabetes, severe kidney disease or kidney dialysis, Raynaud's disease, hyperprolactinaemia (elevated levels of the hormone, prolactin, in the blood), depressive illness. Blood pressure should be checked and pelvic organs and breasts examined regularly before and during the period the drug is being taken. Risk

of thrombosis increases with age, smoking and obesity.

Avoid use: pregnant women, patients with heart or circulatory disease, heart valve disease, history of or at risk of thrombosis, hypertension, hormone-dependent cancers. Also, those with various liver diseases and disorders including liver tumour (adenoma), porphyria, Dublin-Johnson syndrome and Rotor syndrome, abnormal liver function tests. Patients with recent trophoblastic disease, chorea, sickle cell anaemia, undiagnosed vaginal bleeding, ostosclerosis.

Possible interaction: barbiturates, tetracyclines, rifampicin, phenytoin, griseofulvin, carbamazepine, chloral hydrate, glutethimide, ethosuximide dichloralphenazone.

Side effects: cervical erosion and vaginal discharge, pains and leg cramps, loss of libido, feeling of bloatedness due to fluid retention, weight gain, enlargement of breasts, depression, nausea, headaches, breakthrough bleeding.

Manufacturer: Gold Cross.

CONVULEX

Description: an anticonvulsant carboxylic acid preparation produced in the form of soft enteric-coated gelatin capsules of 3 different strengths containing 150mg, 300mg and 500mg of valproic acid.

Used for: epilepsy.

Dosage: adults and children, 15mg per kg of body weight at first in divided doses, gradually increasing by 5–10mg/kg body weight each day as required.

Special care: pregnant women, coagulation tests and liver function tests should be carried out before starting therapy or increasing dose and also at 2-monthly intervals. Urine tests give false positives for ketones.

Avoid use: patients with liver disease.

Possible interaction: alcohol, barbiturates, antidepressants, other antiepileptic drugs, anticoagulants, neuroleptic drugs.

Side effects: gastro-intestinal upset, central nervous system effects, toxic effects on liver coagulation. Rarely, there may be short-lived hair loss, pancreatitis.

Manufacturer: Pharmacia.

CORACTEN

Description: an antianginal and antihypertensive preparation which is a class II calcium antagonist available as sustained-release capsules of 2 different strengths. Grey/pink capsules contain 10mg nifedipine and pink/brown capsules contain 20mg nifedipine. Both are marked with the strength and name.

Used for: prevention of angina, hypertension.

Dosage: adults, 20mg every 12 hours, adjusted according to response within the range of 10–40mg each 12 hours.

Special care: patients with weak hearts, diabetes, liver disease, hypotension, hypovolaemia (abnormally low volume of circulating blood).

Avoid use: children, pregnant women, patients with cardiogenic (heart) shock.

Possible interaction: cimetidine, quinidine, antihypertensive drugs.

Side effects: flushing, headache, dizziness, oedema, lethargy, nausea, rash, pain in eyes, frequency of urination, gum hyperplasia (increase in number of cells); rarely, allergic-type jaundice.

Manufacturer: Evans.

CORDARONE X

Description: a proprietary class III antiarrhythmic preparation produced in the form of tablets of 2 different strengths. White, scored tablets, marked with strength and action potential symbol contain 100mg or 200mg of amiodarone hydrochloride. Also, **CORDARONE X** intravenous injection comprising 50mg per ml of solution in ampoules for injection.

Used for: various heart rhythm disorders especially those which do not respond to other drugs. Tachycardia associated with

Wolfe-Parkinson-White syndrome.
Dosage: adults, 200mg 3 times each day for first week then 200mg twice each day for the following week. Maintenance dose is usually in the order of 200mg each day and the minimum necessary should be used. Children, manufacturer should be consulted.
Special care: pregnancy, heart failure, elderly, liver or kidney disease, enlargement of prostate gland, glaucoma, sensitivity to iodine. Liver, kidney and thyroid function should be tested throughout the course of treatment. Eyes should also be monitored and therapy started under hospital supervision.
Avoid use: breastfeeding, patients with heart block, shock, history of thyroid disease, serious bradycardia.
Possible interaction: other antiarrhythmic drugs, ß-blockers, diuretics, digoxin, phenytoin, calcium antagonists, anticoagulants taken by mouth, anaesthetics.
Side effects: micro-deposits on cornea of eyes, sensitivity to light, effects on eyes, heart, thyroid, liver and nervous system, pulmonary fibrosis or alveolitis (inflammation of alveoli of lungs).
Manufacturer: Sanofi Winthrop.

CORDILOX

Description: an antihypertensive and antiarrhythmic preparation which is a class I calcium antagonist produced as tablets of 3 different strengths and as a solution for intravenous injection. Yellow, film-coated tablets, marked with the name and strength, contain 40mg, 80mg and 120mg of verapamil hydrochloride. **CORDILOX INTRA-VENOUS** contains 2.5mg verapamil hydrochloride per ml in ampoules for injection.
Used for: supraventricular heart arrhythmias, hypertension, angina.
Dosage: adults, heart arrhythmias, 40–120mg 3 times each day; children under 2 years, 20mg 2 or 3 times daily; over 2 years, 40–120mg 2 or 3 times each day. Adults, hypertension, 240–480mg each

day in 2 to 3 divided doses. Adults, angina, 8–120mg 3 times each day.
Special care: patients with weak heart should take digitalis and diuretics; persons with first degree heart block, kidney or liver disease, heart attack, heart conduction disorders, bradycardia, hypotension.
Avoid use: severe bradycardia, second or third degree heart block, heart failure, heart shock, sick sinus syndrome.
Possible interaction: ß-blockers, digoxin, quinidine.
Side effects: flushes and constipation.
Manufacturer: Baker Norton.

CORGUARD

Description: an antihypertensive, non-cardioselective ß-blocker produced in the form of pale blue tablets of 2 different strengths containing either 40 or 80mg of nadolol and marked SQUIBB 207 or SQUIBB 241 respectively.
Used for: heart arrythmias, angina, hypertension, additional therapy in thyroid gland disease (thyrotoxicosis), prevention of migraine.
Dosage: heart arrhythmias, 40mg each day at first increasing as required to maximum of 160mg; angina, 40mg each day at first increasing as required with usual daily dose in the order of 40–240mg; hypotension, 80mg each day at first increasing as needed with usual daily dose in the order of 80–240mg; thyrotoxicosis, 80–160mg once each day; prevention of migraine, 40mg each day at first increasing if necessary to a usual daily dose in the order of 80–160mg.
Special care: pregnancy, breastfeeding, patients with weak hearts should receive diuretics and digitalis, liver or kidney disease, diabetes, metabolic acidosis. Persons undergoing general anaesthesia may need to be withdrawn before planned surgery. Withdraw drug gradually.
Avoid use: children, patients with obstructive airways disease or history of bronchospasm (asthma), various heart

disorders including heart block, heart shock, heart failure, sick sinus syndrome, serious peripheral arterial disease, sinus bradycardia.
Possible interaction: cardiac depressant anaesthetics, antihypertensives, ergotamine, sympathomimetics, verapamil, clonidine withdrawal, CNS depressants, class I antiarrhythmic drugs, cimetidine, reserpine, indomethacin, hypoglycaemics.
Side effects: bradycardia, fatigue on exercise, cold hands and feet, disturbance of sleep, gastro-intestinal upset, bronchospasm, heart failure. Withdraw drug gradually if dry eyes or skin rash occur.
Manufacturer: Sanofi Winthrop.

CORGARETIC 40

Description: a combined antihypertensive, non-cardioselective ß-blocker and thiazide diuretic produced in the form of white, mottled, scored tablets, marked SQUIBB 283, and containing 40mg nadolol and 5mg bendrofluazide. Also, **CORGARETIC 80**, white, mottled, scored tablets marked SQUIBB 284, and containing 80mg nadolol and 5mg bendrofluazide.
Used for: hypertension.
Dosage: adults, 1 to 2 tablets a day (Corgaretic 40), increasing if required to a maximum dose of 2 Corgaretic 80 tablets.
Special care: pregnancy, breastfeeding, weak hearts (should receive digitalis and diuretics), liver or kidney disease, diabetes, metabolic acidosis, gout. Persons undergoing general anaesthesia, may require to be withdrawn before planned surgery. Electrolyte levels should be monitored.
Avoid use: children, patients with obstructive airways disease or history of bronchospasm (asthma), various heart disorders including heart block, heart shock, heart failure, sick sinus syndrome, serious peripheral arterial disease, sinus bradycardia. Severe or progressive kidney failure, anuria.

Possible interaction: cardiac depressant anaesthetics, antihypertensives, ergotamine, sympathomimetics, verapamil, clonidine withdrawal, central nervous system depressants, class I antiarrhythmic drugs, cimetidine, reserpine, indomethacin, hypoglycaemics, lithium, digitalis.
Side effects: bradycardia, fatigue on exercise, cold hands and feet, disturbance of sleep, gastro-intestinal upset, bronchospasm, heart failure, blood changes, sensitivity to light, gout. Withdraw drug gradually if skin rash or dry eyes occur.
Manufacturer: Sanofi Winthrop.

CORLAN

Description: a corticosteroid available as pellets marked CORLAN and GLAXO containing 2.5mg of hydrocortisone (as sodium succinate).
Used for: mouth ulcers.
Dosage: a pellet held in mouth in contact with ulcer and allowed to dissolve.
Special care: pregnant women.
Avoid use: patients with untreated mouth infections.
Manufacturer: Evans.

CORTISTAB

Description: a glucocorticoid-mineralocorticoid (corticosteroid) preparation (corticosteroid hormones are produced by the cortex region of the adrenal glands) available as white, scored tablets containing either 5mg or 25mg of cortisone acetate.
Used for: inflammatory and allergic disorders, rheumatic conditions and collagen diseases, hormonal replacement therapy when adrenal glands have been removed.
Dosage: adults, 12.5–50mg each day, children 5–25mg each day in divided doses.
Special care: pregnancy, liver cirrhosis, glaucoma, epilepsy, diabetes, hypertension, acute glomerulonephritis (inflammation of part of the kidney

tubules), peptic ulcer, active infections, tuberculosis, fungal and viral infections. Patients with osteoporosis, recent intestinal anastomoses, thrombophlebitis, nephritis, secondary cancers, infectious diseases which cause skin spots or rash. Patients should avoid contact with chicken pox or *Herpes zoster* virus while receiving therapy and for 3 months after treatment. In the event of contact or contracting chicken pox, further specialist treatment should be given. Withdraw drug gradually.
Possible interaction: hypoglycaemics, NSAIDs, anticoagulants taken by mouth, anticholinesterases, diuretics, cardiac glycosides, ephedrine, phenytoin, rifampicin, phenobarbitone.
Side effects: hypertension, skin changes, fluid retention, hyperglycaemia, loss of potassium, osteoporosis, peptic ulcer, mood changes—euphoria and depression.
Manufacturer: Boots.

CORTISYL
Description: a glucocorticoid-mineralocorticoid (corticosteroid) preparation produced in the form of white, scored tablets containing 25mg of cortisone acetate.
Used for: replacement therapy following removal of adrenal glands and in Addison's disease (a failure of the cortex of the adrenal glands to produce their hormones).
Dosage: adults, acute attacks, up to 300mg each day with usual maintenance in the order of 12.5mg to 37.5mg daily.
Special care: pregnancy, liver cirrhosis, glaucoma, epilepsy, diabetes, hypertension, acute glomerulonephritis (inflammation of part of the kidney tubules), peptic ulcer, active infections, tuberculosis, fungal and viral infections. Patients with osteoporosis, recent intestinal anastomoses, thrombophlebitis, nephritis, secondary cancers, infectious diseases which cause skin spots or rash. Patients should avoid

contact with chicken pox or *Herpes zoster* virus while receiving therapy and for 3 months after treatment. In the event of contact or contracting chicken pox, further specialist treatment should be given. Withdraw drug gradually.
Avoid use: children.
Possible interaction: hypoglycaemics, NSAIDs, anticoagulants taken by mouth, anticholinesterases, diuretics, cardiac glycosides, ephedrine, phenytoin, rifampicin, phenobarbitone.
Side effects: hypertension, skin changes, fluid retention, hyperglycaemia, loss of potassium, osteoporosis, peptic ulcer, mood changes—euphoria and depression.
Manufacturer: Roussel.

CORWIN
Description: a sympathomimetic heart muscle stimulant which is a partial ß₁-agonist, produced in the form of yellow, film-coated tablets containing 200mg of xamoterol (as fumerate) marked with symbol and CORWIN.
Used for: chronic mild heart failure.
Dosage: adults, start treatment in hsopital with 1 tablet daily in first instance, increasing to 1 tablet twice daily if there is a favourable response.
Special care: withdraw drug if there is a deterioration in the progress of the disease. Patients with obstructive airways disease, disease of heart muscle and a heart valve (aortic stenosis), kidney disease.
Avoid use: children, pregnancy, breastfeeding, more severe forms of heart failure, fatigue when resting and breathlessness, hypotension, tachycardia. Patients with fluid in lungs (pulmonary oedema) or other fluid retention. Those needing ACE inhibitor drugs or taking higher doses of loop diuretics (equivalent to 40mg frusemide).
Side effects: muscle cramps, rash, gastro-intestinal upset, headache, dizziness, palpitations.
Manufacturer: Stuart.

COSMEGEN LYOVAC

Description: a cytotoxic antibiotic drug produced in the form of a powder in vials for reconstitution and injection, containing 0.5mg actinomycin D.
Used for: cancers in children e.g. leukaemia.
Dosage: fast running intravenous infusion at 3 week intervals or as directed by cancer specialist.
Side effects: leakage at injection site causes severe tissue death and damage, vomiting, nausea, baldness, suppression of bone marrow, inflammation of mucous membranes, e.g. in nose and throat.
Manufacturer: M.S.D.

COVERSYL

Description: an antihypertensive preparation which is an ACE inhibitor and is produced as tablets of 2 different strengths. White tablets contain 2mg perindopril tert-butylamine and white, scored oblong tablets contain 4mg.
Used for: additional therapy with digitalis and/or diuretics in congestive heart failure, hypertension.
Dosage: adults, heart failure, treatment should start in hospital under close supervision with 2mg once daily taken in the morning increasing to 4mg once each day. Any diuretic should be withdrawn 3 days before the start of treatment. Hypertension, 2mg once each day before food increasing to daily maintenance dose of 4mg (8mg a day is maximum dose). Elderly persons should take a reduced dose of 2mg each day under close medical supervision. Any diuretic should be withdrawn 3 days before start of treatment.
Special care: patients with kidney disorders or receiving dialysis. Kidney function should be monitored before and during treatment; patients undergoing anaesthesia and surgery.
Avoid use: children, pregnancy, breast-feeding.
Possible interaction: antidepressants, other antihypertensives, lithium, potassium supplements, potassium-sparing diuretics.
Side effects: hypotension, skin rashes and itching, flushing, loss of sense of taste, oedema, headache, malaise, fatigue, nausea, pain in abdomen, weakness, slight cough, blood changes, protein in urine.
Manufacturer: Servier.

CROMOGEN

Description: an anti-inflammatory, non-steroidal, bronchodilator produced in the form of an aerosol for inhalation containing 5mg of sodium cromoglycate per metered dose aerosol. Also, CROMOGEN STERI-NEB, a preservative-free solution containing 10mg sodium cromoglycate per ml, available as a single dose for use with nebuliser.
Used for: prevention of asthma.
Dosage: adults and children, 2 puffs 4 times each day in first instance with a maintenance dose of 1 puff 4 times daily. Cromogen Steri-Neb, 20mg with power-operated nebuliser 4 times each day at 3 to 6 hourly intervals. If necessary frequency can be increased to 5 or 6 times each day and, to be effective, therapy must be continuous.
Side effects: irritation of throat and short-lived cough (due to inhalation of powder). Rarely, short-lived bronchospasm.
Manufacturer: Baker-Norton.

CRYSTAPEN

Description: a preparation of benzylpenicillin or penicillin G, an antibiotic which is inactivated by the penicillinase enzymes produced by certain bacteria. It is inactivated by stomach (gastric) juices and poorly absorbed from the gut and hence is produced as a solution for intravenous or intramuscular injection. Crystapen 600mg benzylpenicillin sodium (unbuffered) as powder in vials for reconstitution and injection.

Used for: gonorrhoea, septicaemia, endocarditis, osteomyelitis, meningitis, respiratory tract, ear, nose and throat, skin and soft tissue infections.
Dosage: adults, 600–1200mg by intravenous or intramuscular injection each day in 2, 3 or 4 divided doses. (For meningitis, up to 14.4g daily in divided doses may be needed). Children, newborns, 30mg per kg of body weight in 2, 3 or 4 divided doses; 1 month to 12 years, 10–20mg per kg each day in 2, 3 or 4 divided doses. For meningitis, age 1 week and under, 60–90mg per kg, in 2 divided doses; 1 week to 1 month, 90–120mg per kg each day in 3 divided doses; 1 month to 12 years, 150–300mg per kg each day in 4, 5 or 6 divided doses. All doses are delivered by intravenous or intramuscular injection.
Special care: history of penicillin allergy or kidney disease.
Avoid use: allergy to penicillin.
Side effects: allergic responses including rash, joint pains, fever, blood changes and anaphylactic shock in hypersensitive persons.
Manufacturer: Britannia.

CYCLIMORPH^{CD}

Description: a strong analgesic preparation which combines an opiate with an anti-emetic and is available as solutions of 2 different strengths in 1ml ampoules for injection. Cyclimorph 10 contains 10mg morphine tartrate and 50mg cyclizine tartrate per ml; CYCLIMORPH 15 contains 15mg morphine tartrate and 50mg cyclizine tartrate per ml.
Used for: acute and chronic intractable pain.
Dosage: adults, Cyclimorph 10, 1ml by subcutaneous, intravenous or intramuscular injection which can be repeated after 4 hours but maximum dose is 3ml in 24 hours. Children, age 1 to 5 years, 0.25–0.5ml as 1 single dose; 6 to 12 years, 0.5–1ml as 1 single dose. Adults, Cyclimorph 15, 1ml by subcutaneous,

intravenous or intramuscular injection which may be repeated after 4 hours but maximum dose is 3ml in 24 hours.
Special care: women in labour, elderly, liver disease or hypothyroidism.
Avoid use: children under 1 year, patients with blocked airways or respiratory depression.
Possible interaction: central nervous system sedatives, MAOIs.
Side effects: drug dependence and tolerance may develop and Chief Medical Officer should be notified in cases of addiction. Rash, constipation, dizziness, nausea.
Manufacturer: Wellcome.

CYCLO-PROGYNOVA

Description: a combined oestrogen/progestogen hormonal preparation available as tablets in 2 different strengths. Cyclo-Progynova 1mg consists of a course of sugar-coated tablets; 11 beige ones contain 1mg oestradiol valerate and 10 brown ones contain 1mg oestradiol valerate and 0.25mg levonorgestrel.
CYCYLO-PROGYNOVA 2mg consist of a course of sugar-coated tablets; 11 white ones contain 2mg oestradiol valerate and 10 brown ones contain 2mg oestradiol valerate and 0.5mg norgestrel (= 0.25mg levonorgestrel).
Used for: menopausal symptoms including the prevention of osteoporosis.
Dosage: 1 oestradiol tablet each day for 11 days (beginning on fifth day of period, if present), followed by 1 combined oestradiol/levonorgestrel tablet for 10 days. Then there are 7 tablet-free days before course is repeated. The lower strength preparation should be tried first.
Special care: women at any risk of thrombosis and those with liver disease. Liver function should be monitored every 2 to 3 months during treatment. Patients with diabetes, porphyria, migraine, epilepsy, hypertension, fibroids in the uterus, multiple sclerosis

ostosclerosis, gallstones, tetany. These persons should be closely monitored. Also, women with a family history of breast cancer or fibrocystic disease of the breast should be carefully monitored. Breasts and pelvic organs should be examined and blood pressure checked regularly before and during the period of treatment.

Avoid use: pregnancy, breastfeeding, endometriosis, undiagnosed vaginal bleeding, hormone-dependent cancers, breast cancer, serious heart, liver or kidney disease, thromboembolism. Also, women with kidney, liver or heart disease and Rotor or Dublin-Johnson syndromes. Drug should be stopped 6 weeks before planned surgery and during any condition which makes thrombosis more likely.

Possible interaction: drugs which induce liver enzymes.

Side effects: breakthrough bleeding, weight gain, tenderness in breasts, gastro-intestinal upset, dizziness, nausea, headache, vomiting. Drug should be stopped immediately in the event of frequent severe headaches, migraine, disturbance of vision, thromboembolism or thrombophlebitis, jaundice or sudden blood pressure rise, pregnancy.

Manufacturer: Schering HC.

CYCLOCAPS

Description: an anti-inflammatory, bronchodilator which is a selective ß₂-agonist produced as a powder in capsules of 2 strengths for inhalation by means of a cyclohaler. Clear/light green capsules, marked with Greek letters and 935, contain 200µg salbutamol (as sulphate). Clear/dark green capsules marked with Greek letters and 945, contain 400µg.

Used for: treatment and prevention of asthma.

Dosage: acute attack, 200 or 400µg as a single dose. Prevention, 400µg as a single dose repeated 3 to 4 times each day. Children, acute attack, 200µg as a single

dose. Prevention, 200µg as a single dose repeated 3 or 4 times each day.

Special care: pregnancy, hypertension, angina, weak hearts, heart arrhythmias, hyperthyroidism.

Possible interaction: sympathomimetics.

Side effects: headache, tremor in muscles, dilation of blood vessels in skin.

Manufacturer: DuPont

CYCLOGEST

Description: a hormonal preparation in the form of suppositories containing either 200mg or 400mg of progesterone.

Used for: premenstrual syndrome, depression following childbirth (but effectiveness is controversial and subject to debate).

Dosage: adults, 200 or 400mg via rectum or vagina once or twice each day from the twelfth or fourteenth day of monthly cycle until period begins.

Special care: use rectally if barrier contraceptives are being used or if patient has thrush infection. Breastfeeding mothers and women with liver, kidney, heart disease, diabetes, hypertension.

Avoid use: women with abnormal and undiagnosed vaginal bleeding or who have a history of, or are at risk from, thromboembolic disorders. Also, those suffering from breast cancer, porphyria, serious arterial disease.

Possible interaction: cyclosporins.

Side effects: gastro-intestinal upset, weight changes, breast tenderness, change in libido, alteration in menstrual cycle, rash, acne.

Manufacturer: Hoechst.

CYKLOKAPRON

Description: an antifibrinolytic preparation produced in the form of tablets, syrup and as a solution for injection. White, oblong, film-coated scored tablets, marked C-Y, contain 500mg tranexamic acid. **CYKLOKAPRON SYRUP** contains 500mg tranexamic acid per 5ml; also

CYKLOKAPRON INJECTION

contains 100mg tranexamic acid per ml in ampoules for injection.

Used for: local or general fibrinolytic disorders, i.e. those characterized by haemorrhage; menorrhagia (abnormally heavy menstrual bleeding or prolonged periods).

Dosage: local fibrinolysis, 15–25mg per kg of body weight 2 or 3 times each day. (For more general fibrinolytic states, as directed by physician). Children, 25mg per kg of body weight 2 or 3 times each day. Adults, menorrhagia, 1 to 1$^1/_2$g 3 or 4 times each day for up to 4 days.

Special care: patients with kidney disorders, haematuria (blood in urine), especially associated with haemophilia. Patients suffering from angioneurotic oedema require eye and liver function tests during the course of long-term treatment.

Avoid use: history of thrombosis.

Side effects: gastro-intestinal upset. If disturbance in colour vision occurs, drug should be withdrawn.

Manufacturer: Pharmacia.

CYMEVENE

Description: an antiviral preparation available as a powder in vials for reconstitution and injection containing 500mg ganciclovir.

Used for: life-threatening viral infections or those which threaten sight, caused by cytomegalovirus in patients with reduced immunity.

Dosage: adults and children, 5mg per kg of body weight given by intravenous infusion over 1-hour period every 12 hours for a period of 14 to 21 days. 6mg per kg of body weight may be required for patients who have sight-threatening infection.

Special care: polythene gloves and safety glasses must be worn while handing the preparation and accidental splashes on skin should be washed off immediately with soap and water. Regular blood counts required due to toxic effects on blood; potential carcinogen. Patients with kidney disease. Should be administered carefully into veins with good bloodflow and patient's fluid level should be maintained after infusion.

Avoid use: pregnant women, lactating mothers should not breastfeed until 72 hours have elapsed since last dose, allergy to ganciclovir or acyclovir. Patients with abnormally low neutrophil (a type of white blood cell) counts.

Possible interaction: other antiviral drugs, zidovudine.

Side effects: effects on blood including anaemia and severe reduction in levels of white blood cells, elevated levels of serum creatinine and blood urea nitrogen. Effects on all body systems and functions, fever, rash, malaise.

Manufacturer: Syntex.

CYPROSTAT

Description: an anti-androgen preparation used to treat prostate cancer, a type which is hormone-dependent and develops under the influence of the male sex hormone, androgen. The drug blocks androgens produced by the adrenal glands and testes. Cyprostat is available in the form of tablets of 2 strengths; white scored tablets, marked BV within a hexagon, contain 50mg cyproterone acetate. White scored tablets, marked LA within a hexagon, contain 100mg cyproterone acetate.

Used for: cancer of the prostate.

Dosage: 300mg each day in 2 or 3 divided doses after food.

Special care: diabetes, liver disease, history of thrombosis, severe depression.

Side effects: weariness, infertility, liver disorders, breast enlargement, anaemia.

Manufacturer: Schering HC.

CYSTRIN

Description: an anticholinergic and antispasmodic preparation available as white tablets containing 3mg oxybutynin hydrochloride and white scored tablets,

marked L11, containing 5mg oxybutynin hydrochloride.
Used for: incontinence, urgency and frequency of urination and night-time bedwetting in children.
Dosage: 5mg 2 or 3 times each day (with a maximum daily dose of 20mg), in divided doses. Elderly persons, 3mg twice each day adjusted according to response. Children, 5 years and over, 3mg twice each day in first instance, adjusted according to response to usual dose in the order of 5mg 2 or 3 times daily. For night-time bedwetting, last dose should be taken at bedtime.
Special care: pregnant women, disease of the autonomic nervous system, liver or kidney disease, heart arrhythmias, heart failure, enlarged prostate, tachycardia, hyperthyroidism, hiatus hernia.
Avoid use: breastfeeding, blocked gastro-intestinal tract or bladder, other intestinal diseases, glaucoma, myasthenia gravis, severe ulcerative colitis.
Possible interaction: other anticholinergics, TCADs, digoxin, levodopa, amantadine, phenothiazines, butyrophenones.
Side effects: facial flushing, anticholinergic effects.

CYTAMEN

Description: a proprietary vitamin B$_{12}$ preparation produced as a solution in 1ml ampoules for injection containing 1000µg cyanocobalamin per ml.
Used for: vitamin B$_{12}$ responsive macrocytic anaemias (characterized by the presence of fragile enlarged red blood cells), megaloblastic anaemia.
Dosage: adults and children, 250–1000µg by intramuscular injection every other day for 1 or 2 weeks and then 250µg once a week until normal blood count is achieved. Usual maintenance dose is 1000µg each month.
Possible interaction: oral contraceptives, chloramphenicol.
Side effects: rarely, allergic reactions.
Manufacturer: Evans

CYTOSAR

Description: a powerful cytotoxic antimetabolite produced as a powder in vials for reconstitution and injection, containing 100mg or 500mg cytarabine.
Used for: to induce remission in acute myeloblastic anaemia.
Dosage: given subcutaneously or intravenously, as directed by physician skilled in cancer chemotherapy.
Special care: requires careful monitoring of blood counts.
Side effects: severe myelosuppression (bone marrow suppression), loss of hair, nausea and vomiting; early menopause in women and sterility in men if therapy is prolonged, local tissue death if there is leakage at the injection site.
Manufacturer: Upjohn.

CYTOTEC

Description: a synthetic form of prostaglandin (a naturally occurring hormone-like substance present in many body tissues) which inhibits the secretion of gastric juice and promotes the healing of ulcers. It is produced in the form of white, hexagonal tablets, containing 200µg misoprostol, and marked SEARLE 1461.
Used for: stomach and duodenal ulcers, ulceration caused by NSAIDs, prevention of NSAID ulceration.
Dosage: adults, 4 tablets each day with meals, in divided doses, with last taken at bedtime for 1 to 2 months. Prevention of ulcers, 1 tablet 2, 3 or 4 times each day during the period that NSAID is being taken.
Special care: women should use effective contraception, patients with circulatory diseases including peripheral or coronary vascular disease and cerebrovascular disease.
Avoid use: children, pregnancy, women planning pregnancy, breastfeeding.
Side effects: gastro-intestinal upset, diarrhoea, pain in abdomen, vaginal bleeding and disturbance of menstrual cycle, dizziness, rash.
Manufacturer: Searle.

DAKTACORT

Description: an antifungal/antibacterial agent with mild steroid, comprising miconazole nitrate (2%) and hydrocortisone (1%). Available as cream and ointment.
Used for: fungal and bacterial (Gram-positive) infections where there is associated inflammation.
Dosage: to be applied 2 or 3 times daily.
Special care: use on face or for children should be limited to 5 days maximum. Withdraw gradually after prolonged use.
Avoid use: on acne, leg ulcers, tuberculous, ringworm or viral skin disease, peri-oral dermatitis, untreated infections whether fungal or bacterial. Extensive or prolonged use during pregnancy.
Side effects: skin atrophy, striae and telangiectasia (permanent widening of superficial blood vessels), suppression of adrenal glands, Cushingoid changes (see Cushing's syndrome).
Manufacturer: Janssen.

DALACIN CREAM

Description: an antibacterial cream (clindamycin phosphate) available as a 2% cream.
Used for: bacterial vaginosis.
Dosage: 1 applicatorful intravaginally each night for 7 days.
Special care: less effectiveness from barrier contraceptives.
Avoid use: in cases of lincomycin sensitivity.
Side effects: vaginal irritation, gastro-intestinal upset. Discontinue with colitis or diarrhoea.
Manufacturer: Upjohn.

DALACIN C

Description: a lincosamide, clindamycin hydrochloride as 75mg (lavender) and 150mg maroon/lavender capsules. Also **DALACIN PAEDIATRIC**, clindamycin palmitate, containing 75mg per 5ml available as 100mg powder.
Used for: serious infections sensitive to clindamycin.
Dosage: 150–450mg every 6 hours. Children under 12 months, 2.5ml every 6 or 8 hours; 1 to 3 years, 2.5–5ml; 4 to 7 years, 5–7.5ml; 8 to 12 years, 7.5–10ml, all every 6 hours.
Also **DALACIN PHOSPHATE**, available as ampoules, 150mg/ml, of clindamycin phosphate.
Dosage: 600mg–2.7g in divided doses each day, by intramuscular injection or intravenous infusion. Children over 1 month, 15–40mg/kg daily in divided doses.
Special care: kidney or liver disease, cease use should colitis or diarrhoea occur.
Avoid use: in cases of lincomycin sensitivity.
Possible interaction: neuromuscular blocking agents.
Side effects: jaundice and blood disorders, gastro-intestinal upsets.
Manufacturer: Upjohn.

DALACIN T

Description: antibiotic clindomycin phosphate in a 10mg/ml solution. Also, **DALACIN T LOTION** available as an aqueous solution in a roll-on bottle.
Used for: moderate to severe acne vulgaris.
Dosage: apply twice daily.
Special care: avoid eyes and mucous membranes.
Avoid use: in cases of lincomycin sensitivity.
Possible interaction: keratolytics (applies to the solution).
Side effects: dermatitis, dry skin, folliculitis (solution). Discontinue should colitis or diarrhoea occur.
Manufacturer: Upjohn.

DALMANE

Description: a long-acting benzodiazepine (hypnotic) prepared as flurazepam hydrochloride in strengths of 15mg (grey/yellow capsules) and 30mg (black/grey capsules) marked with ROCHE and strength.

Used for: short-term treatment of severe or disabling insomnia.

Dosage: 15–30mg at bedtime (elderly, 15mg).

Special care: chronic liver, kidney or lung disease, the elderly. Also during pregnancy, labour or lactation. To be withdrawn gradually. May impair judgement.

Avoid use: acute lung disease, depression of the respiration, obsessional states, chronic psychosis. Not for children.

Possible interaction: anticonvulsants, CNS depressants, alcohol.

Side effects: confusion, vertigo, drowsiness, ataxia, light-headedness, gastro-intestinal upsets, skin rashes, hypotension, disturbance in vision. Urine retention, changes in libido. Dependence is possible.

Manufacturer: Roche.

DANOL

Description: a gonadotrophin release inhibitor, danazol, available in capsules of 100mg (white/grey) and 200mg (white/pink), marked with name and strength.

Used for: menorrhagia (long or heavy menstruation).

Dosage: 200mg daily for 3 months starting on the first day of menstruation.

Also used for: endometriosis and as a pre-operative preparation for endometrial ablation.

Dosage: 400mg daily for 6 to 9 months. 400–800mg daily for 3 to 6 weeks before ablation.

Also used for: severe mastalgia, benign breast cysts, gynaecomastia.

Dosage: 200–400mg daily for up to 6 months depending upon the condition.

Special care: migraine, epilepsy, hypertension, other cardiovascular diseases, diabetes, polycythaemia (increase in

blood erythrocytes), conditions adversely affected by fluid retention.

Avoid use: pregnancy, lactation, porphyria, severe kidney, heart or liver disease, vaginal bleeding, androgen-dependent tumour, thromboembolic disease.

Possible interaction: steroids, anticonvulsants, anticoagulants, cyclosporin, antihypertensives, hypoglycaemics.

Side effects: backache, flushes, muscle spasms, nausea, rashes, male hormone effects, fluid retention, menstrual disturbances, headache, emotional disturbance, cholestatic jaundice (due to blockage of bile flow through any part of the biliary system).

Manufacturer: Sanofi Winthrop.

DANTRIUM

Description: a muscle relaxant, dantrolene sodium, available in capsules (orange with light brown cap) of strength 25mg and 100mg, marked 0030 and 0033 respectively.

Used for: severe or chronic spasticity of skeletal muscle.

Dosage: 25mg daily to start, increasing to a maximum of 100mg 4 times per day.

Special care: lung or heart disease, pregnancy. Liver to be checked before and 6 weeks after the start of treatment.

Avoid use: liver disease, where spasticity is useful for movement.

Possible interaction: CNS depressants, alcohol.

Side effects: diarrhoea, drowsiness, weakness, fatigue.

Manufacturer: Procter & Gamble Pharmaceuticals.

DAONIL

Description: a sulphonylurea, glibenclamide, available as white oblong tablets (5mg) marked LDI with symbol. Also **SEMI-DAONIL** (2.5mg white tablet).

Used for: maturity-onset diabetes (non-insulin-dependent diabetes mellitus).

Dosage: 5mg daily at breakfast increasing by 2.5–5mg weekly to a maximum of 15mg.

Special care: kidney failure, the elderly.
Avoid use: juvenile, growth-onset or unstable brittle diabetes (all now called insulin-dependent diabetes mellitus), severe liver or kidney disease, ketoacidosis, stress, infections, surgery, endocrine disorders. Pregnancy or lactation.
Possible interaction: MAOIs, corticosteroids, corticotrophin, oral contraceptives, alcohol, ß-blockers. Also glucagon, chloramphenicol, rifampicin, sulphonamides, aspirin, phenylbutazone, cyclophosphamide, oral anticoagulants, clofibrate, benzafibrate.
Side effects: sensitivity including skin rash.
Manufacturer: Hoechst.

DARANIDE

Description: a preparation of dichlor-phenamide in yellow tablet form (50mg, marked MSD 49) which is a weak diuretic, reducing fluid in the aqueous humour of the eye.
Used for: treatment of glaucoma.
Dosage: 2 to 4 tablets initially then 2 every 12 hours. Thereafter $^1/_2$ to 1 up to 3 times daily.
Avoid use: with children or with patients suffering from kidney or liver disease, pulmonary obstruction, low sodium or potassium levels. During pregnancy.
Possible interaction: with steroids, local anaesthetics, anticoagulants, anticonvulsants, antidiabetics, salicylates, digitalis, hypoglycaemics and ACTH (adrenocor-ticotrophic hormone).
Side effects: gastro-intestinal upsets, weight loss, frequent urination, headache, lassitude, itching, abnormal blood condition (dyscrasia).
Manufacturer: Merck, Sharp and Dohme.

DDAVP

Description: The acetate of desmo-pressin, an analogue of the hormone vasopressin and an antidiuretic compound.
Used for: it is administered as nose

drops for the treatment of diabetes insipidus and enuresis (bed-wetting, the involuntary passing of urine).
Dosage: adults, 0.1–0.2ml once or twice daily. Children, 0.05–0.2ml at the same rate. (Lower dosage for infants). Also available as white tablets: 0.2–0.4mg at bedtime for adults and children over 5 with enuresin; 0.1mg thrice daily for diabetes insipidus. Injection also available.
Avoid use: in pregnancy and for patients with epilepsy, migraine, asthma or chronic kidney disease.
Side effects: may cause fluid retention, headache, nausea and vomiting.
Manufacturer: Ferring.

DECA-DURABOLIN

Description: a form of the anabolic steroid nandrolone, in ampoules or syringes.
Used for: its protein-building properties (in conjunction with a nourishing diet), particularly after major surgery or debilitating disease. It was administered for osteoporosis but is no longer advocated as its value is dubious. It may be used to treat cancers linked to sex hormones.
Dosage: 50mg every 3 weeks, by intramuscular injection.
Special care: in case of heart, liver or kidney impairment, hypertension, migraine, epilepsy and diabetes.
Possible interaction: with anticoagulants, hypoglycaemics.
Side effects: oedema, hypercalcaemia, some virilization in women (i.e. appearance of male features such as deepening of the voice, growth of body hair and increase in musculature).
Manufacturer: Organon.

DECA-DURABOLIN 100

Description: The same form of the anabolic steroid nandrolene as is found in Deca-Durabolin.
Used for: the treatment of some forms of anaemia, e.g. aplastic anaemia, also post-

cytotoxic therapy anaemia, and anaemia associated with chronic kidney failure.
Dosage: all administered by intramuscular injection: 50–150mg weekly (aplastic); 200mg per week from 2 weeks before cytotoxic therapy until the blood returns to normal; 100mg (females) or 200mg (males) weekly for kidney failure.
Special care: in cases of heart, liver or kidney impairment, hypertension, migraine, epilepsy and diabetes.
Avoid use: in pregnancy, also where there is a known or suspected prostate or mammary cancer in males.
Possible interaction: with anticoagulants, hypoglycaemics.
Side effects: oedema, hypercalcaemia, some virilization in women (i.e. appearance of male features such as deepening of the voice, growth of body hair and increase in musculature).
Manufacturer: Organon.

DECADRON

Description: a corticosteroid preparation available as white (0.5mg) tablets marked MSD 41, or injection.
Used for: treatment of inflammation, particularly in allergic or rheumatic conditions.
Dosage: often a daily dose; magnitude varies with the case.
Special care: to be taken in numerous conditions including nephritis, osteoporosis, peptic ulcer and metastatic carcinoma. Also viral/fungal infections, tuberculosis, hypertension, glaucoma, epilepsy, diabetes, cirrhosis and hypothyroidism. Also pregnancy and stress. To be withdrawn gradually.
Possible interaction: NSAIDs, diuretics, hypoglycaemics, oral anticoagulants, phenobarbitone, ephedrine, phenytoin, anticholinesterases and others.
Side effects: osteoporosis, depression, hyperglycaemia, euphoria, peptic ulceration.
Manufacturer: Merck, Sharp and Dohme.

DECASERPYL

Description: an alkaloid (methoserpidine) compound originally derived from the dried root of the shrub *Rauwolfia serpentina*. It is available in tablet form, 5mg (white) and 10mg (pink), marked D/5 and D/10 respectively, both with RL on reverse.
Used for: treatment of high blood pressure.
Dosage: 10mg 3 times per day initially. This can be increased by 5–10mg daily on a weekly basis up to a maximum of 50mg per dose.
Special care: during pregnancy or lactation.
Avoid use: in patients with a history of mental depression; peptic ulcer, ulcerative colitis or severe kidney disease; Parkinson's disease. It should not be given to children.
Possible interaction: anticonvulsants.
Side effects: vertigo, tremor, lethargy, nasal congestion, and gastro-intestinal upset.
Manufacturer: Roussel.

DECLINAX

Description: The sulphate of debrisoquine available in (white) tablet form marked ROCHE 10 at 10mg strength, and used for moderate to severe hypertension.
Used for: treatment of high blood pressure.
Dosage: 10–20mg once or twice daily to begin with. This may be increased to a daily dose of 120mg.
Special care: with cases of kidney disease.
Avoid use: in cases of recent heart attack; phaeochromocytoma. Not to be used for children.
Possible interaction: sympathomimetics (drugs that stimulate the sympathetic nervous system and whose action resembles noradrenaline), some antidepressants.
Side effects: headache, general malaise, postural hypotension (i.e. low blood pressure on standing) and failure to ejaculate.
Manufacturer: Roche.

DECORTISYL

Description: a corticosteroid containing prednisone, a glucocorticoid steroid. It is available as white tablets (5mg).
Used for: rheumatic and allergic conditions.
Dosage: a divided daily dose of 20–40mg reducing by 2.5/5mg every 3 to 4 days to achieve maintenance daily dosage of 5–20mg. Children 1 to 7 years, quarter to half dose; 7 to 12 years, half to three-quarters dose.
Special care: with numerous conditions including nephritis, osteoporosis, peptic ulcer and metastatic carcinoma. Also viral/fungal infections, tuberculosis, hypertension, glaucoma, epilepsy, diabetes, cirrhosis and hypothyroidism. Also pregnancy and stress. Not to be given to children under 12 months. To be withdrawn gradually.
Possible interaction: NSAIDs, diuretics, hypoglycaemics, oral anticoagulants, phenobarbitone, ephedrine, phenytoin, anticholinesterases and others.
Side effects: osteoporosis, depression, hyperglycaemia, euphoria, peptic ulceration.
Manufacturer: Roussel.

DELTACORTRIL

Description: a corticosteroid preparation containing the glucocorticoid steroid, prednisolone. It is available as 2 enteric-coated tablets, brown (2.5mg) and red (5mg) marked Pfizer.
Used for: allergic conditions, collagen disorders or inflammation.
Dosage: 5–60mg daily, reducing to a minimum for maintenance.
Special care: with numerous conditions including nephritis, osteoporosis, peptic ulcer and metastatic carcinoma. Also viral/fungal infections, tuberculosis, hypertension, glaucoma, epilepsy, diabetes, cirrhosis and hypothyroidism. Also pregnancy and stress. To be withdrawn gradually. Not to be given to children under 12 months.
Possible interaction: NSAIDs, diuretics,

hypoglycaemics, oral anticoagulants, phenobarbitone, ephedrine, phenytoin, anticholinesterases and others.
Side effects: osteoporosis, depression, hyperglycaemia, euphoria, peptic ulceration.
Manufacturer: Pfizer.

DELTASTAB

Description: a corticosteroid preparation containing prednisolone acetate, a glucocorticoid steroid. Available as white tablets (1mg and 5mg) and ampoules of an aqueous solution (25mg/ml).
Used for: (tablets) treatment of inflammation associated with rheumatic and allergic conditions and collagen disorders. Solution injected into joints for rheumatic conditions and intramuscularly for systemic therapy.
Dosage: tablets initially 10–20mg daily (up to 60mg for severe cases), reducing as soon as possible to a maintenance daily dose of 2.5–15mg. Injection of solution in range 5–25mg depending on joint size up to 3 times daily. Intramuscular injection 25–100mg once or twice weekly. Children should receive only minimal doses and for the shortest possible time and even then only when specifically indicated.
Special care: with numerous conditions including nephritis, osteoporosis, peptic ulcer and metastatic carcinoma. Also viral/fungal infections, tuberculosis, hypertension, glaucoma, epilepsy, diabetes, cirrhosis and hypothyroidism. Also pregnancy and stress. To be withdrawn gradually. Not to be given to children under 12 months.
Possible interaction: NSAIDs, diuretics, hypoglycaemics, oral anticoagulants, phenobarbitone, ephedrine, phenytoin, anticholinesterases and others.
Side effects: osteoporosis, depression, hyperglycaemia, euphoria, peptic ulceration.
Manufacturer: Pfizer.

DENTOMYCIN

Description: an antibacterial available as a 2% gel of minocycline hydrochloride.
Used for: periodontitis (disease causing formation of spaces 'pockets' between gums and teeth and loss of bone and connective fibres) where pockets are 5mm or more.
Dosage: using the applicator, the gel is put into the pockets 2 or 3 times at 14-day intervals. After completion of treatment, not to be repeated within 6 months.
Special care: in cases of liver or kidney impairment. Pregnancy, nursing mothers. No intake of food or drink and no rinsing of mouth (including cleaning of teeth) for 2 hours after treatment.
Avoid use: not suitable for children.
Possible interaction: anticoagulants.
Side effects: local irritation.
Manufacturer: Lederle.

DEPIXOL

Description: a thioxanthene antipsychotic drug available in several forms. Yellow tablets (marked LUNDBECK) contain 3mg flupenthixol dihydrochloride. DEPIXOL INJECTION is available as the decanoate of flupenthixol in ampoules, vials and syringes (20mg/ml). DEPIXOL CONC. and DEPIXOL LOW VOLUME are concentrated forms of the decanoate (100mg/ml and 200mg/ml respectively), for injection.
Used for: schizophrenia and other mental disorders, especially for apathetic and withdrawn patients.
Dosage: Depixol—1 to 3 tablets twice daily (6 maximum); Depixol injection—deep intramuscular injection of 20–40mg every 2 to 4 weeks; Depixol Conc. and Depixol Low Volume—50mg 4-weekly up to 300mg every 2 weeks by deep intramuscular injection.
Special care: with the elderly, sufferers of Parkinsonism or kidney, liver, respiratory or cardiovascular disease and anyone with an intolerance to neuroleptic drugs taken orally.

Avoid use: in pregnancy and lactation. Patients who are comatose, excitable or overactive. Not for children.
Possible interaction: alcohol, analgesics and central nervous system depressants. Also anticonvulsants, antidiabetics, levodopa and antihypertensives.
Side effects: muscular spasms, rigidity and tremor, dry mouth and nasal stuffiness, urine retention, increased heart rate, constipation, weight gain, drowsiness, lethargy, fatigue, blood and skin changes, menstrual changes and galactorrhoea.
Manufacturer: Lundbeck.

DEPO-MEDRONE

Description: a corticosteroid preparation containing the glucocorticoid steroid methylprednisolone acetate as vials of 40mg/ml. Also, DEPO-MEDRONE WITH LIDOCAINE, which in addition contains 10mg/ml lignocaine hydrochloride local anaesthetic.
Used for: severe allergic rhinitis, asthma, osteo- and rheumatoid arthritis, collagen disorders and skin diseases (Depo-Medrone). Local use for rheumatic or inflammatory conditions (Depo-Medrone with Lidocaine).
Dosage: by injection into joints or soft tissue, 4–80mg (according to joint size or amount of tissue) repeated 1–5 weekly depending upon response.
Special care: with numerous conditions including nephritis, osteoporosis, peptic ulcer and metastatic carcinoma. Also viral/fungal infections, tuberculosis, hypertension, glaucoma, epilepsy, diabetes, cirrhosis and hypothyroidism. Also pregnancy and stress. To be withdrawn gradually. Not to be given to children under 12 months.
Possible interaction: NSAIDs, diuretics, hypoglycaemics, oral anticoagulants, phenobarbitone, ephedrine, phenytoin, anticholinesterases and others.
Side effects: osteoporosis, depression, hyperglycaemia, euphoria, peptic ulceration.
Manufacturer: Upjohn.

DEPO-PROVERA

Description: a depot-injectable preparation of the progestogen medroxyprogesterone acetate available in vials as a suspension of 150mg/ml and 50mg/ml.

Used for: contraception for women who cannot use other methods and endometriosis. (Also used in treatment of certain types of carcinoma.)

Dosage: for contraception: 50mg by deep intramuscular injection during the first 5 days of the cycle or within 5 weeks of giving birth, repeated 3-monthly; for endometriosis: 50mg weekly or 100mg 2-weekly by intramuscular injection over 6 months and longer if necessary.

Special care: undiagnosed abnormal vaginal bleeding, diabetes or severe depressison. Also, wait 6 weeks after birth if lactating; not for genital malignancy.

Avoid use: pregnancy. Also hormone-dependent carcinoma.

Side effects: temporary fertility with continuous treatment, irregular or heavy vaginal bleeding during early cycles, weight gain, back pain and fluid retention.

Manufacturer: Upjohn.

DEPOSTAT

Description: a depot progestogen available as 2ml ampoules of gestronol hexanoate (100mg/ml).

Used for: benign hyperplasia of the prostate and endometrial cancer.

Dosage: 200–400mg by intramuscular injection every 5 to 7 days for both conditions.

Special care: migraine, epilepsy, asthma and diabetes, kidney disease.

Avoid use: liver disease, severe arterial disease, carcinoma of the breast or genital tract.

Side effects: nausea, fluid retention, weight gain.

Manufacturer: Schering H.C.

DERMOVATE

Description: a potent steroid, clobetasol proprionate, available as 0.05% cream and ointment. Also available as **DERMOVATE SCALP APPLICA-TION** (solution), and **DERMOVATE-NN** which is also an antifungal/antibacterial agent containing, in addition, 0.5% neomycin sulphate and 100,000 units/g nystatin.

Used for: psoriasis, eczemas that are hard to control, inflammatory skin diseases. Dermovate-NN is for such conditions when infection is present or suspected.

Dosage: to be applied sparingly once or twice daily for a maximum of 4 weeks (maximum of 50g weekly for Dermovate-NN), then review.

Special care: limit use of face to 5 days. Withdraw gradually.

Avoid use: on acne, scabies, leg ulcers or prolonged use in pregnancy. Not for children.

Side effects: Cushingoid (see Cushing's syndrome) changes, skin atrophy, telangiectasia (multiple telangiectases, collections of distended blood capillaries).

Manufacturer: Glaxo.

DESERIL

Description: The maleate of methysergide which acts as a serotonin antagonist. Serotonin is active in inflammation (similar to histamine) and also acts as a neurotransmitter and is released by the liver and certain tumours. Available as white tablets of 1mg strength marked DSL.

Used for: diarrhoea associated with carcinoid disease, i.e. a tumour in certai glands in the intestine. For relief of recurring severe migraine, histamine (cluster) headaches and headaches wher other treatments have failed.

Dosage: for diarrhoea: 12 to twenty daily with meals, in divided doses. For migraine: 1 or 2 tablets 3 times per day with meals.

Special care: anyone with a history of peptic ulcer. In treating migraine, 6 months of therapy should be followed b a month's interval and the dosage

reduced 2 to 3 weeks before withdrawal. Patient should be monitored regularly. *Avoid use*: pregnancy or lactation; coronary, peripheral or occlusive vascular disorders; heart or lung disease; severe hypertension; liver or kidney impairment; disease of the urinary tract; poor health, weakness and malnutrition (cachexia); sepsis; phlebitis or cellulitis (skin infection leading to abscess and tissue destruction) of the lower extremities. Not recommended for children.
Possible interaction: vasopressors and vasoconstrictors; ergot alkaloids (alkaloids derived from the fungus *Laviceps purpurea*).
Side effects: dizziness, nausea, oedema, lassitude, leg cramps, drowsiness, weight gain, rashes, hair loss, CNS disturbances, abdominal discomfort, arterial spasm. Discontinue in the event of inflammatory fibrosis.
Manufacturer: Sandoz.

DESFERAL

Description: desferrioxamine mesylate as 500mg powder in a vial for reconstitution and injection. Desferal acts as a chelating agent with the iron, i.e. it locks up the iron chemically, enabling it to be removed from the system.
Used for: iron poisoning, haemochromatoses (excess deposits of iron in the body due to faulty iron metabolism), excess aluminium in dialysis patients.
Dosage: depending upon condition and circumstances—by mouth, intramuscular injection or intravenous infusion.
Special care: kidney dysfunction; pregnancy and lactation; patients with aluminium-related encephalopathy may have seizures (treat first with Clonazepam).
Possible interaction: erythropoietin, prochlorperazine.
Side effects: hypotension if given too rapidly intravenously; cardiovascular, gastro-intestinal and neurological

disturbances; changes in lens and retina; urine has red colouration; leg cramps; liver and kidney dysfunction; blood conditions, e.g. anaemia.
Manufacturer: Ciba.

DESTOLIT

Description: a bile acid, visodeoxycholic acid, available as white tablets (150mg) marked DESTOLIT.
Used for: dissolution of small cholesterol gallstones.
Dosage: 3 to 4 daily in 2 doses after meals, 1 after an evening meal. To be continued for 3 to 4 months after stones have been dissolved.
Avoid use: active gastric or duodenal ulcer; liver and intestine conditions affecting recycling of bile between intestine and liver; if gall bladder not functioning; women if not using contraception (non-hormonal methods ideally). Not for children.
Possible interaction: oestrogens; oral contraceptives; agents lowering cholesterol levels.
Manufacturer: Merrell Dow.

DETECLO

Description: a compound tetracycline preparation containing chlortetracycline hydrochloride (115.4mg), tetracycline hydrochloride (115.4mg) and demeclocycline hydrochloride (69.2mg) in blue film-coated tablets, marked LL, and 5422 on the reverse.
Used for: ear, nose and throat infections; infection of respiratory, gastro-intestinal and urinary tracts and soft tissues; severe cases of acne vulgaris.
Dosage: 1 tablet 12-hourly.
Special care: impaired liver.
Avoid use: during pregnancy and lactation; kidney impairment; SLE.
Possible interaction: penicillins; anticoagulants; oral contraceptives; milk, antacids or mineral supplements.
Side effects: allergic reactions; gastrointestinal upsets; superinfection (i.e. one infection arising during the course of

another); withdraw in the case of
intracranial hypertension.
Manufacturer: Lederle.

DEXA-RHINASPRAY

Description: a metered dose aersol for
nasal inhalation consisting of a
corticosteroid (dexamethasone-21
isonicotinate, 20mg per dose), antibiotic
(neomycin sulphate, 100mg) and the
sympathomimetic (i.e. something that
mimics the effects of organ stimulation
by the sympathetic nervous system)
tramazoline hydrochloride (120mg).
Used for: allergic rhinitis (e.g. hay fever).
Dosage: 1 dose per nostril up to 6 times
per 24 hours. One dose twice daily for
children 5 to 12 years. Not recommended for children under 5 years.
Special care: not to be used over a
prolonged period.
Side effects: nasal irritation.
Manufacturer: Boehringer Ingelheim.

DEXEDRINE^{CD}

Description: a sympathomimetic,
dexamphetamine sulphate, available as a
white tablet (5mg strength), marked
EVANS DB5.
Used for: narcolepsy, untreatable
hyperactivity in children.
Dosage: 1 tablet twice daily increasing
weekly by 10mg to a maximum of 60mg
daily. For the elderly, 5mg daily
increasing by 5mg every week. Not
recommended for children under 3
years; 2.5mg daily increasing by 2.5mg
every week for children aged 3 to 5 and
5–10mg daily for children aged 6 to 12
years, increasing at weekly intervals by
5mg. A maximum of 20mg daily is
customary.
Special care: pregnancy.
Avoid use: glaucoma; hypertension;
hyperexcitability; hyperthyroidism; in
cases of cardiovascular disease; where
there is a history of drug abuse.
Possible interaction: guanethidine,
MAOIs.
Side effects: restlessness and insomnia;

retarded growth; euphoria; dry mouth;
sweating, palpitations; tachycardia;
disturbances of the central nervous
system and stomach; raised blood
pressure. Also, possible dependence.
Manufacturer: Evans.

DEXTROPROPOXYPHENE

Description: an opiate and weak analgesic,
dextropropoxyphene napsylate, available
as capsules (60mg strength).
Used for: mild to moderate pain anywhere
in the body.
Dosage: 3 to 4 capsules per day.
Special care: pregnancy, elderly; liver or
kidney impairment.
Avoid use: in children.
Possible interaction: anticoagulants;
anticonvulsants; alcohol or depressants
of the central nervous system.
Side effects: constipation; rash; nausea
and dizziness; drowsiness. May develop
tolerance and dependence.
Manufacturer: Lilly.

DHC CONTINUS

Description: an opiate, dihydrocodeine
tartrate, available as white capsules for
sustained (prolonged) release and in
strengths of 60, 90 and 120mg, marked
with DHC and strength.
Used for: chronic severe pain e.g. as
associated with cancer.
Dosage: 60-120mg 12-hourly.
Special care: chronic liver disease;
kidney impairment; in pregnancy or the
elderly; allergies; hypothyroidism; raised
intracranial pressure.
Avoid use: depression of respiration;
disease causing obstruction of the airways.
Possible interaction: MAOIs, alcohol
and central nervous system depressants.
Side effects: headache; vertigo; nausea;
constipation.
Manufacturer: Napp.

DIABINESE

Description: a sulphonylurea, and
hypoglycaemic agent containing
chlorpropamide and available as white

tablets of strength 100 and 250mg.
Marked with DIA, strength and Pfizer.
Used for: type II non-insulin dependent
diabetes, adult-onset diabetes mellitus
(when the pancreas is still active to some
extent).
Dosage: usually 100–250mg daily with
breakfast, maximum 500mg.
Special care: the elderly or patients with
kidney failure.
Avoid use: during pregnancy or lactation;
juvenile, growth-onset or unstable brittle
diabetes (insulin-dependent diabetes
mellitus); ketoacidosis; severe kidney or
liver disorders; stress, infections or
surgery; endocrine disorders.
Possible interaction: MAOIs,
corticosteroids, ß-blockers, diuretics,
corticotrophin (ACTH), oral contraceptives, alcohol. Also aspirin, oral
anticoagulants, bezafibrate, clofibrate,
phenylbutazone, cyclophosphamide,
rifampicin, sulphonamides and
chloramphenicol. Also glucagon.
Side effects: skin rash and other
sensitivity reactions. Other conditions
tend to be rare, e.g. hyponatraemia (low
blood sodium concentration) or aplastic
anaemia.
Manufacturer: Pfizer.

DIAMICRON

Description: a sulphonylurea, and
hypoglycaemic agent, containing
gliclazide and available as white tablets
(80mg strength).
Used for: type II non-insulin-dependent
diabetes, adult-onset diabetes mellitus
(when the pancreas is still active to some
extent).
Dosage: half to 1 daily up to a maximum
of 4 (2 divided doses if above 2 tablets).
Special care: the elderly or patients with
kidney failure.
Avoid use: during pregnancy or lactation;
juvenile, growth-onset or unstable brittle
diabetes (insulin-dependent diabetes
mellitus); ketoacidosis; severe kidney or
liver disorders; stress, infections or
surgery; endocrine disorders.

Possible interaction: MAOIs,
corticosteroids, ß-blockers, diuretics,
corticotrophin (ACTH), oral contraceptives, alcohol. Also aspirin, oral
anticoagulants, and the generic drugs
bezafibrate, clofibrate, phenylbutazone,
cyclophosphamide, rifampicin,
sulphonamides and chloramphenicol.
Also glucagon.
Side effects: skin rash and other
sensitivity reactions. Other conditions
tend to be rare, e.g. hyponatraemia (low
blood sodium concentration) or aplastic
anaemia.
Manufacturer: Servier.

DIAMOX

Description: a carbonic anhydrase
inhibitor, acetazolamide, available as
white tablets (250mg strength) marked
LEDERLE 4395.
Used for: congestive heart failure and
oedema; epilepsy; glaucoma.
Dosage: for heart failure, oedema: 250–
375mg to start, each morning or on
alternate days. For premenstrual oedema,
125–375mg in 1 dose 5 to 10 days
before menstruation. For epilepsy: 250–
1000mg each day. Children under 24
months 125mg daily; 2 to 12 years 125–
750mg daily. For glaucoma: 250–1000mg
daily. Children, 125–750mg daily; infants,
125mg daily. All in divided doses.
Also **DIAMOX SR**
Description: as for Diamox, but
available as 250mg strength sustained-
release orange capsule.
Used for: glaucoma.
Dosage: 1 to 2 daily.
Also **DIAMOX PARENTERAL**
Description: as for Diamox, but available
as powder in a vial, 500mg strength.
Used for: congestive heart failure and
oedema; epilepsy; glaucoma.
Dosage: intravenous or intramuscular
injection of equivalent oral dose.
Special care: diabetes, lactation, gout,
potassium supplements may be required.
Monitor blood, electrolytes and fluid.
Also for glaucoma treatment: emphyse-

ma and pulmonary obstruction, any unusual rashes to be reported.
Avoid use: pregnancy, certain kidney conditions, chronic closed angle glaucoma, adrenal insufficiency, hypersensitivity to sulphonamides, depletion of sodium or potassium. Also for glaucoma—liver impairment.
Possible interaction: oral anticoagulants, hypoglycaemics, folic acid antagonists.
Side effects: headache, drowsiness, thirst, flushing, polyuria, blood dyscrasias, rash, excitability, paraesthesia (tingling, "pins and needles").
Manufacturer: Storz.

DIANETTE

Description: the oestrogen/anti-androgen ethinyloestradiol (35µg) with 2mg cyproterone acetate, available as beige tablets.
Used for: severe acne in women; for prolonged oral antibiotic therapy; idiopathic hirsutism.
Dosage: 1 daily for 3 weeks starting on first day of cycle (then 7 days without).
Special care: diabetes, varicose veins, hypertension, Raynaud's disease (numbness in the fingers due to spasm of arteries), asthma, chronic kidney disease (or dialysis), severe depression, multiple sclerosis.
Avoid use: not recommended for children. Also with cardiovascular conditions such as angina, ischaemia, heart valve disease, sickle cell anaemia, those at risk of and with a history of thrombosis. Patients with liver disorders; hormone-dependent carcinoma, undiagnosed vaginal bleeding, pregnancy, chorea, otosclerosis (bone overgrowth in the inner ear causing deafness), haemolytic uraemic syndrome (sudden destruction of red blood cells causing acute kidney failure).
Possible interaction: tetracyclines, barbiturates, phenytoin, griseofulvin, primidone, carbamazepine, rifampicin, chloral hydrate, ethosuximide, glutethimide, dichloralphenazone.

Side effects: leg pains and cramps, depression, enlargement of breasts, fluid retention, headaches, nausea, weight gain, loss of libido, vaginal discharge.
Manufacturer: Schering H.C.

DIAPHINE^{CD}

Description: The analgesic opiate, diamorphine hydrochloride available as powder in ampoules in strengths of 5, 10, 30, 100 and 500mg.
Used for: severe pain.
Dosage: 5–10mg subcutaneously or intramuscularly, to be varied according to patient response.
Special care: liver or kidney impairment, hypotension, hypothyroidism, myxoedema, reduced respiratory capacity, depression of the CNS, toxic psychoses, prostatic hypertrophy, stricture of the urethra, acute alcoholism, delirium tremens, severe diarrhoea, the elderly.
Avoid use: in children. With head injuries, raised intracranial pressure, acute liver disease, acute respiratory depression, diseases causing obstruction of the airways.
Possible interaction: depressants of the central nervous system, MAOIs.
Side effects: shock, cardiac arrest, vomiting, nausea, constipation, depression of respiration. Possible tolerance and dependence.
Manufacturer: Napp.

DIARREST

Description: a combined opiate, antispasmodic and electrolyte containing 5mg codeine phosphate, 2.5mg dicyclomine hydrochloride, 40mg potassium chloride, 50mg sodium chloride, 50mg sodium citrate per 5ml. Avaiiable in 200ml bottles.
Used for: diarrhoea and to maintain levels of electrolytes during attacks.
Dosage: 20ml 4 times per day with water. Children, at the same frequency: 10 to 13 years, 15ml; 6 to 9 years, 10ml; 4 to 5 years, 5ml; under 4 years, contact the manufacturer.

Special care: cardiac failure, liver or kidney malfunction, glaucoma, thyrotoxicosis, ulcerative colitis.
Avoid use: diverticular disease, pseudomembranous colitis (severe colitis occurring in debilitated patients taking broad-spectrum antibiotics).
Possible interaction: MAOIs.
Side effects: sedation.
Manufacturer: Galen.

DIAZEMULS

Description: a long-acting anxiolytic, benzodiazepine, available as an emulsion of 10mg in 2ml.
Used for: severe acute anxiety, delirium tremens; acute muscle spasms; anticonvulsant for status epilepticus (continual seizures resulting in brain damage if not stopped); and as a premedication.
Dosage: 10mg (5mg for elderly) by infusion or intravenous injection at 4-hourly intervals; 0.2mg/kg for children by the same means. As an anticonvulsant, 0.15–0.25mg/kg by intravenous injection, repeated after half to one hour and then up to 3mg/kg over 24 hours by intravenous infusion. For premedication, 0.1–0.2mg/kg by intravenous injection.
Special care: chronic lung insufficiency, chronic liver or kidney disease, the elderly, pregnant, during labour or lactation. Judgement and dexterity may be affected, long-term use is to be avoided. To be withdrawn gradually.
Avoid use: acute lung insufficiency, depression of respiration (escept in cases of acute muscle spasms). Also when treating anxiety, obsessional states or chronic psychosis.
Possible interaction: alcohol and other CNS depressants, anticonvulsants.
Side effects: vertigo, gastro-intestinal upsets, confusion, ataxia, drowsiness, light-headedness, hypotension, disturbance of vision, skin rashes. Also urine retention, changes in libido. Dependence a potential problem.
Manufacturer: Dumex.

DIAZEPAM

Description: an anxiolytic, long-acting benzodiazepine, available as 2, 5 and 10mg tablets and as **DIAZEPAM ELIXIR** (2mg/5ml).
Used for: severe anxiety in the short term, acute alcohol withdrawal, night terrors and sleepwalking in children.
Dosage: 6–30mg daily (elderly 3–15mg); children 1–5mg at bedtime.
Special care: chronic lung insufficiency, chronic liver or kidney disease, the elderly, pregnant, during labour or lactation. Judgement and dexterity may be affected, long-term use is to be avoided. To be withdrawn gradually.
Avoid use: acute lung insufficiency, depression of respiration, obsessional states or chronic psychosis.
Possible interaction: alcohol, other CNS depressants, anticonvulsants.
Side effects: vertigo, gastro-intestinal upsets, confusion, ataxia, drowsiness, light-headedness, hypotension, disturbance of vision, skin rashes. Also urine retention, changes in libido. Dependence is a potential problem.
Manufacturer: non-proprietary.

DIBENYLINE

Description: an anti-adrenaline antihypertensive, phenoxybenzamine hydrochloride, available as 10mg red and white capsules marked SKF. Also as **DIBENYLINE INJECTION** (50mg/ml) in 2ml doses.
Used for: vasodilation to treat high blood pressure associated with phaeochromocytoma.
Dosage: 1 capsule daily increasing by 1 each day to achieve control. Children, 1–2mg/kg daily in divided doses.
Special care: the elderly, kidney disease, cardiovascular or cerebrovascular disease, congestive heart failure.
Avoid use: after myocardial infarction, cerebrovascular accident (i.e. heart attack or stroke).
Side effects: dizziness, tachycardia, low blood pressure on standing, failure

to ejaculate. pinpoint pupils (miosis).
Manufacturer: Forley.

DICLOMAX RETARD

Description: White, sustained-release capsules containing diclofenac sodium (100mg).
Used for: osteoarthritis, rheumatoid arthritis, ankylosing spondylitis, musculoskeletal disorders such as sprains and strains, back pains. Acute gout.
Dosage: 1 tablet daily with food.
Special care: kidney, liver or heart disorders, pregnancy or lactation, the elderly, blood disorders, hepatic porphyria (production of excess porphyrins in the liver producing abdominal pain, neuropathy and photosensitivity), and those with a history of gastro-intestinal lesions. Patients on long-term treatment should be monitored.
Avoid use: active peptic ulcer, asthma, aspirin or anti-inflammatory drug-induced allergy, during last 3 months of pregnancy. Not recommended for children.
Possible interaction: steroids, NSAIDs, anticoagulants, antidiabetics, quinolones, diuretics, salicylates, lithium, digoxin, methotrexate, cyclosporin.
Side effects: headache, oedema, gastro-intestinal upsets, peptic ulcer, liver and kidney malfunction, skin reactions.
Manufacturer: Parke-Davis.

DICONAL^{CD}

Description: an opiate and antiemetic containing cyclizine hydrochloride (30mg) and dipipanone hydrochloride (10mg) and available as a pink tablet, coded WELLCOME F3A.
Used for: moderate to severe pain.
Dosage: 1 initially, then as advised.
Special care: in pregnancy or with severe liver or kidney diseases.
Avoid use: respiratory depression, diseases causing obstruction of the airways. Not suitable for children.

Possible interaction: alcohol, depressants of the central nervous system, MAOIs.
Side effects: dry mouth, drowsiness, blurred vision. Tolerance and dependence may occur.
Manufacturer: Wellcome.

DICYNENE

Description: a haemostatic drug and preparation of ethamsylate, available as ampoules (250mg/2ml) and 500mg white capsules.
Used for: prevention and treatment of periventricular bleeding in low birth weight infants. Also menorrhagia (abnormally heavy menstrual bleeding).
Dosage: for the newly born, 12.5mg/kg body weight 6 hourly within 2 hours of birth given intravenously or intramuscularly, continuing for 4 days. For menorrhagia, one 500mg capsule 4 times per day from the start of bleeding to the end of menstruation.
Side effects: headache, nausea, rash.
Manufacturer: Delandale.

DIDRONEL PMO

Description: a diphosphonate/calcium supplement available as white capsule-shaped tablets containing 400mg etidronate disodium marked NE and 406; with 1250mg calcium carbonate (Cacit) as pink effervescent tablets with an orange taste.
Used for: vertebral osteoporosis.
Dosage: 1 tablet daily for 14 days taken with water in the middle of a 4-hour fast. followed by 1 Cacit tablet daily in water for 76 days. The 90-day cycle is repeated for 3 years.

Also DIDRONEL INJECTION

Description: ampoules of 50mg/ml etidronate disodium.
Used for: hypercalcaemia associated with malignant tumours.
Dosage: slow intravenous infusion of 7.5mg/kg daily for 3 days. Interval of 7 days thereafter.

Also DIDRONEL TABLETS

Description: 200mg of etidronate disodium in white rectangular tablets.
Used for: Paget's disease after treatment for hypercalcaemia of malignancy.
Dosage: 5mg/kg daily taken in the middle of a 4-hour fast over 6 months maximum (for Paget's disease). For hypercalcaemia, 20mg/kg for 30 days.
Special care: pregnancy, lactation, enterocolitis (inflammation of the colon and small intestine). Monitor kidney function and ensure adequate intake of calcium and vitamin D.
Avoid use: severe kidney disease. Not recommended for children.
Side effects: diarrhoea, nausea.
Manufacturer: Procter & Gamble Pharmaceuticals.

DIFLUCAN

Description: a triazole, fluconazole, available as blue and white (50mg), purple and white (200mg) capsules and **DIFLUCON SUSPENSION** (50mg and 200mg/5ml) and **DIFLUCAN INFUSION** (bottles with 2mg/ml). Both capsules marked with FLU, strength and PFIZER.
Used for: candidiasis (thrush) whether oral or vaginal, systemic candidiasis, cryptococcosis (infection, with *Cryptococcus*, of the lungs and possibly the brains and CNS), oral/oropharyngeal candidosis, prevention of fungal infections following cytotoxic radio- or chemotherapy, for maintenance in AIDS sufferers to prevent relapse of cryptococcal meningitis.
Dosage: oral/vaginal candidiasis, 50–100mg daily for 14 to 30 days. Systemic candidiasis, 400mg on first day, and 200–400mg daily thereafter. Oropharyngeal, 50–100mg daily for 7 to 14 days. Maintenance against meningitis, 100–100mg daily. Prevention of fungal infections, 50–100mg daily. Doses delivered orally or by intravenous infusion. For children over 1 year, only in the case of life-threatening infections, 3–6mg/kg daily.

Special care: kidney damage with multiple doses.
Avoid use: during pregnancy or lactation.
Possible interaction: oral sulphonylureas, phenytoin, cyclosporin, rifampicin, theophylline, anticoagulants.
Side effects: gastro-intestinal upsets.
Manufacturer: Pfizer.

DIGIBIND

Description: an antidote for digoxin comprising 40mg of antibody fragments in a vial for reconstitution.
Used for: digoxin overdose.
Dosage: seek advice.
Special care: kidney disease.
Avoid use: allergy to ovine protein.
Side effects: hypokalaemia.
Manufacturer: Wellcome.

DIHYDROCODEINE

Description: an analgesic opiate, dihydrocodeine tartrate, available as tablets (30mg strength). Also as **DIHYDROCODEINE ORAL SOLUTION**, a syrup containing 10mg per 5ml.
Used for: moderate to severe pain.
Dosage: 1 tablet or 5–15ml 4 to 6-hourly, after food and as required. Children, 4 to 12 years, 0.5–1mg/kg body weight, 4 to 6-hourly. Not suitable for children under 4 years.
Also **DIHYDROCODEINE INJECTION** as 50mg/ml in ampoules.
Dosage: up to 50mg by deep subcutaneous or intramuscular injection. Children, same details as for dihydrocodeine/oral solution.
Special care: kidney disease or chronic liver disease, allergies, hypothyroidism. The elderly or pregnant.
Avoid use: respiratory depression, or diseases that cause obstruction of the airways.
Possible interaction: MAOIs, alcohol, depressants of the CNS.
Side effects: nausea, headache, vertigo, constipation.
Manufacturer: Knapp.

DILZEM SR

Description: an antihypertensive/ antianginal calcium ion antagonist prepared as diltiazem hydrochloride. Available as beige sustained-release capsules of strengths 60, 90 or 120mg, marked with strength.
Used for: angina, mild to moderate hypertension.
Dosage: 90mg twice daily initially increasing to 180mg if required. For the elderly 60mg twice daily.
Also DILZEM XL, white capsules of diltiazem hydrochloride available as 120, 180 or 240mg strengths.
Dosage: 180mg daily increasing to 360mg. For the elderly, 120mg daily.
Special care: diabetes, mild bradycardia, impaired left ventricular function, 1st degree AV block or porolonged P-R interval.
Avoid use: pregnancy or lactation, 2nd or 3rd degree AV block, left ventricular failure, bradycardia, liver or kidney disease, sick sinus syndrome (syndromes associated with dysfunction of the sinus (sinoatrial) node, the heart tissue that generates the cardiac electrical impulse).
Possible interaction: infusion of dantrolene, other cardiac depressants or hypertensives, also cyclosporin, digoxin, lithium, diazepam, cimetidine, theophylline, carbamazepine.
Side effects: ankle oedema, nausea, rash, headache, flushes, gastro-intestinal upset, SA or AV block.
Manufacturer: Elan.

DIMETRIOSE

Description: a gonadotrophin release inhibitor, gestrinone, in white capsules (2–5mg).
Used for: endometriosis.
Dosage: 1 twice weekly on the first and fourth day of the cycle, then on the same days of the week throughout the treatment.
Special care: diabetes, hyperlipidaemia.
Avoid use: in pregnancy, lactation. Severe heart, kidney or liver disease,

metabolic or vascular disorders.
Possible interaction: rifampicin, oral contraceptives, anticonvulsants.
Side effects: gastro-intestinal upsets, cramp, hirsutism, depression, voice changes, acne, weight gain.
Manufacturer: Roussel.

DINDEVAN

Description: an anticoagulant, phenindione, of strengths 10 (white, marked D10), 25 (green, marked D25) and 50mg (white, marked D50).
Used for: thromboembolic conditions.
Dosage: 200mg to start, then 100mg the following day and subsequent daily maintenance dose of 50–150mg.
Special care: the elderly, acute illness, vitamin K deficiency. Hypertension, weight changes, kidney disease.
Avoid use: severe liver or kidney disease haemorrhagic conditions, within 24 hours of surgery or labour. Pregnancy or lactation.
Possible interaction: corticosteroids, NSAIDs, sulphonamides, oral hypoglycaemics, quinidine, antibiotics, phenformin, drugs affecting liver enzymes, cimetidine.
Side effects: diarrhoea, hepatitis, kidney damage, urine discoloured, fever, rash, leucopenia, agranulocytosis (abnormal blood condition involving a reduction in the number of granulocytes).
Manufacturer: Goldshield.

DIODERM

Description: a topical steroid, hydrocortisone, available as a 0.1% cream.
Used for: allergic, pruritic or inflammatory skin conditions.
Dosage: to be applied sparingly. Rub in well twice daily.
Special care: maximum 5 days use on face or for children. Withdraw gradually after prolonged use.
Avoid use: acne (and rosacea), scabies, leg ulcers, peri-oral dermatitis, untreated fungal or viral infections, tuberculous, ringworm or viral skin disease.

Extensively or for prolonged period in pregnancy.
Side effects: skin atrophy, striae, telangiectasia (multiple telangiectases, which are collections of distended blood capillaries), Cushingoid changes (see Cushing's syndrome).
Manufacturer: Dermal.

DIPENTUM

Description: a salicylate, olsalazine sodium, available as a 250mg caramel capsule.
Used for: acute mild ulcerative colitis.
Dosage: 4 daily with food to begin, maximum 12 daily (all in divided doses). For maintenance, 2 twice daily with food. Not recommended for children.
Avoid use: pregnancy, severe kidney disease, hypersensitivity to salicylates.
Side effects: headache, rash, arthralgia (joint pain), gastro-intestinal upset.
Manufacturer: Kabi Pharmacia.

DIPRIVAN

Description: a general anaesthetic, propofol, containing 10mg/ml as an emulsion in vials and ampoules. Associated with rapid recovery without a hangover effect.
Used for: general anaesthesia at the start of surgery, and its maintenance.
Dosage: by intravenous injection, 2–2.5mg/kg (less in the elderly) at 20–40mg per 10 seconds; adjusted for children. Maintenance, 4–12mg/kg/hour.
Side effects: occasionally convulsions and brachycardia.
Manufacturer: Zeneca.

DIPROSALIC

Description: a potent steroid and keratolytic (causing shedding of outer skin layer) ointment, containing betamethasone dipropionate (0.05%) and salicylic acid (3%).
Used for: hard skin and dry skin disorders.
Dosage: apply thinly once or twice per day.

Also **DIPROSALIC SCALP APPLICA-TION** comprising betamethasone dipropionate (0.05%), salicylic acid (2%) in solution.
Dosage: apply a few drops to the scalp and rub in, twice daily.
Special care: limit use on face to 5 days. Withdraw gradually after prolonged use.
Avoid use: leg ulcers, scabies, peri-oral dermatitis, untreated fungal or viral infections, tuberculous, ringworm or viral skin diseases, acne. Lengthy or extensive use in pregnancy. Not for children.
Side effects: skin striae and atrophy, telangiectasia (multiple telangiectases, which are collections of distended blood capillaries), Cushingoid changes (see Cushing's syndrome), adrenal gland suppression.
Manufacturer: Schering-Plough.

DIPROSONE

Description: a potent steroid, betamethasone dipropionate, as 0.05% cream and ointment.
Used for: skin diseases that respond to steroid treatment.
Dosage: apply sparingly once or twice per day.
Also **DIPROSONE LOTION**, 0.05% betamethasone dipropionate in alcoholic solution.
Used for: scalp skin diseases
Dosage: apply a few drops twice daily
Special care: limit use on face to 5 days. Withdraw gradually after prolonged use.
Avoid use: leg ulcers, scabies, peri-oral dermatitis, untreated fungal or viral infections, tuberculous, ringworm or viral skin diseases, acne. Lengthy or extensive use in pregnancy. Not for children.
Side effects: skin striae and atrophy, telangiectasia (multiple telangiectases, which are collections of distended blood capillaries), Cushingoid changes (see Cushing's syndrome), adrenal gland suppression.
Manufacturer: Schering-Plough.

DIRYTHMIN SA

Description: an antiarrhythmic, disopyramide phosphate, available as a white 150mg film-coated sustained-release tablet, marked A over DR.
Used for: heart arrhythmias.
Dosage: 2 every 12 hours, maximum 5 per day.
Special care: kidney and liver failure, pregnancy, prostatic hypertrophy, glaucoma, urine retention, hypokalaemia, 1st degree AV block.
Avoid use: cardiomyopathy, cardiogenic shock (low cardiac output), disease of the sinoatrial node when there is no pacemaker, 2nd or 3rd degree AV block. Not recommended for children.
Possible interaction: ß-blockers, other antiarrhythmics in the same class, erythromycin, agents causing potassium reduction, anticholinergics (inhibiting the action of acetylcholine).
Side effects: anticholinergic effects.
Manufacturer: Astra.

DISIPAL

Description: an anticholinergic, orphenadrine hydrochloride, available in yellow, sugar-coated tablets, strength 50mg, marked DISIPAL.
Used for: Parkinsonism.
Dosage: 50mg 3 times per day initially, increased by 50mg every 2 to 3 days. Maintenance 100–300mg per day. Maximum 400mg daily.
Special care: heart disorders, gastro-intestinal obstructions. Withdraw slowly.
Avoid use: prostatic hypertrophy (enlarged prostate), glaucoma, tardive dyskinesia (repetitive muscular movements of the limbs, face or trunk).
Possible interaction: antihistamines, antidepressants, phenothiazines.
Side effects: confusion, agitation, rashes with high dosages, euphoria, anticholinergic effects.
Manufacturer: Brocades.

DISTACLOR MR

Description: a cephalosporin, cefaclor,

available as a blue sustained-release tablet (375mg strength) marked with name and strength.
Used for: infections of the skin, soft tissue and respiratory tract, otitis media, infections of the urinary tract.
Dosage: 1 twice daily or 2 twice daily for the treatment of pneumonia. Not recommended for children.
Also **DISTACLOR CAPSULES** available in white/violet (250mg), violet/grey (500mg) capsules; and Distaclor Suspension (125, 250mg/5ml.)
Dosage: 250mg every 8 hours up to a maximum of 4g per day. Children from 1 month–1 year, 62.5mg; 1 to 5 years, 125mg; over 5 years, 250mg. All 3 times per day to a maximum of 1g.
Special care: pregnancy or lactation. Kidney disease, hypersensitivity to penicillins.
Possible interaction: anticoagulants.
Side effects: gastro-intestinal upsets, hypersensitivity reactions, pseudomembranous colitis (a severe form of colitis).
Manufacturer: Lilly.

DISTALGESIC

Description: an analgesic and compound opiate containing dextropropoxyphene hydrochloride (32.5mg) and paracetamol (325mg), available in white oblong film-coated tablets marked DG.
Used for: mild to moderate pain.
Dosage: 2, 3 or 4 times per day. Not recommended for children.
Special care: kidney or liver disease, pregnancy or the elderly.
Possible interaction: anticonvulsants, anticoagulants, alcohol, depressants of the central nervous system.
Side effects: constipation, drowsiness, dizziness, nausea, rash, tolerance and dependence.
Manufacturer: Dista.

DISTAMINE

Description: a penicillin derivative penicillamine, available as white tablets of strengths 50, 125 (marked DS and

125) and 250mg (marked DM and 250).
Used for: severe active rheumatoid arthritis, heavy metal poisoning, chronic hepatitis, cystinuria (abnormal occurrence of cystine, an amino acid, in the urine), Wilson's disease (a defect in copper metabolism causing deposition of copper in the liver or brain, producing jaundice and cirrhosis, and mental retardation respectively).
Dosage: 125–250mg daily for 4 weeks increasing by 125–2500 mg at intervals of 4 to 12 weeks. Maximum daily dose 1.5g. Maintenance dose 500–750mg.. For the elderly, 50–125mg daily increasing to 500–750mg and a maximum of 1g per day.Children, 50mg per day for 1 month increasing 4-weekly. Maintenance 15–20mg/kg of body weight per day.
Special care: kidney disease, sensitivity to penicillin, blood, urine and functioning of kidneys should be monitored during treatment.
Avoid use: pregnancy, lactation, agranulocytosis (abnormal blood condition involving a reduction in the number of granulocytes), thrombocytopenia, lupus erythematosus (an inflammatory disease affecting the skin and some internal organs, regarded as an autoimmune disease).
Possible interaction: antacids, gold, zinc or iron salts, cytotoxic or antimalarial drugs, phenylbutazone.
Side effects: fever, rash, anorexia, nausea, blood disorders, loss of taste, proteinuria, myasthenia gravis, haematuria, SLE, nephrotic syndrome.
Manufacturer: Dista.

DITROPAN

Description: an anticholinergic/ antispasmodic, oxybutynin hydrochloride, available as blue tablets in strengths 2.5mg and 5mg. All marked with tablet name, strength and company initials.
Also **DITROPAN ELIXIR** as 2.5mg/5ml.
Used for: nocturnal enuresis (involun-

tary urination/bed-wetting), urinary frequency and incontinence, neurogenic bladder instability (often relating to the detrusor muscle of the bladder).
Dosage: 5mg 2 or 3 times per day to a daily maximum of 20g. 5mg twice daily for the elderly. Not recommended for children under 5; 5mg 2 or 3 times per day for children over 5. Last dose to be given at bedtime for nocturnal enuresis.
Special care: liver or kidney disease, hyperthyroidism, congestive heart failure, coronary artery disease, cardiac arrhythmias, tachycardia, hiatus hernia, prostatic hypertrophy, autonomic neuropathy. The frail, elderly or in pregnancy.
Avoid use: bladder or bowel obstruction, severe ulcerative colitis, glaucoma, lactation, myasthenia gravis, intestinal atony (weak), toxic megacolon (a serious complication of ulcerative colitis, involving massive dilatation of the colon).
Possible interaction: levodopa, digoxin, butyrophenones, amantadine, phenothiazines, tricyclic antidepressants, anticholinergics.
Side effects: facial flushes, anticholinergic effects (limit transmission of parasympathetic nerve impulses).
Manufacturer: Smith & Nephew Pharmaceuticals.

DIUMIDE-K CONTINUS

Description: a loop diuretic (a powerful, short-duration drug that acts on the loop of Henle in the kidney) and potassium ion supplement, available as frusemide (40mg) and sustained-release potassium chloride (600mg) in white and orange film-coated tablets marked DK.
Used for: kidney and liver disease where a potassium supplement is required, oedema including that associated with congestive heart failure.
Dosage: 1 tablet per day, taken in the morning.
Special care: diabetes, pregnancy, lactation. Gout, prostatic hypertrophy, liver

or kidney disease, impaired urination.
Avoid use: hyperkalaemia, Addison's disease, precomatose states in cases of liver cirrhosis.
Possible interaction: NSAIDs, cephalosporins, antihypertensives, lithium, digitalis, aminoglycosides, potassium-sparing diuretics.
Side effects: gout. To be discontinued if small bowel appears to be ulcerated or obstructed.
Manufacturer: ASTA Medica.

DIUREXAN

Description: a thiazide-like diuretic, xipamide, available as 20mg, white tablets, marked A.
Used for: oedema, hypertension, congestive heart failure.
Dosage: 1 each morning for hypertension; 2 each morning for oedema initially, then 1 to 4 daily as required. Not recommended for children.
Special care: liver or kidney disease, liver cirrhosis, diabetes, SLE, gout. The elderly, during pregnancy or lactation. Monitor fluid glucose and electrolytes.
Avoid use: severe liver or kidney failure, hypercalcaemia, sensitivity to sulphonamides, Addison's disease.
Possible interaction: NSAIDs, corticosteroids, carbenoxolone, tubocurarine, antidiabetic agents, alcohol, barbiturates, opioids, lithium, cardiac glycosides.
Side effects: gastro-intestinal upset, photosensitivity, rash, blood disorders, pancreatitis, dizziness, impotence, disturbance of electrolytes and metabolism.
Manufacturer: ASTA Medica.

DOBUTREX

Description: a ß₁-antagonist (acts on beta₁ receptors in cardiac muscle) dobutamine hydrochloride available in vials, as a solution of 12.5mg/ml.
Used for: cardiac surgery, cardiomyopathies, septic and cardiogenic shock (low cardiac output with acute myocardial

infarction and congestive heart failure), inotropic (i.e. affecting heart muscle contraction) support in infarction.
Dosage: intravenous infusion of 2.5–10mg/kg/minute varying with response.
Special care: severe hypotension complicating cardiogenic shock.
Side effects: tachycardia, increase in systolic blood pressure indicating overdosage.
Manufacturer: Lilly.

DOLMATIL

Description: a substitute benzamide, sulpiride, available as white tablets (200mg) marked D200.
Used for: chronic schizophrenia.
Dosage: over 14 years, 400–800mg initially per day in divided doses then 200–1200mg twice daily varying with required result. Not recommended for children under 14 years.
Special care: epilepsy, pregnancy, kidney disease, hypomania (a mental state of hyperactivity and irritability).
Avoid use: phaeochromocytoma.
Possible interaction: alcohol, analgesics, depressants of the CNS, antidepressants, antidiabetics, levodopa, anticonvulsants, antihypertensives.
Side effects: muscle spasms, restlessness, rigidity and tremor, urine retention, tachycardia, constipation, dry mouth, hypotension, blurred vision, impotence, weight gain, galactorrhea, hypothermia, amenorrhoea, blood and skin disorders, lethargy, jaundice.
Manufacturer: Delandale.

DOLOBID

Description: a salicylate analgesic and anti-inflammatory drug containing diflurisal and available as peach (250mg) and orange (500mg) film-coated tablets, marked DOLOBID.
Used for: acute and chronic pain; rheumatoid arthritis and osteoarthritis.
Dosage: 500mg twice daily then 250–500mg twice daily for maintenance. For arthritis, 500–1000mg daily, in 1 or 2

doses and varying according to the response. Not recommended for children.
Special care: kidney or liver disease, heart failure, the elderly, a history of gastro-intestinal ulcers or haemorrhage. Kidneys and liver to be monitored during long-term treatment.
Avoid use: pregnancy, lactation, active peptic ulcer, aspirin or anti-inflammatory-induced allergy or asthma.
Possible interaction: anticoagulants, indomethacin.
Side effects: diarrhoea, dyspepsia, headache, rash, tinnitus, dizziness, gastro-intestinal pain.
Manufacturer: Morson

DOLOXENE

Description: an opiate, dextropropoxyphene napsylate, available as pink capsules (60mg) marked LILLY H64.
Used for: mild to moderate pain.
Dosage: 1, 3 or 4 times per day.
Special care: pregnancy, the elderly, kidney or liver disease.
Possible interaction: anticonvulsants, anticoagulants, alcohol, CNS depressants.
Side effects: drowsiness, constipation, nausea, dizziness, rash. Also tolerance and dependence.
Manufacturer: Lilly.

DOLOXENE CO

Description: an analgesic comprising an opiate, salicylate and xanthine containing dextropropoxyphene napsylate (100mg), aspirin (375mg) and caffeine (30mg) and available as red and grey capsules marked H91.
Used for: mild to moderate pain.
Dosage: 1, 3 to 4 times per day.
Special care: kidney or liver disease (monitor during long-term treatment), heart failure, the elderly, anti-inflammatory induced allergies or a history of bronchospasm.
Avoid use: haemophilia, active peptic ulcer, hypoprothrombinaemia (lack of prothrombin in the blood, upsetting clotting function).

Possible interaction: alcohol, CNS depressants, anticonvulsants, anticoagulants, hypoglycaemics, uricosurics (drugs for elimination of uric acid or relief of pain due to gout).
Side effects: nausea, rash, drowsiness, constipation, dizziness. Also tolerance and dependence.
Manufacturer: Lilly.

DOPACARD

Description: a catecholamine, dopexamine hydrochloride, available in ampoules as a solution (50mg/5ml).
Used for: inotropic (i.e. affecting heart muscle contraction) support and vasodilation in heart failure during cardiac surgery.
Dosage: 0.5mg/kg/minute by intravenous infusion which may be increased to 6mg/kg/minute.
Special care: myocardial infarction, recent angina, hyperglycaemia, hypokalaemia. Monitor pulse, blood pressure etc.
Avoid use: thrombocytopenia, phaeochromocytoma, obstruction of the left ventricular outlet.
Side effects: increased heart rate, nausea, vomiting, tremor, anginal pain.
Manufacturer: Porton.

DOPRAM

Description: a respiratory stimulant, doxapram hydrochloride, available in 5ml ampoules (20mg/ml). Also **DOPRAM INFUSION** (2mg/ml).
Used for: ventilatory failure in cases of chronic obstructive airways disease.
Dosage: 1.5–4mg per minute by intravenous infusion, varying according to patient's condition and response.
Special care: epilepsy, liver impairment; used only under precise, expert supervision in hospital.
Avoid use: coronary artery disease, severe hypertension, thyrotoxicosis, status asthmaticus (asthma attack lasting over 24 hours).
Possible interaction: sympathomimetics, theophylline.

Side effects: dizziness, increase in heart rate and blood pressure.
Manufacturer: Wyeth.

DORALESE

Description: a selective a₁ blocker, indoramin, available as pale yellow traingular film-coated tablets (20mg strength).
Used for: obstruction of urine outflow due to benign prostatic hypertrophy.
Dosage: 1 tablet twice daily.
Special care: liver or kidney disease, patients with poor heart function, epilepsy, depression, Parkinsonism.
Avoid use: in cases of heart failure.
Possible interaction: antihypertensives, MAOIs.
Side effects: drowsiness, dry mouth, blocked nose, ejaculation failure, weight gain.
Manufacturer: Bencard.

DOVONEX

Description: an ointment and vitamin D analogue, containing 0.005% calcipotri-ol, also available as **DOVONEX CREAM**.
Used for: mild to moderate psoriasis.
Dosage: to be applied twice daily up to a maximum of 100g per week.
Special care: during pregnancy and lactation. Avoid the face.
Avoid use: calcium metabolism disorders.
Side effects: temporary irritation, facial (including peri-oral) dermatitis.
Manufacturer: Leo.

DOZIC

Description: an antipsychotic drug, butyrophenone available as a liquid preparation of haloperidol in 2 strengths, 1 and 2mg/ml.
Used for: mania, schizophrenia, psychoses, delirium tremens, alcohol withdrawal syndrome, childhood behavioural disorders.
Dosage: psychosis in the elderly: 0.5 0 2mg initially, others 0.5–5mg, both 2 to

3 times per day, increasing as required to a daily maximum of 200mg. This is reduced when control is gained, to a daily dose of 5–10mg. For anxiety, 0.5mg twice daily. For children, 0.05mg/kg daily in 2 divided doses.
Special care: liver or kidney failure, epilepsy, Parkinsonism, pregnancy, thyrotoxicosis and severe cardiovascular disease.
Avoid use: if patient is unconscious.
Possible interaction: alcohol, analgesics, CNS depressants, anticonvulsants, antidiabetics, antidepressants, antihypertensives, levodopa.
Side effects: spasms of eye, face, neck and back muscles, dry mouth, blocked nose, restlessness, tremor and rigidity, tardive dyskinesia (involuntary, repetitious muscle movements), urine retention, tachycardia, constipation, blurred vision, weight gain, impotence, hypothermia, menstrual changes, skin and blood changes, drowsiness, lethargy, sometimes fits.
Manufacturer: R.P. Drugs.

DRICLOR

Description: a 20% solution of aluminium chloride hexahydrate in roll-on bottle.
Used for: very heavy sweating (hyperhidiosis) of hands, feet and armpits.
Dosage: apply at night and wash off in the morning. Reduce applications as sweating lessens. Use only on feet for children.
Special care: area to be treated should be dry and not shaved. Contact with clothes and jewellery to be avoided.
Avoid use: on broken or inflamed skin.
Side effects: skin irritation.
Manufacturer: Stiefel.

DROGENIL

Description: an anti-androgen and form of flutamide available as a 250mg yellow tablet.
Used for: advanced prostatic cancer.
Dosage: 1 tablet 3 times per day.

Special care: fluid retention in patients with heart disease. Liver function tests should be performed periodically.
Possible interaction: warfarin.
Side effects: gynaecomastia, breast tenderness, gastro-intestinal upsets, galactorrhea. Increased appetite, tiredness and insomnia.
Manufacturer: Schering-Plough.

DROLEPTAN

Description: a butyrophenone, droperidol, available as a 10mg yellow tablet marked JANSSEN and D10. Also **DROLEPTAN LIQUID** as 1mg/ml of droperidol.
Used for: the rapid soothing of manic, agitated patients.
Dosage: 5-20mg every 4 to 8 hours. Children 0.5-1mg daily. Adjusted to match response.
Also **DROLEPTAN INJECTION** available as 2ml ampoules (5mg/ml).
Dosage: 5-15mg intravenously or up to 10mg intramuscularly every 4 to 6 hours. Children 0.5-1mg daily, intramuscularly. Adjust to match response.
Also available as 2ml ampoules containing 5mg/ml.
Used for: post-operative or chemothera-y-induced nausea.
Dosage: 5mg intravenously or intramuscularly post-operatively. 1-10mg by the same means 30 minutes before chemotherapy then 1-3mg/hr by continuous intravenous infusion or 1-5mg intramuscularly or intravenously every 1 to 6 hours. Children 0.02-0.075mg/kg by the same means.
Special care: Parkinsonism, epilepsy, pregnancy, lactation, severe liver disease.
Avoid use: severe depression or comatose states.
Possible interaction: alcohol, analgesics, depressants of the CNS, anticonvulsants, antidiabetics, antidepressants, antihypertensives, levodopa.
Side effects: spasms of eye, face, neck and back muscles, dry mouth, blocked nose, restlessness, tremor and rigidity, tardive dyskinesia (involuntary, repetitious muscle movements), urine retention, tachycardia, constipation, blurred vision, weight gain, impotence, hypothermia, menstrual changes, skin and blood changes, drowsiness, lethargy, sometimes fits.
Manufacturer: Janssen.

DTIC-DOME

Description: a cytotoxic drug and preparation of dacarbazine available as powder in vials for reconstitution (100 and 200mg).
Used for: soft tissue sarcomas and in combination for Hodgkin's disease.
Dosage: by intravenous injection.
Special care: an anti-emetic should be given simultaneously to lessen the risk of nausea and vomiting. Kidney function and hearing should be monitored.
Avoid use: again within 4 weeks.
Side effects: severe nausea and vomiting, alopecia, bone marrow suppression (necessitating blood counts), skin irritation.
Manufacturer: Bayer.

DUOVENT

Description: a β_2 agonist and anticholinergic consisting of 100µg ipratropium bromide in a metered dose aerosol. Also **DUOVENT AUTOHALER**.
Used for: obstruction to airways; for bronchodilation.
Dosage: 1 or 2 puffs 3 to 4 times daily. Children over 6, 1 puff 3 times per day. Not recommended for children under 6. Also **DUOVENT UDVS**, 1.25mg fenoterol hydrobromide and 500µg ipratropium bromide per 4ml of solution, in vials.
Used for: acute severe asthma.
Dosage: over 14 years, 1 vial nebulized immediately. Repeat under supervision. Maximum of 4 vials in 24 hours.
Special care: angina, arrhythmias, hyperthyroidism, heart muscle disease,

hypertension, glaucoma, prostatic hypertrophy.
Possible interaction: sympathomimetics.
Side effects: headache, dry mouth, peripheral dilatation.
Manufacturer: Boehringer Ingelheim.

DUPHASTON

Description: a progestogen, dydrogesterone, available as a white tablet (10mg strength) marked DUPHAR 155.
Used for: dysmenorrhoea (painful menstruation), dysfunctional (abnormal) bleeding, endometriosis, premenstrual syndrome (PMS), as part of hormone replacement therapy (HRT), habitual and threatened abortion.
Dosage: 1 twice daily from day 5 to 25 of the cycle (dysmenorrhoea); 1 tablet 2 or 3 times per day from days 5 to 25 or continuously (endometriosis); 1 twice daily from days 12 to 26 (PMS), 1 twice daily for the first 12 to 14 days of the month (HRT).
Special care: high blood pressure, tendency to thrombosis, liver abnormalities, ovarian cysts, migraine, diabetes.
Avoid use: pregnancy, severe heart or kidney disease, previous ectopic pregnancy, benign liver tumours, undiagnosed vaginal bleeding.
Possible interaction: cyclosporin.
Side effects: breast tenderness, irregular menstruation, acne, fluid retention and weight gain.
Manufacturer: Duphar.

DUROMINE^{CD}

Description: a CNS stimulant, phentermine, available as sustained-release capsules, 15mg (green/grey) and 30mg (maroon/grey), both marked with name and strength.
Used for: obesity.
Dosage: 15–30mg daily, at breakfast.
Special care: angina, arrhythmias, hypertension.
Avoid use: pregnancy, lactation, arteriosclerosis, hyperthyroidism, severe hypertension, drug/alcohol

abuse, past psychiatric illness.
Possible interaction: antihypertensives, sympathomimetics, MAOIs, psychotropics (mood-affecting drugs).
Side effects: oedema, tachycardia, raised blood pressure, restlessness, hallucinations. Possible tolerance, dependence, psychoses—avoid prolonged use.
Manufacturer: 3M Health Care.

DYAZIDE

Description: a potassium-sparing thiazide diuretic, consisting of 50mg triamterene and 25mg hydrochlorothiazide in peach tablets coded SKF E93.
Used for: oedema, mild to moderate hypertension.
Dosage: 1 twice daily after meals, falling to 1 daily (oedema), daily maximum of 4. Initially 1 daily for hypertension.
Special care: diabetes, acidosis, gout, pregnancy, lactation, pancreatitis, liver or kidney disease.
Avoid use: Addison's disease, hypercalcaemia, hyperkalaemia, severe liver or kidney failure.
Possible interaction: potassium supplements, potassium-sparing diuretics, lithium, digitalis, NSAIDs, ACE inhibitors, antihypertensives.
Side effects: diarrhoea, nausea, vomiting headache, dry mouth, weakness, cramps rash, hypercalcaemia, hyperglycaemia, low blood pressure.
Manufacturer: Smith, Kline & French.

DYSPAMET

Description: a form of cimetidine in white square chewable tablets (200mg). Also, **DYSPAMET SUSPENSION** (200mg/5ml).
Used for: persistent acid-related dyspeptic conditions.
Dosage: 2 chewed thoroughly (or 10ml) twice daily, at breakfast and bedtime. Minimum recommended course, 4 weeks.
Special care: exclude malignancy first; pregnancy, lactation, impaired kidneys, monitor for long-term treatment.

Possible interaction: phenytoin, theophylline, oral anticoagulants.
Side effects: tiredness, dizziness, rash, diarrhoea, gynaecomastia, confusion.
Manufacturer: Smith, Kline & French.

DYSPORT

Description: a bacterial, botulinum, toxin, type A-haemagglutinin complex (500 units as pellets in vial).
Used for: eyelid and hemifacial spasm.
Dosage: 120 units for affected eye, by subcutaneous injection, spread over 4 sites around the eye (see accompanying literature). Repeat as necessary or every 8 weeks.
Special care: pregnancy, lactation, caution to inject accurately.
Side effects: minor bruising and eyelid swelling, paralysis of mid-facial muscles, reduced blinking giving dry eyes and keratitis (inflammation of the cornea), double vision, eyelid droop (ptosis).
Manufacturer: Porton.

DYTAC

Description: a potassium-sparing diuretic, triamterene, available as 50mg capsules marked SKF.
Used for: oedema in congestive heart failure, liver or kidney disease.
Dosage: 3 to 5 per day in divided doses. Use on alternate days after first week.
Special care: elderly, gout, pregnancy, lactation, liver or kidney disease, acidosis, diabetic nephropathy (kidney disease related to diabetes).
Avoid use: Addison's disease, hyperkalaemia, progessive kidney or liver disease.
Possible interaction: potassium supplements, potassium-sparing diuretics, ACE inhibitors, antihypertensives, indomethacin.
Side effects: weakness, headache, cramps, nausea, diarrhoea, dry mouth, rash, blood dyscrasias (abnormal blood or bone marrow condition e.g. leukaemia), metabolic disturbances.
Manufacturer: Pharmark.

DYTIDE

Description: a potassium-sparing thyazide diuretic comprising 50mg triamterene and 25mg benzthiazide in capsules (clear/maroon) marked SKF.
Used for: oedema.
Dosage: 2 after breakfast and 1 after lunch to begin with, then 1 or 2 on alternate days for maintenance.
Special care: liver or kidney disease, gout, elderly, pregnancy, lactation, diabetes.
Avoid use: severe kidney failure or progressive liver or kidney disease, Addison's disease, hypercalcaemia, diabetic ketoacidosis (acute side effects of uncontrolled diabetes mellitus with electrolyte imbalance, very high blood glucose and acidosis).
Possible interaction: potassium supplements, potassium-sparing diuretics, indomethasin, ACE inhibitors, antihypertensives, digitalis, lithium.
Side effects: weakness, headache, nausea, cramps, diarrhoea, rash, dry mouth, blood dyscrasias (abnormal blood or bone marrow conditions, e.g. leukaemia), metabolic disturbances.
Manufacturer: Pharmark.

ECONACORT

Description: a combined topical steroid and antifungal antibacterial preparation produced in the form of a cream containing 1% hydrocortisone and 1% econazole nitrate.
Used for: Gram-positive bacterial and fungal skin infections with inflammation.
Dosage: massage into affected skin morning and night.
Special care: use in children or on face should be limited to a period of 5 days; short-term use only and withdraw gradually.
Avoid use: continuous or prolonged use

especially in pregnant women, untreated bacterial or fungal infections, infections caused by tuberculosis, viruses or ringworm, acne, leg ulcers, scabies, perioral dermatitis.
Side effects: adrenal gland suppression, thinning of skin, fluid retention.
Manufacturer: Squibb.

EDECRIN

Description: a proprietary loop diuretic (one which acts on part of the loops of Henle of the kidney tubules), in the form of white scored tablets, marked MSD 90, containing 50mg ethacrynic acid. Also **EDECRIN INJECTION** containing sodium ethacrynate equivalent to 50mg ethacrynic acid as powder in vial for reconstitution.
Used for: oedema including that which accompanies liver and kidney diseases and congestive heart failure.
Dosage: adults, 1 tablet daily after breakfast in first instance increasing by half to 1 each day as required. Usual dose is in the order of 1 to 3 tablets daily with maximum of 8 in divided doses. Injection: 50mg given intravenously. Children, 2 to 12 years, half tablet each day after breakfast, increasing by half tablet to the minimum effective dose required.
Special care: pregnancy, gout, enlarged prostate gland, liver disease, diabetes, impaired urination. Electrolyte levels should be monitored and potassium supplements may be needed.
Avoid use: children under 2 years, breast-feeding mothers, patients suffering from anuria, liver cirrhosis, serious kidney failure.
Possible interaction: antihypertensives, corticosteroids, digitalis, lithium, warfarin, aminoglycosides.
Side effects: blood changes, gastro-intestinal upset, jaundice, gout.
Manufacturer: M.S.D.

EFALITH

Description: a proprietary anti-inflammatory preparation produced as an ointment containing 8% lithium succinate and 0.05% zinc sulphate.
Used for: seborrhoeic dermatitis.
Dosage: apply thinly to affected skin and rub in, twice each day in the morning and at night.
Special care: patients with psoriasis; avoid eyes and mucous membranes.
Avoid use: children.
Side effects: local irritation at site of application.
Manufacturer: Searle.

EFAMAST

Description: a fatty acid preparation in soft gelatin, oblong-shaped capsules containing 40mg gamolenic acid.
Used for: mastalgia (breast pain).
Dosage: adults, 3 to 4 capsules twice each day.
Special care: patients suffering from epilepsy. Possibility of breast cancer should be eliminated before treatment begins.
Side effects: headache, nausea.
Manufacturer: Searle.

EFCORTELAN

Description: a topical corticosteroid preparation produced as cream and ointment of different strengths containing 0.5%, 1% or 2.5% hydrocortisone. Mildly potent.
Used for: dermatitis, inflammation and itching in anal and urinogenital areas, neurodermatitis (an itching skin disorder seen in nervous, anxious persons).
Dosage: rub into affected areas 2 or 3 times each day.
Special care: use in children or on face should be limited to 5 days. Short-term use and withdraw gradually.
Avoid use: long-term or extensive use, especially in pregnant women. Untreated fungus or bacterial skin infections or those which are viral or tuberculous in origin, ringworm, acne, leg ulcers, scabies.
Side effects: thinning of skin, adrenal gland suppression, hair growth.
Manufacturer: Glaxo.

EFCORTELAN SOLUBLE

Description: a glucocorticoid-mineralocorticoid preparation produced as a powder in vials for reconstitution and injection and containing 100mg hydrocortisone (as sodium succinate).
Used for: severe shock, adrenal gland failure, status asthmaticus (very severe and prolonged asthma attack which may prove life threatening).
Dosage: adults, 100–500mg by slow intravenous injection repeated according to patient's response. Children up to 1 year, 25mg; 1 to 5 years, 50mg; 6 to 12 years, 100mg, all given by slow intravenous injection.
Special care: pregnancy, hypertension, various inflammatory kidney disorders (nephritis, glomerulonephritis), diabetes, osteoporosis, epilepsy, secondary cancers, recent intestinal anastomoses, liver cirrhosis, thrombophlebitis, peptic ulcer, exanthematous diseases (characterized by rash). Also, stress or psychoses. Contact with chicken pox should be avoided (and specialist care is required for those contracting this disease). Drug should be withdrawn gradually.
Possible interaction: NSAIDs, anticholinesterases, diuretics, anticoagulants taken by mouth, cardiac glycosides, phenobarbitone, phenytoin, rifampicin, ephedrine.
Side effects: hypertension, weakness, depression and euphoria, hyperglycaemia, peptic ulcer, potassium loss, fluid retention, Cushingoid changes (as in Cushing's Syndrome).
Manufacturer: Glaxo.

EFCORTESOL

Description: a glucocorticoid-mineralocorticoid preparation produced as a solution in ampoules for injection, containing 100mg hydrocortisone (as sodium phosphate) per ml. Efcortesol is available in 1ml and 5ml ampoules.
Used for: severe shock, adrenal gland failure, status asthmaticus (very severe and prolonged asthma attack which may prove life-threatening).
Dosage: adults, 100–500mg by slow intravenous injection repeated according to patient's response. Children, up to 1 year, 25mg; 1 to 5 years, 50mg; 6 to 12 years, 100mg, all given by slow intravenous injection.
Special care: pregnancy, hypertension, various inflammatory kidney disorders (nephritis, glomerulonephritis), diabetes, osteoporosis, epilepsy, secondary cancers, recent intestinal anastomoses, liver cirrhosis, thrombophlebitis, peptic ulcer, exanthematous diseases (characterized by rash). Also, patients suffering from stress or psychoses. Contact with chicken pox should be avoided (and specialist care is required for those contracting this disease). Drug should be withdrawn gradually.
Possible interaction: NSAIDs, anticholinesterases, diuretics, anticoagulants taken by mouth, cardiac glycosides, phenobarbitone, phenytoin, rifampicin, ephedrine.
Side effects: hypertension, weakness, depression and euphoria, hyperglycaemia, peptic ulcer, potassium loss, fluid retention, Cushingoid changes (as in Cushing's Syndrome).
Manufacturer: Glaxo.

ELDEPRYL

Description: a proprietary preparation of an anti-Parkinsonism drug which is a monoamine oxidase-B inhibitor (monoamine oxidase B is an enzyme which breaks down dopamine). A deficiency in dopamine accompanies Parkinson's disease and the drug prolongs dopaminergic function in the brain. Eldepryl is produced as white, scored tablets of 2 strengths containing 5mg and 10mg selegiline hydrochloride.
Used for: Parkinsonism; (sometimes given along with levodopa).
Dosage: adults, 10mg daily either as a single morning dose, or in divided doses in the morning and middle of the day; taken with meals.

Special care: if taken with levodopa, side effects of this may be increased and the dosage of levodopa may need to be reduced.

Side effects: nausea, confusion, agitation, vomiting, hypotension.

Manufacturer: Britannia.

ELDISINE

Description: a cytotoxic drug which is a vinca alkaloid produced in the form of a powder in vials for reconstitution and injection. Eldisine contains 5mg vindesine sulphate in vial and in addition, 5ml diluent.

Used for: leukaemia, lymphomas and some other forms of solid tumour, e.g. those which may affect the lung or breast.

Dosage: as directed by physician skilled in cancer chemotherapy.

Special care: precautions must be observed in handling. Powder should be reconstituted by skilled staff wearing protective clothing and gloves under controlled conditions. Contact with skin and eyes should be avoided.

Side effects: vomiting, hair loss, bone marrow suppression, possible early menopause in women, sterility in men.

Manufacturer: Lilly.

ELOCON

Description: a topical and potent steroid produced as an ointment and cream containing 0.1% mometasone furoate. Also ELOCON LOTION (same strength).

Used for: atopic dermatitis (extremely itchy, damaged skin (caused by scratching in allergic individuals), psoriasis including that of the scalp, seborrhoeic dermatitis.

Dosage: apply thinly once each day.

Special care: pregnancy, hypertension, various inflammatory kidney disorders (nephritis, glomerulonephritis), diabetes, osteoporosis, epilepsy, secondary cancers, recent intestinal anastomoses, liver cirrhosis, thrombophlebitis, peptic ulcer, exanthematous diseases (characterized by rash). Also, stress or psychoses.

Contact with chicken pox should be avoided (and specialist care is required for those contracting this disease). Drug should be withdrawn gradually.

Possible interaction: NSAIDs, diuretics, anticholinesterases, anticoagulants taken by mouth, cardiac glycosides, phenobarbitone, phenytoin, rifampicin, ephedrine.

Side effects: hypertension, weakness, depression and euphoria, hyperglycaemia, peptic ulcer, potassium loss, fluid retention, Cushingoid changes (as in Cushing's Syndrome). Any adverse reactions should be reported to Committee on Safety of Medicines.

Manufacturer: Schering-Plough.

ELTROXIN

Description: a preparation of thyroid hormone, thyroxine sodium, produced in the form of tablets of 2 strengths: 50 µg (white, scored) and 100µg (white) both marked with name and strength.

Used for: hypothyroidism in children and adults, including cretinism and myxoedema.

Dosage: adults, 50–100µg each day in first instance increasing every 3 to 4 weeks by 50µg according to response until optimum dose is achieved. Maximum dose is 100–100µg each day. Children 25µg each day in first instance, increasing every 2 to 4 weeks by 25µg according to response. Dose should then be slightly reduced.

Special care: pregnancy, breastfeeding, elderly, patients with weak hearts or with reduced adrenal gland function.

Possible interaction: anticonvulsants, sympathomimetics, antidiabetics, tricyclics, cardiac glycosides, anticoagulants.

Side effects: tachycardia, muscular cramps, chest pains, sweating, flushing, arrhythmias, severe weight loss.

Manufacturer: Goldshield.

ELYZOL

Description: an antibacterial preparation produced in the form of a gel with appli-

cator containing 25% metronidazole.
Used for: additional therapy in severe
periodontal disease.
Dosage: apply gel to affected area and
repeat after 1 week.
Special care: pregnant women.
Avoid use: do not repeat therapy until 6
months have elapsed. Not for children.
Possible interaction: alcohol, disulfiram,
anticoagulants taken orally.
Side effects: local inflammation,
headache.
Manufacturer: Dumex.

EMCOR

Description: an antianginal and antihypertensive preparation, which is a
cardioselective ß-blocker, produced in
the form of heart-shaped, orange, film-
coated tablets containing 10mg
bisoprolol fumerate. Also, **EMCOR LS**
(5mg) which are yellow, scored, film-
coated tablets.
Used for: angina, hypertension.
Dosage: 10mg once each day with a
maximum daily dose of 20mg.
Special care: pregnancy, breastfeeding,
liver or kidney disease, diabetes,
metabolic acidosis, general anaesthesia.
May require to be withdrawn before
planned surgery and should be stopped
gradually. Patients with weak heart
should receive diuretics and digitalis.
Avoid use: children, patients with
obstructive airways disease or history of
bronchospasm, heart and circulatory
diseases including heart block, heart
failure, heart shock, sick sinus
syndrome, sinus bradycardia and
peripheral arterial disease.
Possible interaction: CNS depressants,
cardiac-depressant anaesthetics,
ergotamine, indomethacin, reserpine,
sympathomimetics, some other antihypertensives, clonidine withdrawal,
cimetidine, hypoglycaemic, verapamil,
class I antiarrhythmics.
Side effects: cold feet and hands, fatigue
on exertion, disturbance of sleep, gastro-
intestinal upset, bradycardia, bronchos-

pasm, heart failure. Withdraw gradually
if dry eyes or skin rash appear.
Manufacturer: Merck.

EMESIDE

Description: an anticonvulsant
preparation produced as capsules and as
a flavoured syrup. Orange capsules
contain 250mg ethosuximide and black-
currant or orange-flavoured **EMESIDE
SYRUP** contains 250mg per 5ml.
Used for: epilepsy.
Dosage: adults, 500mg each day in first
instance increasing by 250mg at 5 to 7-
day intervals until condition is
controlled. Maximum daily dose is 2g.
Children under 6 years, 250mg each day
in first instance adjusted every few days
by small amounts until condition is
controlled. Maximum daily dose is 1g.
Children over 6 years receive adult dose.
Special care: pregnancy, breastfeeding;
liver or kidney disease. Drug should be
withdrawn gradually.
Side effects: blood changes, central
nervous system effects, gastro-intestinal
upset, SLE, skin rashes.
Manufacturer: L.A.B.

EMFLEX

Description: an NSAID which is a form
of indomethacin and is produced as
orange/yellow capsules containing 60mg
acemetacin.
Used for: osteoarthritis, rheumatoid
arthritis, pain and inflammation
following surgery and lower back pain.
Dosage: adults, 2 tablets daily in divided
doses taken with meals, a glass of milk,
or with an antacid preparation. The
maximum daily dose is 3 capsules.
Special care: liver or kidney disease,
congestive heart failure, elderly persons,
septic infections, epilepsy, Parkinsonism, psychiatric illness, imbalance in
fluid or electrolyte levels. Patients on
long-term treatment should receive
checks on liver and kidney function,
blood count and eyes.
Avoid use: children, pregnancy, breast-

feeding, certain gastro-intestinal disorders, peptic ulcer, angioneurotic oedema. Also, allergy to NSAID or aspirin.
Possible interaction: thiazides, salcylates, lithium, anticoagulants, frusemide, probenecid, ACE inhibitors, methotrexate, ß-blockers, triamterene haloperidol, quinolones.
Side effects: blood changes, dizziness, blurring of vision, headache, tinnitus, gastro-intestinal upset, oedema.
Manufacturer: Merck.

EMINASE

Description: a fibrinolytic preparation produced in the form of a powder in vials for reconstitution and injection, containing 30 units anistreplase.
Used for: myocardial infarction.
Dosage: adults, one 30-unit dose within 6 hours of myocardial infarction, given over a period of 4 to 5 minutes by slow intravenous injection.
Special care: pregnancy, breastfeeding, heart arrhythmias, risk of bleeding, increased risk of thrombi or emboli.
Avoid use: children, treatment should not be repeated after first 5 days for 12 months, patients who have had surgery within past 10 days, those with menorrhagia, aneurysm, serious hypertension, peptic ulcer, CVA.
Side effects: vomiting, fever, nausea, allergic responses, flushing, hypotension, bleeding, bradycardia.
Manufacturer: Beecham.

EMLA

Description: a local anaesthetic preparation produced in the form of a cream containing 25mg lignocaine, 25mg prilocaine per g.
Used for: local anaesthesia of skin and genital area (removal of genital warts).
Dosage: adults and children, minor surgery, 2g applied to affected area for a minimum of 1 hour and a maximum of 5 hours. For larger areas, 1.5–3g per 10cm² of skin for minimum of 2 hours and maximum of 5 hours. (Cream is

applied as a thick layer under a dressing). Genital warts, 10g applied for 5 to 10 minutes before surgical removal.
Avoid use: infants, patients with atopic dermatitis, on wounds or mucous membranes.
Side effects: local slight skin reactions.
Manufacturer: Astra.

ENDOBULIN

Description: a preparation of human normal immunoglobin (HNIG) available as a concentrate which is freeze-dried plus diluent, for reconstitution and intravenous infusion.
Used for: replacement therapy in patients with deficient immunoglobulins (gamma globulins) which are antibodies present in blood serum.
Dosage: depending upon particular syndrome or disease being treated, in the order of 0.4g to 1g/kg body weight by intravenous infusion for 4 or 5 days, or within first 2 weeks. Some conditions require maintenance doses in the order of 0.1–0.6g/kg body weight each month in 1 or 2 doses.
Special care: pregnant women, patients with diabetes. Monitor closely during infusion for signs of anaphylaxis. Special care in patients with selective immunoglobulin A deficiency who are sensitised and carry antibodies to IGA.
Avoid use: patients known to have certain types of antibody to immunoglobulin.
Possible interaction: live vaccines.
Side effects: fever, chills, headache, fatigue; rarely, anaphylaxis.
Manufacturer: Immuno.

ENDOXANA

Description: an alkylating cytotoxic drug produced as a powder in vials containing 100mg, 200mg, 500mg or 1g of cyclophosphamide, for reconstitution and injection. It is also available as white sugar-coated tablets (50mg).
Used for: malignant diseases e.g. lymphoma, leukaemia and some solid tumours.

Dosage: adults, taken with Uromitexan as directed by physician skilled in cancer chemotherapy.

Special care: patients with diabetes, elderly or debilitated persons.

Avoid use: children.

Possible interaction: sulphonylureas, radiotherapy, doxorubicin.

Side effects: vomiting, hair loss, nausea, bone marrow suppression and suppression of the reticulo-endothelial system, toxic effects on heart and urinary tract, haematuria, male sterility (Azoospermia—a lack of spermaztozoa in the semen), amenorrhoea.

Manufacturer: Asta Medica.

ENGERIX B

Description: a genetically derived suspension of hepatitis B surface antigen (from yeast cells) containing 20 micrograms per ml adsorbed onto aluminium hydroxide, in vials or pre-filled syringes.

Used for: immunisation against the Hepatitis B virus.

Dosage: adults, first dose 1ml by intramuscular injection into the deltoid muscle (upper arm) repeated after an interval of 1 month and 6 months. Children, first dose of 0.5ml by intramuscular injection into the thigh repeated after an interval of 1 month and 6 months.

Special care: pregnant women, patients receiving kidney dialysis or who have a deficient immune system may need to receive additional doses.

Avoid use: severe infections accompanied by fever.

Side effects: slight short-lived soreness at injection site, with inflammation and hardening, dizziness, feverishness, nausea, malaise.

Manufacturer: S.K. & F.

EPANUTIN

Description: an anticonvulsant available as capsules and suspension, which belongs to a group called hydantoins

which are similar in composition to barbiturates. White/purple, white/pink and white/orange capsules contain 25mg, 50mg and 100mg of phenytoin sodium respectively. All marked with capsule name and strength. Also, **EPANUTIN SUSPENSION** containing 30mg phenytoin per 5ml and **EPANUTIN INFATABS** containing 50mg phenytoin in the form of triangular, scored, yellow, chewable tablets.

Used for: prevention and treatment of grand mal (tonic clonic) epileptic seizures, partial (focal) epileptic seizures and seizures which may follow trauma to the brain due to neurosurgery or head injury. Also, trigeminal neuralgia.

Dosage: adults, capsules, 3–4mg/kg body weight in first instance each day, gradually increasing until condition is controlled. Maintenance dose is in the order of 200–500mg in divided doses each day. Suspension: 15ml 3 times each day. Infatabs: 2 tablets 2, 3 or 4 times each day. Children, capsules, (all except newborn babies), 5mg/kg body weight in 2 divided doses, with a maintenance dose in the order of 4–8mg/kg body weight each day. Suspension, under 6 years of age, 5ml twice each day increasing to 5ml 3 or 4 times each day if needed; 6 to 12 years, adult dose. Infatabs: under 6 years of age, half of 1 tablet 2, 3 or 4 times each day; 7 to 12 years, 1 tablet 2, 3 or 4 times each day.

Special care: pregnancy, breastfeeding, liver disease. Adequate intake of vitamin D is necessary and drug should be stopped gradually.

Possible interaction: isoniazid, sulthiame, anticoagulants of the coumarin group, chloramphenicol, oral contraceptives, doxycycline.

Side effects: upset stomach, lack of sleep, allergic effects, blood changes, unsteadiness, swelling of gums and lymph glands; in young persons there may be unusual growth of hair (hirsutism) and motor activity. Rapid abnormal eye movements (nystagmus)

may occur and drug should be withdrawn in the event of skin rash.
Manufacturer: Parke-Davis.

EPANUTIN PARENTERAL

Description: an anticonvulsant and class I antiarrhythmic preparation available in ampoules for injection containing 50mg phenytoin sodium per ml.
Used for: status epilepticus (an emergency situation in which a patient suffers continuous epileptic seizures without regaining consciousness in between. If the convulsions are not halted, the person suffers irreversible brain damage and may die). Also used for prevention of seizures during neurosurgical operations and for heart arrhythmias, particularly those caused by digitalis.
Dosage: adults, status epilepticus, 150–250mg by slow intravenous injection followed by 100–150mg after half an hour if needed. Heart arrhythmias, 3.5–5mg/kg body weight in first instance, by intravenous injection, the rate of which should not be greater than 50mg per minute. This can be repeated once if required. Children for status epilepticus only, dose in proportion to that for a 70kg adult, reduced accordingly.
Special care: pregnant women, breastfeeding mothers, ECG and close monitoring needed; resuscitation equipment should be on hand.
Avoid use: patients with heart block.
Possible interaction: isoniazid, sulthiame, anticoagulants of the coumarin group, chloramphenicol, oral contraceptives, doxycycline.
Side effects: upset stomach, lack of sleep, allergic effects, blood changes, unsteadiness, swelling of gums and lymph glands; in young persons there may be unusual growth of hair (hirsutism) and motor activity. Rapid abnormal eye movements (nystagmus) may occur and drug should be withdrawn in the event of skin rash.
Manufacturer: Parke-Davis.

EPIFOAM

Description: a combined corticosteroid and local anaesthetic produced as a foam in an aerosol. Epifoam contains 1% hydrocortisone acetate and 1% paramoxine hydrochloride.
Used for: injury to the perineum including pain following episiotomy.
Dosage: adults, apply 3 to 4 times each day on non-absorbent sterile dressing for a period not exceeding 7 days.
Avoid use: children, infected skin conditions.
Manufacturer: Stafford-Miller.

EPILIM

Description: an anticonvulsant and carboxylic acid derivative, sodium valproate, available as lilac, enteric-coated tablets containing 200mg or 500mg. **EPILIM CRUSHABLE** white, scored tablets(100mg); **EPILIM SYRUP** (red) contains 200mg per 5ml; **EPILIM LIQUID** (sugar-free, red) contains 200mg per 5ml; **EPILIM CHRONO** sustained-release tablets are lilac-coloured and contain 200mg, 300mg and 500mg as valproate and valproic acid. **EPILIM INTRAVE-NOUS** contains 400mg powder in vial for reconstitution and injection.
Dosage: adults, 600mg each day in 2 divided doses in first instance, then gradually increasing after intervals of 3 days by 200mg until optimum control dose is achieved. Usual maintenance dose is in the order of 1–2g each day with a maximum of 2.5g. Children, less than 20kg body weight, 20mg/kg each day at first; over 20kg, 400mg each day at first. Both in divided doses and both gradually increased until optimum control dose is achieved. Epilim Intravenous (for patients not able to take the oral preparations), adults, 400–800mg each day by slow intravenous injection or infusion with a maximum dose of 2.5g. Children, 20–30mg/kg body weight by slow intravenous injection or infusion.

Special care: pregnant women, children with brain damage, mental retardation or congenital metabolic disorders accompanying severe epilepsy. Patients should be monitored for signs of liver failure and liver function tests should be carried out. Patients having urine tests for diabetes may show false positives for ketones.

Avoid use: patients with liver disorders.

Possible interaction: other anticonvulsant drugs, anticoagulants, antidepressants.

Side effects: liver failure, oedema, pancreatitis, gain in weight, loss of hair, blood changes, effects on nervous system.

Manufacturer: Sanofi Winthrop.

EPOGAM

Description: a fatty acid preparation in the form of gelatin caspsules containing 40mg gamolenic acid and marked Epogam 240. Also, **EPOGAM PAEDIATRIC**, gelatin capsules containing 80mg and marked EPOGAM 60.

Used for: relief of eczema.

Dosage: Capsules are snipped open and contents poured onto food, in drink, or swallowed directly. Adults 4 to 6 capsules twice each day. Epogram paediatric, 2 to 3 capsules each day. Children, over 1 year, 2 to 4 Epogram 240 capsules or 1 to 2 Epogram Paediatric capsules, both twice each day.

Special care: patients with epilepsy.

Avoid use: children under 1 year.

Side effects: headache, nausea.

Manufacturer: Searle.

EPPY

Description: a sympathomimetic preparation available in the form of eye drops containing 1% adrenaline.

Used for: glaucoma (primary open angle and secondary).

Dosage: adults, 1 drop once or twice each day.

Avoid use: children, patients with narrow angle glaucoma or aphakia (absence of all or part of the lens of the eye, usually because it has been surgically removed, e.g. to treat cataracts).

Possible interaction: TCADs, MAOIs.

Side effects: headache, pain in region of eyes and redness due to increased blood flow (hyperaemia), melanosis; rarely, systemic effects.

Manufacturer: Chauvin.

EPREX

Description: a preparation of synthesised human erythropoietin, a glycoprotein hormone, produced by some kidney cells and released into the blood in conditions in which there is a lack of oxygen reaching the tissues. This increases the rate of production of red blood cells (erythropoiesis) which are responsible for transporting oxygen in the circulation. Eprex is produced in vials or pre-filled syringes as a medium for injection and containing epoetin alfa solution.

Used for: anaemia which accompanies chronic renal failure in both dialysis and non-dialysis patients.

Dosage: adults, dialysis patients, (following dialysis), 50iu/kg body weight 3 times each week at first by intravenous or subcutaneous injection. Non-dialysis patients, same dose by subcutaneous injection. Dose increased and adjusted depending upon response and haemoglobin level required. Children, 50iu/kg body weight 3 times each week after dialysis, in first instance. Dose is then adjusted according to patient's condition.

Special care: pregnancy, liver failure, hypertension, ischaemic vascular disease, history of epilepsy. Haemoglobin levels, blood pressure, electrolyte levels and blood count require consistent monitoring. Iron supplements may be needed and treatment for any other causes of anaemia; diet and dialysis treatment may need to be altered.

Avoid use: hypertension which is uncontrolled.

Possible interaction: cyclosporin.
Side effects: headache, rise in blood pressure, feverish flu-like symptoms, skin reactions, seizures, thrombosis.
Manufacturer: Cilag.

EQUAGESIC^{CD}

Description: a compound analgesic preparation which is a controlled drug and combines an opiate, muscle relaxant and salicylate. Three layered pink, white, yellow tablets contain 75mg ethoheptazine citrate, 150mg meprobamate and 250mg aspirin and are marked WYETH on the yellow surface.
Used for: relief of severe muscle and bone pain.
Dosage: adults, 2 tablets 3 or 4 times each day.
Special care: for short-term use only; special care in elderly persons, those suffering from depression or at risk of suicide. Patients with heart failure, liver disease, history of epilepsy.
Avoid use: pregnancy, breastfeeding, children, kidney disease, porphyria, peptic ulcer, alcoholism, haemophilia, allergy to aspirin or other anti-inflammatory drugs.
Possible interaction: anticoagulants, antidiabetic drugs, alcohol, central nervous system sedatives, uricosurics (drugs which lower uric acid levels).
Side efects: blood changes, giddiness, nausea, sleepiness, rash, ataxia.
Manufacturer: Wyeth.

EQUANIL^{CD}

Description: a carbamate tranquillizer which acts as an anxiolytic and a controlled drug. It is available in the form of white, scored tablets of 2 different strengths containing 200mg or 400mg of meprobamate. Both are marked E and WYETH.
Used for: short-term relief of anxiety and muscular tension.
Dosage: adults, 400mg 3 times each day at at night; elderly persons, 200mg 3 times each day.

Special care: pregnancy, breastfeeding, liver or kidney disease, history of depression, epilepsy. Drug should be stopped gradually.
Avoid use: children, patients suffering from alcoholism or acute intermittent porphyria.
Possible interaction: CNS depressants, phenytoin, TCADs, rifampicin, alcohol, anticoagulants of the coumarin type, phenothiazines, griseofulvin, oral contraceptives.
Side effects: addiction may occur and ability to perform skilled tasks such as driving impaired. Gastro-intestinal upset, hypotension, disturbance to central nervous system and excitement, feeling of "pins and needles" (paraesthesia), blood disorders, low blood pressure, allergic reactions.
Manufacturer: Wyeth.

ERADACIN

Description: a 4-quinolone antibiotic preparation produced in the form of yellow/red capsules containing 150mg acrosoxacin.
Used for: treatment of acute gonorrhoea.
Dosage: adults, 1 dose of 2 tablets each day.
Special care: pregnant women, patients with liver or kidney disease.
Avoid use: children.
Side effects: drowsiness, headaches, giddiness, gastro-intestinal upset.
Manufacturer: Sanofi Winthrop.

ERVEVAX

Description: a form of live attenuated virus of Wistar RA27/3 used as a vaccine against Rubella (German measles). It is produced as pink pellets in vials, along with diluent, for reconstitution and injection.
Used for: immunisation against Rubella.
Dosage: 0.5ml by intravenous, intramuscular or subcutaneous injection.
Avoid use: pregnancy, severe fever, altered immunity due to malignant diseases including leukaemia and lymphoma.
Possible interaction: other live vaccines

(with the exception of polio vaccine taken by mouth), transfusions, cytotoxic drugs, immunoglobulins, corticosteroids, irradiation.
Side effects: pains in joints, rash, feverishness, lymphadenopathy (a disease of lymph vessels and nodes).
Manufacturer: S.K. & F.

ERYMAX

Description: an antibiotic preparation of the macrolide, erythromycin, produced as small enteric-coated pellets contained in clear/orange capsules (250mg strength).
Used for: infections sensitive to erythromycin especially in patients with penicillin hypersensitivity. These include legionnaire's disease, campylobacter enteritis, syphilis, chronic prostatitis, pneumonia, non-gonococcal urethritis and acne. Also used as a preventative against whooping cough and diphtheria.
Dosage: adults, for most infections, 250mg at 6-hour intervals or 500mg every 12 hours taken before or with food. For acne, 1 tablet twice each day for 1 month, then 1 tablet daily as maintenance dose. Children, infections, 30–50mg/kg body weight each day in divided doses at 6-hour intervals or twice daily.
Special care: patients with liver disease.
Possible interaction: digoxin, astemizole, anticoagulants taken by mouth, terfenadine, carbamazepine, theophylline.
Side effects: allergic reactions, gastro-intestinal upset, cholestatic jaundice.
Manufacturer: Elan.

ERYTHROCIN

Description: an antibiotic preparation of the macrolide, erythromycin, produced in the form of oblong, white, film-coated tablets, containing 250mg and 500mg (as stearate), all marked with company symbol.
Used for: infections sensitive to erythromycin especially in patients with penicillin hypersensitivity. Acne.

Dosage: adults, 1–2g each day in divided doses.
Special care: patients with liver disease.
Avoid use: children.
Possible interaction: digoxin, anticoagulants taken by mouth, astemizole, theophylline, terfenadine, carbamazepine.
Side effects: allergic reactions, gastro-intestinal upset, cholestatic jaundice.
Manufacturer: Abbott.

ERYTHROMID

Description: an antibiotic preparation of the macrolide, erythromycin, produced in the form of enteric-coated and film-coated orange tablets containing 250mg. Also, **ERYTHROMID DS®** enteric-coated and film-coated orange tablets containing 500mg.
Used for: infections sensitive to erythromycin especially in patients with penicillin hypersensitivity. Acne.
Dosage: adults, 1–2g each day in divided doses with a maximum of 4g in exceptionally severe cases of infection. Children over 8 years, same as adult dose.
Special care: patients with liver disease.
Avoid use: children under 8 years of age.
Possible interaction: digoxin, oral anticoagulants, astemizole, theophylline, terfenadine, carbamazepine.
Side effects: allergic reactions, gastro-intestinal upset, cholestatic jaundice.
Manufacturer: Abbott.

ERYTHOPED A

Description: an antibiotic preparation of the macrolide, erythromycin (as ethyl succinate), produced as oval, film-coated yellow tablets (500mg); **ERYTHROPED A** sachets contain 1g in the form of granules. **ERYTHROPED SACHETS** contain 250mg; **ERYTHROPED SUSPENSION** contains 250mg per 5ml solution. **ERYTHROPED SUGAR-FREE SUSPENSION** contains 125mg per 5ml. **ERYTHROPED FORTE** available as 500mg per 5ml suspension or as granules in sachet. **ERYTHROPED P.I. SUGAR-FREE SUSPENSION**

contains 125mg per 5ml solution.
Used for: infections sensitive to
erythromycin especially in patients with
penicillin hypersensitivity. Acne.
Dosage: adults, 1g twice each day.
Children under 2 years, 250mg; 2 to 8
years, 500mg; over 8 years, 1g. All twice
daily.
Special care: patients with liver disease.
Possible interaction: digoxin, oral
anticoagulants, astemizole, theophylline,
terfenadine, carbamazepine.
Side effects: allergic reactions, gastro-
intestinal upset, cholestatic jaundice.
Manufacturer: Abbott.

ESIDREX

Description: a proprietary thiazide
diuretic preparation produced in the
form of white scored tablets containing
25mg and 50mg of hydrochlorthiazide,
and marked CIBA and UT.
Used for: oedema and hypertension.
Dosage: 25–100mg each morning after
breakfast as a single dose, in first instance.
Dose is then reduced to 25–50mg taken
on alternate days.
Special care: pregnancy, breastfeeding,
elderly persons, diabetes, kidney or liver
disease, gout, cirrhosis of the liver, SLE.
Monitoring of electrolytes, glucose and
fluid levels should be carried out.
Avoid use: patients with serious kidney
or liver failure, sensitivity to sulphonamide drugs, Addison's disease,
hypercalcaemia.
Possible interaction: NSAIDs, alcohol,
opioid and barbiturate drugs, antidiabetic
preparations, corticosteroids, cardiac
glycosides, lithium, carbenoxolone,
tubocurarine.
Side effects: disturbance of metabolism
and electrolyte levels, sensitivity to
light, blood changes, rash, gastro-
intestinal upset, pancreatitis, anorexia,
giddiness, impotence.
Manufacturer: CIBA.

ESKAZOLE

Description: an anthelmintic preparation

designed to act against the larval stages
of 2 species of small parasitic
tapeworms, *Echinococcus granulosus*
and *Echinococcus multilocularis*. It is
produced in the form of oblong, orange,
scored tablets marked SKF, containing
400mg algendazole.
Used for: hydatid cysts.
Dosage: adults over 60kg body weight
800mg each day for 28 days in divided
doses, followed by 14 tablet-free days.
There should be a maximum of 3 cycles
of treatment.
Special care: blood counts and liver
function tests should be carried out.
Avoid use: children, adults under 60kg
bodyweight, women should use non-
hormonal methods of contraception during
treatment and for 1 month afterwards.
Possible interaction: oral contraceptives,
theophylline, anticoagulants, hypoglycaemics taken orally.
Side effects: changes in blood and liver
enzymes, headache, rash, giddiness,
fever, hair loss. Any advere side effects
should be reported.
Manufacturer: Smith-Kline.

ESTRACOMBI

Description: a combined oestrogen,
progestogen preparation in the form of
patches containing either 50µg
oestradiol per 24 hours, or 50µg
oestradiol and 250µg norethisterone
acetate per 24 hours, marked CGDWD
and CGFNF respectively.
Used for: hormone replacement therapy
for menopausal women. Prevention of
osteoporosis after the menopause.
Dosage: oestradiol only patch is applied
to hairless skin below waist twice each
week for 2 weeks, followed by the
combined patch twice weekly for 2
weeks. The patches are changed every 3
to 4 days and placed on a different area
of skin each time.
Special care: patients with a history, or
considered to be at risk, of thrombosis,
those with liver disease. Liver function
should be monitored and breasts and

pelvic organs examined periodically during the period of therapy. Women with any of the following require particularly careful monitoring: diabetes, fibroids in uterus, multiple sclerosis, hypertension, tetany, epilepsy, porphyria, gallstones, migraine, otosclerosis, history of breast cancer.

Avoid use: pregnancy, breastfeeding, thrombosis or thromboembolic disorders, serious heart, kidney or liver disease, endometriosis or vaginal bleeding which is undiagnosed, hormone-dependent cancers such as breast or uterine carcinoma, Dublin-Johnson or Rotor syndrome.

Possible interaction: drugs which induce liver enzymes.

Side effects: enlargement of and soreness in breasts, breakthrough bleeding, vomiting, nausea, gastro-intestinal disturbance, gain in weight, dizziness, headache. Withdraw immediately if frequent severe headaches or migraines occur, disordered vision, pregnancy, rise in blood pressure, signs of thromboembolism, jaundice. Stop before planned surgery.

Manufacturer: CIBA.

ESTRACYT

Description: a preparation of a sex hormone used to treat cancer, which is an oestrogenic alkylating agent, produced in the form of off-white capsules containing 140mg estramustine phosphate (as disodium salt).

Used for: prostatic cancer.

Dosage: adults, 4 capsules each day in divided doses taken 1 hour before meals or 2 hours afterwards, in first instance. Dose is then adjusted according to response of patient's conditioin with an average between 1 and 10 capsules each day. Capsules must not be taken with milk or dairy products.

Special care: bone marrow disorder.

Avoid use: patients with serious heart or liver disease or peptic ulcer.

Possible interaction: milk and dairy products.

Side effects: enlargement of breasts, toxic effects on heart, disturbance of liver function, gastro-intestinal upset.

Manufacturer: Pharmacia.

ESTRADERM

Description: an oestrogen patch containing either 25, 50 or 100µg oestradiol.

Used for: hormone replacement therapy in menopausal women. Prevention of osteoporosis following menopause.

Dosage: for oestrogen replacement; 1 patch is applied to hairless skin below waist and replaced every 3 or 4 days at a different site. The 50µg patch is used for prevention of osteoporosis.

Special care: patients with a history, or at risk, of thrombosis, those with liver disease. Liver function should be monitored and breasts and pelvic organs examined periodically during the period of therapy. Women with any of the following require particularly careful monitoring: diabetes, fibroids in uterus, multiple sclerosis, hypertension, tetany, epilepsy, porphyria, gallstones, migraine, otosclerosis (an hereditary rare disorder of the inner ear), history of breast cancer.

Avoid use: pregnant women, breastfeeding mothers, thrombosis or thromboembolic disorders, serious heart, kidney or liver disease, endometriosis or vaginal bleeding which is undiagnosed, hormone-dependent cancers such as breast or uterine carcinoma, Dublin-Johnson or Rotor syndrome.

Possible interaction: drugs which induce liver enzymes.

Side effects: enlargement of and soreness in breasts, breakthrough bleeding, vomiting, nausea, gastro-intestinal disturbance, gain in weight, dizziness, headache. Withdraw immediately if frequent, severe headaches or migraines occur, disordered vision, pregnancy, rise in blood pressure, signs of thromboembolism, jaundice. Stop before planned surgery.

Manufacturer: CIBA.

ESTRADURIN

Description: a preparation of a sex hormone used to treat cancer and local anaesthetic. It is produced as a powder in vials for reconstitution and injection and contains 80mg polyoestradiol phosphate and 5mg mepivacaine.
Used for: prostate cancer.
Dosage: adults, 80–160mg every 4 weeks given by deep intramuscular injection. Maintenance dose in order of 40–80mg.
Side effects: enlargement of breasts, impotence, oedema, heart disease and thromboembolism, jaundice, nausea.
Manufacturer: Pharmacia.

ESTRAPAK

Description: a combined oestrogen/progestogen preparation available as a patch containing 50µg oestradiol per 24 hours, and as red tablets, marked DG and LK, containing 1mg norethisterone acetate.
Used for: hormone replacement therapy for menopausal women. Prevention of osteoporosis after the menopause.
Dosage: apply patch to hairless skin below waist and replace with new patch in different site every 3 to 4 days. Take 1 tablet each day starting on 15th day through to 26th day of each period of 28 days of oestrogen replacement therapy. Therapy should begin within 5 days of the start of the period if this is present.
Special care: patients with a history, or considered to be at risk, of thrombosis, those with liver disease. Liver function should be monitored and breasts and pelvic organs examined periodically during the period of therapy. Women with any of the following require particularly careful monitoring: diabetes, fibroids in uterus, multiple sclerosis, hypertension, tetany, epilepsy, porphyria, gallstones, migraine, otosclerosis, history of breast cancer.
Avoid use: pregnancy, breastfeeding, thrombosis or thromboembolic disorders, serious heart, kidney or liver disease, endometriosis or vaginal bleeding which is undiagnosed, hormone-dependent cancers such as breast or uterine carcinoma, Dublin-Johnson or Rotor syndrome.
Possible interaction: drugs which induce liver enzymes.
Side effects: enlargement of and soreness in breasts, breakthrough bleeding, vomiting, nausea, gastro-intestinal disturbance, gain in weight, dizziness, headache. Withdraw immediately if frequent, severe headaches or migraines occur, disordered vision, pregnancy, rise in blood pressure, signs of thromboembolism, jaundice. Stop before planned surgery.
Manufacturer: CIBA.

ETHMOZINE

Description: a class I antiarrhythmic preparation, moracizine hydrochloride, available in the form of white, film-coated tablets of different strengths. Round tablets contain 200mg; oval tablets contain 250mg and capsule-shaped tablets contain 300mg. All are marked ROBERTS and with name and strength.
Used for: ventricular arrhythmias (arising in the ventricles of the heart).
Dosage: adults, 200–300mg at 8-hour intervals which may be increased, if required, by 150mg per day every 3 days to a maximum daily dose of 900mg.
Special care: pregnancy, liver or kidney disease, congestive heart failure, sick sinus syndrome. Therapy should be started in hospital and electrolyte levels stabilised before beginning. ECG should be monitored.
Avoid use: breastfeeding, children, patients with heart block, heart shock, recent myocardial infarction.
Possible interaction: cimetidine, theophylline, digoxin.
Side effects: gastro-intestinal upset, chest, muscle and bone pains, disturbance of sleep, blurring of vision, sweating, dry mouth, nervousness, giddiness. If unexplained liver disorder, withdraw drug.
Manufacturer: Monmouth.

EUDEMINE

Description: an antihypertensive (vaso-dilator) and hyperglycaemic produced in ampoules for injection to treat hyper-tension and as tablets for hypoglycae-mia. Ampoules contain 15mg diazoxide/ml and white, sugar-coated tablets contain 50mg diazoxide.

Used for: serious hypertension, especially arising from kidney disease, hypertensive crisis, intractable hypoglycaemia.

Dosage: adults, for hypertension, 300mg by fast, intravenous injection while patient is lying down. Children, 5mg/kg body weight by fast intravenous injection. Adults and children, for hypoglycaemia, 5mg/kg body weight each day at first in 2 or 3 divided doses. Afterwards, adjust according to response.

Special care: pregnancy, serious kidney, heart or cerebral disease, kidney failure, low blood protein levels. Regular checks on blood count, blood pressure, blood glucose levels are required and also monitoring of development and growth in children.

Possible interaction: anticoagulants of coumarin type, other antihypertensives, diuretics.

Side effects: hyperglycaemia, nausea, imbalance electrolyte and fluid levels, tachycardia, vomiting, arrhythmias, orthostatic hypotension (low blood pressure when person is standing), delay in onset of labour, possible coma.

Manufacutrer: Link.

EUGLUCON

Description: an oral hypoglycaemic preparation, glibenclamide, in the form of white tablets of 2 strengths. Tablets marked EU and 2.5 contain 2.5mg and scored, oblong tablets, marked EU-BM, contain 5mg. Glibenclamide belongs to a group of antidiabetic agents called sulphonylureas which enhance the effects of insulin and stimulate its secretion from cells in the pancreas.

Used for: diabetes which develops in adults (maturity-onset or non-insulin dependent type II diabetes).

Dosage: adults, 5mg each day at first, taken at breakfast time, increasing if required by 2.5mg each day at intervals of 1 week. The maximum daily dose is 15mg.

Special care: elderly persons or patients with kidney failure.

Avoid use: pregnancy, breastfeeding, some other types of diabetes (including juvenile, unstable-brittle and growth-onset), patients with infections, hormonal disorders, serious kidney or liver disease, stress, undergoing surgery, ketoacidosis (accumulation of ketones in the body characterized by "pear drops" smell on breath and resulting from diabetes mellitus).

Possible interaction: chloramphenicol, diuretics, anticoagulants taken by mouth, glucagon, chlorpropamide, metiformin, aspirin, MAOIs, oral contraceptives, corticotrophin, corticosteroids, alcohol, phenylbutazone, cyclophosphamide, rifampicin, bezafibrate, diuretics, anticoagulants taken orally.

Side effects: allergic reactions including skin rash.

Manufacturer: Roussel.

EUGYNON 30

Description: a combined oestrogen/pro-gestogen and contraceptive produced in the form of white, sugar-coated tablets containing 30µg ethinyloestradiol and 250µg levonorgestrel.

Used for: oral contraception.

Dosage: 1 tablet each day for 21 days starting on first day of period followed by 7 tablet-free days.

Special care: hypertension, severe kidney disease, dialysis, Raynaud's disease, diabetes, multiple sclerosis, asthma; varicose veins, elevated levels of prolactin (a hormone) in the blood (hyperprolac-taemia). Risk of thrombosis increases with smoking, age and obesity. Blood pressure, breasts and pelvic organs should be checked during period of treatment.

Avoid use: pregnancy, heart and circulatory diseases, angina, sickle cell

anaemia, pulmonary hypertension. Also hormone-dependent cancers, otosclerosis, undiagnosed vaginal bleeding, chorea, liver disease, history of cholestatic jaundice of pregnancy, infectious hepatitis, Dublin-Johnson syndrome, Rotor syndrome, recent trophoblastic disease.
Possible interaction: phenytoin, carbamazepine, tetracyclines, primidone, chloral hydrate, glutehimide, rifampicin, griseofulvin, dichloralphenazone, ethosuximide, barbiturates.
Side effects: feeling of bloatedness due to fluid retention, leg pains, breast enlargement, muscular cramps, weight gain, breakthrough bleeding, depression, vaginal discharge, loss of libido, nausea, brown patches on skin (chloasma). Stop drug immediately if frequent, severe headaches occur or signs of thromboses, rise in blood pressure. Drug should be discontinued before major planned surgery.
Manufacturer: Schering H.C.

EUMOVATE

Description: a moderately potent topical steroid in the form of cream and ointment containing 0.05% clobetasone butyrate.
Used for: dermatitis, eczema and skin conditions responsive to steroids.
Dosage: apply thinly to affected area up to 4 times each day.
Special care: should not be used on face or on children for more than 5 days. Should be stopped gradually.
Avoid use: prolonged or extensive use especially pregnant women or continual use as a preventative. Should not be used to treat acne, leg ulcers, scabies, peri-oral dermatitis, tuberculous skin conditions, skin disorders caused by viruses, ringworm, any untreated bacterial or fungal skin infections.
Side effects: thinning of skin, adrenal gland suppression, hair growth, Cushingoid type symptoms (Cushing's syndrome).
Manufacturer: Glaxo.

EUMOVATE EYEDROPS

Description: Moderately potent steroid eyedrops containing 0.1% clobetasone butyrate. Also **EUMOVATE-N** which additionally contains an antibiotic (0.5% neomycin sulphate as eyedrops).
Used for: drops containing clobetasone butyrate only are used for non-infected inflammatory conditions of the eye. Eumovate-N drops are used for infected inflammatory conditions of the eye.
Dosage: 1 or 2 drops 4 times each day with more severe infections requiring more frequent application every 1 or 2 hours.
Special care: do not use for prolonged periods especially pregnant women and young children.
Avoid use: patients with soft contact lenses, those with tuberculous, fungal or viral infections, glaucoma, dendritic ulcer, infections containing pus.
Side effects: thinning of cornea, cataracts, rise in pressure within eye, fungal infection, sensitisation (patient becomes hypersensitive to drug).
Manufacturer: Cusi.

EVOREL

Description: an oestrogen patch containing 50μg oestradiol per 24 hours.
Used for: hormone replacement therapy in menopausal women.
Dosage: apply patch to hairless area of skin below waist and change for a new patch in a different site after 3 or 4 days. Women who have not had a hysterectomy should also receive a progestogen preparation for 12 out of each 28 day period of treatment.
Special care: patients with history of or considered to be at risk of thrombosis, those with liver disease. Careful monitoring of women with any of the following is required: fibroids in uterus, otosclerosis, porphyria, tetany, epilepsy, gallstones, migraine, multiple sclerosis, hypertension, diabetes. Regular examination of pelvic organs and breasts required during course of therapy,

especially in women with family history of breast cancer.

Avoid use: pregnancy, breastfeeding, women with breast cancer or other cancers which are hormone-dependent, e.g. of genital tract; serious heart, liver or kidney disease, endometriosis, thrombosis, Dublin-Johnson or Rotor syndrome, undiagnosed vaginal bleeding.

Possible interaction: drugs which induce liver enzymes.

Side effects: enlargement and tenderness of breasts, nausea and vomiting, weight gain, breakthrough bleeding, gastro-intestinal upset, headache, giddiness. Withdraw drug immediately if any sign of thrombosis, rise in blood pressure, severe and frequent headaches, migraines, disturbance of vision, jaundice, pregnancy. Stop before planned surgery.

Manufacturer: Ortho.

EXELDERM

Description: an antifungal preparation, an imidazole, produced in the form of a cream containing 1% sulconazole nitrate.

Used for: fungal skin and nail infections.

Dosage: massage in twice each day and continue for 2 to 3 weeks after symptoms have disappeared.

Avoid use: contact with eyes.

Side effects: skin irritation—stop use.

Manufacturer: Zeneca.

EXIREL

Description: a bronchodilator selective $_2$-agonist produced in the form of capsules. Olive/turquoise capsules contain 10mg pirbuterol (as hydrochloride) and beige/turquoise capsules contain 15mg. All are marked with strength, 3M and MXR. Also, **EXIREL INHALER** containing 0.2mg pirbuterol (as acetate) per metered dose delivered by aerosol inhaler.

Used for: bronchial spasm in asthma, emphysema and bronchitis.

Dosage: adults, tablets, 10–15mg 3 or 4 times each day with a maximum dose of 60mg. Inhaler, relief of acute attack, 1 or 2 puffs in 1 dose; prevention, 2 puffs 3 or 4 times each day with a maximum of 12 puffs in 24 hours.

Special care: pregnant women, patients with weak hearts, heart arrhythmias, hypertension, angina, hyperthyroidism.

Avoid use: children.

Possible interaction: sympathomimetics.

Side effects: dilation of peripheral blood vessels, headache, nervousness, tremor.

Manufacturer: 3M Health Care.

EXOCIN

Description: a 4-quinolone antibiotic preparation produced in the form of eyedrops containing 0.3% olfloxacin.

Used for: bacterial eye infections.

Dosage: 1 or 2 drops every 2 to 4 hours into eye during first 2 days of treatment. Then reduce to 1 or 2 drops 4 times daily. Use for a maximum period of 10 days.

Special care: pregnancy, breastfeeding.

Avoid use: patients with soft contact lenses.

Side effects: short-lived eye irritation, rarely headache, dizziness, nausea, numbness.

Manufacturer: Allergan.

EXOSURF NEONATAL

Description: a preparation which acts as a lung surfactant produced as a powder in vials (with diluent) for reconstitution. The powder contains 108mg colfosceril palmitate.

Used for: newborn babies suffering from respiratory distress syndrome who are receiving mechanical ventilation.

Dosage: 67.5mg/kg body weight by means of endotracheal tube; may be repeated after 12 hours.

Special care: for use in babies of a weight greater than 700g; must be continually monitored due to risk of too much oxygen entering blood.

Side effects: tube may become blocked by mucous secretions; risk of pulmonary haemorrhage.

Manufacturer: Wellcome.

EYE-CROM

Description: an anti-inflammatory preparation in the form of eye drops containing 2% sodium cromoglycate.
Used for: allergic conjunctivitis.
Dosage: 1 or 2 drops into eye up to 4 times each day continuing after symptoms have disappeared.
Avoid use: patients with soft contact lenses.
Side effects: passing stinging or burning in eye.
Manufacturer: Norton.

FABROL

Description: a mucolytic preparation produced in the form of granules in sachets for dissolving in water containing 200mg acetylcysteine. It is for cystic fibrosis patients with accompanying abdominal complications.
Used for: bronchitis and infections of the respiratory tract in which a lot of mucus is produced; abdominal problems in cystic fibrosis.
Dosage: respiratory diseases, 3 sachets daily in divided doses; cystic fibrosis, normally 1 or 2 sachets 3 times each day. Children, respiratory diseases, under 2 years, 1 sachet each day; 2 to 6 years, 1 sachet twice each day; over 6 years, as adult dose. Cystic fibrosis, under 2 years, half to 1 sachet 3 times each day; 2 to 6 years, 1 or 2 sachets 3 times each day.
Special care: patients with diabetes.
Side effects: headache, skin rash, vomiting and nausea, gastro-intestinal upset, tinnitus; rarely bronchospasm, anaphylactic reactions (notify Committee on Safety of Medicines).
Manufacturer: Zyma.

FAMVIR

Description: a preparation which interferes with the manufacture of DNA within cells infected by a virus and is a nucleoside analogue produced in the form of white, film-coated tablets containing 250mg famciclovir. The tablets are marked with the strength and name.
Used for: infections caused by herpes zoster virus.
Dosage: adults, 1 tablet 3 times each day for 1 week.
Special care: kidney disease.
Avoid use: children, pregnancy breastfeeding mothers.
Side effects: nausea, headache.
Manufacturer: Smith Kline Beecham.

FANSIDAR

Description: a compound antimalarial preparation, combining a sulphonamide with a diaminopyrimidine drug, produced in the form of quarter-scored white tablets containing 500mg sulfadoxine and 25mg pyrimethamine. The tablets are marked with a hexagon and ROCHE.
Used for: treatment and prevention of malaria (caused by *Plasmodium falciparum*), especially where the disease does not respond to chloroquine.
Dosage: for prevention, adults and children over fourteen years, 1 tablet taken weekly; for treatment, adults and children over fourteen years, 2 to 3 tablets as a single dose. Children, for prevention, under 4 years of age quarter of adult dose; 4 to 8 years, half adult dose; 9 to fourteen years threequarters adult dose. For treatment, under 4 years of age, half tablet; 4 to 6 years, 1 tablet; 7 to 9 years, 1 and a half tablets; 10 to fourteen years, 2 tablets. All ages take tablets as a single dose.
Special care: patients should avoid being out in the sun and regular blood checks are required during long-term preventative treatment.
Avoid use: pregnancy, breastfeeding, newborn babies, patients with serious kidney or liver disease, blood changes o a sensitivity to sulphonamide drugs.
Possible interaction: folate inhibitors.

Side effects: discontinue therapy if pharyngitis (inflammation of pharynx) or pruritis occur. Gastro-intestinal upset, blood changes, skin rash. More rarely, allergic skin conditions.
Manufacturer: Roche.

FARLUTAL

Description: an anticancer drug which is a synthetic version of the female sex hormone, progestogen. It is produced in the form of a suspension in vials for injection, containing 200mg medroxy-progesterone acetate per ml and also in tablets of 3 strengths. White tablets contain 100mg; white scored tablets contain 250mg. Both are marked with tablet strength. White, scored, elongated tablets contain 500mg and are marked FCE 500.
Used for: cancer of breast, endometrium (womb), kidney cells and prostate gland.
Dosage: adults, tablets, breast cancer, 1–1.5g each day; kidney or prostate cancer, 100 -500mg each day.
Special care: patients suffering from epilepsy, diabetes, kidney or heart disease, asthma, migraine.
Avoid use: children, pregnant women, patients with thromboembolism, liver disease, thrombophlebitis (inflamed veins), hypercalcaemia.
Side effects: abnormal menstruation, abnormal production of breast milk, corticoid symptoms.
Manufacturer: Pharmacia.

FASIGYN

Description: an antibacterial preparation which is a nitroimidazole drug effective against certain anaerobic bacteria. It is produced in the form of white, film-coated tablets containing 500mg tinidazole.
Used for: treatment of infections caused by anaerobic bacteria and prevention of such during surgery. Particular sites of such infections are the mouth, gut and vagina (purulent gingivitis, pelvic inflammatory disease, non-specific vaginitis).

Dosage: adults, prevention of infection, 4 tablets taken as 1 dose; treatment, 4 tablets taken as 1 dose at first followed by 2 each day for 5 to 6 days.
Special care: pregnancy, breast-feeding.
Avoid use: children, patients with blood changes or neurological disorders.
Possible interaction: alcohol.
Side effects: unpleasant taste in mouth and furring of tongue, gastro-intestinal upset, nettle rash (urticaria), disturbance of central nervous system, dark-coloured urine, angioneurotic oedema. Rarely, nerve damage and leucopenia if drug is taken long-term.
Manufacturer: Pfizer.

FAVERIN

Description: an antidepressant drug, fluvoxamine, of a type known as 5HT reuptake inhibitors. Faverin is produced in the form of yellow, enteric-coated tablets of 2 strengths containing 50mg, marked DUPHAR and 291, or 100g, marked DUPHAR and 313.
Used for: depression.
Dosage: adults, 100mg taken at night in first instance with a normal maintenance dose in the order of 100–200mg each day in divided doses. The maximum dose is 300mg each day.
Special care: pregnancy, breastfeeding, kidney or liver disease or history of epilepsy.
Avoid use: children.
Possible interaction: alcohol, benzodiazepines, tryptophan, MAOIs, lithium, carbamazepine, propanolol, phenytoin, theophylline, tricyclic antidepressants.
Side effects: gastro-intestinal upset, nausea, diarrhoea, vomiting, nervousness, sleepiness, anorexia, convulsions, tremor.
Manufacturer: Duphar.

FELDENE

Description: a proprietary NSAID and oxicam, piroxicam, which is produced in a number of different forms. Feldene Capsules: blue/maroon capsules, marked FEL 10 and Pfizer, contain 10mg;

maroon capsules, marked FEL 20 and
Pfizer, contain 20mg. **FELDENE
DISPERSIBLE**: scored, white tablets
containing either 10mg or 20mg and
marked FEL 10 and Pfizer or FEL 20
and Pfizer respectively. Higher strength
tablets are oblong in shape. **FELDENE
MELT**: fast dissolving, off-white
coloured tablets containing 20mg;
FELDENE SUPPOSITORIES contain
20mg; **FELDENE INTRAMUSCU-
LAR INJECTION**: solution in
ampoules containing 20mg per ml.
FELDENE GEL: a topical gel
containing 0.5% piroxicam.
Used for: arthritic diseases including
juvenile arthritis, gout, rheumatoid
arthritis, ankylosing spondylitis,
osteoarthritis and other skeletal and
muscle diosrders.
Dosage: adults, preparations taken by
mouth or suppositories depending upon
condition being treated, but about 20–
40mg each day (Melt tablets are
dissolved on tongue and dispersible
tablets dissolved in water or swallowed
whole). Injection, used for acute attacks,
1 dose of 20–40mg by deep intramuscular injection into buttock. Then tablets
should be taken for maintenance.
Feldene Gel is for use by adults only in
patients with tendinitis, musculoskeletal
injuries or joint problems. 3cm gel is
applied to affected area 3 or 4 times each
day for 4 weeks. Children over 6 years
of age, for juvenile arthritis only, usually
dispersible tablets, under 15kg of body
weight, 5mg; 16–25kg of body weight,
10mg; 26–45kg body weight, 15mg;
over 45kg body weight, 20mg. All are
daily doses. Injection and gel are not for
use in children.
Special care: eldery, heart failure, liver
or kidney disease. Feldene gel should not
be applied to broken or infected skin or
eyes, and mucous membranes should be
avoided.
Avoid use: pregnancy, breastfeeding,
patients with allergy to NSAID or
aspirin, peptic ulcers, history of ulcers,

anal inflammation (use suppositories).
Possible interaction: other NSAIDs,
lithium, anticoagulants, hypoglycaemics.
Side effects: gastro-intestinal upset,
oedema, central nervous system
disturbance, malaise, tinnitus,
inflammation at injection site. Gel may
cause skin irritation, rash and itching.
Manufacturer: Pfizer.

FEMODENE

Description: a combined oestrogen/
progestogen hormonal oral contraceptive
in the form of white, sugar-coated tablets
containing 30µg ethinyloestradiol and
75µg gestodene.
Used for: oral contraception.
Dosage: 1 tablet daily, beginning on day
1 of period, for 21 days followed by 7
tablet-free days.
Special care: hypertension, severe
kidney disease receiving dialysis,
Raynaud's disease, diabetes, multiple
sclerosis, asthma, varicose veins,
elevated levels of prolactin (a hormone)
in the blood (hyperprolactaemia). Risk
of thrombosis increases with smoking,
age and obesity. Blood pressure, breasts
and pelvic organs should be checked
during period of treatment.
Avoid use: pregnancy, heart and
circulatory diseases, angina, sickle cell
anaemia, pulmonary hypertension. Also
hormone-dependent cancers, undiagnosed
vaginal bleeding, chorea, liver disease,
history of cholestatic jaundice of
pregnancy, infectious hepatitis,
Dublin-Johnson syndrome, Rotor
syndrome, recent trophoblasic disease.
Possible interaction: phenytoin,
carbamazepine, tetracyclines, primidone,
chloral hydrate, glutethimide, rifampicin,
griseofulvin, dichloralphenazone,
ethosuximide, barbiturates.
Side effects: feeling of bloatedness due
to fluid retention, leg pains, breast
enlargement, muscular cramps, weight
gain, breakthrough bleeding, depression,
vaginal discharge, loss of libido, nausea,
brown patches on skin (chloasma). Stop

drug immediately if frequent, severe headaches occur or signs of thromboses, rise in blood pressure. Drug should be discontinued before major planned surgery.
Manufacturer: Schering H.C.

FEMODENE E.D.

Description: a combined oestrogen/ progestogen hormonal oral contraceptive preparation consisting of 21 white, sugar-coated tablets containing 30µg ethinyloestradiol and 75µg gestodene and 7 white, sugar-coated placebo tablets containing lactose.
Used for: oral contraception.
Dosage: 1 tablet daily starting on first day of period with numbered tablet from red part of pack. Tablets are taken each day without a break, either hormonal or placebo depending upon the time in the cycle.
Special care: hypertension, severe kidney disease receiving dialysis, Raynaud's disease, diabetes, multiple sclerosis, asthma, varicose veins, elevated levels of prolactin (a hormone) in the blood (hyperprolactaemia). Risk of thrombosis increases with smoking, age and obesity. Blood pressure, breasts and pelvic organs should be checked during period of treatment.
Avoid use: pregnancy, heart and circulatory diseases, angina, sickle cell anaemia, pulmonary hypertension. Also hormone-dependent cancers, otosclerosis, undiagnosed vaginal bleeding, chorea, liver disease, history of cholestatic jaundice of pregnancy, infectious hepatitis, Dublin-Johnson syndrome, Rotor syndrome, recent trophoblasic disease.
Possible interaction: phenytoin, carbamazepine, tetracyclines, primidone, chloral hydrate, glutehimide, rifampicin, griseofulvin, dichloralphenazone, ethosuximide, barbiturates.
Side effects: feeling of bloatedness due to fluid retention, leg pains, breast enlargement, muscular cramps, weight gain, breakthrough bleeding, depression,

vaginal discharge, loss of libido, nausea, brown patches on skin (chloasma). Stop drug immediately if frequent, severe headaches occur or signs of thromboses, rise in blood pressure. Drug should be discontinued before major planned surgery.
Manufacturer: Schering H.C.

FEMULEN

Description: a hormonal preparation which is a progestogen only contraceptive in the form of white tablets containing 500µg ethinodiol diacetate marked with manufacturer's name.
Used for: oral contraception.
Dosage: 1 tablet at same time each day starting on first day of period and continuing without a break.
Special care: patients with history of, or considered to be at risk of thrombosis, hypertension, cysts on ovaries, hormone dependent cancer, liver disease. Blood pressure, breasts and pelvic organs should be checked regularly during the course of treatment.
Avoid use: pregnancy, previous ectopic pregnancy, history of heart or arterial disease or stroke, liver tumour, recent trophoblastic cancer, undiagnosed vaginal bleeding.
Possible interaction: meprobamate, chloral hydrate, ethosuximide, barbiturates, carbamazepine, chlorpromazine, griseofulvin, dichloralphenazone, pyrimidone, rifampicin, phenytoin, glutethimide.
Side effects: headache, breast tenderness, ovarian cysts, acne, disruption to normal pattern of menstrual bleeding, acne. Discontinue immediately if jaundice, signs of thrombosis or thrombophlebitis occur.
Manufacturer: Gold Cross.

FENBID SPANSULE

Description: a proprietary NSAID which is a propionic acid produced in the form of sustained-release spansules. Maroon/ pink capsules contain off-white pellets consisting of 300mg ibuprofen.

Used for: pain and arthritic conditions including ankylosing spondylitis, rheumatoid arthritis, osteoarthritis and other disorders of the skeleton and joints.
Dosage: 2 capsules twice each day at first increasing to 3 capsules twice daily if required. The maintenance dose is in the order of 1 or 2 capsules twice each day.
Special care: pregnancy, breastfeeding, elderly, asthma, disease of the gastro-intestinal tract, heart, liver or kidney disorders. Patients taking the drug long-term require careful monitoring.
Avoid use: children, patients with allergy to aspirin or other anti-inflammatory drugs, peptic ulcer.
Possible interaction: thiazide diuretics, quinolones, anticoagulant drugs.
Side effects: rash, gastro-intestinal upset and possibly bleeding, thrombocytopenia (If a patient contracts aseptic meningitis, it must be reported to the Committee on the Safety of Medicines).
Manufacturer: Goldshield.

FENOPRON

Description: a proprietary NSAID and propionic acid, fenoprofen (as calcium salt), produced in the form of tablets of 2 different strengths. Oval-shaped, orange tablets, coded DISTA 4019, contain 300mg ; oblong-shaped orange tablets coded DISTA 4021, contain 600mg.
Used for: pain and arthritic conditions including ankylosing spondylitis, rheumatoid arthritis and osteoarthritis.
Dosage: 300–600mg 3 to 4 times daily with a maximum daily dose of 3g.
Special care: pregnancy, breastfeeding, elderly, liver or kidney disease, heart failure, asthma, a history of disorders involving gastro-intestinal bleeding. Patients taking the drug long-term should receive careful monitoring.
Avoid use: children, patients with ulcers, allergy to aspirin or anti-inflammatory drugs, serious kidney disorders.
Possible interaction: aspirin, quinolones, loop diuretics, anticoagulants, hydantoins, phenobarbitone, sulphonylureas.

Side effects: allergic responses, intolerance of gastro-intestinal tract, blood changes, kidney and liver disorders.
Manufacturers: Dista.

FENTAZIN

Description: a potent antipsychotic preparation and group III phenothiazine (a piperazine), produced as tablets of 2 strengths. White, sugar-coated tablets, coded 1C, contain 2mg perphenazine; white, sugar-coated tablets coded 2C contain 4mg.
Used for: various serious psychiatric disorders including schizophrenia, psychoses, anxiety, nervous stress, vomiting and nausea.
Dosage: adults, 12mg each day in divided doses with a maximum of 24mg daily; elderly persons, quarter to half the full dose.
Special care: pregnancy, breastfeeding, epilepsy, glaucoma, Parkinson's disease, liver disease, hypothyroidism, myasthenia gravis, cardiovascular disease, phaeochromocytoma, enlarged prostate gland.
Avoid use: children, patients with depressed bone marrow or in comatose states.
Possible interaction: alcohol, anti-arrhythmic drugs, anaesthetics, antidepressants, antacids, rifampicin, sulphonylureas, antihypertensives, antiepileptic and antidiabetic drugs.
Side effects: allergic responses, effects on liver and jaundice, changes in menstruation, breasts, weight gain, impotence, effects on heart rhythm (tachycardia), blurred vision, dry mouth, difficulty with urination, blocked nose, constipation, drowsiness, pallor, apathy, insomnia, hypotension, convulsions, effects on eyes and skin colouration with higher doses.
Manufacturer: Forley.

FERFOLIC SV

Description: a combined mineral and vitamin preparation with a haematinic

(iron) and vitamin B component. It is produced in the form of pink, sugar-coated tablets containing 4mg folic acid, 250mg ferrous gluconate and 10mg ascorbic acid.
Used for: anaemias and conditions characterized by deficiency of iron and folic acid. Also used as a preventative to reduce the risk of neural tube defects in a foetus, when a mother known to be at risk is planning a pregnancy.
Dosage: adults, for deficiency, 1 tablet 3 times each day. Prevention of neural tube defects, 1 tablet each day when conception is planned and continuing during first 3 months of pregnancy.
Avoid use: children, patients with megaloblastic anaemia.
Possible interaction: tetracycline antibiotics.
Side effects: constipation, nausea.
Manufacturer: Sinclair.

FERTIRAL

Description: a hormonal preparation of gonadotrophin-releasing hormone, produced in the form of a solution in ampoules for infusion containing 500 micrograms gonadorelin per ml.
Used for: amenorrhoea and certain types of infertility in women.
Dosage: determined individually.
Special care: maximum period of treatment is 6 months and should be discontinued in the event of pregnancy.
Avoid use: patients with cysts in the ovaries or lining of the womb.
Side effects: headache, nausea, abdominal pain, pain at infusion site, menorrhagia (abnormally long or heavy menstrual periods).
Manufacturer: Hoechst.

FILAIR

Description: an anti-inflammatory corticosteroid preparation containing 50 or 100µg beclomethasone dipropionate delivered by metered dose aerosol. Also, FILAIR FORTE containing 250µg.
Used for: reversible obstructive airways disease (asthma).

Dosage: adults, 100µg, 3 or 4 times each day or 200µg twice each day. In extremely severe conditions 600–800µg in divided doses, with a maximum of 1mg, may be taken. Filair Forte, 500µg twice each day or 250µg 4 times each day. Children, Filair only, 50–100µg 2, 3 or 4 times each day.
Special care: pregnancy, history of or active pulmonary tuberculosis, those transferring from other (systemic) steroid drugs.
Side effects: hoarse voice, candidiasis (yeast-like fungal infection) of throat and mouth.
Manufacturer: 3M Health Care.

FLAGYL

Description: an antibacterial preparation and nitroimidazoles, which is effective against anaerobic bacteria and certain other infective organisms. It is produced in a variety of forms: Flagyl tablets, off-white, film-coated tablets contain 200mg and 400mg metronidazole, the higher strength being capsule-shaped. Both are marked with strength and tablet name. FLAGYL-S SUSPENSION contains 200mg metronidazole (as benzoate) per 5ml liquid. FLAGYL SUPPOSITORIES contain 500mg and 1g metronidazole. FLAGYL COMPAK consists of fourteen off-white, film-coated, capsule-shaped tablets containing 400mg metronidazole, marked with name and strength and also fourteen pale yellow coloured pessaries containing 100,000 units nystatin. FLAGYL INTRAVENOUS INFUSION contains 5mg metronidazole per ml in ampoules for intravenous infusion.
Used for: infections caused by anaerobic bacteria, amoebic dysentery, abscess of liver, trichomoniasis (of urogenital tract), vaginosis of bacterial origin, dental infections and severe ulcerative gingivitis. Prevention of infection before surgery.
Dosage: depending upon condition being treated, adults, in the order of 400mg–1g every 8 hours in first instance, then

reduced doses. Period of treatment is usually 1 week. Children receive reduced doses usually in the order of 7.5mg/kg body weight. In cases of vaginosis, sexual partner should also receive therapy at same time.

Special care: pregnancy, breastfeeding, patients with disorders of central nervous system, hepatic encephalopathy (a liver disease in which toxic substances normally removed by the liver interfere with the function of the brain).

Possible interaction: phenobarbitone, alcohol, lithium, anticoagulant drugs taken orally.

Side effects: central nervous system effects, dark coloured urine, unpleasant taste in mouth and furring of tongue, gastro-intestinal upset, rash, angioneurotic oedema, leucopenia. Long-term therapy may cause neuropathy (nerve disorders) and epileptic-type fits.

Manufacturer: Theraplix.

FLAMAZINE

Description: an antibacterial cream containing 1% silver sulphadiazine.

Used for: burns, skin wounds, pressure sores, infected leg ulcers, areas where skin has been removed for grafting.

Dosage: apply a layer of cream 3–5mm thick beneath dressing which should be changed daily for burns and 3 times each week for ulcers.

Special care: patients with liver or kidney disorders.

Avoid use: pregnancy, newborn babies.

Possible interaction: wound-cleaning agents with enzyme action, phenytoin, hypoglycaemic drugs taken orally, sulphonamides.

Manufacturer: S.N.P.

FLAXEDIL

Description: a muscle relaxant produced as a solution in ampoules for injection, containing 40mg gallamine triethiodide per ml.

Used for: to produce paralysis during surgical operations after the patient has

become unconscious and for seriously ill patients receiving prolonged artificial ventilation in intensive care.

Dosage: given by intravenous injection. Adults, 80–120mg and then 20–40mg as needed. Child, 1.5mg/kg body weight; newborn baby, 600µg/kg body weight.

Special care: kidney disorder.

Avoid use: serious kidney disease.

Possible interaction: some antiarrhythmic drugs, some antibacterial drugs, propranolol, verapamil, nifedipine, some cholinergics, magnesium salts, lithium.

Side effects: tachycardia.

Manufacturer: Rhône-Poulenc Rorer.

FLEMOXIN

Description: an antibiotic preparation which is a broad-spectrum penicillin. Flemoxin is produced as white, scored, dissolvable tablets of 2 strengths containing 375mg (marked gbr 183) and 750mg (marked gbr 185) amoxycillin (as trihydrate).

Used for: soft tissue, respiratory tract, urinary tract and ear, nose and throat infections.

Dosage: depending upon type of infection; adults in the order of 375mg–3g, usually twice each day. Tablets may be dissolved in water or swallowed whole. Children, 2–5 years of age, 750mg twice each day; 5 to 10 years, half adult dose; over 10 years, adult dose.

Special care: patients with lymphatic leukaemia, glandular fever.

Side effects: allergic reactions, rash, gastro-intestinal upset.

Manufacturer: Paines and Byrne.

FLEXIN CONTINUS

Description: a NSAID available as continuous-release tablets of thee strengths, all of which are capsule-shaped and marked with strength and 1C. Green, red and yellow tablets contain 25mg, 50mg and 75mg indomethacin respectively.

Used for: arthritic disorders of joints

nd skeleton including osteoarthritis,
nkylosing spondylitis, rheumatoid
rthritis, degenerative disease of the
ip joint, other musculo-skeletal and
ack disorders which cause pain,
ysmenorrhoea (period pain).
Dosage: adults, 25–200mg each day in
or 2 divided doses taken with food,
nilk or antacid preparation.
Special care: elderly persons, patients
vith heart failure, liver or kidney
isease, disorders of the central nervous
ystem. Those taking the drug long-term
equire careful monitoring and eye tests.
Avoid use: pregnancy, breastfeeding,
llergy to aspirin or anti-inflammatory
rug, defects in blood coagulation,
tomach ulcer or ulcer of gastro-
ntestinal lesions.
Possible interaction: corticosteroids, ß-
lockers, quinolones, diuretics,
nethotrexate, salicylates, lithium,
robenecid, anticoagulants.
Side effects: rash, blood changes, effects
n central nervous system, giddiness,
isual disturbance, corneal deposits,
lood in urine, adverse kidney effects
nephrotoxicity), tinnitus, inflammation
f small blood vessels (angitis). Drug
nould be discontinued if recurring
eadaches or gastro-intestinal bleeding
ccur.
Manufacturer: Napp.

FLIXONASE

Description: a corticosteroid nasal spray
0 μg fluticasone propionate per
netered dose.
Used for: prevention and treatment of
llergic rhinitis (hay fever), nasal
ongestion.
Dosage: adults, 2 sprays into each nostril
the morning, with a maximum of 4
prays into both nostrils daily. Children,
ver 4 years of age, 1 spray (maximum
f 2) into each nostril daily.
Special care: pregnancy, breastfeeding,
ansferring from other (systemic)
eroid drugs taken orally.
Avoid use: children under 4 years of age.

Side effects: nosebleed, irritation of
nose, interference with sense of taste
and smell.
Manufacturer: A & H.

FLIXOTIDE

Description: a corticosteroid preparation
containing fluticasone propionate for use
with diskhaler and inhaler. 50, 100, 250
and 500μg fluticasone propionate disks
are for use with breath-operated
diskhaler delivery system. Also, 25, 50,
125 and 250μg fluticasone propionate
per dose are for use with metered dose
aerosol delivery system.
Used for: prevention of bronchial
asthma.
Dosage: adults, 100–1000μg twice
each day; children over 4 years of age,
50–100μg twice each day.
Special care: pregnancy, transferring
from other (systemic) steroid drugs
taken orally, those with history of or
with active tuberculosis.
Avoid use: children under 4 years of age.
Side effects: candidiasis (a yeast-like
fungal infection) of throat and mouth,
hoarseness, occasional unexplained
bronchospasm
Manufacturer: A & H.

FLOLAN

Description: an anticoagulant
prostaglandin preparation produced in
the form of a powder containing 500μg
epoprostenol (as sodium salt) with a
diluent for reconstitution and infusion.
Used for: prevention of blood clotting
during and following heart surgery;
kidney dialysis (with heparin).
Dosage: according to manufacturer's
literature.
Special care: if being given with heparin
in kidney dialysis, anticoagulant
monitoring must be carried out. Must be
given by continuous intravenous infusion.
Side effects: vasodilation, flushing,
hypotension, headache, pallor,
bradycardia, sweating.
Manufacturer: Wellcome.

FLORINEF

Description: a corticosteroid mineralocorticoid preparation produced in the form of scored, pink tablets coded 429 and marked SQUIBB, containing 0.1mg fludrocortisone acetate. Mineralocorticoids regulate the salt/water balance in the body.

Used for: treatment of salt-losing adrenogenital syndrome and to partially replace hormones in Addison's disease.

Dosage: adults, 0.05–3mg each day; children, according to body weight, age and condition being treated.

Special care: pregnancy, hypertension, epilepsy, kidney inflammation (nephritis, glomerulonephritis), diabetes, inflamed veins, stomach ulcer. Patients with glaucoma, secondary cancers, osteoporosis, liver cirrhosis, tuberculosis and other bacterial, viral or fungal infections, recent surgical bowel anastomoses, those suffering from psychoses or stress. Contact wtht chicken pox should be avoided and medical advice sought in the event of this occurring. Withdraw drug gradually.

Possible interaction: anticoagulants taken orally, diuretics, ephedrine, phenytoin, cardiac glycosides, NSAIDs, phenobarbitone, hypoglycaemics, rifampicin, anticholinesterases.

Side effects: fluid retention, hypertension, weakness in muscles, loss of potassium, Cushingoid changes (as in Cushing's syndrome).

Manufacturer: Squibb.

FLOXAPEN

Description: a penicillinase-resistant form of penicillin. (Penicillinase is an enzyme produced by some bacteria that renders penicillin inactive, hence the infection being treated will be resistant to the antibiotic). Floxapen is produced in several forms: black/caramel-coloured capsules of 2 strengths containing 250mg and 500mg flucloxacillin sodium, each marked with strength and name. **FLOXAPEN SYRUP** contains 125mg

flucloxacillin (as magnesium salt) per 5ml, supplied as powder for reconstitution with water to make 100ml.

FLOXAPEN SYRUP FORTE contains 250mg per 5ml, supplied as powder to make 100ml. **FLOXAPEN INJECTION** is supplied as powder in vials for reconstitution at strengths of 250mg, 500mg and 1g flucloxacillin (as sodium salt).

Used for: ear, nose, throat, soft tisssue, skin infections and other infections including those caused by staphylococci bacteria resistant to penicillin.

Dosage: capsules and syrup, 250mg 4 times each day taken 1 hour to half an hour before meals. Injection, 250mg–1g given intravenously 4 times each day. Children, capsules, syrup and injection, age 2 years and under, quarter of adult dose; age 2 to 10 years, half adult dose; over 10 years, adult dose.

Avoid use: allergy to penicillin.

Side effects: gastro-intestinal upset, allergic responses, rarely cholestatic jaundice.

Manufacturer: Beecham.

FLUANXOL

Description: an antidepressant preparation and a thioxanthene, available as red, sugar-coated tablets of 2 strengths, containing 0.5mg and 1mg of flupenthixol (as dihydrochloride), both marked LUNDBECK.

Used for: short-term treatment of depression which may be accompanied by symptoms of anxiety.

Dosage: adults, 1–2mg as a single dose taken in the morning with a maximum daily amount of 3mg in divided doses. Elderly persons, 0.5mg as a single morning dose with a daily maximum of 2g in divided doses.

Special care: patients with serious heart circulatory, liver or kidney disease, arteriosclerosis, Parkinsonism, elderly persons in confused states.

Avoid use: children, overactive, excitable persons, those with very severe depression.

Possible interaction: other antidepressants, central nervous system sedatives, antihypertensives, anticonvulsants, levodopa, alcohol, antidiabetic drugs.
Side effects: dry mouth, blocked nose, visual disturbances, muscular spasms and Parkinsonism-like symptoms, hypotension, tiredness and lethargy. Weight gain, sleepiness, constipation, difficulty passing urine, enlargement of breasts and abnormal production of milk, dermatitis, blood changes, tachycardia and effects on ECG, jaundice, fits.
Manufacturer: Lundbeck.

FLUVIRIN

Description: a vaccine against influenza containing inactivated surface antigens of 3 strains of influenza virus produced in the form of 15 μs of each strain per 0.5ml solution in pre-filled syringes.
Used for: immunisation against influenza.
Dosage: adults, 0.5ml by intramuscular or deep subcutaneous injection. Children over 4 years of age, 0.5ml followed by a further 0.5ml after 1 month to 6 weeks.
Special care: pregnant women.
Avoid use: children under 4 years of age, patients with allergy to chicken or egg protein (as vaccines are cultivated on these).
Side effects: feverishness, headache, malaise, soreness at injection site, all uncommon and transient.
Manufacturer: Evans.

FLUZONE

Description: a vaccine against influenza containing inactivated split virion of 3 strains of influenza virus. Produced in the form of pre-filled syringes containing 15 μs of each strain per 0.5ml.
Used for: immunisation against influenza.
Dosage: adults, 0.5ml by subcutaneous or intramuscular injection; children 6 months to 3 years, 0.25ml followed by further 0.25ml after 1 month; 3 years to 12 years, 0.5ml followed by further

0.5ml after 1 month; over thirteen years as adult.
Avoid use: patients with feverish illness, those with allergy to egg protein.
Side effects: feverishness, headache, malaise, soreness at injection site (of transient nature).
Manufacturer: Servier.

FML

Description: an anti-inflammatory corticosteroid in the form of eyedrops containing 0.1% fluorometholone. Also **FML NEO** corticosteroid and aminoglycoside eyedrops containing 0.1% fluorometholone and 0.5% neomycin sulphate.
Used for: FML—eye inflammation in which there is an absence of infection. FML Neo—eye inflammation in which infection is present.
Dosage: adults, 1 to 2 drops 2, 3 or 4 times daily directly into eye; children over 2 years of age, as adult dose.
Special care: glaucoma; prolonged use in young children or pregnant women.
Avoid use: infections with tuberculous, viral or fungal origin and those in which pus is present; soft contact lenses.
Side effects: rise in pressure within eye, thinning of cornea, secondary fungal infection, cataract.
Manufacturer: Allergan.

FOLICIN

Description: a haematinic and mineral supplement available in the form of white, sugar-coated tablets containing 2.5mg folic acid, 2.5mg manganese sulphate and 200mg dried ferrous sulphate (equivalent to 60mg iron).
Used for: prevention and treatment of anaemia in pregnant women.
Dosage: adults, 1 to 2 tablets each day.
Avoid use: patients with megaloblastic anaemia.
Possible interaction: levodopa, tetracyclines.
Side effects: constipation, nausea.
Manufacturer: Link.

FORCEVAL

Description: a preparation containing minerals, trace elements and vitamins produced in the form of brown/red gelatin capsules marked 6377 and FORCEVAL. Also, **FORCEVAL JUNIOR** available as oval brown gelatin capsules marked 571 and FORCEVAL.
Used for: a dietary supplement to prevent and treat mineral and vitamin deficiencies in patients unable to obtain adequate amounts from food alone. May be used, for example, in patients recuperating from serious illness or surgery, and those on special controlled diets or who have intolerance to foods.
Dosage: 1 capsule daily; children, Forceval Junior only, over 5 years of age, 2 capsules each day.
Avoid use: children under 5 years, patients with disorders of iron absorption and storage (haemochromatosis) or with hypercalcaemia.
Possible interaction: tetracyclines, anticoagulant drugs, phenytoin.
Manufacturer: Unigreg.

FORTAGESIC[CD]

Description: a controlled drug combining a narcotic analgesic with paracetamol, which has analgesic and antipyretic properties (reduces fever). It is produced in the form of white tablets, marked with name and symbol, containing 15mg pentazocine (as hydrochloride) and 500mg paracetamol. Pentazocine is a moderately potent analgesic and is less likely to cause addiction than some other narcotic drugs.
Used for: pain caused by disorders of bone and muscle.
Dosage: 2 tablets up to 4 times each day; children over 7 years, 1 tablet every 3 to 4 hours with a maximum of 4 in 24 hours.
Special care: pregnancy, liver, kidney or respiratory diseases, porphyria.
Avoid use: patients with brain injury or disease, raised intracranial pressure or who are narcotic dependent.

Possible interaction: alcohol, other narcotic drugs, MAOIs.
Side effects: nausea, dizziness, sedation, drug-induced symptoms of psychosis.
Manufacturer: Sanofi Winthrop.

FORTRAL[CD]

Description: a narcotic antagonist and controlled drug, produced in a variety of forms. White, film-coated tablets contain 25mg pentazocine hydrochloride, marked with symbol and name. **FORTRAL CAPSULES** marked FORTRAL 50 and coloured yellow/grey, contain 50mg. **FORTRAL INJECTION** contain 30mg pentazocine (as acetate) per ml in ampoules. **FORTRAL SUPPOSITORIES** contain 50mg.
Used for: relief of pain.
Dosage: adults, tablets or capsules, 25–100mg after meals every 3 to 4 hours; injection, 30–60mg by intravenous, intramuscular or subcutaneous injection every 3 to 4 hours; suppositories, 1 when required with a maximum of 4 in 24 hours. Children, tablets or capsules, 6 to 12 years, 25mg every 3 to 4 hours. Injection, children 1 to 12 years, either a maximum of 1mg/kg body weight as single dose by subcutaneous or intramuscular injection, or 0.5mg/kg body weight given intravenously as single dose.
Special care: pregnancy, liver, kidney or respiratory diseases.
Avoid use: children under 1 year of age, patients with brain injury or disease, raised intracranial pressure, narcotic dependent or who have porphyria.
Possible interaction: other narcotic drugs, alcohol, MAOIs.
Side effects: nausea, dizziness, sedation, drug-induced symptoms of psychosis.
Manufacturer: Sterwin.

FORTUM

Description: a cephalosporin antibiotic preparation produced in the form of powder in vials for reconstitution and

injection, containing 250mg 500mg, 1g, 2g and 3g ceftazidime (as pentahydrate).
Used for: urinary and gastro-intestinal tract infections, infections of ear, nose and throat, joints, bones, soft tissues, skin, meningitis, septicaemia and infections in patients who are immunocompromised.
Dosage: adults, 1g every 8 hours or 2g at 12 hour intervals. If infection is extremely severe, 2g every 8 to 12 hours. Single doses above 1g should be given intravenously, lower doses by intravenous injection or infusion or intramuscularly. Children, 2 months and under, 25–60mg/kg body weight in 2 divided doses each day; over 2 months, 30–100mg/kg body weight each day in 2 or 3 divided doses. A dose of up to 150mg/kg body weight may be given in cases of meningitis or if immunocompromised. In children, the intravenous route should be used. Elderly persons, a maximum dose of 3g each day depending upon type and severity of infection.
Special care: pregnant women, patients with allergy to penicillin (about 10% of whom are also allergic to cephalosporins), kidney disease.
Possible interaction: loop diuretics, aminoglycosides.
Side effects: gastro-intestinal upset, pain at injection site, blood changes involving white blood cells, candidiasis (infection caused by yeast-like fungus), allergic reactions, positive Coombs test, rise in level of blood urea and liver enzymes.
Manufacturer: Glaxo.

FOSCAVIR

Description: an antiviral preparation containing 24mg foscarnet sodium hexahydrate per ml produced as bottles of isotonic infusion.
Used for: life-threatening infections of viral origin particularly those of the eyes in patients with AIDS (cytomegalovirus retinitis).
Dosage: adults, 20mg/kg body weight by intravenous infusion over half an hour,

then 21–200mg/kg body weight each day for 2 to 3 weeks. (Dose depending upon kidney function).
Special care: patients with kidney disease, hypocalcaemia. Blood tests are required during therapy and patient should receive adequate fluids.
Avoid use: patients with severe kidney disease, pregnancy, breastfeeding.
Side effects: rash, nausea, headache, vomiting, tiredness, disturbance of kidney function including kidney failure, decreased haemoglobin and calcium levels. Rarely, convulsions, inflamed veins, hypoglycaemia.
Manufacturer: Astra.

FRAGMIN

Description: an anticoagulant preparation which is a low molecular weight heparin produced as a solution in ampoules for injection and which contain 2500 units or 10,000 units dalteparin sodium per ml. **FRAGMIN PRE-FILLED SYRINGES** contain 2500 units or 5000 units dalteparin sodium per 0.2ml.
Used for: prevention of thrombosis during and after surgery and clotting in extracorporeal circulation during dialysis treatment.
Dosage: dependent upon condition being treated (i.e. surgery or dialysis) and if patient is at high or low risk of bleeding (dialysis).
Special care: pregnancy, breastfeeding, liver disease, those at high risk of bleeding or in whom therapeutic effects of drug occur in narrow dose range. Careful monitoring and blood checks required.
Possible interaction: cardiac glycosides, other anticoagulant and antiplatelet drugs, indomethacin, tetracyclines, probencid, antihistamines, dextran, sulphinpyrazone, aspirin, ethacrynic acid, vitamin K antagonists, cytostatics, dipyradamole, cardiac glycosides.
Side effects: bleeding if dose is high.
Manufacturer: Pharmacia.

FRISIUM

Description: an anxiolytic and anticonvulsant which is a long-acting benzodiazepine produced in the form of blue capsules containing 10mg clobazum and marked FRISIUM.

Used for: anxiety and tense and agitated states; additional therapy in the treatment of epilepsy.

Dosage: adults, 20–30mg each day in divided dose or as single bedtime dose with a maximum of 60mg daily. Elderly persons, 20 mg each day. Children, age 3 to 12 years, half adult dose.

Special care: pregnancy, women in labour, breastfeeding, elderl, liver or kidney disease. Short-term use and withdraw gradually.

Avoid use: patients with breathing difficulties, lung diseases and respiratory depression, those suffering from phobic, psychotic or obsessional psychiatric illnesses. Children under 3 years.

Possible interaction: other central nervous system depressant drugs, anticonvulsants, alcohol.

Side effects: gastro-intestinal upset, light-headedness, disturbance of vision, vertigo, sleepiness, hypotension, confusion, rash, urine retention, reduced libido, ataxia. Rarely there may be blood changes and jaundice. Performance of skilled tasks and judgement is impaired, risk of dependence with higher doses and longer term therapy.

Manufacturer: Hoechst.

FROBEN

Description: an analgesic preparation which is a proprionic acid produced in the form of tablets of 2 strengths. Yellow, sugar-coated tablets contain 50mg and 100mg flurbiprofen, marked F50 and F100 respectively. Also FROBEN SR which are yellow, sustained-release capsules marked FSR containing 200mg flurbiprofen. FROBEN SUPPOSITORIES contain 100mg flurbiprofen

Used for: pain including dysmenorrhoea (period pain) (Froben tablets); musculoskeletal diseases, osteoarthritis and ankylosing spondylitis (Froben SR and Suppositories).

Dosage: adults, tablets, 100–200mg each day in divided doses with a maximum daily dose of 300mg. SR Capsules, 1 each day after evening meal. Suppositories, 150mg—200mg each day as divided doses with a daily maximum of 300mg.

Special care: pregnancy, breastfeeding, elderly, liver or kidney disease, heart failure, asthma. Those taking the drug long-term require careful monitoring.

Avoid use: children, patients with allergy to aspirin or anti-inflammatory drugs, those with stomach ulcer or gastro-intestinal bleeding.

Possible interaction: anticoagulant drugs, frusemide, quinolones.

Side effects: rash, intolerance of gastro-intestinal system, rarely thrombocytopenia, jaundice.

Manufacturer: Boots.

FRU-CO

Description: a potassium-sparing and loop diuretic produced in the form of scored, orange tablets containing 40mg frusemide amd 5mg amiloride hydrochloride (co-amilofuse), marked FRO-CO.

Used for: oedema accompanying kidney or liver disease, heart failure.

Dosage: adults, 1 or 2 tablets taken in the morning.

Special care: pregnancy, breastfeeding, elderly, liver or kidney disease, enlarged prostate gland, difficulty in urination, gout, diabetes, acidosis.

Avoid use: children, hyperkalaemia, coma resulting from cirrhosis of the liver, progressive kidney failure.

Possible interaction: other potassium-sparing diuretics and potassium supplements, hypoglycaemics, aminoglycosides, cephalosporins, lithium, antihypertensives, digitalis, NSAIDs, non-depolarising muscle relaxants (anaesthetics), ACE inhibitors.

Side effects: rash, gastro-intestinal upset, malaise; rarely, blood changes.
Manufacturer: Baker Norton.

FRUMIL

Description: a preparation which is a loop and potassium-sparing diuretic produced in the form of scored, orange tablets containing 40mg frusemide and 5mg amiloride hydrochloride (co-amilofruse) marked FRUMIL. Also FRUMIL LS, orange tablets containing 20mg frusemide and 2.5mg amiloride hydrochloride, marked LS. FRUMIL FORTE, orange scored tablets containing 80mg frusemide and 10mg amiloride hydrochloride, marked DS.
Used for: oedema accompanying kidney or liver disease and heart failure.
Dosage: adults, Frumil tablets, 1 or 2 taken in morning; Frumil LS and Frumil Forte, 1 tablet taken in morning.
Special care: elderly, liver or kidney disease, enlarged prostate gland, difficulty in urination, gout, diabetes, acidosis.
Avoid use: children, pregnancy, breastfeeding, hyperkalaemia, coma resulting from cirrhosis of the liver, progressive kidney failure.
Possible interaction: other potassium-paring diuretics and potassium supplements, ACE inhibitors, hypogly-aemics, antihypertensives, non-depolarising muscle relaxants anaesthetics), cardiac glycosides, NSAIDs, aminoglycosides, lithium, cephalosporins.
Side effects: rash, gastro-intestinal upset, malaise; rarely, blood changes.
Manufacturer: Theraplix.

FRUSENE

Description: a potassium-sparing and loop diuretic produced in the form of scored yellow tablets containing 40mg frusemide and 50mg triamterene.
Used for: oedema accompanying liver or heart disease, congestive heart failure.
Dosage: adults, half to 2 tablets each day

with a daily maximum of 6 (in divided doses).
Special care: pregnancy, breastfeeding mothers, gout, enlarged prostate gland, difficulty in urination, acidosis, liver or kidney disease, diabetes.
Avoid use: children, patients with coma resulting from liver cirrhosis, hyperka-laemia, progressive kidney failure.
Possible interaction: other potassium-sparing diuretics and potassium supplements, aminoglycosides, cardiac glycosides, neuromuscular blocking drugs, lithium, theophylline, NSAIDs, cephalosporins.
Side effects: rash, gastro-intestinal upset, malaise; rarely, blood changes.
Manufacturer: Fisons.

FUCIBET

Description: a potent steroid and antibacterial agent in the form of a cream containing 0.1% betmethasone valerate and 2% fusidic acid
Used for: eczema in which bacterial infection is likely to be present.
Dosage: apply thinly 2 or 3 times each day to affected skin and reduce dose when condition improves.
Special care: short-term use only (maximum of few weeks when lower potency substitute should be tried, if needed), withdraw gradually.
Avoid use: children, extensive or longer-term use in pregnant women, infections due to ringworm, virus, tuberculosis, untreated bacterial and fungal infections, leg ulcers, scabies, acne.
Side effects: adrenal gland suppression, skin thinning, abnormal hair growth, skin changes as in Cushing's syndrome.
Manufacturer: Leo.

FUCIDIN H

Description: an antibacterial agent and mildly potent corticosteroid. It is available as ointment, cream or gel, all containing 2% sodium fusidate and 1% hydrocortisone.
Used for: dermatitis in which bacterial

infection is likely to be present.
Dosage: apply thinly 2 or 3 times each day to affected skin and reduce dose when condition improves.
Special care: limit use in children or on face to a maximum period of 5 days.
Avoid use: extensive or long-term use especially in pregnant women, infections due to ringworm, virus, tuberculosis, untreated bacterial and fungal infections, leg ulcers, scabies, acne.
Side effects: adrenal gland suppression, skin thinning, abnormal hair growth, skin changes as in Cushing's syndrome.
Manufacturer: Leo.

FUCITHALMIC

Description: an antibacterial preparation produced in the form of an eye gel which becomes liquid when in contact with eye, containing 1% fusidic acid.
Used for: conjunctivitis where bacteria, especially staphylococci, are cause of infection.
Dosage: apply 1 drop into eye twice each day.
Side effects: allergic reaction, local irritation of short-lived nature.
Manufacturer: Leo.

FULCIN

Description: an antifungal preparation produced in the form of tablets of 2 strengths and as a solution. Scored, white tablets, marked ICI, contain 125mg and 500mg griseofulvin.
FULCIN SUSPENSION contains 125mg griseofulvin per 5ml of suspension.
Used for: fungal infections of scalp, skin and nails where ointments and creams have been ineffective or are not considered to be appropriate.
Dosage: adults, 125mg 4 times each day or a single dose of 500mg. Children, 10mg/kg body weight in divided doses or as a single dose.
Avoid use: pregnancy, serious liver disease or porphyria.
Possible interaction: oral contraceptives,

alcohol, barbiturates, anticoagulants of the coumarin group.
Side effects: allergic responses and rash, sensitivity to light, headache, stomach upset, blood changes involving white blood cells; rarely, a collagen disease.
Manufacturer: ICI.

FUNGILIN

Description: an antifungal preparation and polyene antibiotic, amphotericin, effective against filamentous and yeast-like fungi and which does not produce drug resistance. Fungilin is produced in the form of scored brown tablets containing 100mg and marked SQUIBB 430.
FUNGILIN SUSPENSION coloured yellow and containing 100mg per ml of solution. **FUNGILIN LOZENGES** coloured yellow containing 10mg and marked SQUIBB 929.
Used for: candidiasis of the intestine, vagina and skin (thrush) and prevention of infection. Lozenges are used for mouth infections.
Dosage: adults, 1 to 2 tablets or 1–2ml suspension each day; lozenges, 1 dissolved slowly in mouth 4 to 8 times each day. Children, suspension, 1ml 4 times each day.
Side effects: gastro-intestinal upset if dose is high.
Manufacturer: Squibb.

FUNGIZONE

Description: an antifungal preparation and polyene antibiotic, effective against filamentous and yeast-like fungi and which does not produce drug resistance. It is produced as a powder in vials for reconstitution and injection containing 50mg amphotericin sodium desoxycholate complex.
Used for: serious, life-threatening systemic fungal infections.
Dosage: by intravenous infusion, 250 μs/kg body weight each day increasing to 1mg in cases of severe infection, if drug is tolerated. Maximum dose is 1.5mg/kg body weight each day or every other day

Special care: produces toxic side effects when given in this way, hence patients require close monitoring of liver and kidney function, blood counts, electrolyte levels in blood plasma.
Special care: pregnancy, breastfeeding. Change injection site frequently.
Side effects: irritation at injection site, rash, vomiting, diarrhoea, nausea, headache, abdominal pain, anorexia, pain in muscles and joints, fever, adverse effects on liver, kidneys, heart, nerves, convulsions, loss of hearing, anaphylactic-type allergic reactions.
Manufacturer: Squibb.

FURADANTIN

Description: an antibacterial preparation which is of a type known as nitofurans (synthetic antibiotic drugs). It is produced in the form of scored, yellow pentagonal-shaped tablets of 2 strengths containing 50mg and 100mg nitrofurantoin both marked with strength and name. Also **FURADANTIN SUSPENSION** containing 25mg nitrofurantoin per 5ml suspension.
Used for: treatment and prevention of genital and urinary tract infections, (c.g. in patient undergoing surgery or exploratory procedure), pyelitis.
Dosage: adults, depending upon condition being treated, in the order of 50–100mg 4 times each day for 1 week (or once a day at bedtime if for prevention of infection on longer term basis), Children, age 3 months to 10 years, in the order of 3mg/kg body weight 4 times each day for 1 week or 1mg/kg once daily if for prevention. Over 10 years, same as adult.
Special care: children under 3 months, breastfeeding, elderly, patients with diabetes, vitamin B deficiency or who are debilitated, anaemia, imbalance of electrolyte (salt) levels. Patients should receive monitoring of liver and lung function if undergoing long-term treatment.
Avoid use: women at end of pregnancy,

kidney disorder, anuria or oliguria.
Possible interaction: probenecid, quinolones, magnesium trisilicate, sulphinpyrazone.
Side effects: gastro-intestinal upset, blood changes, allergic reactions. Drug should be stopped immediately if signs of peripheral nerve damage, lung disorder, breakdown of red blood cells (haemolysis), hepatitis occur.
Manufacturer: P. & G.P.

FYBOGEL MEBEVERINE

Description: a bulking agent and antispasmodic preparation, produced in the form of effervescent granules in sachets for dissolving in water, containing 135mg mebeverine hydrochloride, 3.5g ispaghula husk.
Used for: irritable bowel syndrome, diverticular disease, constipation due to insufficient dietary fibre.
Dosage: adults, 1 sachet every morning and evening half an hour before meals in water. Additional sachet before midday meal may also be taken.
Avoid use: patients with intestinal obstruction, serious heart, circulatory and kidney disorders.
Manufacturer: Reckitt and Colman.

GALENAMET

Description: a preparation that is an H_2-receptor antagonist which acts to reduce the secretion of stomach acid, thereby promoting the healing of ulcers. It is available in tablets of 3 strengths containing 200mg, 400mg and 800mg cimetidine.
Used for: gastro-intestinal ulcers, Zollinger-Ellison syndrome, reflux oesophagitis.
Dosage: for ulcers, 400mg twice each day morning and night, or 800mg taken

at night; occasionally, 400mg 4 times each day may be required with an absolute maximum of 2.4g daily in divided doses (in rare cases of stress ulceration). Zollinger-Ellison syndrome and reflux oesophagitis 400mg 4 times each day. Children, 20–30mg/kg body weight each day in divided doses.
Special care: pregnancy, breastfeeding, liver or kidney disease.
Possible interaction: phenytoin, warfarin, theophylline, some antidepressants, sulphonylureas, carbamazepine, some antifungal drugs, quinine, chloroquine, some antipsychotic drugs, benzodiazepines, ß-blockers, calcium channel blockers, cyclosporin, fluorouracil, flosequinan.
Side effects: rash, dizziness, fatigue, headache, confusion, change in bowel habit, lowered blood count, liver effects, allergic responses, bradycardia, pancreatitis, nephritis (inflammation in kidney), gynaecomastia, heart block. All are rare, but have been reported and may be more likely with higher doses.
Manufacturer: Galen.

GALENAMOX

Description: an antibiotic preparation of amoxicillin, a broad-spectrum penicillin but one which is inactivated by the penicillinase enzymes produced by some bacteria. Hence some infections do not respond as the bacteria causing them are resistant. Galenamox is available in the form of capsules of 2 strengths containing 250mg and 500mg amoxycillin (as trihydrate). Also as **GALENAMOX SUSPENSION** containing 125mg or 250mg per 5ml solution.
Used for: middle ear infections, secondary infections in chronic bronchitis, urinary tract infections, gonorrhoea, typhoid fever, prevention of endocarditis.
Dosage: depending upon type of infection but in the order of 250mg–500mg every 8 hours with higher doses of 3g every 12 hours sometimes being required. Children, depending upon

condition being treated but in the order of 125mg–250mg every 8 hours (up to 10 years of age). Higher doses may sometimes be needed.
Manufacturer: Galen.

GAMANIL

Description: a TCAD preparation available as scored, maroon-coloured, film-coated tablets containing 70mg lofepramine (as hydrochloride).
Used for: depression.
Dosage: adults, 1 tablet in morning and either 1 or 2 at night. Reduced doses for elderly patients.
Special care: elderly, breastfeeding, glaucoma, urinary retention, hyperthyroidism, diabetes, adrenal gland tumour, epilepsy, certain psychiatric disorders or at risk of suicide. Regular blood tests should be carried out.
Avoid use: pregnancy, heart block, heart attack, serious liver disease.
Possible interaction: other antidepressants, antihypertensives, barbiturates, alcohol, MAOIs, cimetidine, local anaesthetics containing noradrenaline or adrenaline, oestrogens.
Side effects: blurred vision, hypotension, sweating, anxiety, dizziness, sleeplessness, ataxia, muscle weakness, drowsiness, palpitations, dry mouth, tachycardia, constipation, gastrointestinal upset, weight changes, allergic responses including skin rash, blood changes, loss of libido or impotence, enlargement of breasts, abnormal milk production, jaundice. Also psychiatric effects especially in the elderly.
Manufacturer: Merck.

GAMMABULIN

Description: a preparation of 16% human normal immunoglobulin (HNIG) as a solution for intramuscular injection.
Used for: immunisation against hepatitis A, measles, rubella in pregnant women, antibody deficiency syndrome.
Dosage: prevention of hepatitis A, adults and children, 0.02–0.04ml/kg body

weight and possibly 0.06–0.12ml/kg body weight if risk is great. Prevention of measles, 0.2ml/kg body weight. Prevention of rubella in pregnant women, 20ml. All given by intramuscular injection.
Possible interaction: live vaccines.
Manufacturer: Immuno.

GANDA
Description: an adrenergic neurone blocker with a sympathomimetic produced in the form of drops to reduce pressure within the eye. It is available in 2 strengths: **GANDA 1 + 0.2** contains 1% guanethidine monosulphate and 0.2% adrenaline; **GANDA 3 + 0.5** contains 3% guanethidine monosulphate and 0.5% adrenaline.
Used for: glaucoma.
Dosage: 1 drop into eye once or twice each day.
Special care: examination of eye for signs of damage to cornea and conjunctiva is required during long-term therapy, and drops should be withdrawn if this occurs.
Avoid use: narrow angle glaucoma, aphakia (a condition in which all or part of the lens of the eye is absent, usually due to surgical removal of a cataract).
Possible interaction: MAOIs.
Side effects: headache, discomfort in eye, skin reactions, melanosis (over-production of the pigment melanin), initial rise in pressure within eye; rarely, other whole body (systemic) effects.
Manufacturer: Chauvin.

GARAMYCIN
Description: an antibiotic preparation available in the form of drops containing 0.3% gentamicin (as sulphate).
Used for: external ear and eye infections.
Dosage: 3 to 4 drops 3 to 4 times each day.
Special care: patients with perforated ear drum (if being used to treat ear infections).
Avoid use: infections of viral, tuberculous or fungal origin or in which pus is present.
Side effects: superinfection, possible

mild irritation of short-lived duration, blurred vision (eye infections).
Manufacturer: Schering-Plough.

GASTROBID CONTINUS
Description: an antidopaminergic preparation used to treat gastro-intestinal upset and available as white, sustained-release tablets containing 15mg metoclopramide hydrochloride marked with strength and NAPP.
Used for: hiatus hernia, reflux oesophagitis (where there is a backflow of acid stomach juice) duodenitis and gastritis (inflammation of duodenum and stomach), dyspepsia. Also, nausea and vomiting including that which may result from chemotherapy for cancer.
Dosage: adults over 20 years of age, 1 tablet twice each day.
Special care: pregnancy, breastfeeding, kidney disease.
Avoid use: children and young adults under 20 years, recent surgery of gastro-intestinal tract, those with breast cancer which is prolactin-dependent or phaeochromocytoma.
Possible interaction: anticholinergic drugs, butyrophenones, phenothiazines.
Side effects: elevated prolactin levels in blood, extrapyramidal responses (concerned with reflex muscle movements of a stereotyped nature, e.g. knee jerk).
Manufacturer: Napp.

GASTROMAX
Description: an antidopaminergic preparation used to treat gastro-intestinal upset and available as yellow/orange sustained-release capsules containing 30mg metoclopramide hydrochloride.
Used for: gastro-intestinal disturbance and upset, nausea and vomiting including that which may be drug-induced (cancer chemotherapy).
Dosage: adults over 20 years of age and elderly persons, 1 tablet each day taken before a meal.
Special care: elderly persons and patients with kidney disease.

Avoid use: children and young adults under 20 years of age, pregnancy, breastfeeding, phaeochromocytoma.
Possible interaction: anticholinergic drugs, butyrophenones, phenothiazines.
Side effects: raised prolactin levels in blood, extrapyramidal responses (concerned with reflex muscle movements of a stereotyped nature, e.g. knee jerk).
Manufacturer: Pharmacia.

GASTROZEPIN

Description: an anticholinergic preparation (a selective antimuscarine drug) which acts to reduce the production and secretion of acid stomach juices. It is produced in the form of scored white tablets containing 50mg pirenzepine marked G over 50 and with manufacturer's logo.
Used for: stomach and duodenal ulcers.
Dosage: adults, 1 tablet twice each day taken thirty minutes before meals for a period of 1 month to 6 weeks. Maximum of 3 tablets each day in divided doses.
Special care: kidney disease.
Avoid use: children, pregnancy, closed angle glaucoma, enlarged prostate gland, paralytic ileus (a condition in which there is a reduction or absence of movement along the gastro-intestinal tract, which may result from a number of different causes), pyloric stenosis.
Side effects: disturbance of vision and dry mouth; rarely, blood changes.
Manufacturer: Boots.

GENOTROPIN

Description: a preparation of the synthetic human growth hormone, somatotropin, produced as a powder containing 4 units in vials (along with ampoules of solution for reconstitution). Various other preparations are available, e.g. **GENOTROPIN MULTIDOSE, GENOTROPIN CARTRIDGES, GENOTROPIN KABIVIAL MULTIDOSE and GENOTROPIN KABIQUICK**.
Used for: children in whom growth is

stunted due to absence or reduced amount of pituitary growth hormone, Turner's syndrome.
Dosage: growth hormone deficiency, usual dose in the order of 0.5–0.7 units/kg body weight each week by subcutaneous injection. Turner's syndrome, 1 unit/kg body weight each week by subcutaneous injection.
Special care: patients with diabetes mellitus.
Avoid use: patients with closed epiphyses.
Manufacturer: Pharmacia.

GENTICIN

Description: an antibiotic and aminoglycoside preparation in the form of drops containing 0.3% gentamicin (as sulphate).
Used for: ear and eye bacterial infections.
Dosage: ear, 2, 3 or 4 drops 3 or 4 times each day; eye, 1 to 3 drops 3 or 4 times each day.
Special care: with ear infections in patients with perforated eardrum.
Side effects: superinfection (secondary infection); eye infections, slight irritation of eye which is short-lived, blurring of vision.
Manufacturer: Roche.

GENTISONE HC

Description: a compound antibiotic and corticosteroid in the form of eardrops containing 0.3% gentamicin (as sulphate) and 1% hydrocortisone acetate.
Used for: external and middle ear infections.
Dosage: 2 to 4 drops placed in ear 3 or 4 times each day and at bedtime. As an alternative, wicks dipped in the solution may be placed in the ear to deliver the dose.
Special care: pregnancy, limit use in young children, patients with perforated eardrum.
Side effects: superinfection (secondary infection).
Manufacturer: Roche.

GESTANIN

Description: a hormonal preparation of a progestogen produced in the form of white tablets containing 5mg allyloestrenol and coded ORGANON and GK4.

Used for: recurrent or threatened miscarriage, threatened premature labour.

Dosage: recurrent miscarriage, 1 tablet 3 times each day as soon as there is confirmation of the pregnancy continuing until 1 month beyond the end of the risk period; threatened premature labour, up to 8 tablets each day according to response.

Avoid use: patients with liver disease.

Side effects: nausea.

Manufacturer: Organon.

GESTONE

Description: a hormonal preparation of a progestogen produced in ampoules for injection in 2 strengths, containing 25mg and 50mg progesterone/ml. Also, as 2ml ampoules containing 100mg progesterone.

Used for: maintenace of pregnancy in early stages in women with history of spontaneous abortion.

Dosage: adults, 25–100mg each day by deep intramuscular injection from fifteenth day of pregnancy to eighth to sixteenth week.

Special care: patients with migraine, epilepsy, diabetes.

Avoid use: patients with breast cancer, history of thrombosis, liver disease, vaginal bleeding which is undiagnosed.

Manufacturer: Paines and Byrne.

GLAUCOL

Description: a ß-blocker produced in the form of an eye solution in single dose vials of 2 strengths containing 0.25% and 0.5% timolol (as maleate).

Used for: open angle glaucoma, secondary glaucoma, hypertension within the eye.

Dosage: adults, 1 drop of lower strength solution twice each day increasing to higher strength if necessary.

Special care: pregnancy, breastfeeding, elderly. Withdraw drops gradually.

Avoid use: patients with heart block, bradycardia, asthma, history of obstructive lung disease.

Possible interaction: antihypertensive drugs, adrenaline, verapamil.

Side effects: irritation of eye, absorption into blood may cause other systemic (whole body) ß-blocker side effects, e.g. disturbance of sleep, cold hands and feet, fatigue on exercise, bradycardia, gastro-intestinal upset, heart failure, bronchospasm.

Manufacturer: Baker Norton.

GLIBENESE

Description: a sulphonylurea drug produced in the form of scored, oblong, white tablets containing 5mg glipizide and marked Pfizer and GBS/5.

Used for: maturity onset diabetes.

Dosage: adults, 2.5mg–5mg each day taken either before breakfast or lunch. Dose may be increased if required by 2.5–5mg daily every third, fourth or fifth day with a maximum of 40mg each day. Doses in excess of 15mg daily should be taken before meals as divided doses. Usual maintenance dose is in the order of 2.5–30mg depending upon response.

Special care: elderly, kidney failure.

Avoid use: children, pregnancy, breastfeeding, other forms of diabetes including unstable brittle diabetes, growth-onset diabetes, juvenile diabetes, ketoacidosis (an accumulation of ketones within the body due to diabetes), infections, serious kidney or liver disease. Also, patients suffering from stress, infections or undergoing suregery.

Possible interaction: sulphonamides, anticoagulants taken orally, corticotrophin, corticosteroids, aspirin, rifampicin, glucagon, oral contraceptives, MAOIs, alcohol, chloramphenicol, ß-blockers, clofibrate, bezafibrate, diuretics, chloropropamide, metformin, acetohexamide.

Side effects: allergic reactions, skin rash.

Manufacturer: Pfizer.

GLUCAGON

Description: a hyperglycaemic preparation produced as a powder in vials along with diluent for reconstitution and injection. Glucagon is produced by Lilly as 1.09mg glucagon hydrochloride and by Novo as 1mg glucagon hydrochloride.

Used for: patients in whom blood sugar level has fallen to seriously low levels (e.g. diabetics taking insulin) and who have become unconscious.

Dosage: 0.5mg–1mg by intravenous, intramuscular or subcutaneous injection in patients who cannot be roused enough to take glucose or sucrose by mouth. If patient still does not wake up, an intravenous dose of glucose should be given.

Special care: pregnancy, breastfeeding.

Avoid use: phaeochromocytoma, pancreatic tumours (glucagonoma or insulinoma).

Possible interaction: warfarin.

Side effects: gastro-intestinal upset, diarrhoea, nausea, vomiting, allergic responses, hypokalaemia.

Manufacturer: Lilly and Novo.

GLUCOBAY

Description: an oral hypoglycaemic preparation which acts to inhibit the activity of the digestive enzyme, alpha-glucosidase, which breaks down carbohydrates. It is produced in the form of off-white tablets of 2 strengths containing 50mg and 100mg acarbose and marked G50 or G100 respectively and with Bayer logo.

Used for: additional therapy (or on its own) in diabetes which is non-insulin dependent and is not completely controlled by diet or oral hypoglycaemics.

Dosage: adults, 50mg 3 times each day at first for 6 to 8 weeks increasing to 100mg 3 times daily if required. The maximum dose is 200mg 3 times each day.

Special care: with maximum dose, the level of liver enzyme, hepatic transaminase, should be carefully monitored. Also monitor patients receiving hypoglycaemics.

Avoid use: pregnancy, breastfeeding, various disorders of the gastro-intestinal tract including inflammation of the bowel, obstruction of intestine, ulceration of colon, disorders of absorption.

Possible interaction: pancreatic enzymes, adsorbent agents, cholestyramine, neomycin.

Side effects: flatulence, feeling of bloatedness, diarrhoea, pain in abdomen.

Manufacturer: Bayer.

GLUCOPHAGE

Description: a biguanide antidiabetic drug available as white, film-coated tablets of 2 strengths containing 500mg and 850mg of metformin hydrochloride and marked with strength and GL.

Used for: additional therapy with sulphonylureas in maturity-onset diabetes, or on its own. Also, as additional therapy in insulin-dependent diabetes, particularly in overweight patients.

Dosage: 500mg twice each day in first instance or 850mg taken with meals. Dose may be gradually increased if needed to a daily maximum of 3g and then should be reduced for maintenance. Normal maintenance dose is in the order of three 500mg or two 850mg doses each day.

Special care: elderly, kidney failure.

Avoid use: pregnancy, breastfeeding, other forms of diabetes including growth-onset, juvenile, unstable brittle diabetes, ketoacidosis (excess amount o ketones in body), infections, hormonal disorders, stress, serious kidney or liver disease, patients undergoing surgery.

Possible interaction: MAOIs, sulphonamides, anticoagulants taken by mouth, corticotrophin, corticosteroids, aspirin, rifampicin, glucagon, oral contraceptives, alcohol, chloramphenicol, ß-blockers, clofibrate, bezafibrate, diuretics, chloro-propamide, metformin acetohexamide.

Side effects: allergic reactions, skin ras

Manufacturer: Lipha.

GLURENORM

Description: sulphonylurea available as scored, white tablets containing 30mg gliquidone and marked G.
Used for: maturity-onset diabetes.
Dosage: in the order of 45–600mg each day in divided doses before meals. Maximum dose is 180mg each day.
Special care: elderly persons, patients with kidney failure.
Avoid use: pregnancy, breastfeeding, other forms of diabetes including growth-onset, juvenile, unstable brittle diabetes, ketoacidosis (excess amount of ketones in body as a result of diabetes detected by smell of acetone on breath), infections, hormonal disorders, stress, serious kidney or liver disease, patients undergoing surgery.
Possible interaction: MAOIs, sulphonamides, anticoagulants taken by mouth, corticotrophin, corticosteroids, aspirin, rifampicin, glucagon, oral contraceptives, alcohol, chloramphenicol, ß-blockers, clofibrate, bezafibrate, diuretics, chloropropamide, metformin, acetohexamide.
Side effects: allergic reactions, skin rash.
Manufacturer: Sanofi Winthrop.

GLYPRESSIN

Description: a vasopressin analogue, produced as a powder in vials containing 1mg terlipressin, along with diluent for reconstitution and injection.
Used for: bleeding varicose veins in the oesophagus.
Dosage: adults, 2mg given by intravenous bolus injection (a dose given all at once) followed by further 1 or 2mg doses 4, 5 or 6 hours later for a maximum period of 72 hours.
Special care: patients with various heart conditions including weak heart, arrhythmias, and also serious atherosclerosis or hypertension. Blood levels of electrolytes (salts), fluid balance and blood pressure require careful monitoring.
Avoid use: pregnancy.

Side effects: hypertension, paleness, headache, cramps in abdomen.
Manufacturer: Ferring.

GONADOTROPHIN L.H.

Description: a hormonal preparation available as a powder in ampoules, with solvent for reconstitution and injection. It is available at various strengths containing 500 units, 1000 units and 5000 units of chorionic gonadotrophin.
Used for: in males, delayed puberty, failure of the testes to descend into the scrotum (cryptorchidism), a reduced amount of spermatozoa in the semen (oligospermia), a cause of infertility. In females, infertility caused by a lack of ovulation.
Dosage: boys, 7 to 10 years, 500 units 3 times each week given by injection for a period of 6 to 10 weeks. Adults, as directed by physician. Women, 10,000 units by injection in middle of monthly cycle following therapy to stimulate maturation of ovarian follicles.
Special care: heart or kidney disease, asthma, migraine or epilepsy.
Side effects: fatigue, headache, oedema, allergic reactions; young boys may become sexually precocious.
Manufacturer: Paines and Byrne.

GOPTEN

Description: an antihypertensive preparation and ACE inhibitor available as capsules of 3 strengths. Yellow/red, orange/red and red/red capsules contain 0.5mg, 1mg and 2mg trandolapril respectively.
Used for: hypertension.
Dosage: adults, 0.5mg once each day in first instance, then doubling at 2 to 4 week intervals. The maximum single dose is 4mg each day with a maintenance dose of 1–2mg once daily.
Special care: any diuretics should be stopped 2 or 3 days before treatment begins. Special care in patients udergoing anaesthesia or surgery, those with congestive heart failure, liver or

kidney disease, having kidney dialysis. Kidney function should be monitored before starting and during therapy.
Avoid use: children, pregnancy, breastfeeding, obstruction of heart outflow or aortic stenosis. Those with angioneurotic oedema, caused by previous treatment with ACE inhibitors.
Possible interaction: NSAIDs, potassium-sparing diuretics.
Side effects: headache, cough, rash, giddiness, weakness, palpitations, hypotension. Rarely there may be depression of bone marrow, blood changes (agranulocytosis—characterized by serious deficiency of certain white blood cells), angioneurotic oedema.
Manufacturer: Knoll.

GRANEODIN

Description: a broad-spectrum aminoglycoside antibiotic preparation available as an ointment containing 0.25% neomycin sulphate and 0.025% gramicidin.
Used for: minor bacterial infections of the skin and prevention of infection during minor surgery.
Dosage: apply ointment to affected area 2, 3 or 4 times daily.
Special care: dressings should not be used and ointment is not suitable for large areas of damaged skin.
Avoid use: persistent, more deep-rooted infections.
Side effects: toxic effects on tissues and organs, sensitisation.
Manufacturer: Squibb.

GRANOCYTE

Description: a drug containing recombinant granulocyte stimulating factor produced as a powder in vials, along with solution, for reconstitution and injection. It contains 263 µg lenograstim (recombinant human granulocyte-colony stimulating factor).
Used for: neutropenia in patients who have had bone marrow transplants, or cytotoxic cancer chemotherapy.

Dosage: adults, bone marrow transplant patients, 150 micrograms/m^2 body surface by subcutaenous infusion over half-hour period each day. Therapy should begin the day after transplantation and continue until conditon improves, for a maximum period of 28 days. Cancer therapy, 150 micrograms/m^2 body surface each day by subcutaneous injection, starting the day after chemotherapy has finished. Continue until condition improves for a maximum period of 28 days. Children over 2 years, same as adult dose.
Special care: pregnancy, breastfeeding, pre-cancerous myeloid (bone marrow) conditions, serious kidney or liver disease. Regular blood counts and checks should be carried out.
Avoid use: children under 2 years of age, patients with myeloid growths.
Side effects: pain at injection site and in bones.
Manufacturer: Chugai Pharma UK Limted/Rhône-Poulenc Rorer Limited.

GREGODERM

Description: an antibacterial, antifungal and mildly potent steroid preparation available in the form of an ointment containing 2,720 units neomycin sulphate, 100,000 units nystatin, 100,000 units polymixin B sulphate and 10mg hydrocortisone/g.
Used for: inflammation of the skin where infection is also present, psoriasis, itching in anal and urogenital areas.
Dosage: apply ointment 2 or 3 times each day to affected area.
Special care: use should be limited in children, infants and on face to a maximum period of 5 days. Should be gradually withdrawn after longer-term use.
Avoid use: extensive or long-term use in pregnancy or for prevention of skin conditions. Patients with acne, or skin infections with tuberculous or viral origin, leg ulcers, ringworm, scabies, dermatitis in region of mouth, any untreated bacterial or fungal infections.

Side effects: skin thinning, suppression of adrenal glands, abnorml hair growth, changes as in Cushing's syndrome.
Manufacturer: Unigreg.

GRISOVIN

Description: an antifungal preparation available in the form of white, film-coated tablets of 2 strengths containing 125mg and 500mg griseofulvin both marked with name, strength and manufacturer's name.
Used for: fungal infections of nails, skin and scalp, especially those not suitable for treatment with topical preparations.
Dosage: adults, 500mg–1g each day in divided doses after meals. Dose should not fall below 10mg/kg body weight. Children, 10mg/kg body weight each day as divided doses.
Special care: pregnancy, long-term use.
Avoid use: patients with serious liver disease, porphyria, SLE (a rare collagen disease).
Possible interaction: anticoagulants of the coumarin type, oral contraceptives, alcohol, barbiturates.
Manufacturer: Glaxo.

GYNO-DAKTARIN 1

Description: an antifungal and antibacterial preparation, miconazole nitrate, produced in a variety of forms: white, soft vaginal capsules contain 200mg ; GYNO-DAKTARIN PESSARIES contain 100mg per pessary; GYNO-DAKTARIN COMBIPAK consists of 14 pessaries plus cream; GYNO-DAKTARIN CREAM contains 2% per 78g with applicator.
Used for: candidiasis (thrush) of the vagina or vulva.
Dosage: adults, capsules, 1 at night, inserted into vagina as single dose. Pessaries, 1 inserted twice each day for 7 days. Combipak, 1 pessary and 1 application of cream inserted twice each day. Cream, 1 applicatorful of cream inserted twice each day for 7 days. Male sexual partner should also

apply cream twice daily for 7 days.
Side effects: slight burning or discomfort of short-lived nature.
Manufacturer: Janssen.

GYNO-PEVARYL 1

Description: an antifungal preparation available as vaginal pessaries or cream or a combination of both, all containing econazole nitrate. GYNO-PEVARYL PESSARIES contain 150mg; GYNO-PEVARYL CREAM contains 1% in 15g. Also available, GYNO-PEVARYL 1 COMBIPAK (1 pessary and 15g cream); GYNO-PEVARYL COMBI-PAK (3 pessaries, 15g cream).
Used for: vulvitis (inflammation of vulva), vaginitis (inflammation of vagina), treatment of sexual partner in order to prevent reinfection.
Dosage: adults, pessaries, 1 inserted at night as single dose or for 3 consecutive nights; cream, apply twice each day for 2 weeks.
Side effects: slight burning or discomfort of short-lived nature.
Manufacturer: Cilag.

HAELAN

Description: a moderately potent steroid preparation available as cream and ointment containing 0.0125% flurandrenolone. Also, HAELAN C (combining the steroid with an antibacterial/antifungal agent), which also contains 3% clioquinol as cream and ointment. HAELAN TAPE is a clear, adhesive polythene film impregnated with 4 µg/cm².
Used for: inflammatory skin conditions which are responsive to steroids. Haelan C is used when infection is present.
Dosage: cream or ointment, apply 2 or 3 times each day to clean skin.

Tape, apply to affected area and leave in place for 12 hours.

Special care: Haelan C may stain clothing and skin; use in children or on face should be limited to a maximum period of 5 days. Short-term use and withdraw slowly if use has been more prolonged.

Avoid use: extensive or prolonged use in pregnancy or continuous use as preventative measure, patients with untreated bacterial or fungal infections, acne, leg ulcers, scabies, skin disease of tuberculous or viral origin, ringworm, dermatitis in area of mouth. (Haelan C is, however, used for some infected conditions).

Side effects: adrenal gland suppression, skin thinning, abnormal hair growth, skin changes as in Cushing's syndrome.

Manufacturer: Dista.

HALCIDERM

Description: a very potent topical steroid preparation available in the form of a cream containing 0.1% halcinomide.

Used for: inflammatory skin conditions responsive to steroids.

Dosage: apply to affected area 2 or 3 times each day.

Special care: should not be used for more than 5 days, short-term use only and a milder substitute should be tried as soon as possible.

Avoid use: children, extensive or prolonged use, especially in pregnancy or as a preventative measure. Avoid use in patients with untreated bacterial or fungal infections, acne, leg ulcers, scabies, skin disease of tuberculous or viral origin, ringworm, dermatitis in area of mouth.

Side effects: adrenal gland suppression, skin thinning, abnormal hair growth, skin changes as in Cushing's syndrome.

Manufacturer: Dista.

HALDOL DECANOATE

Description: an antipsychotic drug, haloperidol (as decanoate), which is a depot butyrophenone available in ampoules for injection at 2 strengths containing 50mg/ml and 100mg/ml. Also, **HALDOL TABLETS** of 2 strengths, blue, coded H5, containing 5mg and yellow, coded H10, containing 10mg. Both are marked Janssen and also scored. **HALDOL ORAL LIQUID** containing 2mg/ml and 10mg/ml and **HALDOL INJECTION** containing 5mg/ml.

Used for: Haldol decanoate, long-term sedative treatment for various forms of psychiatric illness including psychoses, schizophrenia, disturbed behaviour. Other preparations: mania, schizophrenia, psychoses, symptoms precipitated by alcohol withdrawal; delirium tremens. Also used as pre-anaesthetic sedative for anxiety, vomiting and nausea and disturbed behaviour in children.

Dosage: Haldol decanoate, adults only, usual dose in order of 50mg–300mg by deep intramuscular injection once each month. Other oral preparations, adults, 0.5mg–5mg 2 or 3 times each day depending upon condition being treated. Dose may be gradually increased if needed to a daily maximum of 200mg and then should be reduced for maintenance. Haldol injection, for psychoses, 2–30mg by intramuscular injection followed by further dose of 5mg at 1 to 8 hour intervals until condition improves. Children, oral preparations, 0.05mg/kg body weight each day in 2 divided doses.

Special care: pregnancy, breastfeeding, serious heart and circulatory disease, kidney or liver failure, Parkinsonism, epilepsy.

Avoid use: patients in states of coma.

Possible interaction: rifampicin, carbamazepine, lithium, alcohol.

Side effects: hypotension, pallor, drowsiness, tachycardia, palpitations, nightmares, hypothermia, disturbance of sleep, depression, dry mouth, blocked nose, difficulty in urination, blurring of vision, changes in menstruation, breasts and weight, blood changes, ECG and EEG changes, jaundice, skin reactions.

Manufacturer: Janssen.

HALFAN

Description: an antimalarial preparation which is a phenanthrene drug, produced in the form of scored, capsule-shaped, white tablets, marked HALFAN, containing 250mg halofantrine hydrochloride.

Used for: treatment of malaria caused by *Plasmodium vivax* and *Plasmodium falciparum*.

Dosage: adults, 6 tablets taken at 6 hour intervals in 3 divided doses. The dose is repeated 1 week later in patients who are not immune. Tablets should not be taken with meals. Children, over 37kg in weight, same as adult.

Special care: women who may become pregnant, patients with malarial complications or malaria affecting the brain.

Avoid use: pregnancy, breastfeeding, children under 37kg in weight, patients with some forms of heart disease. Not to be used as a preventative for malaria.

Possible interaction: TCADs, antiarrhythmic drugs, astemizole, neuroleptic drugs, terfenadine, chloroquine, quinine, mefloquine.

Side effects: heart arrhythmia, pain in abdomen, gastro-intestinal upset, a short-lived rise in transaminase enzymes in the blood.

Manufacturer: S.K. & F.

HAMARIN

Description: a xanthine oxidase inhibitor produced in the form of scored, white tablets containing 300mg allopurinol and marked with name, strength and triangle symbol. Allopurinol acts on the enzyme xanthine oxidase which converts the substances xanthine and hypoxanthine into uric acid. Hence the levels of uric acid in the blood are reduced and there is less likelihood of an attack of gout.

Used for: treatment of gout, prevention of stones formed from uric acid or calcium oxalate.

Dosage: adults, usual single dose in the order of 100mg–300mg each day increasing for prevention to a maintenance dose in the range 200–600mg daily.

Special care: pregnancy, elderly, liver or kidney disease. When treatment starts, an anti-inflammatory drug or colchicine should be taken for 4 weeks and the patient should drink plenty of fluids.

Avoid use: children, acute gout.

Possible interaction: chlopropamide, azanthioprine, mercatopurine, anticoagulant drugs.

Side effects: acute gout, nausea, drug should be stopped in the event of skin rash occurring.

Manufacturer: Roche.

HARMOGEN

Description: a hormonal oestrogen preparation produced in the form of long, peach-coloured, scored tablets containing 1.5mg piperazine oestrone sulphate and marked LV.

Used for: hormonal replacement therapy in menopausal women and prevention of osteoporosis following menopause.

Dosage: adults, 1 to 2 tablets each day, along with a progestogen preparation for the last 10 to 13 days of each 28 day cycle in women who have not had a hysterectomy.

Special care: patients considered to be at risk of thrombosis or with liver disease. Women with any of the following disorders should be carefully monitored: fibroids in the womb, multiple sclerosis, diabetes, tetany, porphyria, epilepsy, liver disease, hypertension, migraine, otosclerosis, gallstones. Breasts, pelvic organs and blood pressure should be checked at regular intervals during the course of treatment.

Avoid use: pregnancy, breastfeeding, women with conditions which might lead to thrombosis, thrombophlebitis, serious heart, kidney or liver disease, breast cancer, oestrogen-dependent cancers including those of reproductive system, endometriosis, vaginal bleeding which is undiagnosed.

Possible interaction: drugs which induce liver enzymes.

Side effects: tenderness and enlargement of breasts, weight gain, breakthrough bleeding, giddiness, vomiting and nausea, gastro-intestinal upset. Treatment should be halted immediately if severe headaches occur, disturbance of vision, hypertension or any indications of thrombosis, jaundice. Also, in the event of pregnancy and 6 weeks before planned surgery.
Manufacturer: Upjohn.

HAVRIX MONODOSE

Description: a preparation of inactivated hepatitis A virus HM available in pre-filled syringes containing 1440 ELISA units/ml adsorbed on aluminium hydroxide. **HAVRIX ORIGINAL**, pre-filled 1ml syringes containing 720 ELISA units/ml of hepatitis A virus HM 175 strain adsorbed on aluminium hydroxide. Also, **HAVRIX JUNIOR**, pre-filled 0.5ml syringes containing 720 ELISA units/ml of hepatitis A virus HM 175 strain adsorbed on aluminium hydroxide.
Used for: immunisation against hepatitis A virus.
Dosage: adults and children age 16 and over, Havrix Monodose, primary immunisation, 1 intramuscular injection of 1ml followed by repeated dose 6 to 12 months later. Havrix original, primary immunisation, 1 intramuscular injection of 1ml followed by repeated doses after 2 to 4 weeks and 6 to 12 months. Children under 16 years, Havrix junior only, age 1 to 15 years, primary immunisation, 0.5ml by intramuscular injection followed by repeated doses 2 to 4 weeks and 6 to 12 months later.
Special care: pregnancy, breastfeeding, infections, dialysis or with lowered immunity. Patients with bleeding disorders may need subcutaneous injection.
Avoid use: patients with severe fever, children under 1 year.
Possible interaction: nausea, fatigue, malaise, soreness and skin reactions at injection site, appetite loss.
Manufacturer: Smith Kline Beecham.

HEMABATE

Description: a prostaglandin preparation produced in ampoules for injection containing 250µg carboprost as trometamol salt/ml.
Used for: haemorrhage following childbirth in patients who have not responded to other drugs (oxytocin and ergometrine).
Dosage: 1 deep intramuscular injection of 250 micrograms which may be repeated after 1 1/2 hours. If condition is very severe, repeat dose can be given after 15 minutes. Maximum total dose is 12mg.
Special care: patients with hypertension, hypotension, history of glaucoma or hypertension in eye, diabetes, asthma, jaundice, epilepsy, previous uterine injury (high doses may cause rupture of uterus).
Avoid use: patients with heart, liver, kidney or lung disease, pelvic inflammatory disease.
Side effects: gastro-intestinal upset, vomiting, nausea, diarrhoea, flushing, high temperature (hyperthermia), bronchospasm. Rarely, chills, headache, fluid in lungs, sweating, giddiness, pain and skin changes at injection site.
Manufacturer: Upjohn.

HEMINEVRIN

Description: a hypnotic, sedative preparation produced in the form of capsules and as a syrup. Grey-brown capsules contain 192mg chlormethiazole in miglyol, 1 capsule being equivalent to 5ml of syrup. Syrup contains 250mg chlormethiazole edisylate/5ml.
Used for: insomnia in elderly persons, short-lived therapy only. Sedation in elderly patients with senile psychosis, anxiety, confusion, disturbance of sleep, tension, alcohol withdrawal.
Dosage: adults, capsules, 2 at bedtime or 1 three times each day for sedation. Syrup, 10ml in drink at bedtime or three 5ml doses through day for sedation. For alcohol withdrawal symptoms, 3 capsules 4 times each day reducing over 6 days to nil.

Special care: lung, liver or kidney disease.

Avoid use: breastfeeding, children, serious lung disease.

Possible interaction: other central nervous system sedatives, alcohol.

Side effects: blocked and sore nose, sore eyes, gastro-intestinal upset, sedation, judgement and performance of skilled tasks (e.g. driving) is impaired, confusion, agitation, anaphylactic type allergic reactions.

Manufacturer: Astra.

HEMINEVRIN I-V INFUSION

Description: an anticonvulsant sedative preparation available as a solution for infusion containing 8mg chlormethiazole edisylate/ml.

Used for: status epilepticus (a life-threatening condition characterized by continuous convulsions which can cause irreversible brain damage and a dangerous imbalance in the level of salts in the body), pre-eclamptic toxaemia (an abnormal condition which may arise in pregnancy).

Dosage: adults, 60 drops per minute until patient is sedated and then 10–15 drops per minute. Status epilepticus, 40–100ml over a period of 5 to 10 minutes, all by rapid infusion. Children, status epilepticus, 80 µg/kg body weight (0.01ml) per minute at first, with increase if required every 2 to 4 hours until condition is under control. Then dose is gradually reduced unless seizures recur.

Special care: patients with lung disorder or history of obstructive lung disease.

Avoid use: breastfeeding, patients with severe lung disorders.

Possible interaction: central nervous system, sedatives, alcohol.

Side effects: blocked and sore nose, sore eyes, sedation, confusion, agitation, gastro-intestinal upset. Judgement and the ability to perform skilled tasks is impaired.

Manufacturer: Astra.

HERPID

Description: an antiviral preparation available as a solution containing 5% idoxuridine in dimethyl sulphoxide.

Used for: skin infections caused by *herpes zoster* and *herpes simplex*.

Dosage: adults, apply solution (with applicator brush) 4 times each day for a period of 4 days.

Avoid use: pregnancy, breastfeeding.

Manufacturer: Yamanouchi.

HIBTITER

Description: a preparation of inactivated surface antigen consisting of polysaccharide from the capsule of *H. influenzae* type B joined to diphtheria protein.

Used for: immunisation against meningitis, epiglottitis and other diseases caused by *H. influenzae* type B.

Dosage: children only, aged 2 months to 1 year, 3 intramuscular injections of 0.5ml at 4 week intervals, normally along with diphtheria, tetanus, polio immunisation.

Special care: same vaccine must be used throughout course of immunisation.

Avoid use: children with acute infections.

Side effects: possible skin reaction (reddening) at injection site.

Manufacturer: Lederle.

HONVAN

Description: a hormonal oestrogen preparation available in ampoules for injection and also in the form of tablets, both containing tetrasodium fosfesterol which is converted to stilboestrol by enzyme activity. The ampoules contain 276mg tetrasodium fosfesterol/5ml and white tablets contain 100mg.

Used for: cancer of the prostate gland.

Dosage: adults, injection, 552–1104mg by slow intravenous injection daily for a minimum of 5 days. Then 276mg 1 to 4 times each week for maintenance. Tablets, for maintenance, 100–200mg 3 times each day then reducing to 100–300mg in divided doses as daily dose.

Special care: patients with liver disease.
Side effects: thrombosis, oedema, nausea, gynaecomastia, impotence, pain in perineal area.
Manufacturer: Asta Medica.

HORMONIN

Description: a hormonal oestrogen preparation available in the form of scored, pink tablets containing 0.27mg oestriol, 1.4mg oestrone and 0.6mg oestradiol.
Used for: hormone replacement therapy in women with menopausal symptoms, prevention of osteoporosis after menopause.
Dosage: 1 to 2 tablets each day, with a progestogen for last 12 or 13 days of 28 day cycle unless patient has had a hysterectomy.
Special care: women at risk of thrombosis or with liver disorder—liver function should be monitored. Women with any of the following should also receive careful monitoring: otosclerosis, porphyria, fibroids in the uterus, epilepsy, migraine, multiple sclerosis, diabetes, hypertension, tetany, gallstones. Blood pressure, pelvic organs and breasts should be checked regularly during the course of treatment.
Avoid use: pregnancy, breastfeeding, breast cancer, cancer of reproductive system or any hormone-dependent cancer, serious heart, liver or kidney disease, any conditions likely to lead to thrombosis, Rotor or Dublin-Johnson syndrome, endometriosis or vaginal bleeding of unknown cause.
Possible interaction: drugs which induce liver enzymes.
Side effects: breast enlargement and soreness, weight gain, nausea, vomiting, gastro-intestinal upset, headache, giddiness, breakthrough bleeding.
Manufacturer: Shire.

HUMATROPE

Description: a synthetic growth hormone available as powder in ampoules, with diluent for reconstitution and injection,

containing 4 units or 16 units of somatropin (rbe).
Used for: failure of growth in children due to lack of growth hormone, Turner's syndrome.
Dosage: children, deficiency of growth hormone, either 0.07 units/kg body-weight each day or 0.16 units/kg body-weight 3 times each week, all by intramuscular or subcutaneous injection. Turner's syndrome, 0.8–0.9 units/kg body-weight each week in 6 or 7 doses given by intramuscular or subcutaneous injection.
Special care: children with diabetes, intracranial lesion (damaged tissue within cranium), a deficiency of ACTH (adrenocorticotrophic hormone—an adrenal gland hormone). Thyroid function should be monitored during the course of therapy.
Avoid use: patients with tumour, fused epiphyses, pregnancy, breastfeeding.
Manufacturer: Lilly.

HUMEGON

Description: a combined preparation of human menopausal gonadotrophins (HMG) available as powder in ampoules with solvent in 2 strengths. 75 units HMG (equivalent to 75 units of follicle-stimulating hormone (FSH) and 75 units luteinizing hormone (LH)) and 150 units HMG (equivalent to 150 units FSH and 150 units LH).
Used for: male and female infertility due to a lack of gonadotrophin resulting in insufficient stimulation of the gonads (sex organs). Also, for stimulation of ovaries to produce excess eggs for IVF (*in vitro* fertilization).
Dosage: males and females, by intramus-cular injection, according to individual's requirements as directed by physician.
Special care: males and females, exclude all other causes of infertility. Females, monitor size of ovaries and levels of oestrogen during the course of therapy.
Avoid use: tumours of the pituitary gland, testes and ovaries.

Side effects: skin rashes, risk of miscarriage and multiple pregnancy.
Manufacturer: Organon.

HYDERGINE

Description: a cerebral activator-ergot alkaloid available as scored, white tablets containing 1.5mg or 4.5mg codergocrine mesylate both marked with strength and name.
Used for: additional therapy in the treatment of moderate dementia in elderly persons.
Dosage: adults, 4.5mg each day.
Special care: severe bradycardia.
Avoid use: children.
Side effects: blocked nose, rash, flushing, headache, pain in abdomen, giddiness, hypotension, when rising from lying down (postural hypotension).
Manufacturer: Sandoz.

HYDREA

Description: a DNA reactive cytotoxic drug available as pink/green capsules containing 500mg hydroxyurea marked SQUIBB and 830.
Used for: treatment of chronic myeloid leukaemia
Dosage: 20–30mg/kg body weight each day or 80mg/kg body weight every third day.
Side effects: nausea, vomiting, skin rashes, bone marrow suppression.
Manufacturer: Squibb.

HYDRENOX

Description: a thiazide diuretic preparation available as scored white tablets containing 50mg hydroflumethiazide marked H inside a hexagon shape.
Used for: hypertension, oedema.
Dosage: adults, for oedema, 50–200mg as a single dose taken in the morning, in first instance, then reducing to a 25mg–50mg maintenance dose taken on alternate days. For hypertension, 25mg–50mg each day. Children, 1mg/kg body weight each day.
Special care: pregnancy, breastfeeding,

elderly, kidney or liver disease, liver cirrhosis, SLE, diabetes, gout. Glucose, fluid and electrolyte (salt) levels should be monitored during the course of therapy.
Avoid use: patients with hypercalcaemia, serious kidney or liver disease, a sensitivity to sulphonamide drugs, Addison's disease.
Possible interaction: NSAIDs, barbiturates, alcohol, opiod drugs. Cardiac glycosides, lithium, carbenoxolone, corticosteroids, tubocurarine.
Side effects: gastro-intestinal upset, blood changes, sensitivity to light, disturbance of electrolyte balance and metabolism, skin rash, pancreatitis, anorexia, dizziness, impotence.
Manufacturer: Boots.

HYDROCAL

Description: a topical, mildly potent corticosteroid preparation available as cream or ointment containing 1% hydrocortisone acetate and calamine.
Used for: irritated skin conditions responsive to steroids.
Dosage: apply to affected skin 2 or 3 times each day.
Special care: use in children or on face should be limited to a period not exceeding 5 days. Stop gradually if preparation has been used for a long period.
Avoid use: extensive or long-term use, especially in pregnant women or for prevention of skin conditions. Patients with bacterial or fungal infections which are untreated. Skin disease of viral or tuberculous origin or due to ringworm, acne, dermatitis in mouth area, leg ulcers, scabies.
Side effects: thinning of skin, suppression of adrenal glands, abnormal hair growth, skin changes as in Cushing's syndrome.
Manufacturer: Bioglan.

HYDROCORTISTAB CREAM

Description: a mildly potent topical steroid preparation available as cream or ointment containing 1% hydrocortisone acetate.

Used for: irritated skin conditions responsive to steroids.
Dosage: apply thinly to affected skin 2 or 3 times each day.
Special care: use in children or on face should be limited to a period not exceeding 5 days. Stop gradually if preparation has been used for a long period.
Avoid use: extensive or long-term use, especially in pregnant women or for prevention of skin conditions. Patients with bacterial or fungal infections which are untreated. Skin disease of viral or tuberculous origin or due to ringworm, acne, dermatitis in mouth area, leg ulcers, scabies.
Side effects: thinning of skin, suppression of adrenal glands, abnormal hair growth, skin changes as in Cushing's syndrome.
Manufacturer: Boots.

HYDROCORTISTAB TABLETS

Description: a corticosteroid (gluco-corticoid and mineralocorticosteroid) preparation available as scored, white tablets containing 20mg hydro-cortisone.
Also **HYDROCORTISTABL INJECTION** available in ampoules containing 25mg hydrocortisone acetate/ml.
Used for: tablets, hormone replacement therapy, emergency treatment or asthma attack, anaphylaxis, allergic drug response, serum sickness, angioneurotic oedema. Injection, directly into joints in rheumatic diseases and soft tissue injuries.
Dosage: adults, tablets, replacement therapy, 20–30mg each day; emergency treatment, as directed by physician according to patient's condition. Injection, 5–50mg each day directly into joint with a maximum of 3 injections daily. Children, tablets, replacement therapy, 10–30mg each day in divided doses; emergency treatment as directed by physician according to patient's condition. Injection, 5–30mg each day directly into joint with a maximum of 3 injections daily.

Special care: pregnancy, hyperthyroidism, liver cirrhosis, inflammation in kidneys (glomerulonephritis, nephritis), inflammation of veins, peptic ulcer, hypertension. Also, diabetes, recent surgical anastomoses of gastro-intestinal tract, epilepsy, osteoporosis, infectious diseases characterized by skin rash, other infections, tuberculosis, those of fungal or viral origin. Patients with psychoses or suffering from stress. Drug should be gradually withdrawn and patients in contact with *Herpes zoster* virus or chicken pox should seek medical advice and treatment.
Possible interaction: anticoagulants taken orally, diuretics, NSAIDs, cardiac glycosides, anticholinesterases, rifampicin, hypoglycaemics, phenytoin, ephedrine, phenobarbitone.
Side effects: peptic ulcer, skin changes, osteoporosis, depression and euphoria, hyperglycaemia.
Manufacturer: Boots.

HYDROCORTISYL

Description: a mildly potent topical steroid preparation available as cream or ointment containing 1% hydrocortisone acetate.
Used for: irritated skin conditions responsive to steroids.
Dosage: apply thinly to affected skin 2 or 3 times each day.
Special care: use in children or on face should be limited to a period not exceeding 5 days. Stop gradually if preparation has been used for a long period.
Avoid use: extensive or long-term use, especially in pregnant women or for prevention of skin conditions. Patients with bacterial or fungal infections which are untreated. Skin disease of viral or tuberculous origin or due to ringworm, acne, dermatitis in mouth area, leg ulcers, scabies.
Side effects: thinning of skin, suppression of adrenal glands, abnormal hair growth, skin changes as in Cushing's syndrome.
Manufacturer: Roussel.

HYDROCORTONE

Description: a corticosteroid (gluco-corticoid and mineralocorticoid) available as quarter-scored, white tablets containing 10mg or 20mg hydrocortisone and coded MSD 619, MSD 625 respectively.

Used for: hormone replacement therapy due to reduced production of hormones from the adrenal cortex (adrenal glands).

Dosage: 20–30mg each day in divided doses or as directed by physician.

Special care: pregnancy, hyperthyroidism, liver cirrhosis, inflammation in kidneys (glomerulonephritis, nephritis), thrombophlebitis, peptic ulcer, hypertension. Also, diabetes, recent surgical anastomoses of gastro-intestinal tract, epilepsy, osteoporosis, infectious diseases characterized by skin rash, other infections, tuberculosis, those of fungal or viral origin. Patients with psychoses or suffering from stress. Drug should be gradually withdrawn and patients in contact with *Herpes zoster* virus or chicken pox should seek medical advice and treatment.

Possible interaction: anticoagulants taken orally, diuretics, NSAIDs, cardiac glycosides, anticholinesterases, rifampicin, hypoglycaemics, phenytoin, ephedrine, phenobarbitone.

Side effects: peptic ulcer, skin changes as in Cushing's syndrome, osteoporosis, depression and euphoria, hyperglycaemia.

Manufacturer: M.S.D.

HYDROMET

Description: a compound antihypertensive preparation combining a central alpha-agonist and thiazide diuretic. It is available as pink, film-coated tablets containing 250mg methyldopa and 15mg hydrochlorothiazide, marked MSD 423.

Used for: hypertension.

Dosage: adults, 1 tablet twice each day at first gradually increasing at intervals of 2 days. The maximum daily dose is 12 tablets.

Special care: pregnancy, breastfeeding, diabetes, kidney or liver disease, gout, history of liver disease, haemolytic anaemia, undergoing anaesthesia. A potassium supplement may be needed.

Avoid use: patients with serious liver disease, severe kidney failure, phaeochromocytoma, depression.

Possible interaction: antidiabetic substances, TCADs, ACTH (adrenocorticotrophic hormone), corticosteroids, MAOIs, tubocurarine, sympathomimetics, phenothiazines, digitalis, lithium.

Side effects: blocked nose, dry mouth, gastro-intestinal upset, headache, blood changes, sedation, depression, weakness, bradycardia.

Manufacturer: M.S.D.

HYDROSALURIC

Description: a thiazide diuretic preparation available as scored, white tablets of 2 strengths containing 25mg and 50mg of hydrochlorthiazide and marked MSD 42 and MSD 105 respectively.

Used for: hypertension, oedema.

Dosage: adults, oedema, 25mg–100mg once or twice each day or when needed with a maximum daily dose of 200mg. Hypertension, 25–50mg as a single or divided dose each day at first, then adjusting but with a maximum daily dose of 100mg. Children, 6 months and under, 3.5mg/kg body weight each day; 6 months to 2 years, 12.5–37.5mg each day; 2 to 12 years, 27.5–100mg each day. All are in 2 divided doses.

Special care: pregnancy, liver or kidney disease, gout, electrolyte (salts) imbalance, SLE, diabetes. Patients may also require a potassium supplement.

Avoid use: breastfeeding mothers, patients with serious liver or kidney disease, anuria, hypercalcaemia, Addison's disease.

Possible interaction: NSAIDs, antihypertensives, central nervous system depressants, muscle relaxants, corticosteroids, ACE inhibitors, digitalis, lithium.

Side effects: blood changes, fatigue, sensitivity to light, gout, hypokalaemia.

Manufacturer: M.S.D.

HYGROTON

Description: a proprietary, thiazide-like diuretic preparation produced in the form of scored, pale yellow tablets containing 50mg chlorthalidone marked GEIGY and coded ZA.

Used for: hypertension, oedema.

Dosage: adults, hypertension, 25mg–50mg each day as a single dose with breakfast. Oedema, 50mg each day or 100–200mg every other day reducing to a maintenance dose in the order of 50–100mg 3 times each week. Children, up to 2mg/kg body weight each day.

Special care: pregnancy, breastfeeding, elderly, kidney or liver disease, liver cirrhosis, SLE, gout, diabetes. Glucose, fluid and electrolyte (salts) levels should be carefully monitored during the course of therapy.

Avoid use: patients with serious kidney or liver failure, sensitivity to sulphonamide drugs, hypercalcaemia, Addison's disease.

Possible interaction: NSAIDs, barbiturates, antidiabetic substances, corticosteroids, alcohol, tubocurarine, opiods, carbenoxolone, lithium, cardiac glycosides.

Side effects: gastro-intestinal upset, blood changes, skin rash, upset of electrolyte balance and metabolism, sensitivity to light, anorexia, impotence, disturbance of vision, pancreatitis, dizziness.

Manufacturer: Geigy.

HYPNOMIDATE

Description: a reparation which induces general anaesthesia produced in ampoules for injection containing 2mg etomidate/ml. Also, **HYPNOMIDATE CONCENTRATE** containing 125mg etomidate/ml (diluted before use).

Used for: induction of general anaesthesia.

Dosage: by slow intravenous injection, 100–300µg/kg body weight/minute, dose depending upon patient's condition.

Special care: best used following premedication.

Avoid use: porphyria.

Possible interaction: anxiolytics, hypnotics, antidepressants, antihypertensives, antipsychotics, calcium-channel blockers, ß-blockers.

Side effects: muscle movement and pain with injection (lessened with pre-medication). Repeated doses may cause adrenal gland suppression.

Manufacturer: Janssen.

HYPNOVEL

Description: a benzodiazepine drug which has hypnotic, anxiolytic effects, available as a solution in ampoules for injection containing 10mg midazolam/ml.

Used for: sedation in patients undergoing minor surgery, those in intensive care, premedication in patients who are to receive general anaesthesia, induction of anaesthesia.

Dosage: adults, for sedation, 2mg (1–1.5mg in elderly persons) given by intravenous injection over thirty seconds. Then 0.5–1mg at 2 minute intervals if needed. Usual dose range is in the order of 2.5–7.5mg (1–2mg in elderly persons). Sedation of intensive care patients, 30–300µg/kg body weight by intravenous infusion over 5 minutes followed by 30–200µg/kg body weight every hour. Reduced doses may be indicated, especially if another drug (opioid analgesic) is also being given. Premedication, 70–100µg/kg body weight 1 hour to half an hour before general anaesthetic, given by intramuscular injection. Usual dose is in the order of 5mg (2.5mg in elderly persons).

Special care: breastfeeding, elderly, liver or kidney disease, lung disorders, myasthenia gravis, personality disorder. If use has been prolonged (as with intensive care patients) the drug should be gradually withdrawn.

Avoid use: patients with serious lung disorders, depressed respiration or in the last 3 months of pregnancy.

Possible interaction: central nervous system depressants, cimetidine, alcohol, erythromycin, anticonvulsant drugs.

Side effects: pain at injection site, dizziness, headache, circulatory changes, temporary halt in breathing (apnoea), hiccoughs.
Manufacturer: Roche.

HYPOVASE

Description: an antihypertensive preparation which is a selective alpha$_1$-blocker. It is produced as tablets of various strengths all containing prazosin hydrochloride. White 500µg tablets marked Pfizer; scored, orange 1mg tablets marked HYP/1; scored, white 2mg tablets marked HYP/2; scored, white 5mg tablets marked HYP/5 and Pfizer.
Used for: congestive heart failure, hypertension, Raynaud's disease, additional therapy in the treatment of urinary tract obstruction when the cause is benign enlargement of the prostate gland.
Dosage: adults, congestive heart failure, 500µg in first instance increasing to 1mg 3 or 4 times each day. Then a usual maintenance dose in the order of 4–20mg in divided doses. Hypertension, 500µg as evening dose at first, followed by 500µg 2 or 3 times each day for a period of 3 days to 1 week. Then, 1mg 2 or 3 times each day for 3 days to 1 week. The dose may be further increased gradually as required with a daily maximum of 20mg. Raynaud's disease, 500µg twice each day at first, then a maintenance dose of 1 or 2mg twice each day. Additional therapy in urine obstruction, 500µg twice each day at first increasing to a maintenance dose of 2mg twice each day.
Special care: heart failure, patients suffering from congestive heart failure caused by stenosis; urinary tract obstruction, patients liable to fainting during urination.
Possible interaction: other antihypertensive drugs.
Side effects: dry mouth, dizziness on rising from lying down, sudden short-lived loss of consciousness, weariness, skin rash, blurring of vision.
Manufacturer: Invicta.

HYTRIN and HYTRIN BPH

Description: an antihypertensive preparation which is a selective alpha$_1$-blocker produced as tablets of 4 different strengths, all containing terazosin (as hydrochloride). White 1mg, yellow 2mg, brown 5mg and blue 10mg tablets are all marked with triangle-shaped symbols and logo.
Used for: hypertension, urine obstruction caused by benign enlargement of prostate gland.
Dosage: 1mg taken at bedtime at first then gradually increased at weekly intervals. The usual maintenance dose is in the order of 2–10mg taken once each day.
Special care: in patients liable to fainting.
Possible interaction: other antihypertensive drugs.
Side effects: initial dose may cause fainting, hypotension on rising from lying down, dizziness, weariness, fluid retention and swelling of lower limbs.
Manufacturer: Abbott.

IDOXENE

Description: an antiviral preparation available as an eye ointment containing 0.5% idoxuridine.
Used for: herpetic keratitis (an inflammation and infection of the cornea caused by *Herpes simplex* virus).
Dosage: apply 4 times each day and at bedtime and continue for 3 to 5 days after condition has cleared. Maximum period of treatment is 3 weeks.
Special care: pregnancy.
Possible interaction: boric acid, corticosteroids.
Side effects: local irritation in eye and pain, swelling due to oedema.
Manufacturer: Spodefell.

IDURIDIN

Description: an antiviral skin preparation available as a solution with applicator in 2 strengths, containing 5% and 40% idoxuridine, both in dimethyl sulphoxide.
Used for: viral skin infections caused by *Herpes zoster* and *Herpes simplex*.
Dosage: adults and children over 12 years, apply 5% solution to infected area 4 times daily for 4 days. For severe *Herpes zoster* infections (shingles) only, the 40% solution should be used, applied on lint and changed every 24 hours, for a period of 4 days.
Special care: preparation may stain clothing.
Avoid use: children under 12 years, pregnancy, breastfeeding.
Manufacturer: Ferring.

ILOSONE

Description: a macrolide antibiotic preparation available as red/ivory capsules containing 250mg erythromycin estolate and marked DISTA. Also **ILOSONE TABLETS**, oblong, pink, containing 500mg; **ILOSONE SUSPENSION** contains 125mg erythromycin estolate/5ml; **ILOSONE SUSPENSION FORTE** contains 250mg/5ml.
Used for: respiratory and urinary tract infections, soft tissue, skin, dental infections, infections of the middle ear, acne.
Dosage: adults, 250mg every 6 hours with a maximum of 4g each day. Children 20–50mg/kg body weight each day in divided doses.
Avoid use: patients with liver disease or disorder, history of jaundice.
Possible interaction: anticoagulants taken orally, probenecid, carbamazepine, ergotamine, cyclosporin, lincomycin, theophylline, dihydroergotamine, alfentanil, clindamycin, triazolam, bromocriptine, digoxin.
Side effects: gastro-intestinal upset, allergic responses, cholestatic jaundice.
Manufacturer: Dista.

ILUBE

Description: a lubricant eye preparation available in the form of drops containing 5% acetylcysteine and 0.35% hypromellose.
Used for: dry eyes caused by insufficient secretion of tears or abnormal mucus production.
Dosage: 1 or 2 drops into affected eye 3 or 4 times each day.
Avoid use: patients with soft contact lenses.
Manufacturer: Cusi.

IMDUR

Description: an antianginal nitrate preparation available in the form of scored oval, yellow, film-coated, sustained-release tablets containing 60mg isosorbide mononitrate marked A/ID.
Used for: prevention of angina.
Dosage: adults, 1 tablet each day taken in the morning increasing to 2 daily if necessary, as a single dose. If headache occurs, reduce to half a tablet each day.
Avoid use: children.
Side effects: nausea, headache, dizziness.
Manufacturer: Astra.

IMIGRAN

Description: a preparation which is a seratonin agonist available as capsule-shaped, white, film-coated tablets containing 100mg sumatriptan (as succinate), marked with name and company. Also, **IMIGRAM SUBJECT INJECTION**, pre-filled syringes containing 6mg sumatriptan/0.5ml with auto-injector.
Used for: acute attacks of migraine which may be accompanied by aura.
Dosage: tablets, 1 tablet as soon as possible after attack starts which may be repeated if condition improves, but should not exceed 3 tablets in 24 hours. If migraine does not respond in first instance, a repeat dose should not be taken. Injection, 6mg by subcutaneous injection as soon as possible after attack begins which may be repeated after 1 hour if condition improves. The

maximum dose is 12mg in 24 hours.
Special care: pregnancy, breastfeeding,
liver, kidney or heart disease,
indications of coronary artery disease;
persons who have misused other
migraine preparations. Patients should
exercise care if driving or operating
machinery.
Avoid use: children, elderly persons,
patients with history of heart attack,
heart spasm, uncontrolled hypertension,
heart disease, Prinzmetal's angina.
Possible interaction: ergotamine, 5-HT
re-uptake inhibitors (an antidepressant
group), lithium, MAOIs.
Side effects: blood pressure rise, pain at
injection site, tiredness, feeling of
heaviness and pressure, dizziness,
sleepiness, slight disturbance of liver
function. Drug should be withdrawn if
there is pain in chest or throat and cause
investigated.
Manufacturer: Glaxo.

IMMUKIN

Description: a preparation of recombinant human interferon gamma-1b
available as a solution in vials for
injection at a strength of 200 micro-
grams/ml.
Used for: additional treatment (with
antibiotics) to lessen the incidence of
serious infections acquired by patients
with chronic granulomatous disease (any
1 of a number of diseases giving rise to
masses of granulation tissue, known as
granulomata, e.g. tuberculosis and
leprosy).
Dosage: adults and children with body
surface area exceeding $0.5m^2$, $50 \mu g/m^2$
by subcutaneous injection 3 times each
week. Children with body surface area
less than $0.5m^2$, $1.5 \mu g/kg$ body weight 3
times each week.
Special care: patients with serious liver
or kidney disease, heart disease
(congestive heart failure, arrhythmia,
ischaemic heart disease), seizures,
central nervous system disorders. Blood,
liver and kidney function tests and urine

analysis must be carried out during the
course of therapy.
Avoid use: children under 6 months.
Possible interaction: alcohol.
Side effects: headache, chills, pain, fever,
rash, nausea and vomiting, pain at
injection site, ability to perform skilled
tasks, e.g. driving and operating
machinery may be impaired.
Manufacturer: Boehringer-Ingelheim.

IMUNOVIR

Description: an antiviral preparation and
immunopotentiator produced in the form
of white tablets containing 500mg
inosine pranobex.
Used for: infections of mucous
membranes and skin caused by *Herpes
simplex* virus, (type I and/or II) e.g.
genital warts, subacute inflammation of
the brain.
Dosage: *Herpes simplex* infections, 1g 4
times each day for 1 to 2 weeks;
inflammation of the brain, 50–100mg/kg
body weight each day in divided doses.
Special care: patients with abnormally
high blood levels of uric acid (hyperuricaemia), gout, kidney disease.
Avoid use: children
Side effects: raised uric acid levels.
Manufacturer: Leo.

IMURAN

Description: a cytotoxic immunosuppressant preparation, azathioprine,
produced in the form of film-coated
tablets of 2 strengths. Orange tablets
(25mg) are marked Imuran 25; yellow
tablets (50mg) are marked Imuran 50.
Also, **IMURAN INJECTION**
containing 50mg azathioprine (as
sodium salt) produced as powder in vials
for reconstitution.
Used for: to suppress organ or tissue
rejection following transplant
operations; some diseases of the auto-
immune system especially when
treatment with corticosteroids alone has
proved to be inadequate.
Dosage: tablets and/or injection,

prevention of rejection of transplant, usually up to 5mg/kg body weight at first and then a maintenance dose in the order of 1–4mg/kg body weight each day. Auto-immune diseases, up to 3mg/kg body weight each day at first reducing to 1–3mg/kg body weight daily as maintenance dose.

Special care: the injection is an irritant and hence should only be used if tablets cannot be taken. Special care in pregnant women, patients should avoid excessive exposure to sun, persons with kidney or liver disease or suffering from infections. Blood counts and other monitoring for toxic effects should be carried out.

Possible interaction: skin rashes, bone marrow suppression, gastro-intestinal upset, toxic effects on liver.

Manufacturer: Wellcome.

INDERAL

Description: a preparation which is a non-cardioselective ß-blocker produced as pink, film-coated tablets containing 10mg, 40mg and 80mg propranolol hydrochloride all marked with name, strength and ICI. Also, **INDERAL INJECTION** containing 1mg/ml in ampoules for injection.

Used for: heart arrhythmias, prevention of second heart attack, angina, enlarged and weakened heart muscle. Fallot's tetralogy (a congenital defect of the heart), phaeochromocytoma, situational and generalised anxiety.

Dosage: heart attack, 40mg 4 times each day for 2 or 3 days starting from 5 to twenty-1 days after first attack. Then a maintenance dose of 80mg twice each day. Arrhythmias, 10–40mg 3 or 4 times each day. Angina, 40mg 2 or 3 times each day at first increasing at weekly intervals if required to a usual dose in the order of 120–240mg daily. Hypertension, 80mg twice each day at first increasing at weekly intervals if required to usual dose in the order of 160–320mg daily. Phaeochromocytoma,

60mg each day taken along with an alpha-blocker for 3 days before operation for removal. If tumour is inoperable, a 30mg daily dose should be taken. Situational anxiety, 40mg twice each day, generalised anxiety, the same dose by increasing to 3 times each day if needed. Children, arrhythmias, 0.25–0.5mg/kg body weight 3 to 4 times each day. Fallot's tetralogy, up to 1mg/kg body weight 3 or 4 times each day. Phaeochromocytoma, 0.25–0.5mg/kg body weight 3 or 4 times each day.

Special care: pregnancy, breastfeeding, patients underoing planned surgery, those with liver or kidney disease, diabetes, metabolic acidosis. Patients with weak hearts may require diuretics and digitalis. Drug should be gradually withdrawn.

Avoid use: patients with history of bronchospasm, obstructive airways disease, heart block, heart shock, disease of peripheral arteries, sinus bradycardia, uncompensated heart failure.

Possible interaction: sympathomimetics, cimetidine, heart depressant anaesthetics, indomethacin, clonidine withdrawal, hypoglycaemics, class I antiarrhythmics, ergotamine, verapamil, reserpine, antihypertensives.

Side effects: bradycardia, cold hands and feet, tiredness with exercise, gastro-intestinal upset, disturbance of sleep, bronchospasm, heart failure. Drug should be gradually withdrawn if skin rash or dry eyes occur.

Manufacturer: Zeneca.

INDERAL LA

Description: an antianginal, antihypertensive and anxiolytic preparation which is a non-cardioselective ß-blocker. It is produced as pink/purple sustained-release capsules containing 160mg propanolol hydrochloride marked ICI and INDERAL LA. Also, **HALF-INDERAL LA**, pink/purple sustained-release capsules containing 80mg propanolol hydrochloride marked ICI and HALF-INDERAL LA.

Used for: angina, hypertension, additional therapy in thyrotoxicosis, also treatment of symptoms of anxiety.

Dosage: angina, 80mg or 160mg each day with a maximum daily dose of 240mg. Hypertension, 160mg each day at first increasing by 80mg gradually if needed until condition is controlled. Thyrotoxicosis, 80mg or 160mg each day with a maximum daily dose of 240mg. Situational anxiety, 80mg each day, generalised anxiety, 80–160mg each day.

Special care: pregnancy, breastfeeding, patients undergoing planned surgery, liver or kidney disease, diabetes, metabolic acidosis. Patients with weak hearts may require diuretics and digitalis. Drug should be gradually withdrawn.

Avoid use: children, patients with history of bronchospasm, obstructive airways disease, heart block, heart shock, disease of peripheral arteries, sinus bradycardia, uncompensated heart failure.

Possible interaction: sympathomimetics, cimetidine, heart depressant anaesthetics, indomethacin, clonidine withdrawal, hypoglycaemics, class I antiarrhythmics, ergotamine, verapamil, reserpine, antihypertensives

Side effects: bradycardia, cold hands and feet, tiredness with exercise, gastrointestinal upset, disturbance of sleep, bronchospasm, heart failure. Drug should be gradually withdrawn if skin rash or dry eyes occur.

Manufacturer: Zeneca.

INDERETIC

Description: an antihypertensive preparation combining a non-cardioselective ß-blocker and thiazide diuretic, available as white capsules containing 80mg propanolol hydrochloride and 2.5mg bendrofluazide.

Used for: hypertension.

Dosage: adults, 1 tablet twice each day.

Special care: pregnancy, breastfeeding, patients undergoing general anaesthesia or planned surgery, liver or kidney disease, gout, diabetes, metabolic acidosis. Patients with weak hearts may require diuretics and digitalis. Potassium supplements may be needed and patient's electrolyte levels should be monitored.

Avoid use: children, patients with heart block, heart shock, sinus bradycardia, peripheral disease of the arteries, sick sinus syndrome, uncompensated heart failure, obstruction of heart outflow, aortic stenosis (narrrowing of aorta). Those with history of breathing difficulties, bronchospasm, obstructive airways disease.

Possible interaction: sympathomimetics, class I antiarrhythmics, indomethacin, cimetidine, clonidine withdrawal, antihypertensives, ergot alkaloids, heart depressant anaesthetics, depressants, reserpine, hypoglycaemics. Digitalis, potassium-sparing diuretics, potassium supplements, lithium.

Side effects: bradycardia, cold hands and feet, fatigue on exertion, disturbance of sleep, gastro-intestinal upset, heart failure, bronchospasm. Blood changes, sensitivity to light, gout, muscular weakness.

Manufacturer: Zeneca.

INDEREX

Description: an antihypertensive preparation which combines a non-cardioselective ß-blocker and thiazide diuretic. It is available as grey/pink sustained-release capsules containing 160mg propanolol and 80mg bendrofluazide marked ICI and Inderex.

Used for: hypertension.

Dosage: adults, 1 twice each day.

Special care: pregnancy, breastfeeding, patients undergoing general anaesthesia or planned surgery, liver or kidney disease, gout, diabetes, metabolic acidosis. Patients with weak hearts may require diuretics and digitalis. Potassium supplements may be needed and patient's electrolyte levels should be monitored.

Avoid use: children, patients with heart block, heart shock, sinus bradycardia,

peripheral disease of the arteries, sick sinus syndrome, uncompensated heart failure, obstruction of heart outflow, aortic stenosis (narrrowing of aorta). Those with history of breathing difficulties, bronchospasm, obstructive airways disease.
Possible interaction: sympathomimetics, class I antiarrhythmics, indomethacin, cimetidine, clonidine withdrawal, antihypertensives, ergot alkaloids, heart depressant anaesthetics, central nervous system depressants, reserpine, hypoglycaemics. Digitalis, potassium-sparing diuretics, potassium supplements, lithium.
Side effects: bradycardia, cold hands and feet, fatigue on exertion, disturbance of sleep, gastro-intestinal upset, heart failure, bronchospasm. Blood changes, sensitivity to light, gout, muscular weakness.
Manufacturer: Zeneca.

INDOCID

Description: an NSAID and indole available in a variety of forms: capsules are ivory-coloured and contain 25mg and 50mg indomethacin both marked with name and strength. **INDOCID SUSPENSION** contains 25mg/5ml; **INDOCID SUPPOSITORIES** contain 100mg indomethacin. **INDOCID-R** are blue/yellow sustained-release capsules containing 75mg indomethacin marked INDOCID-R 693.
Used for: diseases of skeleton and joints including ankylosing spondylitis, osteoarthritis, lumbago, rheumatoid arthritis, degenerative disease of hip joint, acute joint disorders, acute gout (except Indocid-R). Also, dysmenorrhoea.
Dosage: adults, capsules and suspension, 50–200mg each day in divided doses with meals. Indocid-R, 1 tablet once or twice each day, suppositories, 1 at night and 1 in the morning if needed.
Special care: elderly persons, patients with heart failure, disorders of central nervous system, liver or kidney disease. Patients taking drug long-term should receive careful monitoring.

Avoid use: children, pregnancy, breastfeeding, history of gastro-intestinal ulcer or peptic ulcer, allergy to anti-inflammatory drug or aspirin, angioneurotic oedema, recent proctitis (inflammation of the rectum and anus).
Possible interaction: methotrexate, anticoagulants, corticosteroids, quinolones, probenecid, aminoglycosides, salicylates, ß-blockers, lithium, diuretics.
Side effects: blood changes, effects on central nervous system, gastro-intestinal intolerance, disturbance of vision and corneal deposits. If recurring headaches or gastro-intestinal bleeding occur, drug should be withdrawn. Eye tests should be carried out during the course of long-term therapy.
Manufacturer: Morson.

INDOCID PDA

Description: a prostaglandin synthetase inhibitor produced as a powder in vials for reconstitution and injection containing 1mg indomethacin (as sodium trihydrate).
Used for: patent ductus arteriosus (PDA in premature babies (a condition in which there is a connection between the aorta and pulmonary artery, the ductus arteriosus, which normally closes after birth).
Dosage: 3 intravenous injections, at intervals of 12 to 24 hours depending upon baby's age, condition and urinary output.
Special care: kidney function and plasma levels of electrolytes should be monitored.
Avoid use: babies with serious kidney disorders, untreated infection, bleeding, disorders of blood coagulation.
Possible interaction: frusemide, aminoglycosides, digitalis.
Side effects: bleeding, disturbance in urine production, elevated creatine leve in blood, imbalance in electrolyte (salts levels. If liver disease develops, drug should be withdrawn.
Manufacturer: Morson.

INDOMOD

Description: an NSAID Indole preparation available in the form of capsules of 2 strengths containing enteric-coated, continuous-release pellets. Orange capsules, marked AB27, contain 25mg and brown capsules, marked AB26, contain 75mg indomethacin respectively.
Used for: joint and bone disorders, including ankylosing spondylitis, rheumatoid arthritis, osteoarthritis, tenosynovitis, tendinitis, bursitis, gout.
Dosage: adults, 50–75mg as single or 2 doses each day increasing once a week by 25 or 50mg to a maximum daily dose of 200mg.
Special care: elderly persons, patients with heart failure, liver or kidney disease, disorders of central nervous system. Patients taking drug long-term require careful monitoring and eye tests.
Avoid use: pregnancy, breastfeeding, history of ulcers or active ulcer, allergy to NSAID or aspirin.
Possible interaction: salicylates, probenecid, ß-blockers, corticosteroids, lithium, diuretics, quinolones, anticoagulants.
Side effects: disturbance of vision, deposits in cornea; if recurrent headaches or gastro-intestinal bleeding occur, drug should be withdrawn.
Manufacturer: Indomod.

INFLUVAC

Description: a preparation of inactivated surface antigen obtained from 4 strains of influenza virus. It is produced in pre-filled syringes containing 15µg of each strain of influenza virus/0.5ml suspension.
Dosage: adults, 0.5ml by deep subcutaneous or intramuscular injection. Children, aged 4 to 13 years, 0.5ml then repeated dose 4 to 6 weeks later.
Avoid use: children under 4 years, patients with allergy to poultry, eggs or feathers, chick embryos used to culture virus strains). Patients with feverish conditions.
Side effects: tiredness, headache, feverishness, pain at injection site.
Manufacturer: Duphar.

INNOHEP

Description: an anticoagulant preparation which is a low molecular weight heparin produced as solutions in ampoules or pre-filled syringes for injection. Syringes contain 3500 units activity of anti-factor Xa tinzaparin/0.3ml. Ampoules contain 5000 units activity of anti-factor Xa tinzaparin/0.5ml.
Used for: prevention of thrombosis in patients having orthopaedic or general surgical operations.
Dosage: orthopaedic surgery, 50 units/kg body weight 2 hours before operation by subcutaneous injection then same dose once each day for next 7 to 10 days. General surgery, 3500 units 2 hours before operation by subcutaneous injection then same dose once each day for next 7 to 10 days.
Special care: pregnancy, breastfeeding, asthma, severe liver or kidney disease.
Avoid use: children, patients liable to bleeding, active peptic ulcer, serious hypertension which is uncontrolled, septic endocarditis.
Possible interaction: drugs which affect blood coagulation or platelets.
Side effects: risk of haemorrhage, slight bruising, skin rash, blood changes, short-lived rise in liver enzymes.
Manufacturer: Leo.

INNOVACE

Description: an antihypertensive preparation which is an ACE inhibitor produced as tablets of different strengths, all marked INNOVACE and containing enalapril maleate: white, round 2.5mg tablets; white, scored 5mg tablets; red, triangular 10mg tablets; peach, triangular 20mg tablets.
Used for: congestive heart failure, with digitalis and potassium-sparing diuretics. Prevention of heart attack and progression of disease in left ventricle of heart.
Dosage: adults, 2.5mg once each day at first increasing to a usual maintenance dose in the order of 20mg, maximum is

40mg. Treatment should normally begin in hospital and diuretics discontinued or reduced before therapy starts.
Special care: breastfeeding, patients undergoing anaesthesia, those with kidney disease and hypertension associated with this, patients have kidney dialysis, serious congestive heart failure. Kidney function should be monitored during course of therapy.
Avoid use: children, pregnancy, patients with obstruction to outflow of heart or aortic stenosis (narrowing of aorta).
Possible interaction: potassium supplements or potassium-sparing diuretics, other antihypertensives, lithium.
Side effects: tiredness, headache, dizziness, cough, gastro-intestinal upset, oedema, hypotension.
Manufacturer: M.S.D.

INNOZIDE

Description: an antihypertensive preparation combining an ACE inhibitor and thiazide diuretic produced in the form of scored, yellow tablets containing 20mg enalapril maleate and 12.5mg hydrochlorthiazide marked MSD 718.
Used for: mild to moderate hypotension in patients who have become accus-tomed to the same components taken individually.
Dosage: adults, 1 tablet each day with a maximum of 2 if needed.
Special care: breastfeeding, imbalance in levels of electrolytes (salts) or fluid, kidney or liver disease, heart disease or disease of the blood vessels of the brain. Patients receiving kidney dialysis, suffering from gout, diabetes or undergoing anaesthesia.
Avoid use: children, pregnancy, angio-neurotic oedema resulting from previous treatment with ACE inhibitor, anuria.
Possible interaction: hypoglycaemics, tubocurarine, corticosteroids, potassium supplements, potassium-sparing diuretics, NSAIDs, central nervous system depressants, lithium.
Side effects: cough, tiredness, headache,

skin rash, hypotension, pain in chest, dizziness, weakness, kidney failure, impotence, angioneurotic oedema.
Manufacturer: M.S.D.

INSTILLAGEL

Description: a preparation which has disinfectant and local anaesthetic properties produced in the form of a gel in disposable syringes. It contains 2% lignocaine hydrochloride, 0.25% chlorhexidine gluconate, 0.06% methyl hydroxybenzoate, 0.025% propyl hydroxybenzoate.
Used for: to disinfect and lubricate catheters during insertion and as local anaesthetic.
Dosage: 6–11ml into urethra.
Special care: patients with serious, local haemorrhage.
Manufacturer: CliniMed.

INTAL SYNCRONER

Description: a bronchodilator and NSAID, sodium cromoglycate, produced in a variety of different forms: **INTAL METERED DOSE AEROSOL** with spacer device, delivers 5mg/dose. **INTAL IHHIALER** also delivers 53mg/dose and is a metered dose aerosol. **INTAL SPINCAP**, clear yellow spincaps contain 20mg and are marked INTAL P and FISONS. **INTAL NEBULISER SOLUTION** contains 10mg/2ml in ampoules for use with nebuliser. **INTAL FISONAIRE**, a metered dose aerosol with spacer device within chamber delivering 5mg/dose.
Used for: prevention of bronchial asthma.
Dosage: adults and children, inhaler, 2 puffs 4 times each day reducing to 1 puff for maintenance. Spincaps, 4 each day in spinhaler taken at regular times. Nebuliser, 20mg 4 to 6 times each day continuously.
Side effects: irritated throat, short-lived cough; rarely, bronchospasm.
Manufacturer: Fisons.

INTRAVAL SODIUM

Description: a general anaesthetic preparation produced as a powder for reconstitution containing 0.5 and 2.5g thiopentone sodium.
Used for: induction of general anaesthesia.
Dosage: (in fit persons who have received premedication), 100–150mg over 10 to 15 seconds by intravenous injection; may be repeated after half a minute if required. Or, up to 4mg/kg body weight may be given. Children, 2–7mg/kg body weight.
Special care: depression of respiration and heart may occur if dose is too high.
Possible interaction: alcohol.
Side effects: sedative effects and slow metabolism for up to 24 hours. Ability to perform skilled tasks, e.g. driving, may be impaired.
Manufacturer: Theraplix.

INTRON A

Description: a single-subtype recombinant interferon preparation produced as a powder in vials with solution for reconstitution and injection, in different strengths of 1, 3, 5, 10, 25 and 30 megaunits interferon alfa-2b (rbe).
Used for: leukaemia, maintenance of remission in multiple myeloma, non-Hodgkins lymphoma, AIDS-related Kaposi's sarcoma.
Dosage: according to individual need as directed by physician.
Avoid use: pregnant women.
Possible interaction: theophylline.
Side effects: weariness, depression, influenza-like symptoms, bone marrow suppression, rash; seizures and coma (with higher doses especially in elderly persons).
Manufacturer: Schering-Plough.

INTROPIN

Description: a potent sympathomimetic drug which is an intropic agent produced in ampoules for injection containing 40mg dopamine hydrochloride/ml.
Used for: cardiogenic shock following heart attack and heart failure in cardiac surgery.
Dosage: 2–5 µg/kg body-weight/minute by intravenous infusion but dose is critical.
Special care: hypovalaemia (abnormally low volume of circulating blood) should be corrected.
Avoid use: patients with phaeochromocytoma, fast arrhythmia.
Possible interaction: antidepressants.
Side effects: tachycardia, hypo and hypertension, constriction of peripheral blood vessels, vomiting and nausea.
Manufacturer: DuPont.

IODOFLEX

Description: a preparation which is absorbent and antibacterial available as a paste with removable gauze, containing cadexomer iodine.
Used for: chronic leg ulcers.
Dosage: adults and children over 2 years, apply up to 50g to ulcer and cover with additional dressing; renew when dressing is saturated or 3 times each week. Dose should not exceed 150g in any week and use should be restricted to a period of 3 months.
Special care: patients with disorders of the thyroid gland.
Avoid use: children under 2 years, pregnancy, breastfeeding, patients with thyroid disorders (Grave's disease, Hashimoto's thyroiditis, non-toxic nodular goitre).
Possible interaction: sulphafurazoles, lithium, sulphonylureas.
Manufacturer: Perstop.

IODOSORB

Description: an adsorbent and antibacterial available as a powder in sachets containing cadexomer iodine.
Also **IODOSORB OINTMENT** containing cadexomer iodine.
Used for: leg ulcers, bedsores and moist wounds.

Dosage: adults, apply a layer at least 3mm thick and cover with sterile dressing. Change when dressing is saturated. Ointment, (for chronic leg ulcers), as above but no more than 150g should be used in any 1 week and course of therapy should not exceed 3 months.
Special care: patients with disorders of the thyroid gland.
Avoid use: children, pregnancy, breastfeeding, patients with thyroid disorders (Grave's disease, Hashimoto's thyroiditis, non-toxic nodular goitre).
Possible interaction: sulphafurazoles, lithium, sulphonylureas.
Manufacturer: Perstop.

IONAMIN^{CD}

Description: a central nervous system stimulant which acts as an appetite-suppressant. It is available as sustained-release capsules of 2 strengths: yellow/grey containing 15mg phentermine as resin complex and yellow, containing 30mg phentermine as resin complex. Both are marked with name and strength.
Used for: obesity.
Dosage: adults, 15–30mg each day before breakfast.
Special care: angina, hypertension, heart arrhythmias. For short-term use only.
Avoid use: children, pregnancy, breastfeeding, hyperthyroidism, serious hypertension, arteriosclerosis. Those with history of drug or alcohol abuse or psychiatric illnesses.
Possible interaction: methyldopa, sympathomimetics, guanethidine, MAOIs, psychotropic drugs.
Side effects: drug dependence and tolerance, dry mouth, rise in blood pressure, agitation and nervousness, palpitations, psychiatric disturbances.
Manufacturer: Lipha.

IOPIDINE

Description: an eye solution which is an alpha,-agonist available in single dose

(0.25ml) ampoules containing 1.15% apraclonidine hydrochloride.
Used for: control and prevention of any rise in pressure within the eye following anterior segment laser surgery.
Dosage: 1 drop into eye 1 hour before laser treatment and 1 drop immediately after surgery is completed.
Special care: pregnancy, breastfeeding, serious heart and circulatory disease, hypertension, history of fainting. If there is a great reduction in the pressure within the eye, this should receive careful monitoring.
Avoid use: children.
Possible interaction: MAOIs, sympathomimetics, TCADs.
Side effects: blanching of conjunctiva of eye and retraction of eyelids, dilation of pupil. Possible effects on heart and circulation due to absorption of drug.
Manufacturer: Alcon.

IPRAL

Description: a sulphonamide antibiotic preparation which is a folic acid inhibitor available as white tablets containing 100mg and 200mg trimethoprim, marked SQUIBB 513 and SQUIBB 514 respectively.
Used for: prevention and treatment of infections of the urinary tract; treatment of respiratory tract infections.
Dosage: adults, treatment, 200mg twice each day; prevention of urinary tract infections, 100mg taken at night. Children, over 6 years of age, 100mg twice each day.
Special care: patients with kidney disorder or folate deficiency. Regular blood tests are required during long-term treatment.
Avoid use: children under 6 years, pregnancy, serious kidney disease.
Side effects: gastro-intestinal upset, skin reactions, folate deficiency if drug is taken long-term.
Manufacutrer: Squibb.

ISMELIN

Description: an antihypertensive preparation, guanethidine sulphate, which is an adrenergic neurone blocker, available as white tablets containing 10mg and pink tablets containing 25mg. Both are marked with strength and name. Also **ISMELIN INJECTION** containing 10mg/ml in ampoules.
Used for: hypertension.
Dosage: adults, 10mg each day at first increasing by 10mg once a week if needed to a usual dose in the order of 25–50mg.
Special care: pregnancy, kidney disease, asthma, peptic ulcer, arteriosclerosis, anaesthesia.
Avoid use: patients with heart or kidney failure, phaeochromocytoma.
Possible interaction: sympathomimetics, MAOIs, hypoglycaemics, digitalis, contraceptive pill, TCADs, antiarrhythmics, antipsychotics, other antihypertensives.
Side effects: blocked nose, blood changes, oedema, failure to reach sexual climax (males), bradycardia, diarrhoea, hypotension when rising from lying down.
Manufacturer: Ciba.

ISOPTO ATROPINE

Description: lubricant and anticholinergic eyedrops containing 1% atropine sulphate and 0.5% hypromellose.
Used for: to produce long-lasting mydriasis (the drug is mydriatic)—fixed dilation of the pupil of the eye, and cycloplegia (cycloplegic)—paralysis of the ciliary muscles. This is in order to allow detailed examination of the eye to be carried out.
Dosage: adults, for uveitis (inflammation of the uveal tract), 1 drop 3 times each day; for refraction, 1 to 2 drops 1 hour before eye is examined. Children, uveitis, 1 drop 3 times each day; refraction, 1 drop twice each day for 1 to 2 days before eye is examined.
Special care: infants, pressure should be applied over lachrymal (tear) sac for 1 minute.

Avoid use: patients with soft contact lenses, narrow angle glaucoma.
Side effects: dry mouth, sensitivity to light, stinging in eye, blurring of vision, headache, tachycardia. Also changes in behaviour and psychotic responses.
Manufacturer: Alcon.

ISOPTO CARBACHOL

Description: lubricant and cholinergic eyedrops containing 3% carbachol and 1% hypromellose.
Used for: glaucoma.
Dosage: adults, 2 drops 3 times each day.
Avoid use: children, patients with severe iritis (inflammation of the iris), abrasion of the cornea, wearing soft contact lenses.
Manufacturer: Alcon.

ISOPTO CARPINE

Description: lubricant and cholinergic eyedrops available at different strengths containing 0.5%, 1%, 2%, 3% and 4% pilocarpine all with 0.5% hypromellose.
Used for: glaucoma.
Dosage: adults, 2 drops 3 times each day.
Avoid use: children, patients with severe iritis (inflammation of the iris), wearing soft contact lenses.
Manufacturer: Alcon.

ISOTREX

Description: a topical preparation of vitamin A derivative available as a gel containing 0.05% isotretinoin.
Used for: acne vulgaris.
Dosage: apply thinly once or twice each day for at least 6 to 8 weeks.
Special care: avoid mucous membranes, mouth, angles of nose, eyes, damaged or sunburnt areas. Ultra-violet light should be avoided.
Avoid use: pregnancy, breastfeeding, family history or history of epithelioma of skin (abnormal growth which may or may not be malignant).
Possible interaction: keratolytics.
Side effects: local skin irritation.
Manufacturer: Stiefel.

ISTIN

Description: an antianginal and anti-hypertensive preparation which is a class II calcium antagonist. It is available as 5mg and 10mg white tablets containing amlodipine besylate, marked Pfizer and ITN 5 and ITN 10 respectively.
Used for: angina in myocardial ischaemia, hypertension.
Dosage: adults, 5mg once each day; maximum dose, 10mg daily.
Special care: pregnancy, breastfeeding, children, liver disease.
Side effects: oedema, headache, dizziness, tiredness, nausea, flushing.
Manufacturer: Pfizer.

JECTOFER

Description: a haematinic compound available in ampoules for injection containing iron sorbitol and citric acid (equivalent to 50mg of iron/ml).
Used for: anaemia caused by iron deficiency.
Dosage: adults and children over 3kg in weight by intramuscular injection as a single dose. The maximum dose for each injection is 100mg.
Avoid use: patients with certain other types of anaemia (hypoplastic or aplastic), seriously damaged kidney or liver, acute leukaemia.
Side effects: heart arrhythmias.
Manufacturer: Astra.

JEXIN

Description: a non-depolarizing (or competitive) muscle relaxant preparation used in anaesthesia produced in ampoules for injection containing 10mg tubocurarine chloride/ml.

Used for: production of muscle relaxation during surgery and for patients in intensive care units receiving long-term assisted ventilation.
Dosage: adults, 15–30mg by intravenous injection at first then 5–10mg as needed. Children, 300–500µg/kg body weight at first, then 60–100µg/kg, as needed. Newborn babies, 200–250µg/kg body weight at first then 40–50µg/kg, as needed.
Special care: kidney disease or damage, those in whom hypotension would be undesirable.
Avoid use: patients with myasthenia gravis.
Possible interaction: aminoglycosides, clindamycin, azlocillin, colistin, verapamil, nifedipine, cholinergics, magnesium salts.
Side effects: short-lived hypotension, skin rash.
Manufacturer: Evans.

JUNIFEN

Description: an NSAID produced as a sugar-free, orange-flavoured suspension containing 100mg ibuprofen/5ml.
Used for: relief of pain and reduction of fever in children.
Dosage: children, 1 to 2 years, 2.5ml; 3 to 7 years, 5ml; 8 to 12 years, 10ml. All given 3 to 4 times each day.
Special care: pregnancy, breastfeeding, patients with liver, kidney or heart disease or damage, asthma, gastro-intestinal disease, patients receiving long-term therapy require careful monitoring.
Avoid use: children under 1 year and those less than 7kg body weight, allergy to aspirin or NSAID, peptic ulcer.
Possible interaction: thiazide diuretics, anticoagulants, quinolones.
Side effects: rash, thrombocytopenia, gastro-intestinal upset or haemorrhage.
Manufacturer: Boots.

KABIGLOBULIN

Description: a preparation of human normal immunoglobulin (IINIG) available as a 16% solution in ampoules for injection.

Used for: prevention of hepatitis A infection, prevention of measles, prevention of rubella in pregnancy, burns, antibody deficiency conditions.

Dosage: prevention of hepatitis A, adults and children, usual dose 0.02ml 0 0.04ml/kg body weight or 0.06–0.12 ml if risk is greater. Prevention of measles, 0.02ml/kg body weight or 0.04ml/kg body weight to allow mild attack. Rubella in pregnancy, adults, 20ml to prevent clinical attack. All doses given by Intramuscular injection.

Possible interaction: live vaccines.

Manufacturer: Pharmacia.

KABIKINASE

Description: a fibrinolytic preparation available as a powder in vials for reconstitution and injection in 3 strengths, containing 250,000 units, 750,000 units and 1.5 million units streptokinase.

Used for: to disperse blood clots in life-threatening conditions as in pulmonary embolism, heart attack, deep vein thrombosis, arterial thromboembolism, clots during haemodialysis (kidney dialysis).

Dosage: adults, up to 600,000 units given over thirty minutes by intravascular route (into blood vessel), in first instance. Maintenance dose, 100,000 units every hour for 3 to 6 days. Heart attack, 1.5 million units by intravenous infusion over 1 hour then 150mg of aspirin each day for a minimum of 4 weeks. Children, 1300–1400 units/kg body weight each hour for 3 to 6 days. Other conditions may require different doses.

Special care: patients with pancreatitis, ensure no pre-existing clot which on dissolution might cause embolism. Special care with follow-on anti-coagulant therapy.

Avoid use: pregnancy, patients with recent haemorrhage, surgery or injury, bleeding disorders. Also coagulation disorders, serious hypertension, streptococcal infections, serious liver or kidney damage or disease, peptic ulcer, endocarditis caused by bacteria. Patients with known allergy to streptokinase or who have received treatment with this or anistreplase during the previous 5 days to 6 months.

Possible interaction: drugs acting on blood platelets, anticoagulants.

Side effects: haemorrhage, fever, hypotension, heart arrhythmias; rarely, anaphylaxis (shock).

Manufacturer: Pharmacia.

KALSPARE

Description: a compound diuretic preparation with thiazide-like activity and also potassium-sparing, available in the form of film-coated orange tablets, containing 50mg chlorthalidone and 50mg triamterene, scored on 1 side and marked A on the other.

Used for: hypertension, oedema.

Dosage: adults, hypertension, 1 tablet every morning increasing to 2 as single daily dose if required. Oedema, 1 tablet every morning increasing to 2 daily as single dose if condition has not improved after 7 days.

Special care: pregnancy, breastfeeding, liver or kidney disease or damage, diabetes, gout, acidosis.

Avoid use: patients with serious or worsening kidney failure, anuria, hyperkalaemia.

Possible interaction: potassium-sparing diuretics, potassium supplements, ACE inhibitors, lithium, antihypertensives, digitalis.

Side effects: sensitivity to light, cramps, skin rash, blood changes, gout.
Manufacturer: Cusi.

KALTEN

Description: a compound hypertensive preparation combining a cardio-selective ß-blocker, thiazide and potassium-sparing diuretic. It is available as cream/red capsules containing 50mg atenolol, 25mg hydrochlorothiazide and 2.5mg amiloride hydrochloride marked with logo and KALTEN.
Used for: hypertension.
Dosage: adults, 1 tablet each day.
Special care: pregnancy, breastfeeding, general anaesthesia, liver or kidney disease, diabetes, gout, metabolic acidosis. Patients with weak hearts may require treatment with diuretics and digitalis.
Avoid use: obstructive airways disease or history of bronchospasm, heart block, heart shock, heart failure, disease of peripheral arteries, sick sinus syndrome, serious or worsening kidney failure, anuria.
Possible interaction: sympathomimetics, heart depressant anaesthetics, central nervous system depressants, ergotamine, class I antiarrhythmics, indomethacin, verapamil, hypoglycaemics, clonidine withdrawal, reserpine, cimetidine, clonidine withdrawal. Potassium supplements, potassium-sparing diuretics, digitalis, lithium.
Side effects: gastro-intestinal upset, cold hands and feet, disturbance of sleep, fatigue on exertion, bronchospasm, bradycardia. Sensitivity to light, gout, blood changes, muscle weakness. If unexplained skin rash or dry eyes occur, therapy should be stopped. Withdraw drug gradually.
Manufacturer: Stuart.

KANNASYN

Description: a broad-spectrum aminoglycoside antibiotic preparation available as a powder in vials for reconstitution and injection containing 1g kanamycin (as acid sulphate).
Used for: serious infections such as meningitis and septicaemia, especially where there is resistance to other antibiotics.
Dosage: adults, 1g by intramuscular injections each day in 2, 3 or 4 divided doses for a maximum period of 6 days. Children, 15mg/kg body weight by intramuscular injections in 2, 3 or 4 divided doses each day for a maximum period of 6 days.
Special care: patients with kidney disorders, Parkinsonism, myasthenia gravis; careful control of blood levels and dosage is required.
Avoid use: pregnancy, breastfeeding.
Possible interaction: anaesthetics, frusemide, neuromuscular blocking drugs, ethacrynic acid.
Side effects: damage to hearing and balance, harmful effects on kidneys.
Manufacturer: Sanofi Swinthrop.

KAPAKE

Description: a compound analgesic preparation available in the form of scored, white oval tablets containing 500mg paracetamol and 30mg codeine phosphate, marked KAPAKE.
Used for: severe pain.
Dosage: adults, 1 or 2 tablets every 4 hours with a maximum of 8 in 24 hours.
Special care: elderly, kidney or liver disease, inflammation or obstruction of the bowel, enlargement of the prostate gland, Addison's disease, hypothyroidism.
Avoid use: children, pregnancy, breastfeeding, breathing difficulties, obstructive airways disease, raised pressure inside cranium, alcoholism.
Possible interaction: MAOIs, central nervous system depressants.
Side effects: drug dependence and tolerance, dry mouth, dizziness, nausea, blurring of vision, constipation, nausea, sleepiness.
Manufacturer: Galen.

KEFADOL

Description: a cephalosporin antibiotic preparation available as a powder in vials for reconstitution and injection containing 1g cefamandole (as nafate).
Used for: life-threatening, severe infections.
Dosage: adults, 500mg–2g given by intramuscular or intravenous injection every 4 to 8 hours with a maximum dose of 12g every 24 hours. Children over 1 month, 50—100mg/kg body weight each day every 4 to 8 hours, with a maximum dose of 150mg/kg body weight daily.
Special care: patients with kidney disease or sensitivity to penicillin.
Avoid use: children under 1 month.
Possible interaction: aminoglycosides, loop diuretics.
Side effects: gastro-intestinal upset, blood changes (reduction in levels of white blood cells), thrombocytopenia. Also, allergic reactions, rise in level of blood urea and liver enzymes, cholestatic jaundice, short-lived hepatitis, positive Coomb's test (a test for rhesus antibodies).
Manufacturer: Dista.

KEFLEX

Description: a cephalosporin antibiotic preparation, cephalexin monohydrate, produced in a number of different forms. White/dark green capsules contain 250mg , and dark green/pale green capsules contain 500mg coded LILLY H69 and LILLY H71 respectively. **KEFLEX TABLETS**, peach-coloured containing 250mg coded LILLY U57 and peach, oval tablets containing 500mg coded LILLY U49. Also, **KEFLEX SUSPENSION** in 2 strengths containing 125mg and 250mg/ 5ml solution.
Used for: urinary tract infections, inflammation of middle ear, infections of respiratory tract, skin, bone, soft tissue. Also dental infections.
Dosage: adults, 1–4g each day in divided doses. Children, 25–50mg/kg body weight each day in divided doses.

Special care: patients with kidney disorder and allergy to penicillins.
Possible interaction: loop diuretics.
Side effects: gastro-intestinal upset, allergic reactions.
Manufacturer: Lilly.

KEFZOL

Description: a cephalosporin antibiotic preparation available as a powder in vials for reconstitution and injection, at 2 strengths, containing 500mg and 1g cephazolin (as salt).
Used for: septicaemia, endocarditis, skin, soft tissue, respiratory, urinary tract infections.
Dosage: adults, 500mg–1g every 6 to 8 hours by intramuscular or intravenous injection. Children, over 1 month in age, 25–50mg/kg body weight each day by intramuscular or intravenous injection in divided doses.
Special care: kidney disease or disorder, hypersensitivity to beta-lactam antibiotics. In beta-haemolytic infections, treatment should be given for a minimum period of 10 days.
Avoid use: children under 1 month.
Possible interaction: aminoglycosides, loop diuretics, probenecid.
Side effects: gastro-intestinal upset, blood changes involving white blood cells, candidosis (thrush), pain at injection site, seizures. A rise in levels of blood urea and liver enzymes, positive Coomb's test (a test for rhesus antibodies).
Manufacturer: Lilly.

KELFIZINE W

Description: a sulphonamide antibiotic preparation available as white tablets containing 2g sulfametopyrazine, marked weekly dose on 1 side and name on the reverse.
Used for: treatment and prevention of chronic bronchitis, urinary tract infections.
Dosage: adults, 1 tablet each week.
Special care: patients with kidney or liver disease or damage. Persons taking

drug over long period should receive regular blood checks.
Avoid use: children, women in late pregnancy, nursing mothers.
Possible interaction: hypoglycaemics taken orally, folate antagonists.
Side effects: gastro-intestinal upset, skin rashes, haemolytic anaemia, inflammation of the tongue, blood changes if taken long-term.
Manufacturer: Pharmacia.

KELOCYANOR

Description: a chelating agent (1 which binds to a metal) available as a solution in ampoules for injection containing 1.5% dicobalt edetate in glucose.
Used for: as an antidote in patients with cyanide poisoning.
Dosage: adults and children, 20ml (300mg) by intravenous injection over 1 minute followed straight away by 50ml dextrose intravenous infusion 50%. Both may be repeated once or twice as required.
Side effects: tachycardia, vomiting, short-lived hypotension, toxic effects from cobalt.
Manufacturer: Lipha.

KEMADRIN

Description: an anticholinergic preparation available as scored white tablets containing 5mg procyclidine hydrochloride marked WELLCOME S3A. Also, KEMADRIN INJECTION available as 2ml ampoules containing 2mg procyclidine hydrchloride.
Used for: Parkinsonism, especially drug-induced symptoms.
Dosage: adults, 2.5mg 3 times each day after meals, in first instance, then increasing every second or third day by 2.5–5mg. The usual maximum daily dose is 30mg. Injection, 10–20mg each day by intramusucular or intravenous injection.
Special care: heart disease, enlarged prostate gland, obstruction of gastro-intestinal tract, narrow angle glaucoma. Drug should be gradually withdrawn.

Avoid use: children, patients with tardive dyskinesia (a movement disorder especially affecting elderly people).
Possible interaction: antihistamines, phenothiazines, antidepressants.
Side effects: anticholinergic side effects, confusion with higher doses.
Manufacturer: Wellcome.

KEMICETINE SUCCINATE

Description: a chloramphenicol antibiotic available as a powder in vials for reconstitution and injection containing 1g chloramphenicol (as sodium succinate).
Used for: serious, life-threatening infections including *H. influenzae*, meningitis and typhoid.
Dosage: adults, 1g by intravenous injection every 6 to 8 hours. Children, newborn babies, 25mg/kg body weight each day; others, 50mg/kg body weight daily. All given intravenously every 6 hours in divided doses.
Special care: patients with liver or kidney disease or damage.
Possible interaction: hypoglycaemics, anticoagulants, phenytoin.
Side effects: gastro-intestinal upset, dry mouth, disturbance of vision, rash, Grey syndrome in babies. Drug causes serious blood changes such as aplastic anaemia and is reserved for use in conditions in which no effective alternative is available, and patient's life is at risk. Regular blood tests should be performed.
Manufacturer: Pharmacia.

KENALOG

Description: an anti-inflammatory corticosteroid (glucocorticoid) preparation available in pre-filled syringes and vials for injection, containing 40mg triamcinolone acetonide/ml.
Used for: pain in joints, stiffness and swelling due to rheumatoid arthritis, osteoarthritis. Inflammation of connective tissue (bursa) around joint (bursitis), tendon sheath (tenosynovitis), inflammation of the elbow joint (epicondylitis). Also used for collagen disorders, deficiency of

hormones of adrenal cortex, serious dermatitis, allergic disorders.
Dosage: adults by intramuscular injection, 40mg by deep injection into gluteal muscle; further doses according to patient's condition. For allergic states, e.g. hay fever, 40–100mg as single dose. Joint disorders, 5–40mg by intra-articular injection (directly into joint) according to joint size. Maximum dose if more than one joint is being treated is 80mg. Children, age 6 to 12 years, in proportion to adult dose according to age, severity of condition, bodyweight and joint size.
Special care: pregnancy, inflammation of kidneys, osteoporosis, infections, viral or fungal conditions, tuberculosis, diabetes. Also, glaucoma, recent surgical anastomoses, thrombophlebitis, epilepsy, liver cirrhosis, hypertension, hyperthyroidism. Patients with osteoporosis, secondary cancers, disease characterized by skin rash (exanthematous disease) e.g. measles, psychoses, suffering from stress. Patients should avoid contact with *Herpes zoster* virus or chicken pox and should seek medical help if inadvertently exposed. Drug should be gradually withdrawn.
Avoid use: children under 6 years.
Possible interaction: cardiac glycosides, NSAIDs, phenytoin, anticoagulants taken orally, anticholinesterases, phenobarbitone, hypoglycaemics, rifampicin, ephedrine, diuretics.
Side effects: skin changes as in Cushing's syndrome, peptic ulcer, osteoporosis, hyperglycaemia, euphoria and depression.
Manufacturer: Squibb.

KERLONE

Description: an antihypertensive preparation which is a cardioselective ß-blocker available as scored, white, film-coated tablets containing 20mg betaxolol hydrochloride marked KE 20.
Used for: hypertension.
Dosage: adults, 1 tablet each day, (half for elderly persons in first instance).
Special care: pregnancy, breastfeeding,

diabetes, liver or kidney disease, metabolic acidosis, undergoing general anaesthesia. Drug should be gradually withdrawn. Patients with weak hearts may require digitalis and diuretic treatment.
Avoid use: children, patients with history of bronchospasm, obstructive airways disease, heart block, heart failure, heart shock, peripheral disease of the arteries, sick sinus syndrome.
Possible interaction: CNS depressants, indomethacin, clonidine withdrawal, ergotamine, sympathomimetics, class I antiarrhythmics, cimetidine, verapamil, other antihypertensives, reserpine, hypoglycaemics.
Side effects: bradycardia, cold hands and feet, fatigue on exertion, disturbance of sleep, gastro-intestinal upset, bronchospasm, heart failure. Withdraw if dry eyes or skin rash occur.
Manufacturer: Lorex.

KETALAR

Description: a general anaesthetic available as a solution in vials for injection at strengths of 10mg, 50mg and 100mg/ml, containing ketamine (as hydrochloride).
Used for: induction and maintenance of general anaesthesia especially in children requiring repeated anaesthesia.
Dosage: by intravenous injection or infusion depending upon period of time for which general anaesthesia is required.
Avoid use: patients prone to hallucination, those with hypertension.
Possible interaction: ACE inhibitors, TCADs, antipsychotics, ß-blockers, antihypertensives, anxiolytics and hypnotics.
Side effects: hallucinations (but incidence is reduced if used with diazepam and is less of a problem in children), possible tachycardia and rise in arterial blood pressure. Relatively slow recovery time.
Manufacturer: Parke-Davis.

KETOVITE

Description: a multivitamin preparation available as yellow, sugar-free tablets containing 1mg thiamine hydrochloride,

0.5mg acetomenaphthone, 1mg riboflavine, 0.33mg pyridoxine hydrochloride, 3.3mg nicotinamide, 16.6mg ascorbic acid, 50mg inositol, 1.16mg calcium pantothenate, 0.25mg folic acid, 0.17mg biotin, 5mg tocopheryl acetate. Also **KETOVITE LIQUID**, a pink, sugar-free vitamin supplement, containing 150mg choline chloride, 12.5 micrograms cyanocobalamin, 400 units vitamin D, 2500 units vitamin A, all/5ml.
Used for: dietary supplement for patients on synthetic diets due to disorders of amino acid or carbohydrate metabolism.
Dosage: 1 tablet 3 times each day and 5ml of solution once daily.
Possible interaction: levodopa.
Manufacturer: Paines and Byrne.

KINIDIN DURULES

Description: a class I antiarrhythmic preparation available as white, sustained-release tablets containing 250mg quinidine bisulphate.
Used for: disorders of heart rhythm including types of tachycardia, atrial fibrillation and extrasystoles.
Dosage: adults, 1 tablet each day at first increasing to 2 to 5 daily.
Special care: patients with tachycardia, hypotension, hypokalaemia, congestive heart failure.
Avoid use: children, pregnancy, heart block, myas-thenia gravis, inflammation or damage of heart muscle, uncompensated heart failure, toxic effects of digitalis.
Possible interaction: digitalis, cimetidine, anticoagulants taken orally, vasodilators, non-depolarising substances, antihypertensives.
Side effects: hepatitis, allergic responses, cinchonism (a condition resulting from overdose of quinine and quinidine characterized by ringing in the ears, deafness, headache, brain congestion).
Manufacturer: Astra.

KLARICID

Description: a macrolide antibiotic preparation, available in a variety of forms: oval, yellow, film-coated tablets containing 250mg clarithromycin marked with logo; **KLARICID PAEDIATRIC SUSPENSION** containing 125mg/5ml solution; **KLARICID INTRAVENOUS INJECTION** containing 500mg clarithromycin as powder in vials for reconstitution.
Used for: infections of respiratory tract, middle ear, soft tissue and skin.
Dosage: adults, and children over 12 years, tablets, 1 twice each day for 1 week; serious infections, 2 tablets daily for up to 2 weeks. Injection, 1g by intravenous infusion in 2 divided doses each day for 5 days. Children, use paediatric suspension under 1 year, 7.5mg/kg body weight, 1 to 2 years, 2.5ml; 3 to 6 years, 5ml; 7 to 9 years, 7.5ml; 10 to 12 years, 10ml. All twice each day in divided doses.
Special care: pregnancy, breastfeeding, liver or kidney disease.
Possible interaction: anticoagulants taken by mouth, carbamazepine, theophylline, terfenadine, digoxin.
Side effects: gastro-intestinal upset, vomiting, diarrhoea, nausea, pain in abdomen, short-lived central nervous system effects, headache, skin rash, pain and skin reactions at injection site.
Manufacturer: Abbott.

KONAKION

Description: a vitamin A derivative available as a solution in ampoules for injection containing 1mg phytomenadione/0.5ml, and as white, sugar-coated tablets containing 10mg phytomenadione.
Used for: hypoprothrombinaemia (an abnormally low level of prothrombin clotting factor II in the blood, characterized by bleeding and loss of blood clotting ability). Also, haemorrhagic disease of the newborn (a bleeding disorder of newborn infants caused by vitamin K deficiency).
Dosage: adults, 10–20mg by intramuscular or slow intravenous injection, or as tablets. The maximum dose is 40mg in 24 hours. Newborn babies, 1mg given

intramuscularly; babies over 3 months,
5–10mg each day.
Side effects: sweating, flushing, lack of
oxygen in blood (cyanosis) causing
bluish tinge to skin and mucous
membranes. Symptoms of analphylaxis
may occur with injection.
Manufacturer: Roche.

KYTRIL

Description: an anti-emetic preparation
which is a 5HT$_3$-antagonist that acts to
block vomiting and nausea reflexes
which occur when 5HT$_3$ receptors in the
gut are stimulated. It is available as
triangular, white, film-coated tablets
containing 1mg granisetron as
hydrochloride. Also, **KYTRIL
INJECTION** available as a solution in
ampoules containing 1mg/ml.
Used for: prevention and treatment of
vomiting and nausea caused by cytotoxic
drug therapy.
Dosage: 1 tablet 1 hour before chemotherapy begins followed by 1 every 12 hours.
Injection, 3mg diluted in 20–50ml infusion
fluid given over 5 minutes by intravenous
route. Can be repeated if required at 10
minute intervals with a maximum dose of
9mg in 24 hours.
Special care: pregnant women, patients
with obstruction of intestine.
Avoid use: children, breastfeeding.
Side effects: constipation, headache,
short-lived rise in level of liver enzymes.
Manufacturer: Smith Kline Beecham.

LACTITOL

Description: an osmotic laxative, lactitol
monohydrate (10g) as powder in a sachet.
Used for: constipation, acute or chronic
portal systemic encephalopathy, PSE
(hepatic coma-toxic waste not neutralized
in the liver, reaching the brain or

substances required for brain function
not synthesized in the liver).
Dosage: 1 sachet mixed with food or
drink morning or evening. For
constipation, adults, 2 sachets reducing
to 1 daily; children 1 to 6 years, quarter
to half sachet; 6 to 12 years half to 1
sachet; 12 to 16 years, 1 to 2 sachets; all
daily. Not for children under 12 months.
For PSE, 0.5–0.7g/kg weight per day in
3 divided doses with meals.
Special care: pregnancy. Maintain fluid
intake and monitor electrolyte in long-
term treatment of elderly or debilitated.
Avoid use: obstruction of intestine,
galactosaemia (accumulation of
galactose in the blood in children who
cannot utilize this sugar due to inborn
lack of the appropriate enzyme).
Possible interaction: antacids, neomycin
for those with PSE.
Side effects: flatulence, bloating, gastro-
intestinal discomfort, chronic itching
around the anus.
Manufacturer: Zyma.

LAMICTAL

Description: a triazine, lamotrigine,
available as yellow tablets of strength
25mg, 50mg and 100mg marked with
name and strength.
Used for: anticonvulsant.
Dosage: 50mg daily for 2 weeks, then
50mg twice daily for 2 weeks increasing
to maintenance dose of 200–400mg daily
in 2 divided doses. If sodium valproate
is being taken, 25mg on alternate days
for 2 weeks then 25mg daily for 2 weeks
up to a maintenance dose of 100–200mg
daily in 1 or 2 doses. Not recommended
for children or the elderly.
Special care: pregnancy, lactation. Monitor
liver, kidney and clotting in patients
developing fever, flu, rash, drowsiness or
deterioration of seizure control. Withdraw
gradually over 2 weeks.
Avoid use: liver or kidney disease.
Possible interaction: sodium valproate,
primidone, phenobarbitone, phenytoin,
carbamazepine.

Side effects: dizziness, blurred vision, headache, drowsiness, gastro-intestinal upsets, rash, Stevens-Johnson syndrome, angioneurotic oedema.
Manufacturer: Wellcome.

LAMISIL

Description: an allylamine antifungal, terbinafine hydrochloride, as white 250mg tablets marked LAMISIL.
Used for: fungal infections of skin and nails.
Dosage: 1 daily for 2 to 6 weeks (athlete's foot); groin infection, 2 to 4 weeks; body infection 4 weeks and 6 to 12 weeks for nail infections. Not for children.
Also **LAMISIL CREAM**, a 1% cream.
Used for: fungal and yeast infections of the skin.
Dosage: apply to infected area 1 or 2 times per day for 1 to 2 weeks. Not for children.
Special care: pregnancy, lactation, chronic liver disorder, impaired kidney function.
Possible interaction: any drug affecting liver enzymes.
Side effects: headache, myalgia, arthralgia, allergic skin reaction, gastro-intestinal upset.
Manufacturer: Sandoz.

LAMPRENE

Description: a phenazine, clofazimine, available as 100mg strength in brown gelatin capsules marked GEIGY AND GM.
Used for: leprosy.
Dosage: as advised, but often as part of a 3-drug treatment when 300mg once a month given by the physician and 50mg daily, self-administered. Treatment may be prolonged (over 2 years).
Special care: pregnancy, lactation, diarrhoea, abdominal pain, liver or kidney disease.
Side effects: dry skin, pruritis, discolouration of hair, skin and secretions, gastro-intestinal upsets. Dosage can be reduced accordingly.
Manufacturer: Geigy.

LANOXIN

Description: a cardiac glycoside, digoxin, available as 250µg white tablet marked WELLCOME Y3B. Also **LANOXIN-PF**, 62.5µg blue tablet marked WELLCOME USA, **LANOX-IN-PG ELIXIR**, 50µg/ml and **LANOXIN INJECTION**, 250µg/ml digoxin in 2ml ampoules.
Used for: digitalis treatment, especially congestive heart failure.
Dosage: maintenance dose: adults, 125–750µg daily; elderly, 62.5–250µg daily; for children, see literature.
Special care: acute myocardial infarction, atrio-ventricular block, thyroid disorder, severe lung disease, kidney impairment.
Avoid use: hypercalcaemia, ventricular tachycardia, hypertrophic obstructive cardiomyopathy.
Possible interaction: calcium tablets or injections, cardiac glycosides, potassium-depleting agents, lithium, quinidine, antacids, antibiotics.
Side effects: changes in heart rhythm, gastro intestinal upsets, visual disturbances.
Manufacturer: Wellcome.

LANVIS

Description: a cytotoxic preparation of thioguanine available as 40mg yellow tablets marked WELLCOME U3B.
Used for: treatment of acute leukaemias.
Dosage: 2–2.5mg/kg daily at the outset.
Special care: interference with production of red blood cells in the bone marrow, causing some loss of immunity to infection. Monitor blood regularly.
Side effects: nausea, vomiting, gastro-intestinal upsets, hair loss.
Manufacturer: Wellcome.

LARGACTIL

Description: a group I phenothiazine, chlorpromazine hydrochloride available in 10, 25, 50 and 100mg white tablets marked with LG and strength. Also, **LARGACTIL SYRUP** (25mg/5ml), **LARGACTIL FORTE SUSPENSION**,

chlorpromazine carbonate equivalent to 100mg chlorpromazine hydrochloride per 5ml and **LARGACTIL INJECTION**, 25mg/ml chlorpromazine hydrochloride in 2ml ampoules.
Used for: disturbances of the CNS that require sedation, schizophrenia, nausea and vomiting (of terminal illness), induction of hypothermia, mood disorders.
Dosage: 25mg 3 times per day, increasing by 25mg per day. Maintenance dose 75–300mg daily. See literature for children.
Injection: 25–50mg by deep intra-muscular injection in a single dose. Can be repeated after 6 to 8 hours; to be followed by oral therapy as soon as possible.
Special care: pregnancy, lactation.
Children: use in severe cases only.
Avoid use: heart failure, epilepsy, Parkinsonism, liver or kidney disorder, hypothyroidism, elderly, glaucoma, enlarged prostate, unconscious patients, depression of bone marrow function.
Possible interaction: depressants of the CNS, alcohol, antidepressants, anticonvulsants, antidiabetics, levodopa, analgesics, antihypertensives.
Side effects: muscle spasms (eye, neck, back, face), restlessness, rigidity and tremor, tardive dyskinesia (repetitious muscular movements), dry mouth, blocked nose, difficulty in passing urine, tachycardia, blurred vision, hypotension, constipation, weight gain, impotence, galactorrhoea, gynaecomastia, amenorrhoea, blood and skin changes, lethargy, fatigue, ECG irregularities.
Manufacturer: Rhône-Poulenc Rorer.

LARIAM

Description: a 4-aminoquinolone, mefloquine hydrochloride, as 250mg white tablets.
Used for: treatment and prevention of malaria.
Dosage: prevention: 1 tablet weekly; children, 15–19kg quarter tablet; 20–30kg, half tablet; 31–45kg three-quarters tablet. Not recommended under 15kg. For visits up to 3 weeks, dose to be taken weekly on the same day for a minimum of 6 weeks starting 1 week before departure and continuing for 4 weeks after return. For stays over 3 weeks, weekly dose on the same day during the stay starting 1 week before and continuing for 4 weeks after return. Do not use for more than 3 months. For treatment dosages, see literature.
Special care: patients with heart conduction disorders. Women must use reliable contraception during and for 3 months after the stay.
Avoid use: liver or kidney damage, pregnancy, lactation, history of convulsions or psychiatric disorders.
Possible interaction: sodium valproate; typhoid vaccination, delay use for at least 12 hours after quinine.
Side effects: in treatment: dizziness, nausea, vomiting, appetite loss, gastro-intestinal upset.
Manufacturer: Roche.

LARODOPA

Description: the dopamine precursor, levodopa, as 500mg white tablets marked ROCHE in a hexagon.
Used for: Parkinsonism.
Dosage: over 25 years, 125mg twice daily after food increasing after 1 week to 125mg 4 to 5 times per day and further at weekly intervals by 375mg daily, the total in 4 or 5 divided doses. Maintenance dose of 2.5–8g. Not recommended for anyone under 25.
Special care: cardiovascular, liver, kidney, lung or endocrine disease, glaucoma, pregnancy, peptic ulcer. Monitor blood, and liver, kidney and cardiovascular function.
Avoid use: glaucoma, severe psychoses, history of malignant melanoma.
Possible interaction: MAOIs, antihypertensives, sympathomimetics, pyridoxine, ferrous sulphate.
Side effects: anorexia, nausea, vomiting, involuntary movements, heart and CNS disturbances, urine discolouration, low blood pressure when standing up.
Manufacturer: Cambridge.

LASIKAL

Description: a loop diuretic and potassium supplement comprising 20mg frusemide and 750mg potassium chloride in a sustained release matrix, forming a white/yellow two-layered tablet marked LK.

Used for: oedema with the need of a potassium supplement.

Dosage: 2 daily as 1 morning dose increasing to 4 if necessary (in 2 divided doses) or reducing to 1 daily.

Special care: diabetes, enlarged prostate or impaired urination, liver or kidney disease, pregnancy, lactation, gout.

Avoid use: Addison's disease, hyperkalaemia, cirrhosis of the liver.

Possible interaction: digitalis, lithium, NSAIDs, aminoglycosides, antihypertensives, cephalosporins, potassium-sparing diuretics.

Side effects: rash, gout, gastro-intestinal upset. Discontinue if ulceration or obstruction of small bowel occurs.

Manufacturer: Hoechst.

LASILACTONE

Description: a loop and potassium-sparing diuretic consisting of 20mg frusemide and 50mg spironolactone in a blue/white capsule.

Used for: oedema that has not responded to other therapy, hypertension of certain types.

Dosage: 1 to 4 daily, not recommended for children.

Special care: liver or kidney disease, impaired urination, enlarged prostate, diabetes, pregnancy, lactation, gout. Not to be used long-term for young patients.

Avoid use: kidney failure, liver cirrhosis, hyperkalaemia, Addison's disease.

Possible interaction: potassium supplements, potassium-sparing diuretics, antihypertensives, lithium, digitalis, ACE inhibitors, NSAIDs, cephalosporins, aminoglycosides.

Side effects: rash, gout, blood changes, gynaecomastia, gastro-intestinal upsets.

Manufacturer: Hoechst.

LASIX

Description: a loop diuretic, frusemide, available as 20mg white tablets marked DLF and 40mg white tablets marked DLI, both also marked with manufacturer's symbol.

Used for: oedema, mild to moderate hypertension.

Dosage: 20–80mg in 1 dose daily or every other day. Children 1–3mg/kg per day. Also **LASIX 500**, 500mg frusemide in yellow tablet form marked with the manufacturer's symbol and DIX on the reverse.

Used for: acute or chronic kidney insufficiency (used under hospital supervision).

Dosage: see literature. Also **LASIX PAEDIATRIC LIQUID**, 1mg/ml frusemide.

Dosage: 1–3mg/kg daily. Also, **LASIX INJECTION**, 10mg/ml frusemide in 2, 5 and 25ml ampoules.

Dosage: 20–50mg intramuscularly or slow intravenous injection. Children, 0.5–1.5mg/kg daily.

Special care: gout, diabetes, enlarged prostate, liver or kidney disease, impaired urination, pregnancy, lactation. Potassium supplements may be necessary.

Avoid use: liver cirrhosis.

Possible interaction: NSAIDs, antihypertensives, cephalosporins, aminoglycosides, lithium, digitalis.

Side effects: gout, rash, gastro-intestinal upset.

Manufacturer: Hoechst.

LASIX + K

Description: A loop diuretic and potassium supplement, frusemide, available in 40mg white tablets marked with the manufacturer's symbol and DLI on the reverse; and 750mg potassium chloride as pale yellow sustained-release tablets.

Used for: diuretic therapy where potassium is required.

Dosage: 1 frusemide tablet in the morning

and 1 potassium chloride tablet at midday and in the evening. Not for children.
Special care: liver or kidney disease, diabetes, gout, enlarged prostrate (prostatic hypertrophy) or impaired urination, pregnancy, lactation.
Avoid use: liver cirrhosis, Addison's disease, hyperkalaemia.
Possible interaction: NSAIDs, cephalosporins, antihypertensives, digitalis, lithium, aminoglycosides, potassium-sparing diuretics.
Side effects: rash, gout, gastro-intestinal upset. Discontinue if ulceration or obstruction of small bowel occurs.
Manufacturer: Hoechst.

LASORIDE

Description: a loop and potassium-sparing diuretic comprising 40mg frusemide and 5mg amiloride hydrochloride in yellow tablets.
Used for: rapid diuretic treatment and conservation of potassium.
Dosage: 1 to 2 tablets in the morning, adjust for elderly. Not for children.
Special care: enlarged prostate, impaired urination, diabetes, gout, pregnancy, lactation, elderly. Electrolyte and fluid levels should be checked regularly.
Avoid use: liver cirrhosis, kidney failure, Addison's disease, hyperkalaemia, electrolyte imbalance.
Possible interaction: NSAIDs, digitalis, antidiabetic drugs, antihypertensives, lithium, ototoxic or nephrotoxic antibiotics, potassium supplements, potassium-sparing diuretics, certain muscle relaxants.
Side effects: gastro-intestinal upset, itching, blood changes, malaise, reduced alertness, calcium loss. Occasionally minor mental disturbances, pancreatitis, altered liver function.
Manufacturer: Hoechst.

LEDCLAIR

Description: a chelating agent, sodium calcium edetate as 200mg/ml in 5ml ampoules.

Used for: treatment of poisoning with lead and other heavy metals.
Dosage: up to 40mg/kg twice daily by intravenous drip or intramuscular injection for adults and children. To diagnose poisoning, 25mg/kg intramuscularly 3 times per day. See literature in both cases.
Special care: impaired kidney function.
Side effects: nausea, cramp, kidney damage on overdosage.
Manufacturer: Sinclair.

LEDERCORT

Description: a glucocorticoid, triamcinolone, in strengths of 2mg (blue, oblong tablet marked LL11) and 4mg (white, oblong tablet marked LL 9352).
Used for: rheumatoid arthritis, allergies.
Dosage: 2–24mg daily but see literature.
Special care: thrombophlebitis, psychoses, recent intestinal anastomoses, chronic nephritis, certain cancers, osteoporosis, peptic ulcer, skin eruption/rash related to a disease, viral, fungal or active infections, tuberculosis. Hypertension, glaucoma, epilepsy, acute glomerulonephritis (inflammation of kidney glomerulus), diabetes, cirrhosis, hypothyroidism, pregnancy, stress. To be withdrawn gradually.
Possible interaction: NSAIDs, oral anticoagulants, phenytoin, ephedrine, phenobarbitone, rifampicin, diuretics, cardiac glycosides, anticholinesterases, hypoglycaemics.
Side effects: osteoporosis, depression, euphoria, hyperglycaemia, peptic ulcers, Cushingoid changes.
Also available as triamcinolone acetonide, 0.1% cream.
Used for: inflamed skin disorders.
Dosage: use sparingly 3 or 4 times per day.
Special care: maximum 5 days use on face or for children. Withdraw gradually.
Avoid use: acne, scabies, leg ulcers, perioral dermatitis; tuberculous, viral skin or ringworm infections, untreated bacterial or fungal infections. Do not use extensively or for a prolonged period in pregnancy.

Side effects: skin striae and atrophy,
Cushingoid changes (see Cushing's
syndrome), adrenal gland suppression,
telangiectasia (collections of distended
blood capillaries).
Manufacturer: Lederle.

LEDERFEN

Description: propionic acid as fenbufen
in light blue tablet marked LEDERFEN
(300mg), and light blue oblong tablet
marked LEDERFEN 450 (450mg). Also,
LEDERFEN CAPSULES, 300mg
fenbufen in dark blue capsules marked
LEDERFEN.
Used for: osteoarthritis, rheumatoid
arthritis, ankylosing spondylitis and
acute muscle/bone disorders.
Dosage: 300mg in the morning with
600mg at night, or 450mg twice daily.
Not for children.
Also **LEDERFEN F**, fenbufen as white
effervescent tablets (450mg).
Dosage: 1 dissolved in water, twice per
day. Not for children.
Special care: heart failure, kidney or
liver disease, pregnancy, lactation,
elderly. Monitor those on long-term
treatment.
Avoid use: active peptic ulcers or history
of gastro-intestinal lesions, allergy
induced by aspirin or anti-inflammatory
drug.
Possible interaction: anticoagulants,
salicylates, quinolones.
Side effects: gastro-intestinal intolerance,
rash.
Manufacturer: Lederle.

LEDERFOLIN

Description: folinic acid (as calcium
folinate), 350mg strength, powder in a
vial. Also, **LEDERFOLIN SOLUTION**
as 10mg/ml in a 35ml ampoule.
Used for: alongside 5-fluorouracil in
treatment of advanced colorectal cancer.
Dosage: see literature.
Special care: toxicity of 5-fluorouracil
increased.
Manufacturer: Lederle.

LEDERMYCIN

Description: a tetracycline, demeclocycline hydrochloride available as dark
red/light red capsules marked LEDERLE
9123 (150mg strength).
Used for: respiratory and soft tissue
infections.
Dosage: 300mg twice per day or 150mg
4 times. Not for children.
Special care: liver and kidney disease.
Avoid use: pregnancy, lactation.
Possible interaction: milk, mineral
supplements, antacids, oral contraceptives.
Side effects: sensitivity to light, gastro-
intestinal upset, further infections.
Manufacturer: Lederle.

LEDERSPAN 20mg

Description: a glucocorticoid,
triamcinolone hexacetonide in vials,
20mg/ml.
Used for: local inflammation of joints
and soft tissues in arthritis, tendinitis and
bursitis (inflammation of the connective
tissue surrounding a joint).
Dosage: 2–30mg depending upon
condition and size of joint or synovial
space at 3 to 4 weekly intervals.
Also **LEDERSPAN 5mg**
Description: triamcinolone hexacetonide
in a vial (5mg/ml).
Used for: skin conditions.
Dosage: 0.5mg (or less) per square inch
of affected skin.
Special care: thrombophlebitis,
psychoses, recent intestinal anastomoses,
chronic nephritis, certain cancers,
osteoporosis, peptic ulcer, skin eruption/
rash related to a disease, viral, fungal or
active infections, tuberculosis.
Hypertension, glaucoma, epilepsy, acute
glomerulonephritis (inflammation of
kidney glomerulus), diabetes, cirrhosis,
hypothyroidism, pregnancy, stress. To be
withdrawn gradually.
Possible interaction: NSAIDs, oral
anticoagulants, phenytoin, ephedrine,
phenobarbitone, rifampicin, diuretics,
cardiac glycosides, anticholinesterases,
hypoglycaemics.

Side effects: osteoporosis, depression, euphoria, hyperglycaemia, peptic ulcers, Cushingoid changes.
Manufacturer: Lederle.

LENTARON

Description: an aromatase inhibitor, formestane, available as a powder (250mg strength) in a vial with 2ml diluent.
Used for: advanced stages of breast cancer occurring after the menopause.
Dosage: 250mg intramuscularly every 2 weeks in gluteal muscle (buttock). Site of injection alternated.
Special care: avoid making injection into vein or sciatic nerve.
Avoid use: pregnancy, lactation, pre-menopausal women.
Side effects: pain and irritation at site of injection, vaginal bleeding or irritation, hot flushes, arthralgia, pelvic or muscular cramps, oedema, thrombophlebitis, sore throat, upset in the CNS or gastro-intestinal tract.
Manufacutrer: Ciba.

LENTIZOL

Description: a tricyclic antidepressant, amitriptyline hydrochloride available as sustained-release pink capsules (25mg) or pink/red capsules (50mg) both with white pellets and marked with LENTIZOL and the capsule strength.
Used for: treatment of depression when sedation is required.
Dosage: 50–100mg at night, up to a maximum of 200mg per day. Elderly, 25–75mg daily. Not for children.
Special care: liver disorders, hyperthyoidism, glaucoma, lactation, epilepsy, diabetes, adrenal tumour, heart disease, urine retention. Psychotic or suicidal patients.
Avoid use: heart block, heart attacks, severe liver disease, pregnancy.
Possible interaction: MAOIs (or within 14 days of their use), alcohol, anti-depressants, barbiturates, anticholinergics, local anaesthetics that contain adrenaline or noradrenaline, oestrogens, cimetidine,

antihypertensives.
Side effects: constipation, urine retention, dry mouth, blurred vision, palpitations, tachycardia, nervousness, drowsiness, insomnia. Changes in weight, blood and blood sugar, jaundice, skin reactions, weakness, ataxia, hypotension, sweating, altered libido, gynaecomastia, galactorrhoea.
Manufacturer: Parke-Davis.

LESCOL

Description: a suppressant of cholesterol production and sodium salt of fluvastatin available as red-brown/pale yellow (20mg strength) or red-brown/orange-yellow (40mg strength) capsules, marked with XU, the strength and the company logo.
Used for: hypercholesterolaemia (high blood cholesterol levels) for patients where levels cannot be controlled by diet.
Dosage: over 18 years, 20–40mg once per day in the evening. Adjust to response, monitor lipid levels. Not for children.
Special care: history of liver disease, or high alcohol intake (test liver function), myalgias or muscle weakness particularly with fever or if generally unwell. Any condition predisposing to rhabdomyolysis.
Avoid use: kidney or liver disease, pregnancy, lactation.
Possible interaction: immunosuppressive drugs, rifampicin, erythromycin, nicotinic acid, gemfibrozil.
Side effects: flatulence, abdominal pain, sinusitis, insomnia, nausea, dyspepsia, hypoaesthesia (some loss of sense of touch), infection of the urinary tract, disorders of the teeth.
Manufacturer: Sandoz.

LEUCOMAX

Description: a recombinant human granulocyte macrophage-colony stimulating factor (GM-CSF) available as molgramostim in the form of powder in vials. There are 3 strengths: 150, 300 and 700µg (equivalent to 1.67, 3.33 and 7.77 million-unit).

Used for: reduction in neutropenia and therefore risk of infection associated with cytotoxic chemotherapy, speeding up bone marrow recovery after transplantation of same, neutropenia in patients on gamciclovir in AIDS-related cytomegalovirus retinitis.
Dosage: chemotherapy, 60,000–110,000 units/kg/day (by subcutaneous injection) for 7 to 10 days commencing 24 hours after last chemotherapy; bone marrow transplantation, 110,000 units/kg/day (by intravenous infusion) commencing 24 hours after transplantation and until white cell count is at required level (maximum 30 days treatment); in ganciclovir treatment, 60,000 units/kg/day by subcutaneous injection for 5 days, then adjust to response.
Special care: full blood monitoring necessary, monitor those with lung disease, pregnancy and lactation, history of autoimmune disease. Not recommended for those under 18 years.
Avoid use: bone marrow cancer.
Side effects: anorexia, nausea, vomiting, diarrhoea, shortness of breath, weakness, rash, rigors, fever, muscle and bone pains, local reaction at site of injection. Anaphylaxis, cardiac failure, convulsions, hypotension, heartbeat abnormalities, pericarditis, pulmonary oedema.
Manufacturer: Sandoz/Schering Plough.

LEUKERAN

Description: an alkylating agent and cytotoxic drug, chlorambucil, available as yellow tablets (2 and 5mg strengths), marked WELLCOME C2A and H2A respectively.
Used for: ovarian cancer, Hodgkin's disease, chronic lymphocytic leukaemia.
Dosage: 100–200µg/kg daily for 4 to 8 weeks, but see literature.
Special care: kidney disease.
Avoid use: porphyria.
Side effects: bone marrow suppression, rashes.
Manufacturer: Wellcome.

LEVOPHED

Description: a vasoconstrictor and sympathomimetic amine, noradrenaline (as the acid tartrate) as 1mg/ml, in ampoules for dilution. Also, **LEVOPHED SPECIAL**, 0.1mg/ml.
Used for: cardiac arrest, acute hypotension.
Dosage: intravenous infusion of 8 µg/ml at a rate of 2.3ml/minute initially, adjusted to the response. By intracardiac or rapid intravenous injection, 0.5–0.75ml of a solution with 200 µg/ml .
Special care: extravasation at site of injection (escape of fluid, e.g. blood into tissues) may cause localized necrosis.
Avoid use: pregnancy, myocardial infarction.
Possible interaction: anaesthetics, tricyclics, ß-blockers, dopexamine.
Side effects: headache, uneven heartbeat.
Manufacturer: Sanofi Winthrop.

LEXOTAN

Description: an anxiolytic benzodiazepine for intermediate-acting use, bromazepam, available as lilac and pink tablets (1.5mg and 3mg strengths respectively) marked with L and the strength.
Used for: short-term treatment of severe or disabling anxiety, with or without insomnia.
Dosage: 3–18mg per day (elderly, 1.5–9mg) in divided doses. Not for children.
Special care: chronic kidney or liver disease or lung insufficiency, pregnancy, labour, lactation, elderly. May impair judgement. Avoid long-term use and withdraw gradually.
Avoid use: acute lung disorders, depression of respiration, phobias, chronic psychosis.
Possible interaction: anticonvulsants, alcohol, depressants of the CNS.
Side effects: gastro-intestinal upset, vertigo, ataxia, confusion, drowsiness, light-headedness, hypotension, skin reactions and visual changes, urine retention, changes in libido. Dependence a risk with high doses and long treatment.
Manufacturer: Roche.

LEXPEC

Description: a haematinic (haemoglobin-increasing drug), folic acid, available as a syrup containing 2.5mg/5ml.
Used for: megaloblasic anaemia caused by a deficiency of folic acid.
Dosage: 20–40 ml per day for 14 days, then 5–20ml per day. Children, 10–30ml per day.
Also, **LEXPEC WITH IRON**, a combination of folic acid (2.5mg) with ferric ammonium citrate (400mg)/5ml of syrup; and **LEXPEC WITH IRON-M**, 0.5mg folic acid and 400mg of ferric ammonium citrate/5ml of syrup.
Used for: anaemia during pregnancy caused by iron and folic acid deficiency.
Dosage: 5–10ml per day before food for the pregnancy and 1 month after.
Avoid use: megaloblastic anaemia due to vitamin B_{12} deficiency.
Possible interaction: tetracyclines.
Side effects: nausea, constipation, discolouration of teeth (syrup should be drunk through a straw).
Manufacturer: R.P. Drugs.

LI-LIQUID

Description: Lithium salt (the citrate) available as a sugar-free liquid in concentrations of 5.4mmol and 10.8mmol/5ml.
Used for: mania, hypomania (excitable, hyperactive and irritable), self-mutilation, extreme mood changes.
Dosage: 10.8–32.4mmol per day initially in 2 divided doses. Lithium levels in serum to be maintained, see literature.
Special care: start treatment in hospital and maintain salt and fluid levels. Record kidney, heart and thyroid functions.
Avoid use: Addison's disease, pregnancy, lactation, hypothyroidism, kidney or heart insufficiency, sodium imbalance.
Possible interaction: NSAIDs, phenytoin, diuretics, carbamazepine, diazepam, flupenthixol, methyldopa, haloperidol, tetracyclines, metoclopramide.
Side effects: hand tremor, weak muscles, diarrhoea, nausea, oedema, weight gain,

disturbances to CNS and in ECG, skin changes, polyuria, polydipsia, hypo- or hyperthyroidism.
Manufacturer: R.P. Drugs.

LIBRIUM

Description: a long-acting benzodiazepine, chlordiazepoxide, available in 3 strengths: 5mg (yellow-green tablets), 10mg (light blue-green) and 25mg (dark blue-green), all marked with LIB and the strength. Also, **LIBRIUM CAPSULES**, as green-yellow (5mg) and green/black (10mg) capsules marked with LIB and the strength.
Used for: treatment of severe anxiety over the short-term, with or without insomnia, symptoms of acute alcohol withdrawal.
Dosage: 30mg per day initially to a maximum of 100mg. For insomnia, 10–30mg at bedtime. For alcohol withdrawal, 25–100mg repeated in 2 to 4 hours if necessary. Elderly, 5mg per day to begin with. Not for children.
Special care: chronic kidney or liver disease or lung insufficiency, pregnancy, labour, lactation, the elderly. May impair judgement. Avoid long-term use and withdraw gradually.
Avoid use: acute lung disorders, depression of respiration, phobias, chronic psychosis.
Possible interaction: anticonvulsants, alcohol, depressants of the CNS.
Side effects: gastro-intestinal upset, vertigo, ataxia, confusion, drowsiness, light-headedness, hypotension, skin reactions and visual changes, urine retention, changes in libido. Dependence a risk with high doses and long treatment.
Manufacturer: Roche.

LIMCLAIR

Description: a chelating agent, trisodium edetate, available in ampoules (strength 200mg/ml).
Used for: parathyroidism, digitalis arrhythmia, hypercalcaemia, corneal opacities.
Dosage: up to 70mg/kg daily by slow

intravenous infusion, but see literature. For children, up to 60mg/kg daily by same means.
Special care: tuberculosis.
Avoid use: kidney disease.
Manufacturer: Sinclair.

LINGRAINE

Description: an ergot-derived alkaloid ergotamine tartrate available as green tablets, strength 2mg.
Used for: migraine and headache.
Dosage: 1 under the tongue at the start of the attack, repeat 30–60 minutes later if required; maximum 3 in 24 hours and 6 in 1 week. Not for children.
Avoid use: liver or kidney disease, severe hypertension, sepsis; coronary, peripheral or occlusive vascular disease; pregnancy, lactation, porphyria, hyperthyroidism.
Possible interaction: ß-blockers, erythromycin.
Side effects: leg cramps, stomach pain, nausea.
Manufacturer: Sanofi Winthrop.

LIORESAL

Description: a gamma-amino-butyric acid (GABA) derivative, baclofen, available as a white tablet (strength 10mg), marked CG and KJ. Also **LIORESAL LIQUID** , a sugar-free liquid containing 5mg/5ml.
Used for: muscle relaxant, for cerebral palsy, meningitis, spasticity of voluntary muscle due to cerebrovascular accidents, multiple sclerosis, spinal lesions.
Dosage: 5mg 3 times per day to begin with, increasing by 5mg 3 times per day at intervals of 3 days. Maximum 100mg per day. For children, see the literature.
Special care: epilepsy, pregnancy, cerebrovascular accidents, the elderly, psychosis, hypertonic (abnormally increased tone or strength) bladder sphincter, liver or kidney disorders, defective respiration. Withdraw gradually.
Avoid use: peptic ulcer.
Possible interactions: lithium, antihypertensives, tricyclic antidepres-

sants, depressants of the CNS, alcohol, fentanyl, levodopa, carbidopa, ibuprofen.
Side effects: sedation and drowsiness, nausea, disturbances of the central nervous system, muscle fatigue, hypotension, disturbance of the heart, lung or circulatory system, frequent and painful urination (dysuria).
Manufacturer: Ciba.

LIPANTIL

Description: an isobutyric acid derivative, fenofibrate, for lowering of lipids. Available as a white capsule, 100mg strength.
Used for: certain types of hyperlipidaemia (high levels of fat in the blood) resistant to the influence of diet.
Dosage: 3 tablets per day initially, in divided doses with food. 2 to 4 tablets per day for maintenance. For children, 5mg/kg body weight/day.
Special care: in cases of kidney impairment.
Avoid use: severe liver or kidney disorder, pregnancy, lactation, disease of the gall bladder.
Possible interaction: oral hypoglycaemics, anticoagulants, phenylbutazone.
Side effects: headache, tiredness, vertigo, gastro-intestinal upsets, rashes.
Manufacturer: Fournier.

LIPOSTAT

Description: a preparation of pravastratin (as the sodium salt) available as pink oblong tablets in 10 and 20mg strengths, marked with the company name and 154 or 178.
Used for: hypercholesterolaemia (high levels of blood cholesterol) which does not respond to other treatments (levels above 7.8mmol/l of cholesterol).
Dosage: 10mg at night to begin with, adjusting to the response at intervals of weeks. Usually 10–40mg as 1 dose, daily, at night. Not for children.
Special care: history of liver disease. Liver function tests to be undertaken during treatment.

Avoid use: pregnancy, lactation, liver disease.
Possible interaction: gemfibrozil and similar derivatives of isobutyric acid, to be taken 1 hour before or 4 hours after colestipolor cholestyramine.
Side effects: muscle pain, headache, rashes, nausea, vomiting, tiredness, diarrhoea, chest pains not related to the heart.
Manufacturer: Squibb.

LISKONUM

Description: a sedative, available as white, oblong, controlled-release tablets containing 450mg lithium carbonate (equivalent to 12.2mmol of lithium ions, Li⁺).
Used for: acute mania, hypomania, prevention of the recurrence of manic depression.
Dosage: blood lithium levels to be kept in the range 0.8–1.5mmol/l (for mania or hypomania) and 0.5–1.0mmol/l for prevention. Not for children.
Special care: commence treatment in hospital, salt and fluid intake to be kept up. Thyroid and kidney functions to be checked. Any symptoms of intoxication should be reported.
Avoid use: pregnancy, lactation, Addison's disease, kidney or heart disease, hypothyroidism, sodium imbalance.
Possible interaction: NSAIDs, diuretics, flupenthixol, fluoxetine, methyldopa, carbamazepine, fluvoxamine, haloperidol, phenytoin, metoclopramide.
Side effects: muscle weakness, hand tremor, diarrhoea, nausea, disturbances to heart and brain, oedema, weight gain, hypo- or hyperthyroidism, intense thirst, frequent urination, changes in kidney, skin reactions.
Manufacturer: Smith, Kline & French.

LITAREX

Description: a white, oval, controlled-release tablet containing 564mg lithium citrate (equivalent to 6mmol of lithium ions, Li⁺).
Used for: acute mania, prevention of recurrence of emotional disorders.

Dosage: 1 morning and evening to begin with. Blood lithium level should then be kept in the range 0.8–1.0mmol/l.
Special care: commence treatment in hospital, salt and fluid intake to be kept up. Thyroid and kidney functions should be checked. Any symptoms of intoxication should be reported.
Avoid use: pregnancy, lactation, Addison's disease, kidney or cardiovascular disease, the elderly, hypothyroidism, conditions altering sodium balance.
Possible interaction: NSAIDs, diuretics, flupenthixol, methyldopa, carbamazepine, haloperidol, phenytoin, antidepressants, metoclopramide.
Side effects: muscle weakness, diarrhoea, nausea, hand tremor, heart and brain disturbances, oedema, weight gain, hypo- or hyperthyroidism, intense thirst, frequent urination, skin reactions.
Manufacturer: CP Pharmaceuticals.

LIVIAL

Description: a white tablet containing 2.5mg tibolone (a gonadomimetic), marked MK2, ORGANON and *.
Used for: vasomotor symptoms (affecting blood vessel constriction or dilatation) associated with the menopause.
Dosage: a tablet daily for a minimum of 3 months.
Special care: kidney disorder or history of same, migraine, diabetes, epilepsy, high blood cholesterol levels. Menstrual bleeding may occur irregularly if commenced within 1 year of last period. Treatment to be stopped if liver disorder, cholestatic jaundice or thromboembolic disorders occur.
Avoid use: undiagnosed vaginal bleeding, hormone-dependent tumours, pregnancy, lactation, severe liver disease, cardio- or cerebrovascular disorder.
Possible interaction: carbamazepine, phenytoin, anticoagulants, rifampicin.
Side effects: headache, dizziness, vaginal bleeding, bodyweight changes, seborrhoeic

dermatitis (eczema associated with oil-sebum-secreting glands), abnormal liver function, gastro-intestinal upset, hair growth, oedema in front of the tibia.
Manufacturer: Organon.

LOBAK

Description: a muscle relaxant and analgesic, comprising 100mg chlormezanone and 450mg paracetamol available as white tablets marked LOBAK.
Used for: relief of painful muscle spasms.
Dosage: 1 or 2 three times per day, up to a maximum of 8. Half dose for the elderly not recommended for children.
Special care: pregnancy, lactation, kidney or liver disease.
Avoid use: porphyria.
Possible interaction: MAOIs, depressants of the central nervous system, alcohol.
Side effects: dizziness, drowsiness, reduced alertness, dry mouth, rash, jaundice.
Manufacturer: Sanofi Winthrop.

LOCABIOTAL

Description: an antibiotic and anti-inflammatory, fusafungine available as a metered dose aerosol (125µg per dose).
Used for: inflammation and infection of the upper respiratory tract.
Dosage: 5 oral sprays or 3 sprays in each nostril, 5 times per day. Children: over 12 years, 4 oral sprays 3 times per day or 3 sprays in each nostril 5 times per day; 6 to 12 years, 3 oral sprays 3 times per day or 2 sprays in each nostril 5 times per day; 3 to 5 years, 2 oral sprays 3 times per day or 1 spray in each nostril 5 times per day. Not recommended for children under 3 years.
Manufacturer: Servier.

LOCERYL

Description: an antifungal cream, containing 0.25% amorolfine hydrochloride.
Used for: microscopic fungal or ringworm skin infestation.
Dosage: apply daily in the evening,

usually for 2 to 3 weeks. Continue for 3 to 5 days after cure. Not for children.
Also, **LOCERYL LACQUER**, 5% amorolfine hydrochloride as a lacquer.
Used for: microscopic fungal, yeast and mould nail infestation.
Dosage: apply once or twice per week; review every 3 months. Not for children.
Special care: do not allow to come into contact with eyes, ears or mucous membranes.
Avoid use: pregnancy, lactation.
Side effects: sometimes pruritus (itching), temporary burning sensation.
Manufacturer: Roche.

LOCOID

Description: a strong steroid, hydro-cortisone 17-butyrate, available as a 0.1% cream and ointment.
Used for: eczema, psoriasis, skin disorders.
Dosage: apply 2 or 3 times per day.
Also, **LOCOID LIPOCREAM**, 0.1% hydrocortisone 17-butyrate in a base containing 70% oil.
Used for: skin disorders.
Dosage: apply 2 or 3 times per day.
Also **LOCOID SCALP LOTION**, 0.1% hydrocortisone 17-butyrate in an alcoholic solution.
Used for: seborrhoea of the scalp.
Dosage: apply twice daily.
Also, **LOCOID C**, a strong steroid 0.1% hydrocortisone 17-butyrate with an antifungal and antibacterial, 3% chlorquinaldol, available as cream and ointment.
Used for: eczema, psoriasis, and skin disorders when there is also infection.
Dosage: apply 2 to 4 times per day.
Special care: maximum 5 days use on face, withdraw gradually after prolonged use.
Avoid use: acne, dermatitis around the mouth, leg ulcers, scabies, viral skin disease, ringworm or tubercular infection, untreated infections caused by fungi or bacteria. Avoid prolonged or extensive use during pregnancy. Children.

Side effects: suppression of adrenal glands, skin striae and atrophy, telangiectasia (multiple telangiectases — collections of distended blood capillaries), Cushingoid changes.
Manufacturer: Brocades.

LOCORTEN-VIOFORM

Description: an antibacterial and corticosteroid, comprising 1% clioquinol and 0.02% flumethasone pivalate, as drops.
Used for: inflammation of the outer ear where there may be secondary infection.
Dosage: 2 to 3 drops twice daily for 7 to 10 days for all but children under 2 years of age.
Special care: lactation.
Avoid use: primary infections of the outer ear, perforated eardrum.
Side effects: skin irritation, discolouration of hair.
Manufacturer: Zyma.

LODINE

Description: a NSAID, pyranocarboxylate, available as 200mg etodolac in dark grey/light grey capsules with 2 red bands and marked LODINE 200, and 300mg etodolac in light grey capsules with 2 red bands and marked LODINE 300. Also, **LODINE TABLETS**, 200mg etodolac in brown, film-coated tablets marked LODINE 200.
Used for: osteoarthrosis, rheumatoid arthritis.
Dosage: 200 or 300mg twice per day, or 400 or 600mg as 1 dose if response is better. Maximum daily dose of 600mg. Not for children.
Also, **LODINE SR**, 600mg etodolac as grey, sustained-release tablets, marked LODINE and SR 600.
Dosage: 1 daily. Not for children.
Special care: liver, kidney or heart disorder, heart failure, elderly. Monitor those on long-term treatment.
Avoid use: active or history of peptic ulcer, history of gastro-intestinal bleeding, aspirin or anti-inflammatory induced allergy, pregnancy, lactation.

Possible interaction: hypoglycaemics, anticoagulants, quinolones.
Side effects: gastro-intestinal upset or bleeding, nausea, epigastric (upper central abdomen) pain, headache, dizziness, nephritis, rash, tinnitus, angioneurotic oedema.
Manufacturer: Wyeth.

LOESTRIN 20

Description: an oestrogen/progestogen, ethinyloestradiol (20mg) with norethisterone acetate (1.5mg) in green tablets. Also **LOESTRIN 30**, which contains 30mg ethinyloestradiol.
Used for: oral contraception.
Dosage: 1 tablet daily for 21 days, commencing on the fifth day of menstruation, then 7 days without tablets.
Special care: hypertension, Raynaud's disease (reduced blood supply to an organ of the body's extremities), asthma, severe depression, diabetes, varicose veins, multiple sclerosis, chronic kidney disease, kidney dialysis. Blood pressure, breasts and pelvic organs to be checked regularly; smoking not advised.
Avoid use: history of heart disease, infectious hepatitis, sickle cell anaemia, porphyria, liver tumour, undiagnosed vaginal bleeding, pregnancy, hormone-dependent cancer, haemolytic uraemic syndrome (rare kidney disorder), chorea, otosclerosis.
Possible interaction: barbiturates, tetracyclines, griseofulvin, rifampicin, primidone, phenytoin, chloral hydrate, ethosuximide, carbamazepine, glutethimide, dichloralphenazone.
Side effects: fluid retention and bloating, leg cramps/pains, breast enlargement, depression, headaches, nausea, loss of libido, weight gain, vaginal discharge, cervical erosion (alteration of epithelial cells), chloasma (pigmentation of nose, cheeks or forehead), breakthrough bleeding (bleeding between periods).
Manufacturer: Parke-Davis.

LOGIPARIN

Description: an anticoagulant, and low molecular weight heparin (LMWH), tinzaparin sodium available as 11,700 units of anti-Factor Xa (a blood coagulation factor) per ml in syringes.
Used for: prevention of thromboembolism during general or orthopaedic surgery.
Dosage: general surgery—3,500 units injected subcutaneously 2 hours before an operation then 3,500 once daily for 7 to 10 days. Orthopaedic surgery—2,500 units (body weight under 60kg), 3,500 units (60–80kg), 4,500 units (over 80kg), all injected subcutaneously before the operation and repeated once daily for a further 7 to 10 days. Not for children.
Special care: pregnancy, lactation, asthma, severe liver or kidney disorder.
Avoid use: tendency to haemorrhage, peptic ulcer, severe hypertension, endocarditis.
Possible interaction: drugs that affect coagulation or platelet function.
Side effects: increased haemmorhage risk, bruising, skin rashes, thrombocytopenia, temporary increase in liver enzymes.
Manufacturer: Novo Nordisk.

LOGYNON

Description: an oestrogen/progestogen contraceptive comprising ethinyloestradiol and levonorgestrel in the combinations: 30µg/50µg (6 brown tablets), 40µg/75µg (5 white tablets), 30µg/125µg (10 ochre tablets).
Used for: oral contraception.
Dosage: 1 tablet daily for 21 days starting on the first day of menstruation, then 7 days without tablets.
Special care: hypertension, Raynaud's disease (reduced blood supply to an organ of the body's extremities), asthma, severe depression, diabetes, varicose veins, multiple sclerosis, chronic kidney disease, kidney dialysis. Blood pressure, breasts and pelvic organs to be checked regularly; smoking not advised.

Avoid use: history of heart disease, infectious hepatitis, sickle cell anaemia, porphyria, liver tumour, undiagnosed vaginal bleeding, pregnancy, hormone-dependent cancer, haemolytic uraemic syndrome (rare kidney disorder), chorea, otosclerosis.
Possible interaction: barbiturates, tetracyclines, griseofulvin, rifampicin, primidone, phenytoin, chloral hydrate, ethosuximide, carbamazepine, glutethimide, dichloralphenazone.
Side effects: fluid retention and bloating, leg cramps/pains, breast enlargement, depression, headaches, nausea, loss of libido, weight gain, vaginal discharge, cervical erosion (alteration of epithelial cells), chloasma (pigmentation of nose, cheeks or forehead), breakthrough bleeding (bleeding between periods).
Manufacturer: Schering H.C.

LOGYNON ED

Description: an oestrogen/progestogen contraceptive comprising ethinyloestradiol and levonorgestrel in the combinations: 30µg/50µg (6 brown tablets), 40µg/75µg (5 white tablets), 30µg/125µg (10 ochre tablets) plus 7 white tablets containing inert lactose.
Used for: oral contraception.
Dosage: 1 tablet daily for 28 days starting on the first day of the cycle.
Special care: hypertension, Raynaud's disease (reduced blood supply to an organ of the body's extremities), asthma, severe depression, diabetes, varicose veins, multiple sclerosis, chronic kidney disease, kidney dialysis. Blood pressure, breasts and pelvic organs to be checked regularly; smoking not advised.
Avoid use: history of heart disease, infectious hepatitis, sickle cell anaemia, porphyria, liver tumour, undiagnosed vaginal bleeding, pregnancy, hormone-dependent cancer, haemolytic uraemic syndrome (rare kidney disorder), chorea, otosclerosis.
Possible interaction: barbiturates, tetracyclines, griseofulvin, rifampicin,

primidone, phenytoin, chloral hydrate, ethosuximide, carbamazepine, glutethimide, dichloralphenazone.
Side effects: fluid retention and bloating, leg cramps/pains, breast enlargement, depression, headaches, nausea, loss of libido, weight gain, vaginal discharge, cervical erosion (alteration of epithelial cells), chloasma (pigmentation of nose, cheeks or forehead), breakthrough bleeding (bleeding between periods).
Manufacturer: Schering H.C.

LOMOTIL

Description: an opiate and anticholinergic, diphenoxylate hydrochloride (2.5mg) and atropine sulphate (25µg) in a white tablet marked SEARLE. Also, **LOMOTIL LIQUID** (5ml is equivalent to 1 tablet).
Used for: diarrhoea.
Dosage: 4 tablets or 20ml to begin with then half this dose every 6 hours until control is achieved. Children: 13 to 16 years, 2 tablets or 10ml 3 times per day; 9 to 12 years, 1 tablet or 5ml 4 times per day; 4 to 8 years, 1 tablet or 5ml 3 times daily. Not recommended below 4 years.
Special care: pregnancy, lactation, liver disorder, do not use if there is severe dehydration or imbalance of electrolytes.
Avoid use: acute ulcerative colitis, obstruction in the intestines, jaundice, pseudomembranous colitis (a severe form of colitis).
Possible interaction: depressants of the CNS, MAOIs.
Side effects: allergic reactions, gastrointestinal upset, disturbances of the CNS, anticholinergic effects.
Manufacturer: Gold Cross (Searle).

LONITEN

Description: a vasodilator and antihypertensive, minoxidil, available as white tablets (2.5mg, 5mg and 10mg) marked with the tablet strength and on the reverse with U.
Used for: severe hypertension.
Dosage: 5mg per day initially in 1 or 2 divided doses, increasing at intervals of 3 days, to 10mg and thereafter by increases of 10mg daily to a maximum of 50mg. Children: 0.2mg/kg to begin with daily in 1 or 2 divided doses, increasing by 0.1–0.2mg/kg at intervals of 3 days to a maximum of 1mg/kg body weight daily.
Special care: heart attack. Antihypertensives (other than diuretics and ß-blockers) should be withdrawn gradually before starting treatment. Diuretics and sympathetic suppressants to be given at the same time.
Avoid use: phaeochromocytoma.
Side effects: oedema, tachycardia, hairgrowth.
Manufacturer: Upjohn.

LOPID

Description: an isobutyric acid derivative, gemfibrozil, available as white/maroon capsules (300mg strength) marked LOPID 300. Also **LOPID TABLETS**, 600mg gemfibrozil in white oval tablets marked LOPID.
Used for: prevention of coronary heart disease through lowering high levels of cholesterol or other fats in the blood.
Dosage: 600mg twice per day to a maximum of 1500mg per day.
Special care: blood count, liver function and lipid profile tests before treatment and blood counts over the first year of treatment. Annual check on eyes, period check on serum lipids. To be stopped in cases of persistent abnormal liver function.
Avoid use: gallstones, alcoholism, pregnancy, lactation, liver disorder.
Possible interaction: anticoagulants, simvastatin, pravastatin.
Side effects: headache, dizziness, blurred vision, muscle pain, painful extremities, skin rash, impotence, gastro-intestinal upset.
Manufacturer: Parke-Davis.

LOPRAZOLAM

Description: an intermediate-acting benzodiazepine hypnotic, loprazolam mesylate, available in 1mg tablets.
Used for: treatment of insomnia or

waking at night over the short-term.
Dosage: 1 or 2 at bedtime; up to 1 for the elderly. Not for children.
Special care: chronic kidney or liver disease, lung insufficiency, pregnancy, labour, lactation, elderly. May cause impaired judgement. Avoid prolonged use and withdraw gradually.
Avoid use: acute lung disease, psychotic, phobic or obsessional states, depression of respiration.
Possible interaction: depressants of the CNS, alcohol, anticonvulsants.
Side effects: ataxia, confusion, light-headedness, drowsiness, gastro-intestinal upset, changes in vision and libido, skin rash, hypotension, retention of urine. Dependence risk increases with prolonged treatment or higher dosages.
Manufacturer: Roussel.

LOPRESOR

Description: a ß-blocker, metoprolol tartrate, available as pink tablets (50mg strength) and light blue tablets (100mg strength), marked GEIGY.
Used for: prevention of mortality after myocardial infarction (MI), arrhythmias.
Dosage: see literature for initial dosage after MI, 200mg per day for maintenance. Arrhythmias, 50mg twice or 3 times per day to a daily maximum of 300mg.
Also used for: angina.
Dosage: 50–100mg 2 or 3 times per day.
Also **LOPRESOR SR**, 200mg metoprolol tartrate in a yellow, sustained-release capsule-shaped tablet marked CG/CG and CDC/CDC on the reverse.
Dosage: 1 per day; up to 2, once per day if necessary.
Also used for: hypertension, additional therapy in thyrotoxicosis.'
Dosage: hypertension, 100mg daily to begin with increasing if necessary to 200mg in 1 or 2 divided doses.
Thyrotoxicosis, 50mg, 4 times per day. Or 1 tablet of Lopresor SR in the morning.
Also used for: migraine.
Dosage: 100–200mg per day in divided doses.

Special care: history of bronchospasm and certain ß-blockers, diabetes, liver or kidney disease, pregnancy, lactation, general anaesthesia. Withdraw gradually. Not for children.
Avoid use: heart block or failure, slow heart rate (bradycardia), sick sinus syndrome (associated with sinus node disorder), certain ß-blockers, severe peripheral arterial disease.
Possible interaction: verapamil, hypoglycaemics, reserpine, clonidine withdrawal, some antiarrhythmics and anaesthetics, antihypertensives, depressants of the CNS, cimetidine, indomethacin, sympathomimetics.
Side effects: bradycardia, cold hands and feet, disturbance to sleep, heart failure, gastro-intestinal upset, tiredness on exertion, bronchospasm.
Manufacturer: Geigy.

LOPRESORETIC

Description: a ß-blocker and thiazide diuretic, metoprolol tartrate (100mg) and chlorthalidone (12.5mg), available as an off-white tablet marked GEIGY 56.
Used for: hypertension.
Dosage: 1 daily to begin with in the morning increasing if required to 3 or 4 per day in single or divided doses. Not for children.
Special care: history of bronchospasm and certain ß-blockers, diabetes, liver or kidney disease, pregnancy, lactation, general anaesthesia, gout, check electrolyte levels, K^+ supplements may be required depending on the case. Withdraw gradually. Not for children.
Avoid use: heart block or failure, slow heart rate (bradycardia), sick sinus syndrome (associated with sinus node disorder), certain ß-blockers, severe peripheral arterial disease, pregnancy, lactation, severe kidney failure, anuria, hepatic cornea.
Possible interaction: verapamil, hypoglycaemics, reserpine, clonidine withdrawal, some antiarrhythmics and anaesthetics, antihypertensives,

depressants of the CNS, cimetidine, indomethacin, sympathomimetics, lithium, potassium supplements with potassium-sparing diuretics, digitalis.
Side effects: bradycardia, cold hands and feet, disturbance to sleep, heart failure, gastro-intestinal upset, tiredness on exertion, bronchospasm, gout, weakness, blood disorders, sensitivity to light.
Manufacturer: Geigy.

LORAZEPAM

Description: an intermediate-acting benzodiazepine, lorazepam, available in tablets strength 1mg.
Used for: moderate to severe anxiety.
Dosage: 1–4mg per day in divided doses, elderly 0.5–2mg. Not for children.
Special care: chronic liver or kidney disease, chronic lung disease, pregnancy, labour, lactation, elderly. May impair judgement. Withdraw gradually and avoid prolonged use.
Avoid use: depression of respiration, acute lung disease; psychotic, phobic or obsessional states.
Possible interaction: anticonvulsants, depressants of the CNS, alcohol.
Side effects: ataxia, confusion, light-headedness, drowsiness, hypotension, gastro-intestinal upsets, disturbances in vision and libido, skin rashes, retention of urine, vertigo. Sometimes jaundice or blood disorders.
Manufacturer: available from Wyeth.

LORMETAZEPAM

Description: an intermediate-acting benzodiazepine, lormetazepam, available in 0.5mg and 1mg tablets.
Used for: insomnia.
Dosage: 1mg at bedtime elderly 0.5mg. Not for children.
Special care: chronic liver or kidney disease, chronic lung disease, pregnancy, labour, lactation, elderly. May impair judgement. Withdraw gradually and avoid prolonged use.

Avoid use: depression of respiration, acute lung disease; psychotic, phobic or obsessional states.
Possible interaction: anticonvulsants, depressants of the CNS, alcohol.
Side effects: ataxia, confusion, light-headedness, drowsiness, hypotension, gastro-intestinal upsets, disturbances in vision and libido, skin rashes, retention of urine, vertigo. Sometimes jaundice or blood disorders.
Manufacturer: available from APS, Cox, Wyeth.

LORON

Description: a diphosphonate, sodium clodronate, available in ampoules as a solution of 30mg/ml.
Used for: hypercalcaemia induced by tumour.
Dosage: 300mg per day initially, by slow intravenous infusion, for a maximum of 10 days. For maintenance use tablets or capsules. Not for children.
Also **LORON TABLETS**, containing 520mg sodium clodronate and in white oblong tablets marked BM E9.
Dosage: 2 to 4 tablets per day in 1, or 2 divided doses 1 hour before or after food. Maximum usage, 6 months. Not for children.
Also, **LORON CAPSULES**, 400mg sodium clodronate, in white capsules marked BM B7.
Dosage: 4 to 8 capsules per day in 1, or 2 divided doses 1 hour before or after food for a maximum period of 6 months. Not for children.
Special care: kidney function, serum calcium and phosphate to be monitored.
Avoid use: pregnancy, lactation, kidney failure, inflammation of the intestines.
Possible interaction: antacids, mineral supplements, other diphosphonates.
Side effects: gastro-intestinal upset. Sometimes allergic reactions, hypocalcaemia. Temporary proteinuria.
Manufacturer: Boehringer Mannheim Pharmaceuticals.

LOSEC

Description: a proton pump inhibitor (limits gastric H⁺), omeprazole, available in pink/brown capsules (20mg) marked A/OM and 20, and brown capsules (40mg) both of which contain enteric-coated granules.
Used for: reflux oesophagitis, duodenal and benign gastic ulcers, Zollinger-Ellison (ZE) syndrome.
Dosage: reflux oesophagitis: 20mg per day for 4 weeks, plus a further 4 to 8 weeks if necessary. In unresponsive (refractory) cases, 40mg once per day. 20mg daily for long-term treatment. Duodenal ulcer: 20mg per day for 8 weeks, and 40mg for severe cases. 20mg daily for long-term treatment. Gastric ulcer: 20mg per day for 8 weeks, increasing to 40mg for severe cases. Z-E syndrome: 60mg per day, modified according to response, maintenance 20–120mg daily (doses over 80mg in 2 divided doses). Not for children.
Special care: for suspected gastric ulcer, malignancy must be excluded prior to treatment.
Avoid use: pregnancy, lactation.
Possible interaction: warfarin, digoxin, phenytoin, diazepam.
Side effects: diarrhoea, headache, nausea, skin rashes, constipation.
Manufacturer: Astra.

LOTRIDERM

Description: a potent steroid and antifungal agent, betamethasone dipropionate (0.05%) and clotrimazole (1%) available as a cream.
Used for: short-term treatment fungal infections of the skin.
Dosage: apply for 2 weeks, morning and evening (4 weeks for treatment of the feet).
Special care: maximum 5 days use on face or for children, withdraw gradually after prolonged use.
Avoid use: acne, dermatitis around the mouth, leg ulcers, scabies, viral skin disease, ringworm or tubercular infection, untreated infections caused by

fungi or bacteria. Avoid prolonged or extensive use during pregnancy. Children.
Side effects: irritation, localized mild burning sensation, hypersensitivity reactions.
Manufacturer: Schering-Plough.

LOXAPAC

Description: a dibenzoxapine, loxapine succinate, available in yellow/green (10mg), light green/dark green (25mg) and blue/dark green (50mg) capsules marked L2, L3 or L4 respectively.
Used for: chronic and acute psychoses.
Dosage: 20–50mg per day, to begin with, in 2 doses and increasing over 7 to 10 days to 60–100mg daily. Maximum, 250mg daily. Not for children.
Special care: cardiovascular disease, epilepsy, urine retention, glaucoma, pregnancy, lactation.
Avoid use: patients in a coma or depression induced by drugs.
Possible interaction: anticholinergics, depressants of the CNS.
Side effects: faintness, muscle twitches, weakness, dizziness, drowsiness, confusion, tachycardia, hyper- or hypotension, skin reactions, nausea, changes in ECG and eye, headache, vomiting, dyspnoea (shortness of breath), anticholinergic effects.
Manufacturer: Novex.

LUDIOMIL

Description: a tetracyclic antidepressant, maprotiline hydrochloride, available as peach tablets (10mg, marked Co), greyish-red tablets (25mg, marked DP), light orange tablets (50mg, marked ER) and brown-orange tablets (75mg, marked FS). All are also marked CIBA.
Used for: depression.
Dosage: 25–75mg per day to start with in 1 or 3 divided doses, modifying after 1 or 2 weeks as required; maximum of 150mg daily. Elderly, 30mg once daily or 3 doses of 10mg per day. Not for children.
Special care: pregnancy, lactation, elderly, cardiovascular disease,

schizophrenia, hyperthyroidism.
Avoid use: severe liver or kidney disease,
narrow-angle glaucoma, mania, history
of epilepsy, urine retention, recent
coronary thrombosis.
Possible interaction: sympathomimetics,
barbiturates, MAOIs, antipsychotics,
alcohol, antihypertensives, anaesthetics,
cimetidine, phenytoin, benzodiazepines.
Side effects: skin rash, convulsions,
impaired reactions, anticholinergic effects.
Manufacturer: Ciba.

LURSELLE

Description: a butylphenol, probucol,
available as white tablets (250mg
strength) marked LURSELLE.
Used for: treatment of high blood levels
of protein-bound lipids (hyperlipoproteinaemia).
Dosage: 2 tablets twice daily accompanying the morning and evening meals.
Not for children.
Special care: heart disorders. Monitor
ECG before starting treatment. Stop
treatment 6 months before a planned
pregnancy.
Avoid use: pregnancy, lactation.
Side effects: diarrhoea, gastro intestinal
upset.
Manufacturer: Merrell Dow.

LUSTRAL

Description: sertraline hydrochloride
available as white, capsule-shaped
tablets in 50 and 100mg strengths and
marked PFIZER with LTL-50 or LTL-
100 respectively.
Used for: depression and the prevention
of relapse or further bouts of depression.
Dosage: 50mg per day at the start, with
food, increasing by 50mg if necessary,
every 2 to 4 weeks to a daily maximum
of 200mg. Maintenance is usually 50–
100mg per day. A dosage of 150mg or
more should not be used for more than 8
weeks. Not for children.
Special care: pregnancy, lactation,
unstable epilepsy, anyone undergoing
electroconvulsive therapy.

Avoid use: kidney or liver disorders.
Possible interaction: lithium, tryptophan, MAOIs.
Side effects: nausea, diarrhoea, tremor,
increased sweating, dyspepsia, dry
mouth, delay in ejaculation.
Manufacturer: Invicta.

MACROBID

Description: a preparation which is a
nitrofuran antibacterial drug available as
yellow/blue modified-release capsules
containing 100mg nitrofurantoin, marked
Eaton BID.
Used for: infections of urinary tract,
prevention of infection during surgical
procedures on genital/urinary tract,
pyelitis.
Dosage: adults, treatment, 1 tablet
twice each day with food; prevention
of infection, 1 tablet twice daily for
4 days starting on day of surgery.
Special care: breastfeeding, patients
with diabetes, deficiency of vitamin B,
debilitation, anaemia, imbalance in
electrolyte
(salts) levels. Elderly patients and those
on long-term treatment require
monitoring of liver, lung and nerve
function.
Avoid use: children, pregnant women at
end of pregnancy, patients with kidney
disease or damage or failure or
reduction in ability to produce urine
(anuria and oliguria).
Possible interaction: probenecid,
quinolones, magnesium trisilicate,
sulphinpyrazone.
Side effects: gastro-intestinal upset,
blood changes, allergic responses,
anorexia. Drug should be withdrawn if
hepatitis, lung reactions, peripheral
nerve damage or haemolysis occur.
Manufacturer: P. & G.P.

MACRODANTIN

Description: an antibacterial nitrofuran drug available as white/yellow capsules containing 50mg nitrofurantoin, and yellow capsules containing 100mg nitrofurantoin.

Used for: treatment and prevention of urinary tract infections (during surgical procedure), pyelitis.

Dosage: adults and children over 10 years, treatment of acute infection, 50mg 4 times each day for 1 week; serious, recurring infection, 100mg 4 times each day for 1 week. Long-term suppression of infection, 50–100mg each day taken as single dose at bedtime. Prevention, 50mg 4 times each day for 4 days beginning on day of prcedure. Children, 3 months to 10 years, acute infection, 3mg/kg body weight in divided doses each day for 1 week. Suppression of infection, 1mg/kg body weight once each day.

Special care: breastfeeding, patients who are debilitated, vitamin B deficiency, anaemia, imbalance in electrolyte (salts) levels, diabetes. Elderly patients and those on long-term treatment require regular monitoring of liver and lung function.

Avoid use: pregnant women at end of pregnancy, patients with kidney disease or damage, anuria and oliguria.

Possible interaction: probenecid, quinolones, sulphinpyrazone, magnesium trisilicate.

Side effects: gastro-intestinal upset, allergic responses, blood changes, anorexia. Drug should be withdrawn if hepatitis, lung reactions, peripheral nerve damage or haemolysis occur.

Manufacturer: P. & G.P.

MADOPAR

Description: a combined preparation of dopamine precursor (levodopa) and an enzyme which is a dopa decarboxylase inhibitor, benserazide (as hydrochloride), available as capsules of different strengths. '62.5' blue/grey capsles contain 50mg and 12.5mg respectively.

'125' blue/pink capsules contain 100mg and 25mg. '250' blue/caramel capsules contain 200mg and 50mg. All capsules are marked ROCHE. Also, **MADOPAR DISPERSIBLE TABLETS**, white scored tablets of 2 different strengths: '62.5' contain 50mg and 12.5mg; '125' contain 100mg and 25mg. Tablets all marked with name and strength. Also, **MADOPAR CR** green/blue continuous-release capsules containing 100mg levodopa and 25mg benserazide (as hydrochloride), marked ROCHE.

Used for: Parkinsonism.

Dosage: adults over 25 years of age not already receiving levodopa, 1 '62.5' tablet 3 or 4 times each day at first taken after meals. Dose may be increased by 1 '125' tablet each day once or twice a week. Usual maintenance dose is in the order of 4 to 8 '125' tablets each day in divided doses. Elderly persons, 1 '62.5' once or twice each day with additional '62.5' tablet every third or fourth day if increase is required. Madopar continuous-release capsules: dose individually determined for each patient, usually 50% more than previous levodopa therapy.

Special care: peptic ulcer, wide angle glaucoma, liver, kidney, heart, lung, circulatory diseases or endocrine (hormonal) disorders. Also, psychiatric disorders, soft bones (osteomalacia). Regular blood checks and monitoring of liver, kidney, heart and circulatory function should be carried out.

Avoid use: children and young adults under 25 years of age, pregnancy, breastfeeding. Patients with history of malignant melanoma (tumours of melanocytes which form the skin pigment, melanin), narrow angle glaucoma, severe psychoses.

Possible interaction: sympathomimetics antihypertensives, other similar preparations, ferrous sulphate, MAOIs; antacids (Madopar CR).

Side effects: heart and central nervous system disturbance, involuntary movements, hypotension when rising

from lying down, anorexia, nausea, vomiting, discoloured urine. Rarely, haemolytic anaemia.
Manufacturer: Roche.

MAGNAPEN

Description: a compound broad-spectrum penicillin and penicillinase-resistant (i.e. resistant to enzymes produced by some bacteria) preparation. Is available as turquoise/black capsules containing 250mg ampicillin and 250mg flucloxacillin and marked MAGNAPEN. Also, **MAGNAPEN SYRUP** containing 125mg ampicillin and 125mg flucloxacillin/5ml.
MAGNAPEN INJECTION containing 500mg or 1g powder in vials for reconstitution and injection, both with equal quantities of ampicillin and flucloxacillin.
Used for: severe and mixed infections where some penicillin-resistant (staphylococci) bacteria are present.
Dosage: adults and children over 10, 1 capsule or 10ml syrup 4 times each day taken thirty minutes to 1 hour before meals. Injection, 500mg 4 times each day. Children, under 10 years, 5ml syrup 4 times each day thirty minutes to 1 hour before meals. Injection, under 2 years, quarter of adult dose; 2 to 10 years, half adult dose.
Special care: patients with glandular fever (infectious mononucleosis).
Side effects: gastro-intestinal upset, allergic reactions; rarely, cholestatic jaundice.
Manufacturer: Beecham.

MALOPRIM

Description: a compound antimalarial preparation combining sulphone and diaminopyrimidine drugs, available as scored white tablets containing 100mg dapsone and 12.5mg pyrimethamine, marked WELLCOME H9A.
Used for: prevention of malaria.
Dosage: adults and children over 10 years, 1 tablet each week. Children, 5 to 10 years of age, 1 half tablet weekly.

Special care: patient should continue to take tablets for 4 weeks after leaving area where malaria is present. Special care in breastfeeding mothers, pregnant women should take folate supplements, patients with liver or kidney disease.
Avoid use: children under 5 years, patients with dermatitis herpetiformis (a type of dermatitis).
Possible interaction: folate inhibitors.
Side effects: severe haemolysis, skin sensitivity, blood disorders.
Manufacturer: Wellcome.

MANERIX

Description: an antidepressant preparation which is a reversible MAO-A inhibitor (monoamine oxidase A inhibitor) which acts to prevent the breakdown of this neuro-transmitter by enzyme, thereby prolonging its activity. It is available as scored, oblong, yellow, film-coated tablets containing 150mg moclobemide, marked ROCHE 150.
Used for: severe depression.
Dosage: adults, 2 tablets each day in divided doses (maximum of 4 daily) taken after meals.
Special care: pregnancy, breastfeeding, serious liver disease, thyrotoxicosis. Also, patients with schizophrenia in which agitation is a predominant symptom. Some foods may need to be avoided.
Avoid use: children, patients with phaeochromocytoma, severe confusional disorders.
Possible interaction: morphine, cimetidine, some sympathomimetic amines, pethidine, fentanyl, some other antidepressants, codeine.
Side effects: headache, giddiness, agitation and restlessness, confusion, nausea, disturbance of sleep.
Manufacturer: Roche.

MAREVAN

Description: a coumarin anticoagulant preparation available as scored tablets of different strengths all containing warfarin sodium; brown 1mg tablets

marked M1, blue 3mg tablets marked M3 and pink 5mg tablets marked M5.
Used for: thromboembolic states.
Dosage: adults, 10mg each day adjusted according to response.
Special care: patients who are seriously ill, have kidney disease or disorder, hypertension, vitamin K deficiency, weight changes and elderly persons.
Avoid use: pregnancy, within 24 hours of labour or surgery, reduced liver or kidney function, haemorrhage or bleeding disorders.
Possible interaction: antibiotics, cimetidine, corticosteroids, hypoglycaemics taken orally, phenformin, sulphonamides, NSAIDs, quinidine, drugs have an effect on liver enzymes.
Side effects: skin rash, diarrhoea, baldness.
Manufacturer: Goldshield.

MARPLAN

Description: an antidepressant MAOI available as scored, pink tablets containing 10mg isocarboxazid, marked ROCHE.
Used for: depression.
Dosage: adults, 30mg each day at first reducing to a usual maintenance dose in the order of 10–20mg daily. Elderly persons, half adult dose.
Special care: elderly persons and patients with epilepsy.
Avoid use: children, patients with congestive heart failure, circulatory disease of arteries of brain (cerebral vascular disease), liver disease, phaeochromocytoma, blood changes, hyperthyroidism, heart disease.
Possible interaction: anticholinergics, barbiturates, alcohol, hypoglycaemics, insulin, reserpine, guanethidine, methyldopa. Also sympathomimetic amines, especially ephedrine, amphetamine, levodopa, methylphenidate, phenylpropanolamine, fenfluramine. Also, pethidine, TCADs, narcotic analgesics. Many foods need to be avoided including: meat extracts (Bovril, Oxo), bananas, yeast extracts (Marmite), broad beans, foods made from textured vegetable proteins,

alcohol, low alcohol drinks, pickled herrings, all foods that are not completely fresh. All these drugs and foods should be avoided for at least 14 days after treatment stops then tried cautiously.
Side effects: allergic responses with certai foods, tiredness, muscle weakness, low blood pressure on rising, dizziness, swelling of ankles. Dry mouth, blurring o vision, gastro-intestinal upset, constipation, difficulty ir urination. Skin rashes, weight gain, blood changes, change in libido, jaundice. Sometimes psychiatric disturbances and confusion.
Manufacturer: Cambridge.

MARVELON

Description: a combined oestrogen/progestogen oral contraceptive preparation available as white tablets containing 30mg ethinyloestradiol and 150 micrograms desogestrel, marked ORGANON, TR over 5 and with *.
Used for: oral contraception.
Dosage: 1 tablet each day for 21 days, starting on first or fifth day of monthly cycle, followed by 7 tablet-free days.
Special care: patients with multiple sclerosis, serious kidney disease or kidne dialysis, asthma, Raynaud's disease, abnormally high levels of prolactin in the blood (hyperprolactinaemia), varicos veins, hypertension. Also, patients suffering from severe depression. Thrombosis risk increases with smokir age and obesity. During the course of treatment, regular checks on blood pressure, pelvic organs and breasts should be carried out.
Avoid use: pregnancy, those at risk of thrombosis, suffering from heart disea pulmonary hyper-tension, angina, sickle cell anaemia. Also, undiagnosed vaginal bleeding, history of cholestatic jaundice during pregnancy, cancers which are hormone-dependent, infectious hepati liver disorders. Also, porphyria, Dubli Johnson and Rotor syndrome, otoscleromesis, chorea, haemolytic uraemic syndrome, recent trophoblastic disease

Possible interaction: barbiturates, ethosuximide, glutethimide, rifampicin, phenytoin, tetracyclines, carbamazepine, chloral hydrate, griseofulvin, dichloralphenazone, primidone.
Side effects: weight gain, breast enlargement, pains in legs, cramps, loss of sexual desire, headaches, depression, nausea, breakthrough bleeding, cervical erosion, vaginal discharge, brownish patches on skin (chloasma), oedema and bloatedness.
Manufacturer: Organon.

MAXIDEX

Description: lubricant and corticosteroid eyedrops containing 0.5% hypromellose and 0.1% dexamethasone.
Used for: inflammation of anterior segment of eye.
Dosage: serious disease, 1 to 2 drops each hour, reducing dose as condition improves. For milder conditions, 1 or 2 drops 4, 5 or 6 times each day.
Special care: long-term use by pregnant women and in babies.
Avoid use: patients with glaucoma, suffering from tuberculous, viral or fungal infections or those producing pus; patients with soft contact lenses.
Side effects: cataract, thinning of cornea, rise in pressure within eye, fungal infection.
Manufacturer: Alcon.

MAXITROL

Description: a compound preparation in the form of eyedrops combining a corticosteroid, aminoglycoside, lubricant and peptide. It contains 0.1% dexamethasone, 0.35% neomycin sulphate, 0.5% hypromellose, 6000 units polymyxin B sulphate/ml. Also **MAXITROL OINTMENT** containing 0.1% dexamethasone, 0.35% neomycin sulphate, 6000 units polymyxin B sulphate/gram.
Used for: infected and inflamed conditions of the eye.
Dosage: apply 3 or 4 times each day.
Special care: long-term use by pregnant women or in babies.

Avoid use: patients with glaucoma, suffering from tuberculous, viral or fungal infections or those producing pus; patients with soft contact lenses.
Side effects: cataract, thinning of cornea, rise in pressure within eye, fungal infection.
Manufacturer: Alcon.

MAXOLON

Description: an anti-emetic, antidopaminergic preparation, metoclopramide hydrochloride, which acts on the gastrointestinal tract and is available in a number of different forms: white, scored tablets containing 10mg marked MAXOLON. **MAXOLON SYRUP** containing 5mg/5ml. **MAXOLON PAEDIATRIC LIQUID** containing 1mg/ml. **MAXOLON INJECTION** as a solution in ampoules for injection containing 10mg/2ml. **MAXOLON SR** clear capsules containing white, sustained-release granules at a strength of 15mg, marked MAXOLON SR 15. **MAXOLON HIGH DOSE** available as a solution in ampoules for injection containing 100mg/20ml.
Used for: indigestion, gastro-intestinal disturbance, backflow of blood. Also, vomiting and nausea due to cytotoxic drug therapy, cobalt therapy, deep X-ray or post-operative sickness.
Dosage: adults, over 20 years of age, 15mg twice each day with a daily maximum of 0.5mg/kg body weight. Children and young adults under 20 years, for vomiting caused by cancer chemotherapy or radiotherapy from 1 to 5mg, 2 or 3 times per day, depending upon body weight.
Special care: pregnancy, breastfeeding, liver or kidney disease/damage, epilepsy.
Avoid use: patients who have recently had operations on gastro-intestinal tract, phaeochromocytoma, breast cancer which is prolactin-dependent.
Possible interaction: phenothiazines, anticholinergics, butyrophenones.
Side effects: diarrhoea, raised levels of prolactin in blood, sleepiness,

extrapyramidal reactions (involuntary muscle movements, changes in posture and muscle tone).
Manufacturer: Beecham.

MAXTREX

Description: a folic acid antagonist available as tablets of 2 strengths. Yellow tablets contain 2.5mg methotrexate and are marked M2.5 on 1 side and F on the other. Yellow, scored tablets contain 10mg and are marked M10.
Used for: abnormal growths and serious psoriasis which has not been controlled by other treatments.
Dosage: individually determined according to patient's condition and response.
Special care: patients with gastro-intestinal diseases and disorders, liver or kidney disease or damage, low blood cell counts, psychiatric illness, elderly or young persons. Patients should be monitored for liver and kidney function and blood checks.
Avoid use: pregnancy, breastfeeding, patients with serious liver or kidney disorder, abnormally low levels of white blood cells and platelets, severe anaemia.
Possible interaction: alcohol, NSAIDs, live vaccines, drugs that bind to proteins, anticonvulsants, folic acid, etretinate.
Side effects: gastro-intestinal upset, skin rashes, liver disorders, depression of bone marrow.
Manufacturer: Pharmacia.

MEDIHALER-EPI

Description: a sympathomimetic preparation available as a metered dose aerosol delivering 0.28mg adrenaline acid tartrate per dose.
Used for: additional treatment in anaphylaxis caused by sensitivity to insect stings or drugs.
Dosage: adults, anaphylaxis only, at least 20 puffs. Children, 10–15 puffs.
Special care: diabetes.
Avoid use: patients with hyperthy-

roidism, serious heart disease, heart arrhythmias, hypertension.
Possible interaction: sympathomimetics, TCADs, MAOIs.
Side effects: palpitations, agitation, dry mouth, stomach pain.
Manufacturer: 3M Health Care.

MEDIHALER-ERGOTAMINE

Description: an NSAID which is an ergot alkaloid available as a metered dose aerosol delivering 0.36mg ergotamine tartrate/metered dose.
Used for: rapid treatment of migraine.
Dosage: adults and children over 10, 1 dose repeated after 5 minutes if needed with a maximum of 6 doses in 24 hours and 15 in any 7 day period.
Avoid use: pregnancy, breastfeeding, children under 10 years, patients with liver or kidney disorder, hypertension, heart disease or disease of peripheral arteries, sepsis.
Possible interaction: ß-blockers, erythromycin.
Side effects: muscle pain, nausea.
Manufacturer: 3M Health Care.

MEDIHALER ISO

Description: a bronchodilator which is a non-selective ß-agonist available as a metered dose aerosol delivering 0.08mg isoprenaline sulphate per dose. Also, MEDIHALER ISO FORTE delivering 0.4mg isoprenaline sulphate per dose by metered dose aerosol.
Used for: severe bronchitis and bronchial asthma.
Dosage: adults, 1–3 puffs which may be repeated after half an hour if required. Maximum dose is 24 puffs in 24 hours.
Special care: pregnancy, diabetes or hypertension.
Avoid use: children, hyperthyroidism or severe coronary disease.
Possible interaction: sympathomimetics, tricyclics, MAOIs.
Side effects: palpitations, agitation, dry mouth.
Manufacturer: 3M Health Care.

MEDRONE

Description: an anti-inflammatory, glucocorticoid corticosteroid preparation available as tablets of different strengths, all containing methylprednisolone. Oval, pink, scored 2mg tablets marked UPJOHN; oval, white, scored 4mg tablets marked UPJOHN; white, scored 16mg tablets, marked UPJOHN 73; light-blue, scored 100mg tablets marked UPJOHN 3379.

Used for: treatment and control of allergic and inflammatory disorders including dermatological, respiratory, neoplastic and collagen diseases and rheumatoid arthritis.

Dosage: 2–40mg each day depending upon patient's condition and response.

Special care: pregnancy, active infections and those of fungal, viral or tuberculous origin, kidney inflammation, diseases characterized by skin rash (exanthematous), hypertension. Also, patients who have recently had surgical anastomoses of intestine, suffering from epilepsy, diabetes, liver cirrhosis, peptic ulcer, hyperthyroidism, secondary cancers. Patients suffering from stress or psychoses, contact with herpes zoster or chicken pox should be avoided and medical help and treatment will be required if this inadvertently occurs.

Possible interaction: cardiac glycosides, phenytoin, rifampicin, NSAIDs, anti-cholinesterases, ephedrine, phenobarbitone, anticoagulants taken orally, diuretics, hypoglycaemics.

Side effects: symptoms as in Cushing's syndrome, osteoporosis, peptic ulcer, hyperglycaemia, depression and euphoria.

Manufacturer: Upjohn.

MEFOXIN

Description: a cephalosporin antibiotic preparation available as a powder in vials for reconstitution and injection, in 2 strengths containing 1g or 2g cefoxitin.

Used for: skin, soft tissue, respiratory tract infections, septicaemia and peritonitis. Prevention of infection in gynaecological and obstetric operations, treatment of post-operative infections. Gonorrhoea and urinary tract infections.

Dosage: adults, 1–2g by intravenous or intramuscular injection at 8 hour intervals. Prevention of infection, 2g 30 minutes to 1 hour before surgery 10 every 6 hours post-operatively for 24 hours. Children, newborn babies up to 1 week, 20–40mg/kg body weight at 12 hour intervals. 1 week to 1 month of age, 20–40mg/kg at 8 hour intervals; 1 month and over, 20–40kg/kg at 6 to 8 hour intervals. Prevention of infection, newborn babies, 30–40mg/kg, 30 minutes to 1 hour before operation then every 8 to 12 hours post-operatively for 24 hours. Older babies and children, 30–40mg/kg at same times as in adults.

Special care: pregnancy, breastfeeding, patients with allergy to penicillin, kidney disorder.

Possible interaction: aminoglycosides, loop diuretics.

Side effects: gastro-intestinal upset, blood changes, (reduction in levels of white blood cells and platelets), allergic reactions, pain at injection site, rise in levels of blood urea and liver enzymes. Positive Coomb's test (a test for detecting rhesus antibodies).

Manufacturer: M.S.D.

MEGACE

Description: a hormonal progestogen preparation available as tablets of 2 strengths: scored, white tablets contain 40mg megestrol acetate marked 40; oval, off-white scored tablets contain 160mg marked 160.

Used for: breast and endometrial cancer.

Dosage: breast cancer, 160mg each day as single or divided doses. Endometrial cancer, 40–320mg each day in divided doses. All taken for at least 2 months.

Special care: patients with inflamed veins (thrombophlebitis).

Avoid use: pregnant women.

Side effects: nausea, nettle rash (urticaria), gain in weight.

Manufacturer: Bristol-Myers.

MELLERIL

Description: a phenothiazine group II antipsychotic drug available as white, film-coated tablets of different strengths containing 10mg, 25mg, 50mg and 100mg thioridazine hydrochloride respectively. All are marked with strength and MEL. Also, **MELLERIL SYRUP** containing 25mg/5ml. **MELLERIL SUSPENSION** in 2 strengths containing 25mg and 100mg thioridazine base/5ml.

Used for: mania, schizophrenia, hypomania, additional short-term therapy in the treatment of psychoneuroses. Symptoms of senility, disturbed behaviour and epilepsy in children.

Dosage: depending upon severity and type of condition, in the order of 30–600mg each day. Children, 1 to 5 years, 1mg/kg body weight each day; over 5 years, 75–150mg/kg daily. Maximum dose in this age group is 300mg each day.

Special care: myasthenia gravis, epilepsy, phaeochromocytoma, enlarged prostate gland, Parkinsonism, heart and circulatory diseases, glaucoma, liver or kidney disorders, respiratory diseases.

Avoid use: pregnancy, breastfeeding, history of blood changes, coma, serious heart or circulatory diseases, severe depression, porphyria.

Possible interaction: alcohol, antiarrhythmics, antacids, tricyclics, antimuscarines, calcium channel blockers, anxiolytics, lithium.

Side effects: hypotension, changes in libido, apathy, depression, insomnia, dry mouth, blocked nose, effects on heart rhythm, disturbance of sleep, constipation, difficulty in passing urine. Blood changes, rashes, jaundice, effects on liver, menstrual changes, breast enlargement, weight gain, abnormal production of breast milk. Rarely, fits, blurring of vision due to deposition of pigment (higher doses).

Manufacturer: Sandoz.

MENGIVAC (A + C)

Description: a vaccine preparation containing inactivated surface antigen of meningitis A and C. It is produced as a powder in vials, with diluent, containing 50 micrograms of both group A and group C polysaccharide antigens of *Neisseria meningitidis*.

Used for: immunisation against meningitis, types A and C.

Dosage: adults and children over eighteen months, 0.5ml by deep subcutaneous or intramuscular injection.

Special care: pregnancy, breastfeeding.

Avoid use: patients with severe infections and feverish illnesses.

Possible interaction: substances which suppress immune system.

Side effects: local skin reactions, slight fever.

Manufacturer: Merieux.

MENOPHASE

Description: a hormonal combined oestrogen/progestogen preparation available as tablets containing mestranol and norethisterone; 5 pink tablets contain 12.5µg mestranol; 8 orange tablets contain 25µg mestranol; 2 yellow tablets contain 50µg mestranol; 3 green tablets contain 25µg mestranol and 1mg norethisterone; 6 blue tablets contain 30µg mestranol and 1.5mg norethisterone; 4 lavender tablets contain 20µg mestranol and 750µg norethisterone.

Used for: treatment of menopausal symptoms and prevention of osteoporosis following menopause.

Dosage: 1 tablet each day starting on a Sunday with pink tablets and continuing in order, as indicated. Treatment should be continuous for 6 months to 1 year.

Special care: patients with history of, or considered to be at risk of thrombosis. Women with any of the following should receive careful monitoring: epilepsy, gallstones, porphyria, multiple sclerosis, otosclerosis, diabetes, migraine, hypertension, tetany, fibroids in the uterus. Blood pressure, breasts and pelvic organs

should be examined regularly during the course of treatment especially in women who may be at risk of breast cancer.
Avoid use: pregnancy, breastfeeding, women with breast cancer, cancer of reproductive system or other hormonally dependent cancer. Women with inflammation of veins or other thromboembolic conditions, endometriosis, undiagnosed vaginal bleeding, serious liver, kidney or heart disease, Dublin-Johnson or Rotor syndromes.
Possible interaction: drugs which induce liver enzymes.
Side effects: soreness and enlargement of breasts, breakthrough bleeding, weight gain, gastro-intestinal upset, dizziness, nausea, headache, vomiting. If frequent, severe, migraine-like headaches, distrubance of vision, rise in blood pressure, jaundice or indications of thrombosis occur, drug should immediately be withdrawn, and also in the event of pregnancy. Drug should be stopped 6 weeks before planned major surgery.
Manufacturer: Syntex.

MENZOL

Description: an hormonal progestogen preparation available in the form of scored, white tablets containing 5mg norethisterone marked NE5, MENZOL 20-day.
Used for: menstrual pain (dysmenorrhoea), menorrhagia, premenstrual syndrome (PMS).
Dosage: 1 tablet 2 or 3 times each day starting at different times in the monthly cycle depending upon condition being treated). Treatment usually continues for several cycles.
Special care: patients with disturbance of liver function.
Avoid use: pregnancy, severe disturbance of liver function, Dublin-Johnson or Rotor syndrome, history of jaundice during pregnancy, severe pruritus (itching) or herpes gestationus (a raised itchy rash which appears in the last 3 months of pregnancy).

Side effects: weight gain, depression, headache, vomiting, breakthrough bleeding, nausea, oedema, masculinizing (androgenic) effects.
Manufacturer: Schwarz.

MEPTID

Description: an analgesic preparation which is an opiate partial agonist available as film-coated orange tablets containing 200mg meptazinol marked MPL-023. Also, **MEPTID INJECTION** containing 100mg meptazinol as hydrochloride/ml.
Used for: short-term relief of pain.
Dosage: adults, 75–100mg by intramuscular injection or 50–100mg intravenously. May be repeated every 2 to 4 hours as required. Obstetric patients, 2mg/kg body weight given intramuscularly.
Special care: patients with liver or kidney disease, serious breathing problems.
Avoid use: children.
Side effects: nausea, dizziness.
Manufacturer: Monmouth.

MERBENTYL

Description: an anticholinergic preparation available as white tablets containing 10mg dicyclomine hydrochloride, marked M within 2 circles; white oval tablets containing 20mg, marked MERBENTYL 20. Also **MERBENTYL SYRUP** containing 10mg/5ml.
Used for: spasm of stomach and gastro-intestinal tract.
Dosage: adults, 10–20mg 3 times each day before or after meals. Children, 6 months to 2 years, 5–10mg 3 or 4 times each day fifteen minutes before food with a maximum of 40mg daily. Over 2 years, 10mg 3 times each day.
Special care: enlarged prostate gland, glaucoma, reflux oesophagitis with hiatus hernia.
Avoid use: children under 6 months of age.
Side effects: thirst, dry mouth, dizziness.
Manufacturer: Merrell Dow.

MERCILON

Description: an hormonal combinal oestrogen/progestogen preparation available as white tablets containing 20µg ethinyloestradiol and 150µg desogestrel, marked TR over 4.

Used for: oral contraception.

Dosage: 1 tablet each day for 21 days starting on first or fifth day of monthly cycle, followed by 7 tablet-free days.

Special care: multiple sclerosis, serious kidney disease or kidney dialysis, asthma, Raynaud's disease, abnormally high levels of prolactin in the blood (hyperprolactinaemia), varicose veins, hypertension. Also, patients suffering from severe depression. Thrombosis risk increases with smoking, age and obesity. During the course of treatment, regular checks on blood pressure, pelvic organs and breasts should be carried out.

Avoid use: pregnancy, those at risk of thrombosis, suffering from heart disease, pulmonary hypertension, angina, sickle cell anaemia. Also, undiagnosed vaginal bleeding, history of cholestatic jaundice during pregnancy, cancers which are hormone-dependent, infectious hepatitis, liver disorders. Also, porphyria, Dublin-Johnson and Rotor syndrome, otosclerosis, chorea, haemolytic uraemic syndrome, recent trophoblastic disease.

Possible interaction: barbiturates, ethosuximide, glutethimide, rifampicin, phenytoin, tetracyclines, carbamazepine, chloral hydrate, griseofulvin, dichloralphenazone, primidone.

Side effects: weight gain, breast enlargement, pains in legs and cramps, headaches, loss of sexual desire, depression, nausea, breakthrough bleeding, cervical erosion, brownish patches on skin (chloasma), vaginal discharge, oedema and bloatedness.

Manufacturer: Organon.

MESTINON

Description: an anticholinesterase preparation which acts to inhibit the enzyme that breaks down acetylcholine so that the effects of the neurotransmitter are prolonged. It is produced in the form of white, quarter-scored tablets containing 60mg pyridostigmine bromide, marked ROCHE.

Used for: myasthenia gravis, paralytic ileus.

Dosage: myasthenia gravis, 5 to 20 tablets each day in divided doses; paralytic ileus, 1 to 4 tablets, as needed. Children, myasthenia gravis, under 6 years, 30mg at first, 6 to 12 years, 60mg at first. Both doses may be gradually increased by 15–30mg each day until condition is controlled.

Special care: patients with epilepsy, Parkinsonism, asthma, recent heart attack, peptic ulcer, kidney disease, bradycardia, hypotension, abnormal over-activity of vagus nerve.

Avoid use: patients with gastro-intestinal or urinary tract obstruction.

Possible interaction: cyclopropane, depolarising muscle relaxants, halothane.

Side effects: over-production of saliva, nausea, diarrhoea, colic-type pain.

Manufacturer: Roche.

METERIX

Description: a thiazide-like diuretic preparation available as blue tablets containing 5mg metolazone marked with strength and symbol.

Used for: oedema, toxaemia of pregnancy, hypertension, ascites (collection of fluid in peritoneal cavity of the abdomen).

Dosage: oedema, 5–10mg as a single daily dose with a maximum of 80mg each day; hypertension, 5mg each day at first reducing after 3 to 4 weeks to this dose taken every second day.

Special care: pregnancy, breastfeeding, elderly, liver or kidney disease, cirrhosis of the liver, gout, diabetes, collagen disease. Fluid, electrolytes (salts), and glucose levels require monitoring during the course of therapy.

Avoid use: children, hypercalcaemia, serious liver or kidney failure, allergy to sulphonamide drugs, Addison's disease.

Possible interaction: NSAIDs, carben-oxolone, lithium, barbiturates, tubo-curarine, alcohol, cardiac glycosides, alcohol, corticosteroids, opioids.
Side effects: gastro-intestinal distur-bance, anorexia, sensitivity to light, disturbance of electrolyte balance and metabolism, pancreatitis, rash, impotence, blood changes, dizziness.
Manufacturer: Hoechst.

METERFOLIC

Description: a haematinic and folic acid preparation available as grey, film-coated tablets containing ferrous fumerate (equivalent to 100mg iron) and 400µg folic acid, marked METERFOLIC.
Used for: prevention of iron and folic acid deficiency during pregnancy. As a supplement taken when pregnancy is planned to prevent neural tube defects in foetus.
Dosage: pregnant women, 1 tablet once or twice each day; prevention of neural tube defects, 1 tablet each day before conception and continuing for at least the first third of pregnancy.
Special care: patients with history of peptic ulcer or haemolytic anaemia.
Avoid use: patients with vitamin B_{12} deficiency.
Possible interaction: tetracyclines.
Side effects: constipation and nausea.
Manufacturer: Sinclair.

METOPIRONE

Description: a diuretic preparation which is an aldosterone inhibitor. Used with glucocorticoids, it acts to eliminate fluid which has accumulated due to increased secretion of the mineralocorti-coid hormone, aldosterone. It is produced as creams containing 250mg metyrapone, coded LN and CIBA.
Used for: in addition to glucocorticoids to treat resistant oedema caused by excess secretion of aldosterone. Also, for Cushing's syndrome.
Dosage: adults, resistant oedema, 250mg–6g each day; Cushing's

syndrome, 2.5–4.5g each day as divided doses.
Special care: patients with decreased function of the pituitary gland.
Avoid use: pregnancy, breastfeeding, children.
Side effects: allergic responses, nausea, vomiting, hypotension.
Manufacturer: Ciba.

METOSYN

Description: a potent topical steroid preparation available as cream and ointment containing 0.05% fluocinonide. Also, METOSYN SCALP LOTION containing 0.05% fluocinonide in an alcholic solution.
Used for: inflamed and allergic skin conditions, those producing pus.
Dosage: apply thinly each morning and night to affected area.
Special care: short-term use only.
Avoid use: children, long-term or extensive use especially in pregnant women, patients with untreated bacterial or fungal infections or skin infections of tuberculous or viral origin or due to ringworm. Also, patients with dermatitis in area of mouth, acne, leg ulcers or scabies.
Side effects: suppression of adrenal glands, skin thinning, abnormal hair growth, changes as in Cushing's syndrome.
Manufacturer: Stuart.

METRODIN HIGH PURITY

Description: an hormonal gonadotrophin preparation available as freeze-dried powder in ampoules, with diluent, for reconstitution and injection, containing 75 units and 150 units urofolitrophin (follicle-stimulating hormone).
Used for: absence or reduced ovulation caused by dysfunction of the hypothala-mus, which regulates the hormonal output of the pituitary gland, in turn producing hormones which control the sex organs. Also, for superovulation in women having fertility treatment (IVF).
Dosage: hypothalamic pituitary gland dysfunction, 75–150 units each day at

first by subcutaneous or intramuscular injection. Subsequent treatment depends on response. Superovulation, 150–225 units each day.
Special care: monitoring is essential hence treatment is usually under close medical supervision. Any hormonal disorders or brain lesions must be corrected before therapy starts.
Avoid use: pregnant women.
Side effects: allergic reactions, over-stimulation of ovaries which may lead to enlargement or rupture, multiple pregnancy.
Manufacturer: Seronon.

METROGEL
Description: a nitroimidazole antibiotic preparation available in the form of a gel, containing 0.75% metronidazole.
Used for: inflammatory conditions relating to acne rosacea.
Dosage: adults, apply thinly twice each day for 8 to 9 weeks.
Avoid use: children, pregnant women.
Side effects: local skin irritation.
Manufacturer: Sandox.

METROTOP
Description: an antibacterial preparation available in the form of a gel containing 0.8% metronidazol.
Used for: to deodorize a tumour producing an unpleasant smell because of fungus infection.
Dosage: apply to clean wound once or twice each day and cover.
Avoid use: pregnancy, breastfeeding.
Side effects: local skin irritation.
Manufacturer: Pharmacia.

MEXITIL
Description: a class I antiarrhythmic preparation, mexiletine hydrochloride, available in a variety of different forms. Purple/red capsules contain 50mg and red capsules contain 200mg both marked with strength and symbol. Also, MEXITIL PERLONGETS, red/turquoise sustained-release capsules

contain 360mg. MEXITIL INJECTION contains 25mg/ml in ampoules for injection.
Used for: arrhythmias originating from ventricles of heart.
Dosage: capsules, 400–600mg at first then a further 200–250mg 2 hours later repeated 3 or 4 times each day. Perlongets, 1 capsule twice each day.
Special care: hypotension, Parkinsonism, liver, kidney or heart failure, conduction defects of the heart, bradycardia.
Avoid use: children.
Side effects: effects on central nervous system, hypotension, gastro-intestinal upset.
Manufacturer: Boehringer Ing.

MFV-JECT
Description: a preparation of inactivated material derived from 3 strains of influenza virus available in pre-filled syringes containing 15 micrograms of each type/5ml suspension.
Used for: immunisation against influenza.
Dosage: adults, 0.5ml by intramuscular or deep subcutaneous injection. Children, 6 months to 3 years, 0.25ml repeated after 1 month to 6 weeks; 3 to 12 years, 0.5ml repeated after 1 month to 6 weeks. All given by intramuscular or deep subcutaneous injection. (Children who have been vaccinated before or infected with influenza require only 1 dose).
Avoid use: patients with feverish illness, allergic to egg protein (used in culture of viruses).
Side effects: malaise, fever.
Manufacturer: Merieux.

MICROGYNON 30
Description: an hormonal oestrogen/progestogen combined preparation in the form of beige, sugar-coated tablets containing 30µg ethinyloestradiol and 150µg levonorgestrel.
Used for: oral contraception.
Dosage: 1 tablet each day starting on first day of period followed by 7 tablet-free days.

Special care: patients with multiple sclerosis, serious kidney disease or kidney dialysis, asthma, Raynaud's disease, abnormally high levels of prolactin in the blood (hyperprolactinaemia), varicose veins, hypertension. Also, patients suffering from severe depression. Thrombosis risk increases with smoking, age and obesity. During the course of treatment, regular checks on blood pressure, pelvic organs and breasts should be carried out.

Avoid use: pregnancy, those at risk of thrombosis, suffering from heart disease, pulmonary hypertension, angina, sickle cell anaemia. Also, undiagnosed vaginal bleeding, history of cholestatic jaundice during pregnancy, cancers which are hormone-dependent, infectious hepatitis, liver disorders. Also, porphyria, Dublin-Johnson and Rotor syndrome, otosclerosis, chorea, haemolytic uraemic syndrome, recent trophoblastic disease.

Possible interaction: barbiturates, ethosuximide, glutethimide, rifampicin, phenytoin, tetracyclines, carbamazepine, chloral hydrate, griseofulvin, dichloralphenazone, primidone.

Side effects: weight gain, breast enlargement, pains in legs and cramps, headaches, loss of sexual desire, depression, nausea, breakthrough bleeding, cervical erosion, vaginal discharge, brownish patches on skin (chloasma), oedema and bloatedness.

Manufacturer: Schering H.C.

MICRONOR

Description: an hormonal progestogen available as white tablets containing 350µg norethisterone, marked C over 035.

Used for: oral contraception.

Dosage: 1 tablet at same time each day starting on first day of cycle and continuing without a break.

Special care: history of or at risk of thrombosis or embolism, liver disease, cancer which is hormone-dependent, ovarian cysts, hypertension, migraine. Blood pressure, breasts and pelvic organs should be checked regularly during the course of treatment.

Avoid use: pregnancy, patients who have previously had a stroke, poor circulation to heart leading to heart disease, diseased arteries, previous ectopic pregnancy. Also, undiagnosed vaginal bleeding, benign tumour (adenoma) of the liver derived from glandular tissue, recent trophoblastic disease.

Possible interaction: chloral hydrate, barbiturates, meprobamate, phenytoin, rifampicin, carbamazepine, griseofulvin, primidone, glutethimide dichloralphenazone, chlorpromazine, ethosuximide.

Side effects: changes in pattern of menstruation, headache, ovarian cysts, sore breasts, acne.

Manufacturer: Ortho.

MICROVAL

Description: an hormonal progestogen available in the form of white tablets containing 30µg levonorgestrel.

Used for: oral contraception.

Dosage: 1 tablet at same time each day starting of first day of monthly cycle and continuing without any break.

Special care: history of or at risk of thrombosis or embolism, liver disease, cancer which is hormone-dependent, ovarian cysts, hypertension, migraine. Blood pressure, breasts and pelvic organs should be checked regularly during the course of treatment.

Avoid use: pregnancy, patients who have previously had a stroke, poor circulation to heart leading to heart disease, diseased arteries, previous ectopic pregnancy. Also, women with undiagnosed vaginal bleeding, benign tumour (adenoma) of the liver derived from glandular tissue, recent trophoblastic disease.

Possible interaction: chloral hydrate, barbiturates, meprobamate, phenytoin, rifampicin, carbamazepine, griseofulvin, primidone, glutethimide dichloralphenazone, chlorpromazine, ethosuximide.

Side effects: changes in pattern of menstruation, headache, ovarian cysts, sore breasts, acne.

Manufacturer: Wyeth.

MICTRAL

Description: a compound preparation combining a quinolone and alkalysing agent available as dissolvable granules in sachets, containing 660mg nalidixic acid, anhydrous citric acid, sodium bicarbonate and sodium citrate (equivalent to 4.1g citrate).
Used for: cystitis and infections of lower urinary tract.
Dosage: adults, 1 sachet in water taken 3 times daily in divided doses for a period of 3 days.
Special care: pregnancy, breastfeeding, liver disease. Sunlight should be avoided.
Avoid use: children, patients with kidney disorders, history of fits, porphyria.
Possible interaction: antibacterials and anticoagulants.
Side effects: sensitivity to light, gastro-intestinal upset, skin rashes, haemolytic anaemia, disturbance of vision, convulsions, blood changes.
Manufacturer: Sanofi Winthrop.

MIDAMOR

Description: a potassium-sparing diuretic preparation available as diamond-shaped, yellow tablets containing 5mg amiloride hydrochloride marked MSD 92.
Used for: used with other diuretics to save potassium.
Dosage: 1 or 2 tablets each day with a daily maximum of 4.
Special care: pregnancy, breastfeeding, kidney or liver disease, acidosis, gout, a tendency to hyperkalaemia due to diabetes.
Avoid use: children, patients with serious or worsening kidney failure, hyperkalaemia, anuria.
Possible interaction: ACE inhibitors, lithium, potassium-sparing diuretics, potassium supplements.
Side effects: skin rash, gastro-intestinal upset.
Manufacturer: Morson.

MIFEGYNE

Description: a preparation which is a progesterone antagonist available as bi-convex, cylindrical-shaped, yellow tablets containing 200mg mifepristone, marked with logo and 167 B.
Used for: termination of early pregnancy, up to 63 days of gestation.
Dosage: adults, 600mg as a single dose under close medical supervision.
Special care: close observation required and patient may require further treatment to complete termination. Patients with obstructive airways disease or asthma, heart disease, replacement heart valves, kidney or liver disease, history of infected endocarditis. Patients should not take NSAIDs or aspirin for at least 12 days.
Avoid use: women with more advanced pregnancy over 64 days, ectopic or suspected ectopic pregnancy, porphyria, haemorrhage or bleeding disorders, women who smoke aged over 35 years. Also, patients receiving anticoagulant therapy or who have had long-term treatment with corticosteroids.
Possible interaction: aspirin, NSAIDs.
Side effects: vomiting, nausea, vaginal bleeding which may be severe, fainting, malaise, womb and urinary tract infections, skin rashes.
Manufacturer: Roussel.

MIGRAVESS FORTE

Description: a compound preparation which is an anti-emetic and analgesic available in the form of effervescent, scored white tablets containing 5mg metoclopramide and 450mg aspirin marked F over F. Also, **MIGRAVESS EFFERVESCENT**, scored, white tablets containing 5mg metoclopramide and 325mg aspirin, marked M over M.
Used for: relief of migraine.
Dosage: adults, 2 tablets in water at start of migraine attack with a maximum daily dose of 6 tablets. Children, 12 to 15 years, half adult dose.
Special care: pregnancy, liver or kidney disease, asthma.
Avoid use: children under 12 years, patients with allergy to aspirin or NSAIDs, peptic ulcer, bleeding disorders.

Possible interaction: anticoagulants, phenothiazines, uricosurics, anticholinergics, hypoglycaemics, butyrophenones.
Side effects: sleepiness, extrapyramidal symptoms (characterized by involuntary and reflex muscle movements and changes in tone of muscles), diarrhoea, rise in levels of prolactin in blood.
Manufacturer: Bayer.

MIGRIL

Description: a compound preparation combining an ergot alkaloid, antihistamine and xanthine produced as scored, white tablets containing 2mg ergotamine tartrate, 50mg cyclizine hydrochloride, 50mg caffeine hydrate, coded WELLCOME A4A.
Used for: relief of migraine.
Dosage: 1 at start of migraine attack followed by ¹/₂ to 1 tablet at 30 minute intervals. Maximum dose is 4 tablets for 1 migraine attack and 6 weekly.
Special care: patients with hyperthyroidism, sepsis, anaemia.
Avoid use: pregnancy, breastfeeding, children, patients with heart or circulatory disease, liver or kidney disorders, serious hypertension.
Possible interaction: ß-blockers, central nervous system depressants, erythromycin.
Side effects: sleepiness, rebound headache, pain in abdomen, dry mouth, peripheral ischaemia.
Manufacturer: Wellcome.

MILDISON LIPOCREAM

Description: a mildly potent topical steroid preparation available in the form of a cream containing 1% hydrocortisone.
Used for: dermatitis and eczema.
Dosage: apply to affected skin 2 or 3 times each day.
Special care: use on face or in children should be limited to a maximum period of 5 days. Stop using gradually after longer-term use.
Avoid use: long-term use or as a preventative especially by pregnant women, patients with untreated bacterial or fungal infections, skin infections of tuberculous or viral origin, scabies or ringworm. Also, leg ulcers, dermatitis in area of mouth, acne.
Side effects: changes as in Cushing's syndrome, skin thinning, abnormal hair growth, suppression of adrenal glands.
Manufacturer: Yamanouchi.

MINIHEP

Description: an anticoagulant preparation available as a solution in pre-filled syringes containing 5000 units sodium heparin/0.2ml. Also, **MINIHEP CALCIUM** solution in pre-filled syringes and ampoules containing 5000 units calcium heparin/0.2ml. Both are for subcutaneous injection only.
Used for: pulmonary embolism and deep vein thrombosis.
Dosage: 15,000 units every 12 hours; children 250 units/kg body weight 12 hourly. Both following on from first doses given by intravenous infusion or injection.
Special care: pregnancy, kidney or liver disease. Drug should be withdrawn gradually if taken for more than 5 days. Platelet counts are required if taken for more than 5 days.
Avoid use: bleeding disorders, haemophilia, serious hypertension, recent operation on eye or nervous system, cerebral aneurysm, serious liver disease, peptic ulcer, allergy to heparin, thrombocytopenia.
Possible interaction: aspirin, dipyridamole, glyceryl trinitrate infusion.
Side effects: allergic reactions, skin necrosis, osteoporosis (if taken long-term). Stop drug immediately if thrombocytopenia occurs.
Manufacturer: Leo.

MINIMS AMETHOCAINE

Description: a topical anaesthetic preparation for the eye, produced in the form of drops in 2 strengths containing 0.5% or 1% amethocaine hydrochloride in single dose units.

Used for: anaesthesia for eye during ophthalmic procedures.
Dosage: adults and children, except newborn babies, 1 drop as required.
Special care: protect eye.
Avoid use: newborn babies.
Possible interaction: sulphonamides.
Side effects: short-lived burning sensation, dermatitis.
Manufacturer: Chauvin.

MINIMS ATROPINE

Description: an anticholinergic preparation for the eye produced in the form of single-dose drops containing 1% atropine sulphate.
Used for: to produce mydnasis (dilation of the pupil of the eye by contraction of certain muscles in the iris) and cytoplegia (paralysis of the muscles of accommodation in the eye along with relaxation of the ciliary muscle). This is to allow examination of eye.
Dosage: adults and children, 1 drop as required.
Special care: patients should not drive for 2 hours.
Avoid use: patients with glaucoma.
Side effects: contact dermatitis, occasionally toxic systemic reactions especially in elderly persons and children. Closed angle glaucoma is possible especially in elderly patients.
Manufacturer: Chauvin.

MINIMS BENOXINATE

Description: a topical anaesthetic preparation for the eye produced in the form of single dose drops containing 0.4% oxybuprocaine hydrochloride.
Used for: anaesthesia of eye during ophthalmic procedures.
Dosage: 1 or more drops as needed.
Manufacturer: Chauvin.

MINIMS CHLORAMPHENICOL

Description: a broad-spectrum antibiotic preparation produced in the form of single dose eyedrops containing 0.5% chloramphenicol.

Used for: bacterial eye infections.
Dosage: adults, 1 or more drops, as needed; children, 1 drop as needed.
Special care: remove contact lenses.
Possible interaction: chymotrypsin.
Side effects: rarely, aplastic anaemia. Stop treatment immediately if local allergic reactions occur.
Manufacturer: Chauvin.

MINIMS CYCLOPEN-TOLATE

Description: an anticholinergic eye preparation produced in the form of single dose eyedrops of 2 strengths containing 0.5% or 1% cyclopentolate hydrochloride.
Used for: mydriasis (dilation of the pupil of the eye by contraction of certain muscles in the iris) and cytoplegia (paralysis of the muscles of accommodation within the eye along with relaxation of the ciliary muscle). This is in order to allow ophthalmic procedures to be carried out.
Dosage: adults and children (except newborn babies), 1 or 2 drops as needed.
Special care: patient with raised pressure within eye.
Avoid use: patients with narrow angle glaucoma.
Side effects: contact dermatitis, rarely toxic systemic effects especially in elderly and children, closed angle glaucoma is possible especially in elderly patients.
Manufacturer: Chauvin.

MINIMS GENTAMICIN

Description: an antibiotic aminoglycoside preparation produced in the form of single dose eye drops containing 0.3% gentamicin as sulphate.
Used for: bacterial infections of the eye.
Dosage: 1 drop as required.
Manufacturer: Chauvin.

MINIMS HOMATROPINE

Description: an anticholinergic eye preparation produced in the form of single dose drops containing 2% homatropine hydrobromide.

Used for: to produce mydriasis (dilation of the pupil of the eye by contraction of certain muscles in the iris) and cytoplegia (paralysis of the muscles of accommodation in the eye along with relaxation of the ciliary muscle).
Used for: narrow angle glaucoma.
Dosage: adults and children, 1 or more drops as needed.
Special care: patients should not drive for 2 hours.
Side effects: contact dermatitis, possibly closed angle glaucoma in elderly patients.
Manufacturer: Chauvin.

MINIMS LIGNOCAINE and FLUORESCEIN

Description: an eye preparation which is a local anaesthetic and stain available in the form of single dose eye drops containing 4% lignocaine hydrochloride and 0.25% fluorescein sodium.
Used for: ophthalmic procedures.
Dosage: adults and children, 1 or more drops as needed.
Manufacturer: Chauvin.

MINIMS METIPRANOLOL

Description: a non-selective ß-blocker produced in the form of single dose eyedrops of 2 strengths containing 0.1% and 0.3% metipranolol.
Used for: control of raised pressure within eye following surgery. Also, for chronic glaucoma in patients wearing soft contact lenses or who are allergic to preservatives.
Dosage: glaucoma, 1 drop into eye twice each day.
Avoid use: patients with obstructive airways disease, asthma, heart failure, bradycardia, heart block.
Possible interaction: verapamil and possibly other drugs following systemic absorption.
Side effects: dry eyes, allergic blepharoconjunctivitis (involving lining of eyelids).
Manufacturer: Chauvin.

MINIMS NEOMYCIN

Description: an aminoglycoside broad-spectrum antibiotic preparation produced in the form of single dose eyedrops containing 0.5% neomycin sulphate.
Used for: bacterial eye infections.
Dosage: adults, 1 or more drops as needed. Children, 1 drop as needed.
Manufacturer: Chauvin.

MINIMS PILOCARPINE

Description: a miotic preparation (one which causes contraction of the pupil) which is a cholinergic agonist and acts to cause constriction of the ciliary eye muscle. This helps to open drainage channels hence reducing pressure within the eye. It is produced as single dose eyedrops in 3 strengths containing 1%, 2% and 4% pilocarpine nitrate.
Used for: emergency treatment of glaucoma. To reverse the effect of weak mydriatic drugs.
Dosage: 1 drop every 5 minutes until the pupil is contracted.
Side effects: headache, blurred vision, bradycardia, colic pains, sweating, over-production of saliva, bronchospasm may occur if systemic absorption (into body) of eyedrops occur.
Manufacturer: Chauvin.

MINIMS PREDNISOLONE

Description: a corticosteroid preparation available as single dose eyedrops containing 0.5% prednisolone sodium.
Used for: inflammation of the eye which is not infected.
Dosage: adults and children, 1 or 2 drops every 1 or 2 hours then reduce frequency when condition improves.
Avoid use: pregnancy, glaucoma or tuberculous, viral or fungal infections or those producing pus. Avoid long-term treatment in babies.
Side effects: thinning of cornea, "steroid cataract" (especially prolonged use and higher doses), rise in pressure within eye, fungal infection.
Manufacturer: Chauvin.

MINIMS TROPICAMIDE

Description: an anticholinergic preparation available as single dose eyedrops in 2 strengths containing 0.5% and 1% tropicamide.

Used for: as a short-term mydriatic and cycloplegic drug. (A mydriatic produces mydriasis—dilation of the pupil of the eye by contraction of certain muscles in the iris. A cyclopleglic produces cycloplegia—paralysis of the muscles of accommodation in the eye along with relaxation of the ciliary muscle). Enables ophthalmic examinations and procedures to be carried out.

Dosage: adults and children, 1 or 2 drops every 5 minutes then repeated after 30 minutes if needed.

Special care: in babies, pressure should be applied over the tear sac for 1 minute. Patients should not drive for 2 hours.

Avoid use: patients with narrow angle glaucoma.

Side effects: stinging on application which is short-lived.

Manufacturer: Chauvin.

MINOCIN

Description: a tetracycline antibiotic available as film-coated orange tablets containing 100mg minocycline as hydrochloride, marked M over 100 on one side and LL on the other. Also, **MINOCIN MR**, yellow/brown modified-release capsules containing 100mg marked 8560 and Lederle. Also **MINOCIN 50**, beige, film-coated tablets containing 50mg marked M50 on one side and LL on the other.

Used for: Minocin: ear, nose and throat, respiratory, soft tissue, skin and urinary tract infections. Minocin MR: acne.

Dosage: adults, Minocin, 100mg twice each day; Minocin MR 1 each day swallowed whole; Minocin 50 1 tablet twice each day for at least 6 weeks.

Special care: patients with liver disorder.

Avoid use: children, pregnancy, breastfeeding, kidney disease.

Possible interaction: mineral supplements, antacids, penicillins.

Side effects: gastro-intestinal upset, superinfections; rarely, disorders of balance, allergic responses.

Manufacturer: Lederle.

MINODIAB

Description: a sulphonylurea available as scored, white tablets of 2 strengths containing 2.5mg and 5mg glipizide.

Used for: maturity-onset diabetes.

Dosage: adults, 2.5mg or 5mg each day at first increasing by 2.5–5mg every week. The usual maintenance dose is 2.5–30mg each day, maximum 40mg. Doses higher than 15mg each day should be divided and taken about 15 minutes before meals.

Special care: elderly, kidney failure.

Avoid use: pregnancy, breastfeeding, children, patients with other types of diabetes (juvenile, unstable-brittle, growth-onset diabetes), serious liver or kidney diseases, hormonal disorders. Also patients with ketoacidosis, infections, stress, undergoing surgery.

Possible interaction: anticoagulants taken orally, bezafibrate, aspirin, corticotrophin, corticosteroids, clofibrate, ß-blockers, alcohol, chlorpropamide, acetohexamide, melformin, MAOIs, oral contrraceptives, sulphonamides, glucagon, diuretics, phenylbutazone, chloramphenicol, cyclophosphamide, rifampicin.

Side effects: allergic reactions including skin rash.

Manufacturer: Pharmacia.

MINTEZOL

Description: an antihelmintic preparation used to treat infestation with various kinds of worm; available as scored, orange, chewable tablets containing 500mg thiabendazole.

Used for: guinea worm, threadworm, hookworm, trichinosis, large roundworm, larva migrans, whipworm.

Dosage: adults and children over 60kg body weight, 1.5g twice each day with meals. Less than 60kg, 25mg/kg twice each day with meals.

Special care: patients with liver or kidney disorder.
Avoid use: pregnancy, breastfeeding.
Possible interaction: xanthine derivatives.
Side effects: disturbances of vision and hearing, reduction in alertness, allergic reactions, liver damage, gastro-intestinal upset, hypotension, central nervous system disturbance, enuresis (incontinence, especially bedwetting).
Manufacturer: M.S.D.

MINULET

Description: an hormonal combined estrogen/progestogen preparation available as sugar-coated white tablets containing 30µg ethinyloestradiol and 75µg gestodene.
Used for: oral contraception.
Dosage: 1 tablet each day for 21 days beginning on first day of period followed by 7 tablet-free days.
Special care: patients with multiple sclerosis, serious kidney disease, kidney dialysis, asthma, Raynaud's disease, abnormally high levels of prolactin in the blood (hyperprolactinaemia), varicose veins, hypertension. Also, patients suffering severe depression. Thrombosis risk increases with smoking, age and obesity. During the course of treatment, regular checks on blood pressure, pelvic organs and breasts should be carried out.
Avoid use: pregnancy, patients considered to be at risk of thrombosis, suffering from heart disease, pulmonary hypertension, angina, sickle cell anaemia. Also, undiagnosed vaginal bleeding, history of cholestatic jaundice during pregnancy, cancers which are hormone-dependent, infectious hepatitis, liver disorders. Also, porphyria, Dublin-Johnson and Rotor syndrome, otosclerosis, chorea, haemolytic uraemic syndrome, recent trophoblastic disease.
Possible interaction: barbiturates, ethosuximide, glutethimide, rifampicin, phenytoin, tetracyclines, carbamazepine, chloral hydrate, griseofulvin, dichloralphenazone, primidone.

Side effects: weight gain, breast enlargement, pains in legs and cramps, headaches, loss of sexual desire, depression, nausea, breakthrough bleeding, cervical erosion, brownish patches on skin (chloasma), vaginal discharge, oedema and bloatedness.
Manufacturer: Wyeth.

MITIIRACIN

Description: a cytotoxic antibiotic preparation available as a powder in vials for reconstitution and injection containing 2.5mg plicamycin.
Used for: hypercalcaemia due to malignancy.
Dosage: 25µg/kg body 8 each day for 3 to 4 days repeated at minimum intervals of 1 week if necessary. Maintenance dose is 25µg/kg 1 to 3 times each week, all by intravenous infusion.
Special care: patients with liver or kidney disease.
Side effects: irritant to tissues, bone marrow suppression, vomiting, nausea, hair loss.
Manufacturer: Pfizer.

MITOXANA

Description: an alkylating cytotoxic drug, available as powder in vials for reconstitution and injection in 2 strengths containing 1g and 2g ifosfamide.
Used for: lymphomas, solid tumours, chronic lymphocytic leukaemia, usually given with mesna (*see* Uromitexan, a drug which lessens or prevents the toxic effects of ifosfamide on the bladder).
Dosage: given intravenously as directed by physician.
Special care: ensure plenty of fluids are taken—3 to 4 litres each day following injection.
Possible interaction: warfarin.
Side effects: bone marrow suppression, nausea, vomiting, hair loss, haemorrhagic cystitis (risk is reduced with increased fluid intake and mesna).
Manufacturer: Asta Medica.

MIVACRON

Description: a short-acting, non-depolarising muscle relaxant available in ampoules for injection containing 2mg mivacurium as chloride/ml.

Used for: muscle paralysis during surgical operations.

Dosage: adults, by intravenous injection, 70–150µg/kg body 8 at first then 100 µg/kg every 15 minutes. By intravenous infusion, to maintain paralysis, 8–10 µg/kg/minute, adjusted if needed to usual dose of 6–7 µg/kg/minute. Children, intravenous injection, age 2 to 12 years, 100–200µg/kg at first then 100 µg/kg every 6 to 7 minutes. Intravenous infusion, 10–15µg/kg/minute.

Special care: patients with heart disease or asthma (slower injection rate required).

Avoid use: patients with myasthenia gravis.

Possible interaction: clindamycin, azlocillin, colistin, verapamil, nifedipine, dantrolene, ecothiopate, demacarium, neostigmine, pyridostiamine, magnesium salts.

Manufacturer: Wellcome.

MMR II

Description: a preparation of measles, mumps and rubella vaccine. It contains measles, mumps and rubella vaccine along with 0.25mg neomycin and is available as powder in vials with diluent.

Used for: immunisation of children (and some adults) against measles, mumps and rubella.

Dosage: children over 12 months, 0.5ml by subcutaneous or intramuscular injection.

Special care: history of convulsions and feverishness, altered immunity states in whom fever is undesirable, patients who have had blood or plasma transfusion within last 3 months.

Avoid use: pregnancy, women should avoid pregnancy for 3 months after vaccination. Acute feverish illnesses, thrombocytopenia, history of symptoms of anaphylaxis to eggs or neomycin (egg protein is used in culture of virus for vaccine). Do not give within 1 month of other live vaccines.

Possible interaction: live vaccines.

Side effects: allergic responses, fever, headache, malaise, skin rash.

Manufacturer: M.S.D.

MOBIFLEX

Description: an NSAID belonging to the Oxicam group available as film-coated, pentagonal brown tablets containing 20mg tenoxicam marked Mobiflex. Also MOBIFLEX MILK granules in sachets containing 20mg; MOBIFLEX EFFERVESCENT tablets containing 20mg. MOBIFLEX INJECTION available as powder in vials for reconstitution containing 20mg.

Used for: rheumatoid arthritis, osteoarthritis, treatment of soft tissue injuries, (short-term only).

Dosage: 1 tablet or sachet in water each day; injection, 20mg by intravenous or intramuscular injection for first 1 or 2 days, then tablets or granules.

Special care: elderly patients, those with liver or kidney disease or heart failure.

Avoid use: pregnancy, children, inflammation of gastro-intestinal tract or bleeding, history of or actual peptic ulcer, allergy to NSAID or aspirin.

Possible interaction: hypoglycaemics taken orally, lithium, anticoagulants, other NSAIDs.

Side effects: headache, blood changes, skin rash, gastro-intestinal upset, rise in level of liver enzsymes, oedema, distubance of vision.

Manufacturer: Roche.

MODALIM

Description: an isobutyric acid derivative used to lower the levels of lipds (fats) in the blood. It is available as capsule-shape white, scored tablets containing 100mg ciprofibrate and marked MODALIM.

Used for: hyperlipidaemias (elevated blood lipid levels) of types IIa, IIb, III and IV which cannot be controlled by diet alone.

Dosage: adults, 1 or 2 tablets as a single daily dose.
Special care: liver or kidney disease; live tests should be carried out during the course of treatment.
Avoid use: pregnancy, breastfeeding, children, severe liver or kidney disease.
Possible interaction: hypoglycaemics taken by mouth, oral contraceptives, anticoagulants.
Side effects: vertigo, gastro-intestinal upset, loss of hair, impotence, muscle pain; rarely, sleepiness, dizziness.
Manufacturer: Sanofi Winthrop.

MODECATE

Description: an antipsychotic preparation which is a depot phenothiazine group III, available in ampoules and disposable syringes containing 25mg fluphenazine decanoate/ml. Also MODECATE CONCENTRATE in ampoules containing 100mg/ml.
Used for: maintenance of certain psychiatric illnesses especially schizophrenia.
Dosage: adults, 12.5mg by deep intramuscular injection (into gluteal muscle) as first test dose in order to see if patient is able to experience extrapyramidal (e.g. involuntary, reflex-type muscle movements) symptoms. Then, usual dose in the order of 12.5mg–100mg, according to response, every 2 to 5 weeks. Elderly receive lower initial test dose of 6.25mg.
Special care: elderly, patients who exhibit extrapyramidal symptoms (reduce dose or use alternative drug), pregnancy, breastfeeding, patients wtih myasthenia gravis. Also heart disease, heart arrhythmias, epilepsy, liver or respiratory diseases, enlarged prostate gland, and underactive thyroid gland, glaucoma, thyrotoxicosis.
Avoid use: children, patients with phaeochromocytoma, liver or kidney failure, severe heart disease, severe atherosclerosis of cerebral arteries, coma. Also those suffering from severe depression.

Possible interaction: alcohol, antacids, TCADs, antihypertensives, calcium-channel blockers, cimetidine.
Side effects: extrapyramidal symptoms, effects on heart and heart rhythm, effects on central nervous system and EEG, sleepiness, apathy, depression, dry mouth, blocked nose, difficulty passing urine, constipation. Hormonal changes, effects on mestruation, enlargement of breasts, abnormal production of breast milk, impotence. Blood changes, skin rashes, jaundice, effects on liver. Effects on eyes, blurred vision, pigmentation of skin and eyes.
Manufacturer: Sanofi Winthrop.

MODITEN

Description: an antipsychotic preparation which is a phenothiazine group III drug available as sugar-coated tablets in 3 strengths all containing fluphenazine hydrochloride; pink 1mg, yellow 2.5mg and white 5mg.
Used for: schizophrenia, paranoia, mania, hypomania, short-term treatment of anxiety, agitation and disordered behaviour.
Dosage: adults, schizophrenia and psychoses, 2.5mg–10mg as 2 or 3 divided doses each day with a maximum of 20mg. Anxiety and agitation, 1–2mg twice each day at first and then according to response. Elderly persons receive lower doses.
Special care: patients who exhibit extrapyramidal reactions (e.g. involuntary reflex-type muscle movements) should receive lower doses or alternative drug; pregnancy, breastfeeding. Myasthenia gravis, enlarged prostate gland, thyrotoxicosis, heart disease, heart arrhythmias, epilepsy, liver or respiratory diseases, underactive thyroid gland, glaucoma.
Avoid use: children, serious heart conditions, phaeochromocytoma, liver or kidney failure, severe atherosclerosis of cerebral arteries, coma. Also, patients who are severely depressed.

Possible interaction: alcohol, antacids, TCADs, antihypertensives, calcium-channel blockers, cimetidine.
Side effects: extrapyramidal symptoms, effects on heart and heart rhythm, effects on central nervous system and EEG, sleepiness, apathy, depression, dry mouth, blocked nose, difficulty passing urine, constipation. Hormonal changes, effects on menstruation, enlargement of breasts, abnormal production of breast milk, impotence. Blood changes, skin rashes, jaundice, effects on liver. Effects on eyes, blurred vision, pigmentation of skin and eyes.
Manufacturer: Sanofi Winthrop.

MODRASONE

Description: a moderately potent topical steroid preparation available as cream and ointment containing 0.05% alclometasone diproprionate.
Used for: skin conditions which respond to steroids.
Dosage: apply thinly 2 or 3 times each day.
Special care: do not use on face or in children for more than 5 days. Withdraw treatment gradually if use has been long-term.
Avoid use: extensive or long-term use, especially pregnant women, or as a preventative. Patients with untreated fungal or bacterial infections, skin conditions with tuberculous or viral origin or ringworm. Also, patients with leg ulcers, acne, scabies, dermatitis in area of mouth.
Side effects: changes as in Cushing's syndrome, skin thinning, suppression of adrenal glands, abnormal hair growth.
Manufacturer: Schering-Plough.

MODRENAL

Description: a preparation of a drug which inhibits the production of corticosteroid hormones by the adrenal glands. It is available as capsules of 2 strengths; black/pink capsules containing 60mg trilostane and yellow/pink

capsules containing 120mg. Both are marked with the strength of the capsules.
Used for: excessive activity of adrenal cortex resulting in excess hormone release as in primary aldosteronism (oversecretion of aldosterone, also called Conn's syndrome) and hypercortisolism. Also for breast cancer in post-menopausal women.
Dosage: adults, 60mg 4 times each day at first then, according to response, adjusted to a usual daily dose in the order of 120mg–480mg as divided doses. The maximum is 960mg each day. Breast cancer, the initial dose is 240mg each day increasing by this amount at 3 day intervals to a maximum 960mg. Glucocorticoid treatment should be given at the same time in these patients.
Special care: eliminate the presence of a tumour producing ACTH (adrenocortico trophic hormone) before treatment begins, patients with kidney or liver disease, suffering from stress. Non-hormonal methods of contraception should be used.
Avoid use: pregnancy, patients with serious liver or kidney disease.
Possible interaction: aldosterone antagonists, potassium supplements, triamterene, amiloride.
Side effects: nausea, diarrhoea, flushing runny nose.
Manufacturer: Wanskerne.

MODUCREN

Description: a compound antihyperten-sive preparation combining a non-cardioselective ß-blocker, a thiazide and potassium-sparing diuretic available as scored, blue tablets containing 25mg hydrochlorthiazide, 2.5mg amiloride hydrochloride and 10mg timolol maleate, marked MODUCREN.
Used for: hypertension.
Dosage: adults, 1 or 2 tablets as a single dose each day.
Special care: pregnancy, breastfeeding, patients with weak hearts may require diuretics and digitalis, those with

diabetes, undergoing general anaesthesia, kidney or liver disorders, gout. Electrolyte (salts) levels may need to be monitored.
Avoid use: history of bronchospasm or obstructive airways disease, heart block, heart shock, uncompensated heart failure, disease of peripheral arteries, bradycardia. Patients with serious or worsening kidney failure or anuria.
Possible interaction: sympathomimetics, class 1 antiarrhythmics, central nervous system depressants, clonidine withdrawal, ergot alkaloids, cardiac depressant anaesthetics, verapamil, reserpine, indomethacin, hypoglycaemics, cimetidine, other antihypertensives. Digitalis, potassium supplements, potassium-sparing diuretics, lithium.
Side effects: cold hands and feet, disturbance of sleep, fatigue on exercise, bronchospasm, bradycardia, gastro-intestinal disturbances, heart failure, blood changes, gout, sensitivity to light, muscle weakness. If skin rash or dry eyes occur, withdraw drug gradually.
Manufacturer: Morson.

MODURET 25

Description: a compound preparation combining a potassium-sparing and thiazide diuretic available as diamond-shaped, off-white tablets containing 2.5mg amiloride hydrochloride and 25mg hydrochlorothiazide, coded MSD 923.
Used for: hypertension, congestive heart failure, liver cirrhosis (accompanied by an abnormal collection of fluid in the abdomen, ascites).
Dosage: adults, 1 to 4 tablets each day in divided doses.
Special care: patients with liver or kidney disorders, diabetes, acidosis and gout.
Avoid use: children, pregnancy, breastfeeding, serious or worsening kidney failure, hyperkalaemia.
Possible interaction: lithium, ACE inhibitors, potassium supplements and potassium-sparing diuretics, antihypertensives, digitalis.
Manufacturer: DuPont.

MODURETIC

Description: a compound preparation combining a potassium-sparing and thiazide diuretic available in the form of diamond-shaped, scored, peach tablets containing 5mg amiloride hydrochloride and 50mg hydrochlorothiazide, marked NSD 917. Also, **MODURETIC SOLUTION** (in 5ml).
Used for: hypertension, congestive heart failure, liver cirrhosis (accompanied by an abnormal collection of fluid in the abdomen, ascites).
Dosage: 1 or 2 tablets or 5–10ml solution each day as single or divided doses. May be increased, if required, to a daily maximum of 4 tablets or 20ml.
Special care: liver or kidney disorders, acidosis, gout, diabetes.
Avoid use: children, pregnancy, breastfeeding, hyperkalaemia.
Possible interaction: lithium, potassium-sparing diuretics, potassium supplements, antihypertensives, digitalis.
Side effects: sensitivity to light, gout, rash, blood changes.
Manufacturer: DuPont.

MOGADON

Description: a long-acting benzodiazepine preparation available as scored, white tablets containing 5mg nitrazepam marked with 2 "eyes" and ROCHE.
Used for: insomnia, short-term only.
Dosage: adults, 5–10mg, elderly persons, 2.5–5mg, with doses taken at bedtime.
Special care: kidney or liver disorders, lung insufficiency, pregnancy, labour, breastfeeding. For short-term treatment as drug dependence and tolerance may develop.
Avoid use: history of drug or alcohol abuse, serious lung insufficiency and depressed respiration. Suffering from psychoses, obsessional or phobic states.
Possible interaction: CNS depressants, alcohol, anticonvulsants.
Side effects: headache, drowsiness, loss of co-ordination (ataxia), confusion, hypotension, gastro-intestinal upset.

Skin rash, retention of urine, changes in libido, vertigo, disturbance of vision. Rarely, jaundice and blood disorders.
Manufacturer: Roche.

MOLIPAXIN

Description: an antidepressant preparation available in a variety of different forms, all containing trazodone hydrochloride. Pink, film-coated, scored tablets (150mg) are marked MOLIPAXIN 150. **MOLIPAXIN CAPSULES** are green/purple (50mg) marked with logo and R365B; fawn/purple (100mg) marked with logo and R365C. **MOLIPAXIN CR**, blue, octagonal-shaped sustained-release tablets (150mg) marked with strength and name. **MOLIPAXIN LIQUID** contains 50mg/5ml.
Used for: depression which may be accompanied by anxiety.
Dosage: 150mg each day as divided doses taken after meals or single night-time dose. After 1 week, dose may be increased to 300mg each day with a maximum of 600mg. Elderly persons, 100mg each day in divided doses after meals or as a single night-time dose. Maximum of 300mg each day.
Special care: serious kidney or liver disease or epilepsy.
Avoid use: children.
Possible interaction: CNS depressants, clonidine, muscle relaxants, MAOIs, some anaesthetics.
Side effects: dizziness, headache, drowsines. Discontinue if priapism (abnormal, persistent erection of penis, which is painful and not associated with sexual arousal) occurs.
Manufacturer: Roussel.

MONASPOR

Description: a cephalosporin antibiotic preparation available as powder in vials for reconstitution and injection containing 1g cefsulodin sodium.
Used for: urinary tract, soft tissue, respiratory and some bone infections. Infections caused by the organism *Pseudomonas aerugginosa*.

Dosage: adults, 1–4g daily in 2, 3 or 4 divided doses by intravenous or intramuscular injection. Children, 20–50mg/kg body weight each day by intravenous or intramuscular injection.
Special care: pregnancy, patients allergic to penicillin, kidney failure. Tests of kidney function and blood counts should be carried out if taking drug long-term.
Possible interaction: aminoglycosides, loop diuretics.
Side effects: blood changes (abnormal reduction in number of blood platelets and white cells), gastro-intestinal upset, candidiasis (thrush), rise in level of blood urea and liver enzymes. Positive Coomb's test (a test for rhesus antibodies).
Manufacturer: Ciba.

MONIT

Description: an antianginal nitrate preparation available as scored, white tablets containing 20mg isosorbide mononitrate marked STUART 20. Also, **MONIT LS**, white tablets containing 10mg and marked STUART 10; **MONIT SR**, white, sugar-coated sustained-release tablets containing 40mg.
Used for: prevention of angina.
Dosage: 1 tablet each day in the morning.
Avoid use: children.
Side effects: flushes, headache, dizziness.
Manufacturer: Lorex.

MONOCLATE-P

Description: a preparation of freeze-dried coagulation factor VIII with antihaemophiliac activities of 250, 500 and 1000 units in vials for injection.
Used for: treatment of haemophilia A.
Dosage: by intravenous infusion according to body weight and severity of condition.
Special care: in patients with blood groups A, B or AB there is a possibility of haemolysis after large or numerous doses.
Side effects: allergic reactions, nausea, chills, pain at injection site. If more pronounced hypersensitivity reactions occur, discontinue treatment.
Manufacturer: Armour.

MONOCUR

Description: an antianginal and anti-hypertensive preparation which is a cardioselective ß-blocker available as pink, scored, film-coated tablets containing 5mg bisoprolol fumerate, marked 5 on one side and LL on the other. Also, white film-coated tablets containing 10mg, marked 10 on one side and LL on the other.

Used for: angina and hypertension.

Dosage: usual dose is 10mg once each day with a maximum of 20mg.

Special care: pregnancy, breastfeeding, patients with weak hearts may require diuretics and digitalis. Also, liver or kidney disease, general anaesthesia, metabolic acidosis, diabetes. Drug should be gradually withdrawn.

Avoid use: obstructive airways disease, history of bronchospasm, heart block, heart shock, uncompensated heart failure, sick sinus syndrome, disease of peripheral arteries, bradycardia.

Possible interaction: CNS depressants, verapamil, indomethacin, reserpine, class I antiarrhythmics, hypoglycaemics, clonidine withdrawal, sympathomimetics, cardiac depressants anaesthetics, ergot alkaloids, antihypertensives.

Side effects: gastro-intestinal upset, fatigue on exercise, cold hands and feet, disturbance of sleep, bronchospasm, bradycardia, heart failure. If skin rash or dry eyes occur, drug should be gradually withdrawn.

Manufacturer: Cyanamid.

MONONINE

Description: a preparation of freeze-dried human coagulation factor IX with slight antihaemophiliac activity. Available as 250, 500 and 1000 unit vials.

Used for: haemophilia B.

Dosage: by intravenous infusion depending upon patient's weight and severity of bleeding.

Special care: risk of thrombosis.

Avoid use: widespread coagulation within blood vessels.

Side effects: allergic reactions, flushing, vomiting and nausea, headache, fever, chills, tingling sensation, tiredness. Possible thromboembolism. If hypersensitivity reactions occur, drug should be withdrawn.

Manufacturer: Armour.

MONPARIN

Description: an anticoagulant preparation of heparin sodium available as 1000, 5000 and 25,000 units/ml in single dose ampoules. Also, MON-OPARIN CA containing 25,000 units heparin calcium/ml.

Used for: treatment of pulmonary embolism and deep vein thrombosis.

Dosage: adults, initial loading dose of 5000 units (10,000 in severe conditions) by intravenous injection followed by continuous infusion at a rate of 1000–2000 units/hour. Or 15,000 units at 12 hour intervals may be given by subcutaneous injection. Small adult or child, lower initial dose then 15–25 units/kg body weight by intravenous infusion/hour or 250 units/kg by subcutaneous injection.

Special care: pregnancy, liver or kidney disorders. If treatment period exceeds 5 days, platelet counts must be carried out.

Avoid use: bleeding disorders or haemophilia, thrombocytopenia, serious liver disease, severe hypertension, peptic ulcer, cerebral aneurysm, recent surgery to central nervous system or eye. Known hypersensitivity to heparin.

Possible interaction: aspirin, antiplatelet drugs, nitrates.

Side effects: hypersensitivity responses, haemorrhage, osteoporosis (after long-term use), skin necrosis. Also, thrombocytopenia, in which case drug should be immediately withdrawn.

Manufacturer: CP Pharmaceuticals.

MONOTRIM

Description: an antibacterial and folic acid inhibitor available in a variety of forms all containing trimethoprim.

MONOTRIM TABLETS in 2 strengths, scored, white containing 100mg coded AE over 2; scored, white containing 200mg coded DE over 5, both marked with symbol. **MONOTRIM SUGAR-FREE SUSPENSION** containing 50mg/5ml. **MONOTRIM INJECTION** containing 20mg as lactate/ml.
Used for: urinary tract infections and others sensitive to trimethoprim.
Dosage: tablets or suspension, 200mg twice each day; injection, 200mg by intravenous injection or infusion every 12 hours. Children, tablets or suspension, age 6 weeks to 5 months, 25mg; 6 months to 5 years, 50mg; 6 to 12 years, 100mg. All doses twice each day. Injection, 8mg/kg body weight each day in 2 or 3 divided doses by intravenous injection or infusion.
Special care: elderly, babies, folate deficiency or kidney disorders. During long-term treatment, regular blood tests should be carried out.
Avoid use: pregnancy, serious kidney disease.
Possible interaction: procainamide, warfarin, nicoumalone, sulphonylureas, phenytoin, maloprim, fansidar, methotrexate.
Side effects: skin rashes, gastro-intestinal upset.
Manufacturer: Duphar.

MONOZIDE 10

Description: a compound preparation combining a cardioselective ß-blocker and thiazide diuretic available as film-coated, white tablets containing 10mg bisoprolol fumerate and 6.25mg hydrochlorothiazide.
Used for: hypertension.
Dosage: adults, 1 tablet each day.
Special care: pregnancy, breastfeeding, liver or kidney disease, diabetes, gout, metabolic acidosis. Patients with weak hearts may require digitalis and diuretics. Electrolyte (salts) levels require regular monitoring. Also, special care in patients undergoing general anaesthesia.

Avoid use: children, obstructive airways disease, history of bronchospasm, uncompensated heart failure, heart block, heart shock, bradycardia, disease of peripheral arteries, sick sinus syndrome. Also, serious or worsening kidney failure, anuria.
Possible interaction: CNS depressants, verapamil, indomethacin, class I antiarrhythmics, sympathomimetics, cardiac depressant anaesthetics, clonidine withdrawal, ergot alkaloids, reserpine, ergot alkaloids, hypoglycae-mics, antihypertensives. Potassium supplements, potassium-sparing diuretics, lithium, digitalis.
Side effects: cold hands and feet, disturbance of sleep, fatigue on exercise, gastro-intestinal upset, bradycardia, heart failure, bronchospasm, gout. Blood changes, muscle weakness, sensitivity to light. Drug should be gradually withdrawn if dry eyes or skin rash occur.
Manufacturer: Lederle.

MONURIL

Description: an antibacterial preparation available as granules in sachets containing 3g fosfomycin as trometamol. Also, **MONURIL PAEDIATRIC** containing 2g fosfomycin as trometamol as granules in sachets.
Used for: lower urinary tract infections and prevention of infection during surgical procedures in this area.
Dosage: adults, treatment, single 3g dose taken 1 to 2 hours after a meal or at night. Prevention, 3g taken 3 hours before procedure, dose is then repeated 24 hours afterwards. Children, treatment, age over 5 years, a single 2g dose taken 1 or 2 hours after a meal or at night.
Special care: pregnancy, breastfeeding, elderly, kidney disease or disorder.
Avoid use: children under 5 years, elderly people over 75 years, patients with serious kidney disease or disorder.
Possible interaction: metoclopramide.
Side effects: rash, gastro-intestinal upset.
Manufacturer: Pharmax.

MOTENS

Description: an antihypertensive preparation which is a class II calcium antagonist available as white, film-coated tablets containing 2mg and 4mg lacidipine, marked 10L and 9L respectively, and with logo.
Used for: hypertension.
Dosage: adults, 2mg once each day as morning dose with breakfast. May be increased after 3 or 4 weeks to 6mg once each day if needed. The maintenance dose is 4mg once each day. Elderly, 2mg once each day increasing if needed to 4mg after 4 weeks.
Special care: weak hearts, liver disease, disturbances of conduction (of electrical nerve impulses).
Avoid use: children, pregnancy, breastfeeding.
Possible interaction: cimetidine.
Side effects: palpitations, flushing, headache, rash, oedema, polyuria, increase in amount of gum tissue. Drug should be withdrawn if chest pain occurs.
Manufacturer: Boehringer Ingelheim.

MOTILIUM

Description: an antidopaminergic preparation available in a number of different forms all containing domperidone. Motilium Tablets are white, film-coated and contain 10mg, marked with the name. **MOTILIUM SUSPENSION** contains 1mg/ml solution; **MOTILIUM SUPPOSITORIES** contain 30mg.
Used for: nausea and vomiting, indigestion (tablets).
Dosage: tablets for indigestion, 10–20mg 2 or 3 times each day. For nausea and vomiting, 10–20mg as tablets or suspension or 1 or 2 suppositories, both every 4 to 8 hours. Children, for nausea and vomiting following cancer therapy only, 0.2–0.4mg/kg body weight as suspension every 4 to 8 hours, or 1 to 4 suppositories each day, dose determined by body weight.
Avoid use: pregnancy.

Side effects: extrapyramidal reactions (characterized by involuntary reflex muscle movements and spasms), skin rash, raised levels of prolactin in blood.
Manufacturer: Sanofi Winthrop.

MOTIPRESS

Description: an anxiolytic and antidepressant combining a phenothiazine group III and TCAD available as triangular, sugar-coated yellow tablets containing 1.5mg fluphenazine hydrochloride and 30mg nortriptyline (as hydrochloride).
Used for: anxiety and depression.
Dosage: 1 tablet each day, preferably taken at bedtime. Maximum treatment period is 3 months.
Special care: breastfeeding, epilepsy, disease of arteries of heart, glaucoma, liver disease, hyperthyroidism, tumours of adrenal glands. Patients with psychoses or at risk of suicide.
Avoid use: pregnancy, damaged liver or kidneys, serious heart disorders, heart attack, heart block, blood changes, history of brain damage or grand mal epilepsy.
Possible interaction: antidepressants, anticonvulsants, alcohol, within 2 weeks of taking MAOIs, barbiturates, adrenaline, noradrenaline, antihypertensives, anticholinergics, oestrogens, cimetidine.
Side effects: sleepiness, vertigo, light-headedness, unsteadiness, disturbance of vision, rash, hypotension, gastro-intestinal upset, changes in libido, retention of urine. Allergic reactions, dry mouth, constipation, sweating, tachycardia, nervousness, heart arrhythmias. Impotence, effects on breasts, weight loss or gain.
Manufacturer: Sanofi Winthrop.

MOTIVAL

Description: an anxiolytic and antidepressant preparation combining a phenothiazine group III and TCAD available as sugar-coated, pink, triangular-shaped tablets containing 0.5mg fluphenazine hydrochloride and 10mg nortriptyline as hydrochloride.

Used for: anxiety and depression.
Dosage: 1 tablet 3 times each day for a maximum period of 3 months.
Special care: breastfeeding, epilepsy, disease of arteries of heart, glaucoma, liver disease, hyperthyroidism, tumours of adrenal glands. Patients with psychoses or at risk of suicide.
Avoid use: pregnancy, damaged liver or kidneys, serious heart disorders, heart attack, heart block, blood changes, history of brain damage or grand mal epilepsy.
Possible interaction: antidepressants, anticonvulsants, alcohol, within 2 weeks of taking MAOIs, barbiturates, adrenaline, noradrenaline, antihypertensives, anticholinergics, oestrogens, cimetidine.
Side effects: sleepiness, vertigo, lightheadedness, unsteadiness, disturbance of vision, rash, hypotension, gastro-intestinal upset, changes in libido, retention of urine. Allergic reactions, dry mouth, constipation, sweating, tachycardia, nervousness, heart arrhythmias. Impotence, effects on breasts, weight loss or gain.
Manufacturer: Sanofi Winthrop.

MOTRIN

Description: an NSAID and proprionic acid, available in the form of film-coated tablets of 4 strengths. Red tablets contain 200mg ibuprofen; orange tablets contain 400mg; oval-shaped, peach-coloured tablets contain 600mg, all marked with a U. Orange, capsule-shaped tablets contain 800mg, marked with strength and name.
Used for: pain, rheumatism and other bone and muscle disorders including osteoarthritis, rheumatoid arthritis and ankylosing spondylitis.
Dosage: adults, 1200–1800mg each day in divided doses, the maximum being 2400mg daily. Children, 20mg/kg body weight each day with a maximum dose of 500mg for children weighing less than 30kg. For juvenile rheumatoid arthritis, 40mg/kg may be given.

Special care: pregnancy, breastfeeding, elderly, liver or kidney disorders, heart disease, asthma, disease of gastro-intestinal tract.
Avoid use: patients with known allergy to NSAID or aspirin, peptic ulcer.
Possible interaction: thiazide diuretics, anticoagulants, quinolones.
Side effects: rash, gastro-intestinal disorder or bleeding, thrombocytopenia.
Manufacturer: Upjohn.

MST CONTINUS^{CD}

Description: an opiate preparation which is a controlled drug available as continuous-release film-coated tablets of different strengths, all containing morphine sulphate. White, 5mg; brown, 10mg; light green, 15mg; purple, 30mg; orange, 60mg; grey, 100mg; green, 200mg; tablets are all marked NAPP and with strength. Also, **CONTINUS SUSPENSION**, produced as granules in sachets for dissolving in water, to make raspberry-flavoured continuous-release suspension containing morphine (equivalent to morphine sulphate). Suspension is available in 20mg, 30mg, 60,mg, 100mg and 200mg strengths.
Used for: long-term relief of severe pain when other drugs have proved inadequate.
Dosage: 30mg every 12 hours at first, then adjusted to dose necessary to provide pain relief for 12 hours according to patient's response. Children, 0.2–0.8mg/kg body weight every 12 hours at first, then adjusted to dose necessary to provide pain relief for 12 hours. (Granules may be dissolved in water or mixed with food).
Special care: elderly, liver or kidney disease; hypothyroidism (underactive thyroid gland).
Avoid use: pregnant women, patients with severe liver disease, obstructive airways disease, depressed respiration.
Possible interaction: central nervous system depressants, MAOIs.
Side effects: nausea, constipation, vomiting, drug tolerance and dependence.
Manufacturer: Napp.

MUCAINE

Description: a combined antacid and local anaesthetic preparation containing 10mg oxethazine, 4.75ml aluminium hydroxide gel and 100mg magnesium hydroxide/5ml suspension.
Used for: hiatus hernia and oesophagitis.
Dosage: adults, 10–20ml 3 times each day after meals and at night.
Avoid use: children.
Manufacturer: Wyeth.

MUCODYNE

Description: a mucolytic preparation available as a syrup containing 250mg carbocisteine/5ml. Also, MUCODYNE CAPSULES, yellow capsules containing 375mg carbocisteine marked MUCO-DYNE 375. MUCODYNE PAEDIATRIC contains 125mg carbocisteine/5ml as a syrup.
Used for: copious, thick mucus, glue ear in children.
Dosage: adults, 750mg, 3 times each day, reducing to 500mg. Children, syrup, aged 2 to 5 years, 2.5–5ml 4 times each day; 5 to 10 years, 10ml 3 times each day.
Special care: pregnancy, history of peptic ulcer.
Avoid use: children under 2 years, patients with peptic ulcer.
Side effects: nausea, gastro-intestinal upset, rash.
Manufacturer: Theraplix.

MULTILOAD

Description: an inter-uterine contraceptive device formed from copper wire on a polyethylene stem. Also, MULTI-LOAD Cu 250 SHORT, and MULTI-LOAD Cu 375.
Used for: contraception.
Special care: diabetes, anaemia, history of endocarditis or pelvic inflammatory disease, epilepsy, hypermenorrhoea (or menorrhagia, long or heavy menstrual periods). Examine after 3 months, then annually.
Avoid use: pregnancy, past ectopic

pregnancy, uterus disorders, infection of vagina or cervix, acute pelvic inflammatory diseases, cervical cancer, abnormal vaginal bleeding, endometrial disease, immunosuppressive therapy, copper allergy, cancer of the genitalia.
Possible interaction: anticoagulants.
Side effects: pain, pelvic infection, perforation of the uterus, abnormal bleeding. On insertion there may be attack of asthma or epilepsy, bradycardia, Remove if persistent bleeding or cramps, perforation of cervix or uterus, pregnancy, persistent pelvic infection.
Manufacturer: Organon.

MULTIPARIN

Description: an anticoagulant preparation of heparin sodium available as 1000, 5000 and 25,000 units/ml in multidose vials.
Used for: treatment of pulmonary embolism and deep vein thrombosis.
Dosage: adults, initial loading dose of 5000 units (10,000 in severe conditions) by intravenous injection followed by continuous infusion at a rate of 1000–2000 units/hour. Or 15,000 units at 12 hour intervals may be given by subcutaneous injection. Small adult or child, lower initial dose then 15–25 units/kg body weight by intravenous infusion/hour or 250 units/kg by subcutaneous injection.
Special care: pregnancy, liver or kidney disorders. If treatment period exceeds 5 days, platelet counts must be carried out.
Avoid use: bleeding disorders or haemophilia, thrombocytopenia, serious liver disease, severe hypertension, peptic ulcer, cerebral aneurysm, having had recent surgery to central nervous system or eye. Known hypersensitivity to heparin.
Possible interaction: aspirin, antiplatelet drugs, nitrates.
Side effects: hypersensitivity responses, haemorrhage, osteoporosis (after long-term use), skin necrosis. Also, thrombocytopenia, in which case drug should be immediately withdrawn and, rarely, baldness.
Manufacturer: CP Pharmaceuticals.

MUMPS VAX

Description: a preparation of mumps vaccine of live attenuated virus of the Jeryl Lynn strain available as powder in single dose vials with diluent, containing the virus and 0.25mg neomycin per dose.

Used for: immunisation against mumps for all ages over 1 year.

Dosage: 1 dose of reconstituted vaccine by subcutaneous injection.

Avoid use: children under 1 year, pregnant women, patients with infections, low levels of gammaglobulins in blood, severe egg allergy.

Possible interaction: live vaccines, immunoglobulins, transfusions, cytotoxic drugs, radiation therapy, corticosteroids.

Manufacturer: Morson.

MYAMBUTOL

Description: an anti-tuberculous drug available as yellow tablets containing 100mg ethambutol and grey tablets containing 400mg ethambutol.

Used for: treatment of tuberculosis along with other antituberculous drugs and prevention of tuberculosis.

Dosage: prevention and treatment, 15mg/kg body weight each day as a single dose. Children, treatment, 25mg/kg each day for 60 days. Prevention, 15mg/kg each day as a single dose.

Special care: breastfeeding, kidney disorders. Visual tests must be carried out.

Avoid use: patients with inflammation of the optic nerve.

Side effects: visual disturbances, blurred vision, distortion of colour vision—drug should be withdrawn.

Manufacturer: Lederle.

MYCOBUTIN

Description: an antimycobacterial ansamycin drug available as brown/red capsules containing 150mg rifambutin.

Used for: as sole therapy in prevention of monobacterial infections in immunocompromised patients (whose immune system is not working properly). Additional treatment of mycobacterial infections.

Dosage: prevention of mycobacterial infections, 2 tablets each day. As additional therapy in non-tuberculous mycobacterial disease, 3 to 4 tablets each day continuing for 6 months after infection has cleared. Pulmonary tuberculosis, 1 to 3 tablets each day as additional therapy for a minimum period of 6 months.

Special care: severe liver or kidney failure. Blood checks and liver enzyme tests should be carried out.

Avoid use: children, patients wearing soft contact lenses, pregnancy, breastfeeding.

Possible interaction: triazole antifungal drugs, hypoglycaemics taken by mouth, oral contraceptives, cyclosporin, macrolides, anticoagulants, dapsone, zidovudine, digitalis, quinidine, analgesics, phenytoin, corticosteroids.

Side effects: anaemia, leucopenia and thrombocytopenia, pain in muscles and joints, discolouration of urine, skin and bodily secretions.

Manufacterer: Pharmacia.

MYDRIACYL

Description: an anticholinergic preparation available as eyedrops containing 0.5% and 1% tropicamide.

Used for: to produce mydriasis (dilation of the pupil of the eye by contraction of certain muscles in the iris) and cytoplegia (paralysis of the muscles of accommodation in the eye along with relaxation of the ciliary muscle).

Dosage: 1 or 2 drops of either strength at intervals between 1 and 5 minutes.

Special care: patients in whom pressure within eye is not known. In infants, pressure should be applied over tear sac for 1 minute.

Avoid use: patients wearing soft contact lenses, those with narrow angle glaucoma.

Side effects: short-lived stinging, sensitivity to light, dry mouth, headache, tachycardia, blurred vision. Also, mental disturbances, behavioural changes, psychoses.

Manufactuer: Alcon.

MYDRILATE

Description: an anticholinergic preparation available in the form of eyedrops in 2 strengths containing 0.5% and 1% cyclopentolate hydrochloride.

Used for: refraction and uveitis (inflamma-tion of the uveal tract which includes the choroid, iris and ciliary body, characterized by impaired vision and can cause blindness).

Dosage: adults, refraction, 1 drop of solution of either strength repeated after 15 minutes if needed. Uveitis, 1 or 2 drops of either strength repeated as needed. Children, refraction, under 6 years, 1 or 2 drops of 1% solution; over 6 years, 1 drop of 1% solution. Uveitis, children over 3 months, same dose as adult.

Special care: eye inflammation, raised pressure within eye.

Avoid use: patients with glaucoma.

Side effects: systemic toxic effects due to absorption of drops, especially elderly persons and children, contact dermatitis.

Manufacturer: Bochringer Ingelheim.

MYLERAN

Description: an alkylating cytotoxic drug available as white tablets in 2 strengths containing 0.5mg and 2mg busulphan, coded F2A and K2A respectively, and WELLCOME.

Used for: chronic myeloid leukaemia.

Dosage: adults, to induce remission, 60µg/kg body weight each day with a maximum daily dose of 4mg. Maintenance dose is 0.5–2mg.

Special care: pregnant women—patients should be treated in hospital. Frequent blood counts are required.

Avoid use: patients with porphyria, children.

Possible interaction: radiotherapy, other cytotoxic drugs.

Side effects: severe bone marrow suppression, nausea, vomiting, hair loss, excessive pigmentation of skin.

Manufacturer: Wellcome.

MYOCRISIN

Description: a long-acting suppressive drug and gold salt available in ampoules for injection containing 10mg, 20mg and 50mg sodium aurothiomalate/0.5ml.

Used for: rheumatoid arthritis, juvenile arthritis.

Dosage: initial test of 10mg by deep intra-muscular injection followed by 50mg each week until condition improves. Children, initial test dose of one tenth to one fifth of ongoing dose which is 1mg/kg bodyweight weekly up to a maximum of 50mg. The interval between doses is gradually increased to 4 weeks depending on response

Special care: elderly, urine tests and blood counts are essential. Eczema, urticaria, colitis (inflamed bowel). No improvement can be expected in adults until 300mg–500mg has been given, and if condition has not changed after 1g total dose, drug should be withdrawn.

Avoid use: pregnancy, breastfeeding, patients with history of blood changes, certain skin disorders, liver or kidney disease, porphyria.

Possible interaction: phenylbutazone, penicillamine.

Side effects: rash, eosinophilia (increased number of eosinophils (a type of white blood cells) in blood, an allergic response), albuminuria (presence of albumin in urine). Patients should report if itching (pruritus), bleeding gums, mouth ulcers, sore throat, sore tongue, diarrhoea, bruising, metallic taste in mouth or heavy menstrual bleeding occur. Also toxic effects on liver, cholestatic jaundice, baldness, lung fibrosis may occur.

Manufacturer: Theraplix.

MYOTONINE

Description: a cholinergic preparation available as scored white tablets containing 10mg bethanechol chloride and white, cross-scored tablets containing 25mg bethanechol chloride.

Used for: total or partial immobility of

the bowel or stomach, large, abnormally extended colon, reflux oesophagitis, retention of urine.

Dosage: adults, 10–25mg 3 to 4 times each day; children, reduced dose in proportion to that for 70kg adult.

Avoid use: pregnancy, epilepsy, recent heart attack, serious hypotension, obstruction of urinary or gastro-intestinal tract, Parkinson's disease, severe bradycardia, asthma, hyperthyroidism, vagotonia (abnormal increase in the activity of the vagus nerve).

Side effects: blurred vision, abdominal pains, nausea, frequency of urination, vomiting, sweating.

Manufacturer: Glenwood.

MYSOLINE

Description: an anticonvulsant pyrimidinedone preparation available as scored, white tablets containing 250mg primidone, marked with 2 lines and ICI. Also, **MYSOLINE SUSPENSION** containing 250mg primidone/5ml.

Used for: epilepsy.

Dosage: 125mg taken at night in first instance increasing every 3 days by 125mg to 500mg each day. Then a further increase every third day of 250mg to a maximum dose of 1.5g daily. Children, same initial dose as adults but increasing by 125mg. Usual daily maintenance doses as follows: up to 2 years, 250–500mg; 2 to 5 years, 500–750mg; 6 to 9 years, 750mg–1g; 9 to 12 years, 750mg–1.5g.

Special care: patients with kidney and liver disorders, serious lung insufficiency.

Avoid use: pregnancy, breastfeeding, elderly, patients who are debilitated, porphyria , pain which is not controlled, history of drug or alcohol abuse.

Possible interaction: CNS depressants, griseofulvin, alcohol, phenytoin, systemic steroids, chloramphenicol, rifampicin, metronidazole, anticoagulants of the coumarin type.

Side effects: headache, respiratory depression, dizziness, unsteadiness, sleepiness, confusion, agitation, allergic responses, megaloblastic anaemia. Drug tolerance and dependence may occur. Drug is metabolized to phenobarbitone.

Manufacturer: Zeneca.

MYSTECLIN

Description: a compound tetracycline and antifungal preparation available as sugar-coated orange tablets containing 250mg tetracycline hydrochloride and 250,000 units nystatin.

Used for: injections and acne susceptible to tetracycline, particularly where candidiasis also occurs.

Dosage: adults 1 or 2 tablets 4 times each day.

Special care: liver or kidney disease.

Avoid use: pregnancy, breastfeeding, children.

Possible interaction: oral contraceptives, antacids, mineral supplements, milk, anticoagulants.

Side effects: allergic responses, gastro-intestinal upset, superinfection. If rise in intracranial pressure occurs, drug should be withdrawn.

Manufacturer: Squibb.

NACTON FORTE

Description: an anticholinergic, poldine methylsulphate, available as orange tablets (4mg strength), marked NACTON 4.

Used for: peptic ulcer, acidity.

Dosage: 4mg 3 times per day and at bedtime. Elderly, half dose. Not for children. Also **NACTON**, 2mg poldine methylsulphate as white tablets marked NACTON 2.

Dosage: see literature. Not for children.

Special care: glaucoma, tachycardia, difficulty in urinating.

Side effects: anticholinergic effects

Manufacturer: Pharmark.

NALCROM

Description: an anti-inflammatory non-steroid, sodium cromoglycate as clear capsules containing white powder (100mg) and marked FISONS and 101.
Used for: food allergy.
Dosage: 2 capsules 4 times per day before meals, maximum 40mg/kg per day. Children over 2 years, 1 capsule 4 times per day. Not recommended for children under 2.
Side effects: rashes, joint pain, nausea.
Manufacturer: Fisons.

NALOREX

Description: a narcotic antagonist, naltrexone hydrochloride, available as mottled orange tablets (50mg strength) and marked DuPont and NTR.
Used for: maintenance treatment for patients detoxified after opioid dependency.
Dosage: 25mg daily to start with and then 50mg per day for at least 3 months. Treatment should be started in a drug addiction centre. Not for children.
Special care: kidney or liver disorder.
Avoid use: a current dependence on opiates, liver failure, acute hepatitis.
Side effects: drowsiness, dizziness, cramps, vomiting, joint and muscle pains.
Manufacturer: DuPont.

NAPRATEC

Description: an NSAID and propionic acid/prostaglandin analogue, available as naproxen, a yellow oblong tablet (500mg) marked Searle N500, and misoprostol, a white hexagonal tablet (200µg) marked Searle 1461.
Used for: osteoarthritis, rheumatoid arthritis, ankylosing spondylitis where the stomach has to be protected against the medication.
Dosage: 1 tablet of each drug taken twice daily with food.
Special care: asthma, liver or kidney damage, elderly, disease of blood vesssels. Effective contraception must be used by women of child-bearing age.

Avoid use: pregnancy, lactation, duodenal or gastric ulcer, allergy induced by aspirin or anti-inflammatory drugs.
Possible interaction: diuretics, anticoagulants, sulphonylureas, quinolones, sulphonamides, hydantoins, lithium, ß-blockers, probenecid, methotrexate.
Side effects: diarrhoea, abdominal pain, gastro-intestinal upset, vaginal bleeding, menorrhagia (long or heavy menstruation), rash, headache, urticaria, dizziness, tinnitus, vertigo, blood changes.
Manufacturer: Searle.

NAPROSYN SR

Description: Propionic acid, naproxen (as the sodium salt) available as 500mg in white, capsule-shaped tablets marked 500.
Used for: osteoarthritis, rheumatoid arthritis, ankylosing spondylitis, musculoskeletal disorders, acute gout.
Dosage: 1 to 2 tablets once per day. Not for children.
Also, **NAPROSYN EC**, naproxen as 250mg, 375mg and 500mg strength white tablets marked with tablet name, the strength and SYNTEX.
NAPROSYN TABLETS, naproxen as 250mg (buff tablets), 375mg (pink tablets) and 500mg (buff tablets) marked with tablet name, strength and SYNTEX.
NAPROSYN SUSPENSION, naproxen as 250mg per 10ml and **NAPROSYN GRANULES**, 500mg naproxen as peppermint-flavoured granules in a sachet.
Dosage: 500–1000mg per day in 2 divided doses or as 1 dose morning or evening. For gout, 750mg to start with and then 250mg every 8 hours. For musculoskeletal disorders, 500mg to start with, then 250mg every 6 to 8 hours as necessary, no more than 1250mg per day after the first 24 hours. Children: for juvenile rheumatoid arthritis, 5 to 16 years, 10mg/kg body weight per day in 2 divided doses. Not for children under 5.
Also, **NAPROSYN SUPPOSITORIES**, naproxen 500mg.

Dosage: 1 at night with another in the morning (or 500mg by mouth) if necessary.

Special care: liver or kidney damage, elderly, heart failure, asthma, pregnancy, lactation, a history of gastro-intestinal lesions.

Avoid use: peptic ulcer, allergy caused by aspirin or anti-inflammatory drugs.

Possible interaction: ACE inhibitors, ß-blockers, lithium, anticoagulants, quinolones, sulphonylureas, hydantoins, frusemide, methotrexate, probenecid.

Side effects: headache, gastro-intestinal intolerance, rash, vertigo, blood changes, tinnitus.

Manufacturer: Syntex.

NARCAN

Description: a narcotic antagonist, naloxone hydrochloride, available as ampoules or pre-filled syringes (0.4mg/ml, 1mg/ml).

Used for: diagnosis of opioid overdosage, reversal of opioid depression including that due to pentazocine and dextropropoxyphone.

Dosage: 0.4–2mg by injection (intravenous, intramuscular or subcutaneous) every 2 to 3 minutes as necessary, or by intravenous infusion (see literature). Post-operative, 0.1–0.2mg intravenously as required. Children 10µg/kg by same means.

Also, **NARCAN NEONATAL**, naloxone hydrochloride as 0.02mg/ml in 2ml ampoules.

Used for: depression of neonatal respiration due to obstetric analgesia.

Dosage: 10µg/kg by injection (intravenous, intramuscular or subcutaneous), repeated as required.

Special care: pregnancy, opioid dependence. Patient should be monitored to determine whether repeat doses are needed.

Manufacturer: DuPont.

NARDIL

Description: an antidepressant and MAOI, phenelzine sulphate, available as orange tablets (15mg strength).

Used for: depression, phobias.

Dosage: 1 tablet 3 times per day initially, reduced gradually for maintenance. Not for children.

Special care: elderly, epilepsy.

Avoid use: liver disease, blood changes, congestive heart failure, brain vascular disease, hyperthyroidism, phaeochromocytoma.

Possible interaction: sympathomimetic amines (e.g. amphetamine and others), TCADs, pethidine and similar analgesics. The effect of barbiturates and alcohol, insulin, hypnotics may be enhanced and the side effects of anticholinergics may be enhanced or increased, antihypertensives. Avoid foods such as cheese, meat extracts (e.g. Oxo or Bovril), yeast extracts (e.g. Marmite), alcohol, broad beans, bananas, pickled herrings, vegetable proteins. Do not use any of these within 14 days of stopping the drug.

Side effects: severe hypertension with certain foods (see above), dizziness, drowsiness, insomnia, weakness, fatigue, postural hypotension, constipation, dry mouth, gastro-intestinal upsets, difficult in urinating, blurred vision, ankle oedema. Skin rashes, blood disorders, weight gain, jaundice, changes in libido.

Manufacturer: Parke-Davis.

NARPHEN^{CD}

Description: an opiate, phenazocine hydrobromide available as white, scored tablets (strength 5mg) marked SNP/2.

Used for: severe, prolonged pain including pancreatic and biliary pain.

Dosage: 1 tablet every 4 to 6 hours, taken by mouth, or beneath the tongue, as necessary. Maximum single dose, 20mg. Not for children.

Special care: hypothyroidism, chronic kidney or liver disease, elderly. In labour or during pregnancy.

Avoid use: coma, epilepsy, acute alcoholism, breathing difficulty, blocked airways.

Possible interaction: depressants of the central nervous system, MAOIs.
Side effects: constipation, dizziness nausea. Danger of tolerance and dependence.
Manufacturer: Napp.

NASEPTIN

Description: an antibacterial cream comprising chlorhexidine hydrochloride (0.1%) and neomycin sulphate (0.5%).
Used for: staphylococcal infections of the nose.
Dosage: small amounts to be applied into each nostril 2 to 4 times per day.
Special care: prolonged use should be avoided.
Side effects: sensitive skin.
Manufacturer: Zeneca.

NATRILIX

Description: a vasorelaxant, indapamide hemihydrate, available as white, film-coated tablets (strength 2.5mg).
Used for: hypertension.
Dosage: 1 tablet in the morning. Not for children.
Special care: pregnancy, severe kidney disease.
Avoid use: lactation, severe liver disease.
Possible interaction: corticosteroids, laxatives, lithium, cardiac glycosides, diuretics, anti-arrhythmics.
Side effects: nausea, headache, hypokalaemia.
Manufacturer: Servier.

NATULAN

Description: a cytostatic agent, procarbazine hydrochloride, available as yellow capsules (strength 50mg).
Used for: Hodgkin's disease, advanced reticoloses (normally malignant overgrowths in the lymphatic or immune system), solid tumours that do not respond to other therapies.
Dosage: see literature but likely to be 50mg per day to begin with, rising to 250–300mg per day in 50mg daily increments. Dose for maintenance (on remission), 50–150mg per day.

Special care: induction therapy should commence in hospital.
Avoid use: pregnancy, severe liver or kidney damage, severe leucopenia, thrombocytopenia.
Possible interaction: alcohol, narcotics, barbiturates, phenothiazines, imipramine-type compounds.
Side effects: nausea, loss of appetite, myelosuppression (reduction in the production of blood cells in the bone marrow).
Manufacturer: Cambridge.

NAVIDREX

Description: a thiazide diuretic, cyclopenthiazide (0.5mg), available as white scored tablets marked CIBA and AO.
Used for: oedema, heart failure, hypertension.
Dosage: 0.25–1mg per day to a maximum of 1.5mg daily, but see manufacturer's literature. For children, contact the manufacturer.
Special care: liver cirrhosis, liver or kidney disease, SLE, gout, the elderly, pregnancy, lactation. Electrolytes, glucose and fluids should be monitored.
Avoid use: hypercalcaemia, Addison's disease, severe liver or kidney failure, if sensitive to sulphonamides.
Possible interaction: corticosteroids, cardiac glycosides, lithium, carbenozolone, tubocurarine, antidiabetic drugs, NSAIDs, opioids, barbiturates, alcohol.
Side effects: gastro-intestinal upset, anorexia, blood changes, rash, sensitivity to light, dizziness, pancreatitis, metabolic and electrolyte upset, impotence.
Manufacturer: Ciba.

NAVISPARE

Description: a thiazide and potassium-sparing diuretic, cyclopenthiazide (0.25mg) with 2.5mg amiloride, available as yellow tablets marked CIBA and RC.
Used for: mild to moderate hypertension.
Dosage: 1 or 2 tablets per day in the morning. Not for children.

Special care: liver or kidney disease, diabetes, hyperlipidaemia, pregnancy, lactation, gout, respiratory or metabolic acidosis.
Avoid use: severe kidney or liver failure, anuria, hyperkalaemia, Addison's disease, hypercalcaemia, hyponatiaemia (low blood sodium levels).
Possible interaction: ACE inhibitors, other antihypertensives, lithium, digitalis, potassium supplements, potassium-sparing diuretics.
Side effects: blood changes, gout, gastro-intestinal upset, fatigue, rash, sensitivity to light.
Manufacturer: Ciba.

NAVOBAN

Description: a 5HT$_3$-antagonist, tropisetron hydrochloride, which blocks vomiting reflexes, available as yellow/white capsules (5mg strength). Also, **NAVOBAN INJECTION**, containing 5mg/5ml in ampoules.
Used for: chemotherapy-induced nausea and vomiting.
Dosage: 5mg by intravenous injection of infusion before therapy and 1 capsule 1 hour before morning food, for 5 days. Not for children.
Special care: uncontrolled hypertension.
Avoid use: pregnancy, breastfeeding.
Possible interaction: drugs that affect liver enzymes.
Side effects: constipation, dizziness, headache, tiredness, stomach upset.
Manufacturer: Sandoz.

NEBCIN

Description: an aminoglycoside, tabramycin sulphate, available as solution in vials containing 20, 40 or 80mg.
Used for: infections of gastro-intestinal and respiratory tract, skin and soft tissue, CNS, urinary tract; septicaemia.
Dosage: 3–5mg/kg per day by intramuscular injection, intravenous injection or infusion in 3 or 4 divided doses. Children: 6–7.5mg/kg daily in divided doses; babies up to 1 month, 4mg/kg per day in 2 doses.

Special care: kidney damage; control dosage and blood levels.
Avoid use: pregnancy, lactation.
Possible interaction: loop diuretics, other aminoglycosides, neuromuscular blocking agents.
Side effects: anaphylaxis, ototoxicity (affecting hearing and balance), nephrotoxicity, raised liver enzymes.
Manufacturer: Lilly.

NEGRAM

Description: a quinolone, nalidixic acid (500mg) available as light brown tablets marked NEGRAM with a symbol on the reverse. Also, **NEGRAM SUSPENSION**, containing 300mg/5ml as a suspension.
Used for: infections of the grastro-intestinal tract by Gram-negative organisms.
Dosage: 500mg–1g 4 times per day. Children up to 12 years, up to 50mg/kg per day. Not for children under 3 months.
Special care: liver or kidney disease, lactation. Avoid sunlight.
Avoid use: history of convulsions.
Possible interaction: probenecid, anticoagulants.
Side effects: rashes, blood changes, convulsions, disturbances in vision and stomach.
Manufacturer: Sanofi Winthrop.

NEO-CORTEF

Description: an antibiotic and cortico-steroid comprising 0.5% neomycin in sulphate and 1.5% hydrocortisone acetate, as drops.
Used for: otitis externa and eye inflammation.
Dosage: 2 to 3 drops 4 times per day (otitis), 1 to 2 drops in each eye up to 6 times per day.
Also, **NEO-CORTEF OINTMENT**
Dosage: apply once or twice per day (otitis), apply 2 or 3 times per day or if drops are used during the day, use at night
Special care: prolonged use on infants during pregnancy.

Avoid use: perforated ear drum, glaucoma, fungal, viral, tuberculous or acute pus-containing infections.
Side effects: sensitization, superinfection, cataract, rise in pressure within the eye.
Manufacturer: Cusi.

NEO-CYTAMEN

Description: vitamin B$_{12}$, hydroxocobalamin, available as 1ml ampoules containing 1000μg per ml.
Used for: megaloblastic anaemia, and other anaemias responsive to B$_{12}$, Leber's disease (a rare hereditary visual defect), tobacco amblyopia (reduced vision although eye structure appears normal).
Dosage: 250–1000μg intramuscularly on alternate days for 7 to 14 days then 250μg once per week until blood count is normal. 1000μg every 2 to 3 months for maintenance. For amblyopia, see literature.
Possible interaction: oral contraceptives, chloramphenicol.
Side effects: some rare hypersensitivity reactions.
Manufacturer: Evans.

NEO-MEDRONE CREAM

Description: a mild steroid and antibacterial, 0.25% methylprednisolone acetate and 0.5% neomycin sulphate, as a cream.
Used for: allergic and inflammatory skin conditions where there is bacterial infection.
Dosage: use 1 to 3 times per day.
Special care: thrombophlebitis, psychoses, recent intestinal anastomoses, chronic nephritis, certain cancers, osteoporosis, peptic ulcer, skin eruption/ rash related to a disease, viral, fungal or active infections, tuberculosis. Hypertension, glaucoma, epilepsy, acute glomerulonephritis (inflammation of kidney glomerulus), diabetes, cirrhosis, hypothyroidism, pregnancy, stress. To be withdrawn gradually.
Possible interaction: NSAIDs, oral anticoagulants, phenytoin, ephedrine,

phenobarbitone, rifampicin, diuretics, cardiac glycosides, anticholinesterases, hypoglycaemics.
Side effects: osteoporosis, depression, euphoria, hyperglycaemia, peptic ulcers, Cushingoid changes.
Manufacturer: Upjohn.

NEO-MERCAZOLE

Description: an antithyroid, carbimazole, available as pink tablets (strengths 5 and 20mg) marked BS with strength on the reverse.
Used for: thyrotoxicosis.
Dosage: 20–60mg per day initially in 2 or 3 divided doses until thyroid functions normally. 5–15mg per day for 6 to 18 months for maintenance, or maintain 20–60mg per day with 50–150μg supplemental thyroxine daily for 6 to 18 months. Children, 5–15mg per day in divided doses.
Special care: pregnancy (but see literature).
Avoid use: lactation, obstruction of the trachea.
Side effects: arthralgia, headache, nausea, rashes. Depression of the bone marrow. Drug should be discontinued if there are mouth ulcers or a sore throat.
Manufacturer: Nicholas.

NEO-NACLEX

Description: a thiazide, bendrofluazide (5mg), available as white, scored tablets marked NEO-NACLEX.
Used for: hypertension, oedema.
Dosage: 1 to 2 tablets once per day for oedema, half or 1 tablet for maintenance periodically. For hypertension, half to 2 once per day. For children, 50–100μg/kg body weight.
Special care: cirrhosis of the liver, liver or kidney disease, diabetes, SLE, gout, pregnancy, breastfeeding, elderly. Monitor glucose, electrolytes and fluids.
Avoid use: hypercalcaemia, severe liver or kidney failure, sensitivity to sulphonamides, Addison's disease.
Possible interaction: lithium, cardiac

glycosides, potassium-sparing diuretics, potassium supplements, corticosteroids, tubocurarine, NSAIDs, carbenoxolone, alcohol, opiods, barbiturates, antidiabetic drugs.
Side effects: rash, blood changes, anorexia, dizziness, pancreatitis, gastrointestinal upset, sensitivity to light, upset to metabolism and electrolytes.
Manufacturer: Goldshield.

NEO-NACLEX-K

Description: a thiazide and potassium supplement, bendrofluazide (2.5mg) with 630mg potassium chloride in a slow-release, two-layer tablet, pink and white, marked NEO-NACLEX-K.
Used for: hypertension and chronic oedema.
Dosage: 1 to 4 per day (hypertension). 2 per day for oedema inreasing to 4 if required, maintenance 1 or 2 periodically. Not for children.
Special care: liver cirrhosis, diabetes, liver or kidney disease, SLE, gout, elderly, pregnancy, lactation. Monitor glucose, fluid and electrolytes.
Avoid use: hypercalcaemia, severe liver or kidney failure, Addison's disease, sensitivity to sulphonamides.
Possible interaction: lithium, corticosteroids, cardiac glycosides, potassium supplements, potassium-sparing diuretics, NSAIDs, tubocurarine, carbenoxolone, alcohol, opioids, barbiturates, antidiabetic drugs.
Side effects: rash, blood changes, gastrointestinal upsets, sensitivity to light, impotence, dizziness, pancreatitis, anorexia, upset to metabolism and electrolytes. Stop if signs of blockage or ulceration of small bowel occur.
Manufacturer: Goldshield.

NEOCON 1/35

Description: an oestrogen/progestogen oral contraceptive containing 35µg ethinyloestradiol and 500µg norethisterone in white tablets marked C over 535.
Used for: oral contraception.

Dosage: 1 per day for 21 days commencing on the fifth day of menstruation, then 7 days without tablets.
Special care: hypertension, Raynaud's disease (reduced blood supply to an organ of the body's extremities), asthma, severe depression, diabetes, varicose veins, multiple sclerosis, chronic kidney disease, kidney dialysis. Blood pressure, breasts and pelvic organs to be checked regularly; smoking not advised.
Avoid use: history of heart disease, infectious hepatitis, sickle cell anaemia, porphyria, liver tumour, undiagnosed vaginal bleeding, pregnancy, hormone-dependent cancer, haemolytic uraemic syndrome (rare kidney disorder), chorea, otosclerosis.
Possible interaction: barbiturates, tetracyclines, griseofulvin, rifampicin, primidone, phenytoin, chloral hydrate, ethosuximide, carbamazepine, glutethimide, dichloralphenazone.
Side effects: fluid retention and bloating, leg cramps/pains, breast enlargement, depression, headaches, nausea, loss of libido, weight gain, vaginal discharge, cervical erosion (alteration of epithelial cells), chloasma (pigmentation of nose, cheeks or forehead), breakthrough bleeding (bleeding between periods).
Manufacturer: Ortho.

NEOGEST

Description: a progestogen-only contraceptive, norgestrel (75µg) available in brown tablets.
Used for: oral contraception.
Dosage: starting on the first day of the cycle, 1 tablet each day at the same time, without a break.
Special care: hypertension, thromboembolic disorders, liver disease, hormone-dependent cancer, ovarian cysts, migraine. Regular checks on blood pressure, breasts and pelvic organs.
Avoid use: previous severe arterial or heart disease, benign liver tumours, undiagnosed vaginal bleeding, pregnancy, past ectopic pregnancy.

Discontinue immediately for pregnancy, jaundice, thrombophlebitis or thromboembolism.
Possible interaction: griseofulvin, rifampicin, meprobamate, chloral hydrate, carbamazepine, primidone, barbiturates, phenytoin, dichloralphenazone, ethosuximide, glutethimide.
Side effects: acne, breast discomfort, headache, ovarian cysts, irregular menstrual bleeding.
Manufacturer: Schering H.C.

NEOSPORIN

Description: a peptide and aminoglycoside, polymyxin B sulphate (5000 units) and neomycin sulphate (1700 units) with gramicidin (25 units/ml), as drops.
Used for: bacterial infections, prevention of infections in the eye before and after surgery, removal of foreign bodies from the eye.
Dosage: 1 or 2 drops 4 or more times per day.
Special care: existing eye defect.
Manufacturer: Cusi.

NEOTIGASON

Description: a vitamin A derivative, acitretin, used only in hospitals and available as brown/white (10mg) and brown/yellow capsules marked ROCHE.
Used for: severe psoriasis, congenital ichthyosis, Darier's disease (skin disease with brown or black wart-like patches).
Dosage: 25–30mg per day initially, for 2 to 4 weeks up to a maximum of 75mg per day. 25–50mg per day for maintenance. Maximum treatment period, 6 months. Not for children.
Special care: teratogenic, effective contraception necessary during treatment and for 2 years after stopping. Diabetes, monitor liver, serum lipids and bone. Do not donate blood for 1 year afterwards.
Avoid use: kidney or liver disease, pregnancy, lactation.
Possible interaction: alcohol, tetracyclines, methotrexate, high doses or vitamin A.

Side effects: hair loss, itching, erythema, dryness, erosion of mucous membranes, nausea, headache, sweating, drowsiness, myalgia, arthralgia, bone thickening, liver disorder.
Manufacturer: Roche.

NEPHRIL

Description: a thiazide diuretic, polythiazide, available as white tablets (1mg) with NEP over 1 marked on one side and Pfizer on the reverse.
Used for: oedema, hypertension.
Dosage: 1–4mg per day for oedema, 500µg–4mg per day for hypertension. Not recommended for children.
Special care: liver or kidney disease, liver cirrhosis, gout, SLE, diabetes, elderly, pregnancy, breastfeeding. Check glucose, electrolytes and fluid.
Avoid use: liver or kidney failure, hypercalcaemia, Addison's disease, sensitivity to sulphonamides.
Possible interaction: NSAIDs, cardiac glycosides, lithium corticosteroids, carbenoxolone, tubocurarine, alcohol, barbiturates, opioids, antidiabetic drugs.
Side effects: rash, blood changes, dizziness, impotence, anorexia, pancreatitis, gastro-intestinal, electrolyte or metabolism upset, sensitivity to light.
Manufacturer: Pfizer.

NERISONE

Description: a potent steroid, diflucortolone valerate (0.1%) available as a cream, oily cream or ointment.
Used for: skin disorders that respond to steroids.
Dosage: apply 2 or 3 times per day reducing to once per day for maintenance. On children under 4, do not use for more than 3 weeks.
Also, **NERISONE FORTE**, a very potent form (0.3%) available as ointment and oily cream.
Used for: initial treatment of resistant, severe skin disorders.
Dosage: apply sparingly 2 or 3 times per day for a maximum of 2 weeks

(maximum total use 60g/week). For maintenance use Nerisone. Not recommended for children under 4.
Special care: thrombophlebitis, psychoses, recent intestinal anastomoses, chronic nephritis, certain cancers, osteoporosis, peptic ulcer, skin eruption/rash related to a disease, viral, fungal or active infections, tuberculosis. Hypertension, glaucoma, epilepsy, acute glomerulonephritis (inflammation of kidney glomerulus), diabetes, cirrhosis, hypothyroidism, pregnancy, stress. To be withdrawn gradually.
Possible interaction: NSAIDs, oral anticoagulants, phenytoin, ephedrine, phenobarbitone, rifampicin, diuretics, cardiac glycosides, anticholinesterases, hypoglycaemics.
Side effects: osteoporosis, depression, euphoria, hyperglycaemia, peptic ulcers, Cushingoid changes.
Manufacturer: Schering H.C.

NETILLIN

Description: an aminoglycoside and anti-bacterial, netilmicin sulphate, available as ampoules containing 10, 50 or 100mg/ml.
Used for: septicaemia, bacteraemia (bacteria in the blood), serious infections of the kidney, urinary tract, skin and soft tissues, respiratory tract. Gonorrhoea.
Dosage: 4–6mg/kg once per day as 2 or 3 divided doses. For life-threatening infections, up to 7.5mg/kg per day in 3 divided doses, all by intramuscular or slow intravenous injection. Children (by the same means): over 2 years, 2–2.5mg/kg 8-hourly; 1 week to 2 years, 2.5–3mg/kg 8-hourly; under 1 week 3mg/kg 12-hourly.
Special care: myasthenia gravis, Parkinsonism. Control total dosage in cases of kidney disease.
Avoid use: pregnancy.
Possible interaction: anaesthetics, etha crynic acid, frusemide, neuromuscular blockers.
Side effects: nephrotoxicity and ototoxicity (affects hearing and balance).
Manufacturer: Schering-Plough.

NEULACTIL

Description: a group II phenothiazine and antipsychotic, pericyazine, available as yellow tablets, marked with name (2.5mg) or marked with name and strength (10mg). Also NEULACTIL FORTE SYRUP, containing 10mg/5ml.
Used for: schizophrenia, severe anxiety and tension, agitation, behavioural disorders, maintenance of sedation for psychotic states.
Dosage: 15–75mg per day initially (elderly 5–30mg), to a maximum of 300mg daily. See literature for children.
Special care: pregnancy, lactation, elderly during very hot or cold weather.
Avoid use: heart failure, epilepsy, Parkinsonism, liver or kidney disorder, hypothyroidism, glaucoma, coma, bone marrow depression, enlarged prostate.
Possible interaction: alcohol, CNS depressants, antihypertensives, analgesics, levodopa, antidepressants, anticonvulsants, antidiabetic drugs.
Side effects: muscle spasms (eye, neck, back, face), restlessness, rigidity and tremor, tardive dyskinesia (repetitious muscular movements), dry mouth, blocked nose, difficulty in passing urine, tachycardia, blurred vision, hypotension, constipation, weight gain, impotence, galactorrhoea, gynaecomastia, amenorrhoea, blood and skin changes, lethargy, fatigue, ECG irregularities.
Manufacturer: R.P.R.

NEUPOGEN

Description: a recombinant human granulocyte colony stimulating factor (G-CSF), filgrastim, available as 30 million units in a single dose vial, for specialist use.
Used for: reduction of neutropenia during cytotoxic chemotherapy and after bone marrow transplantation.
Dosage: chemotherapy, 500,000 units/kg per day by subcutaneous injection or intravenous infusion starting within 24 hours of chemotherapy and continuing until neutrophil count is normal (about

14 days). Bone marrow transplantation —1 million units/kg per day starting within 24 hours.
Special care: risk of bone marrow tumour growth, pre-malignant bone marrow conditions. Monitor platelets, haemoglobin, osteoporosis, pregnancy, lactation.
Side effects: temporary hypotension, urinary abnormalities, musculo-skeletal pain, disturbances in liver enzymes and serum uric acid.
Manufacturer: Amgen, Roche.

NEURONTIN

Description: a GABA analogue, gabapentin, available as capsules: white (100mg), yellow (300mg); orange (400mg), all marked with name and strength.
Used for: added treatment of seizures not controlled by other anticonvulsants.
Dosage: 300mg once, twice and 3 times per day on days 1, 2 and 3 respectively, increasing to 400mg 3 times per day up to a maximum of 800mg. Not for children.
Special care: haemodialysis, pregnancy, kidney disease, elderly, lactation, avoid sudden withdrawal (minimum 1 week).
Possible interaction: antacids.
Side effects: ataxia, dizziness, fatigue, headache, tremor, diplopia, nausea, vomiting, nystagmus (involuntary eye movements) rhinitis, amblyopia (reduced vision in an eye that appears normal structurally).
Manufacturer: Parke-Davis.

NIFENSAR XL

Description: a class II calcium antagonist and antihypertensive, nifedipine, available as yellow, sustained-release tablets (20mg) marked N20.
Used for: mild to moderate hypertension.
Dosage: 2 once per day swallowed with food, adjusted according to response. 1 or 2 once per day for maintenance. Maximum 5 per day. Elderly, 1 per day initially. Not for children.
Special care: diabetes, angina pectoris, kidney disease, weak heart.

Avoid use: pregnancy, breastfeeding, liver disease.
Possible interaction: other antihypertensives, digoxin, climetidine, quinidine, fentaryl.
Side effects: nausea, oedema, headache, flushes, dizziness, ischaemic pain, jaundice, rash, lethargy, enlarged gums.
Manufacturer: R.P.R.

NIMOTOP

Description: a class II calcium antagonist, nimodipine, available as 30mg off-white tablets marked Bayer and SK.
Used for: prevention of ischaemic, neurological defects after a subarachnoid (intracranial) haemorrhage.
Dosage: 2 tablets every 4 hours commencing within 4 days of the haemorrhage and continuing for 21 days.
Also, **NIMOTOP INFUSION**, containing 0.2mg/ml in vial and bottle.
Used for: neurological deficits after subarachnoid haemorrhage.
Dosage: 1mg/hour by intravenous infusion for 2 hours, then 2mg/hour for 5 to 14 days. For bodyweights under 70kg, or for unstable blood pressure, start at 0.5mg/hour. Not for children.
Special care: raised intracranial pressure, cerebral oedema, kidney disease, pregnancy. Check blood pressure. PVC apparatus should not be used—use polyethylene or polypropylene.
Possible interaction: ß-blockers, other calcium antagonists.
Side effects: flushes, headache, hypotension, heart rate changes.
Manufacturer: Bayer.

NIPENT

Description: an adenosine deaminase inhibitor, and cytotoxic drug pentostatin, available as 10mg powder in vial for reconstitution, used in cancer chemotherapy.
Used for: prolonged remission in the treatment of malignancies.
Dosage: intravenously on alternate weeks. For specialist use only.

Side effects: nausea and vomiting, bone marrow suppression, suppression of the immune system, hair loss, teratogenic.
Manufacturer: Lederle.

NIPRIDE

Description: a vasodilator, sodium nitroprusside available as powder (50mg) in ampoules.
Used for: critical hypertension, heart failure, controlled hypotension in surgery.
Dosage: for hypertension, 0.3µg/kg/minute by intravenous infusion to begin then adjust to response, usually 0.5–6µg/kg/minute (maximum 8µg/kg/minute). Lower doses for patients already taking antihypertensives. Lower doses also in surgery (up to 1.5µg/kg/minute). For heart failure, 10–15µg/minute by intravenous infusion increasing at 5 to 10 minute intervals to a maximum of 280µg/minute. Maximum treatment 72 hours, withdraw over 10 to 30 minutes.
Special care: severe kidney disease, hypothyroidism, ischaemic heart disease, elderly, pregnancy, lactation, impaired circulation in the brain. Check blood pressure and concentration of cyanide in plasma.
Avoid use: vitamin B_{12} deficiency, severe liver disease, optic atrophy (causing blindness).
Possible interaction: ACE inhibitors, NSAIDs, alcohol, antipsychotics, antidepressants, ß-blockers, diuretics, anxiolytics and hypnotics, corticosteroids, sex hormones, baclofen, carbenoxolone, levodopa.
Side effects: headache, nausea, dizziness, stomach pain, palpitations, sweating, reeduced platelet count. Also those due to high cyanide concentrations in plasma which *in addition* are tachycardia, metabolic acidosis.
Manufacturer: Roche.

NITOMAN

Description: a dopamine reducing agent, tetrabenazine, available as yellow-buff tablets (25mg) marked ROCHE 120.
Used for: Huntington's chorea, senile chorea, hemiballismus (violent involuntary movement).
Dosage: 25mg 3 times per day initially, increasing by 25mg/day every 3 or 4 days to a daily maximum of 200mg. Not for children.
Special care: pregnancy.
Avoid use: breastfeeding.
Possible interaction: levodopa, MAOIs, reserpine.
Side effects: drowsiness, depression, hypotension on standing, rigidity, tremor.
Manufacturer: Roche.

NITRAZEPAM

Description: a long-acting benzodi-azepine, nitrazepam, available as tablets (5mg). Also, **NITRAZEPAM ORAL SUSPENSION** containing 2.5mg/5ml.
Used for: insomnia over the short-term or when it is severe.
Dosage: 5–10mg at bedtime; elderly, 2.5–5mg. Not for children.
Special care: chronic liver or kidney disease, chronic lung disease, pregnancy, labour, lactation, elderly. May impair judgement. Withdraw gradually and avoid prolonged use.
Avoid use: depression of respiration, acute lung disease; psychotic, phobic or obsessional states.
Possible interaction: anticonvulsants, depressants of the CNS, alcohol.
Side effects: ataxia, confusion, light-headedness, drowsiness, hypotension, gastro-intestinal upsets, disturbances in vision and libido, skin rashes, retention of urine, vertigo. Sometimes jaundice or blood disorders.
Manufacturer: non-proprietary—available from several suppliers.

NITROCINE

Description: a solution of glyceryl trinitrate (1mg/ml) in ampoules and bottles.
Used for: prevention and treatment of angina, left ventricular failure.

Dosage: 10–200µg/minute by
intravenous infusion.
Special care: hypotension, tolerance.
Avoid use: anaemia, cerebral haemorrhage,
head trauma, closed angle glaucoma.
Side effects: flushes, headache, tachycar-
dia, dizziness, hypotension on standing.
Manufacturer: Schwarz.

NITRONAL

Description: a solution of glyceryl
trinitrate (1mg/ml) in ampoules and vials.
Used for: prevention and treatment of
angina, left ventricular failure.
Dosage: 10–200µg/minute by
intravenous infusion.
Special care: hypotension, tolerance.
Avoid use: anaemia, cerebral haemorrhage,
head trauma, closed angle glaucoma.
Side effects: flushes, headache, tachycar-
dia, dizziness, hypotension on standing.
Manufacturer: Lipha.

NIVAQUINE

Description: a suppressive drug and 4-
aminoquinoline, chloroquine sulphate,
available as yellow tablet (150mg)
marked NIVAQUINE 200.
Used for: rheumatoid arthritis, malaria.
Dosage: 1 tablet per day (arthritis); for
malaria prevention, 2 tablets in 1 dose
on the same week day for 2 weeks
before being subjected to possible
infection and for 4 weeks after. Children
should use the syrup.
Also, NIVAQUINE SYRUP, 50mg/5ml
chloroquine sulphate.
Dosage: 3mg/kg per day for arthritis;
prevention of malaria, 5mg/kg at weekly
intervals, for 2 weeks before and 4
weeks after being subjected to possible
infection. For treatment see literature.
Also, NIVAQUINE INJECTION,
40mg/ml in ampoules.
Used for: emergency treatment.
Dosage: see literature.
Special care: porphyria, kidney or liver
disorders, severe gastro-intestinal, blood
or neurological disorders, psoriasis,
pregnancy, lactation, history of epilepsy.

Regular eye tests before and during
treatment.
Side effects: gastro-intestinal upset,
headache, skin eruptions, loss of
pigment, hair loss, blurred vision,
damage to retina, blood disorders,
allergic reactions, opacities in cornea.
Manufacturer: R.P.R.

NIVEMYCIN

Description: an antibiotic and aminoglycoside, neomycin sulphate, available as
500mg tablets. Also, NIVEMYCIN
ELIXIR containing 100mg/5ml.
Used for: preparation before bowel surgery
and an added treatment for hepatic coma.
Dosage: 2 tablets per hour for 4 hours,
then 2 every 4 hours for 2 to 3 days (pre-
operation). Children: over 12 years, 2
tablets; 6 to 12 years, half to 1 tablet; 1
to 5 years, 10–20ml; under 1 year, 2.5–
10ml. All taken 4 hourly for 2 to 3 days
pre-operatively.
Special care: Parkinsonism, hepatic
coma, kidney disease.
Avoid use: bowel obstruction.
Side effects: gastro-intestinal upset.
Manufacturer: Boots.

NIZORAL

Description: an imidazole and
antifungal, ketoconazole, available as
white tablets (200mg) marked JANSSEN
and K over 200. Also, NIZORAL
SUSPENSION containing 100mg/5ml.
Used for: systemic fungal infections,
prevention of infections in patients with
reduced immune response, chronic
vaginal thrush and infections of the
gastro-intestinal tract not responding to
other teatment, skin and mucous
membrane fungal infections.
Dosage: 200–400mg daily with meals
continuing 1 week after symptoms have
ceased. For vaginal thrush 400mg once per
day for 5 days. Children 3mg/kg daily.
Also, NIZORAL CREAM, 2%
ketoconazole.
Used for: candidal vulvitis.
Dosage: apply once or twice per day

Avoid use: liver disease or liver abnormalities, pregnancy, hypersensitivity to other imidazoles.
Possible interaction: antacids, anticoagulants, phenytoin, rifampicin, cyclosporin, astemizole, terfenadine, anticholinergics, H₂ antagonists.
Side effects: hypersensitivity, rashes, headache, gastro-intestinal disturbances, hepatitis, thrombocytopenia (reduction in blood platelets), rarely breast enlargement.
Nizoral Cream *also used for*: ringworm infections, skin infection, seborrhoeic dermatitis.
Dosage: apply once or twice per day.
Side effects: skin irritation.
Also **NIZORAL SHAMPOO**, 20mg ketoconazole per ml of liquid.
Used for: seborrhoeic dermatitis, dandruff, scaly skin rash (pityriasis).
Dosage: dermatitis, use shampoo twice weekly for 2 to 4 weeks, and once every 1 or 2 weeks for prevention. Pityriasis, shampoo once per day for 5 days; prevention once daily for 3 days maximum.
Side effects: skin irritation.
Manufacturer: Janssen.

NOBRIUM

Description: a long-acting benzodiazepine and anxiolytic medazepam, available as yellow/orange capsules (5mg) marked with strength and ROCHE.
Used for: treatment of severe or disabling anxiety over the short-term whether it occcurs alone or with insomnia.
Dosage: 15–40mg in divided doses; elderly 5–20mg. Not for children.
Special care: chronic liver or kidney disease, chronic lung disease, pregnancy, labour, lactation, elderly. May impair judgement. Withdraw gradually and avoid prolonged use.
Avoid use: depression of respiration, acute lung disease; psychotic, phobic or obsessional states.
Possible interaction: anticonvulsants, depressants of the CNS, alcohol.
Side effects: ataxia, confusion, lightheadedness, drowsiness, hypotension,

gastro-intestinal upsets, disturbances in vision and libido, skin rashes, retention of urine, vertigo. Sometimes jaundice or blood disorders.
Manufacturer: Roche.

NOCTEC

Description: a sedative and hypnotic chloral hydrate, available as liquid-filled red capsules containing 500mg.
Used for: insomnia.
Dosage: 500mg–1g with water 15 to 30 minutes before bedtime. Daily maximum, 2g. Not for children.
Special care: porphyria, lactation, impaired judgement and dexterity.
Avoid use: gastritis, pregnancy, severe liver, heart or kidney disease.
Possible interaction: anticoagulants, CNS depressants, alcohol.
Side effects: headache, skin allergies, ketonuria, excitement, delirium.
Manufacturer: Squibb.

NODS TROPICAMIDE

Description: an anticholinergic, tropicamide (125µg), available as sterile ophthalmic applicator strips.
Used for: a short-acting dilator of the pupil and paralyser of the ciliary muscle of the eye.
Dosage: 1 unit in lower conjunctival sac, repeating after 30–45 minutes if required.
Special care: if driving or operating machinery.
Avoid use: narrow angle glaucoma.
Manufacturer: Chauvin.

NOLVADEX-D

Description: an antioestrogen and infertility drug, tamoxifen citrate, available as white octagonal tablets (20mg) marked NOVADEX-D and ICI.
Also, **NOLVADEX FORTE**, as white elongated octagonal tablets (40mg) marked NOLVADEX FORTE and ICI.
Also, **NOLVADEX**, 10mg white tablets marked NOLVADEX and ICI.
Used for: infertility.
Dosage: 20mg per day on 4 consecutive

days starting on second day of menstruation, increasing to 40mg and 80mg for later courses, if necessary.
Avoid use: pregnancy.
Possible interaction: warfarin.
Side effects: vaginal bleeding, hot flushes, dizziness, gastro-intestinal upset. Stop if there are disturbances to vision.
Manufacturer: Zeneca.

NOOTROPIL

Description: a GABA analogue, piracetam, available as white, oblong tablets (800 and 1200mg strengths) marked N. Also, **NOOTROPIL SOLUTION**, containing 333mg/ml.
Used for: additional treatment for cortical myoclonus (sudden muscular spasms).
Dosage: 7.2g per day initially, increasing by 4.8g daily at 3 or 4 day intervals to a maximum of 20g per day in 2 or 3 divided doses. Not for children under 16 years.
Special care: kidney disease, elderly. Withdraw gradually.
Avoid use: severe kidney dysfunction, liver disease, pregnancy, breastfeeding.
Possible interaction: thyroid hormones.
Side effects: insomnia, nervousness, weight gain, depression, diarrhoea, rash, hyperactivity.
Manufacturer: UCB.

NORCURON

Description: a muscle relaxant, vercuronium bromide (10mg) as powder in vials with water for injections.
Used for: short to medium duration muscle relaxant.
Dosage: 80–100µg/kg by intravenous injection and 20–30µg/kg for maintenance. Infants over 5 months as for adult; up to 4 months 10–20µg/kg then increase gradually to obtain response. 50–80µg/kg/hour by intravenous infusion after initial injection of 40–100µg/kg.
Special care: respiration should be assisted, reduce dose in kidney disease.
Possible interaction: some cholinergics, nifedipine, verapamil.
Manufacturer: Organon-Teknika.

NORDITROPIN

Description: a growth hormone, somatropin, available as a powder in a vial (12 units) plus diluent.
Used for: failure of growth in children due to growth hormone deficiency, Turner's syndrome.
Dosage: 0.07–0.1 units/kg body weight 6 to 7 times per week by subcutaneous injection (growth failure). For Turner's syndrome, 0.1 units/kg.
Also, **NORDITROPIN PENSET**, 12 and 24 units somatropin as powder in vials with 2ml of solvent.
Dosage: as above.
Special care: diabetes, deficiency of ACTH (adrenocorticotrophic hormones), intracranial lesion. Check thyroid function.
Avoid use: pregnancy, lactation, tumour, closure of epiphyses.
Side effects: oedema, hypothyroidism, pain at injection site.
Special care: chronic liver or kidney disease, chronic lung disease, pregnancy, labour, lactation, elderly. May impair judgement. Withdraw gradually and avoid prolonged use
Avoid use: depression of respiration, acute lung disease; psychotic, phobic or obsessional states.
Possible interaction: anticonvulsants, depressants of the CNS, alcohol.
Side effects: ataxia, confusion, lightheadedness, drowsiness, hypotension, gastro-intestinal upsets, disturbances in vision and libido, skin rashes, retention of urine, vertigo. Sometimes jaundice or blood disorders.(Move site of injection to avoid lipoatrophy).
Manufacturer: Novo Nordisk.

NORDOX

Description: a tetracycline, doxycycline, available in green capsules (100mg) marked NORDOX 100.
Used for: infections of the respiratory tract including bronchitis and sinusitis. Acne. Infections of the genito-urinary tract.
Dosage: 200mg on the first day, then

100mg per day with food or drink. Not for children.
Special care: liver disease.
Avoid use: pregnancy, breastfeeding.
Possible interaction: mineral supplements, antacids.
Side effects: allergic reactions, gastro-intestinal upset, superinfections. Stop if there is intracranial hypertension.
Manufacturer: Panpharma.

NORFLEX
Description: an anticholinergic, orphenadrine citrate, available in ampoules (30mg/ml).
Used for: musculoskeletal pain.
Dosage: 60mg by intramuscular or slow intravenous injection, repeated every 12 hours if required. Not for children.
Special care: pregnancy, tachycardia.
Avoid use: glaucoma, lactation, myasthenia gravis, urine retention.
Side effects: nausea, blurred vision, dizziness, dry mouth, confusion, tremor.
Manufacturer: 3M Health Care.

NORGESTON
Description: a progestogen-only contraceptive, levonorgestrel, available in white tablets (30µg).
Used for: oral contraception.
Dosage: 1 at the same time each day without a break, starting on the first day of the cycle.
Special care: hypertension, thromboem-bolic disorders, liver disease, hormone-dependent cancer, ovarian cysts, migraine. Regular checks on blood pressure, breasts and pelvic organs.
Avoid use: previous severe arterial or heart disease, benign liver tumours, undiagnosed vaginal bleeding, pregnancy, past ectopic pregnancy. Discontinue immediately for pregnancy, jaundice, thrombophlebitis or thromboembolism.
Possible interaction: griseofulvin, rifampicin, meprobamate, chloral hydrate, carbamazepine, primidone, barbiturates, phenytoin, dichloralphena-zone, ethosuximide, glutethimide.

Side effects: acne, breast discomfort, headache, ovarian cysts, irregular menstrual bleeding.
Manufacturer: Schering H.C.

NORIDAY
Description: a progestogen-only contraceptive, norethisterone, available as white tablets (350µg) marked NORIDAY and SYNTEX.
Used for: oral contraception.
Dosage: 1 at the same time each day without a break, starting on the first day of the cycle.
Special care: hypertension, thromboem-bolic disorders, liver disease, hormone-dependent cancer, ovarian cysts, migraine. Regular checks on blood pressure, breasts and pelvic organs.
Avoid use: previous severe arterial or heart disease, benign liver tumours, undiagnosed vaginal bleeding, pregnancy, past ectopic pregnancy. Discontinue immediately for pregnancy, jaundice, thrombophlebitis or thromboembolism.
Possible interaction: griseofulvin, rifampicin, meprobamate, chloral hydrate, carbamazepine, primidone, barbiturates, phenytoin, dichloralphena-zone, ethosuximide, glutethimide.
Side effects: acne, breast discomfort, headache, ovarian cysts, irregular menstrual bleeding.
Manufacturer: Schering H.C.

NORIMIN
Description: a combined oestrogen/progestogen contraceptive containing 35µg ethinyloestradiol and 1mg norethisterone in a peach tablet marked C over 135.
Used for: oral contraception.
Dosage: 1 per day for 21 days, starting on the fifth day of menstruation, then 7 days without tablets.
Special care: hypertension, Raynaud's disease (reduced blood supply to an organ of the body's extremities), asthma, severe depression, diabetes, varicose veins, multiple sclerosis, chronic kidney disease, kidney dialysis. Blood pressure, breasts

and pelvic organs to be checked regularly; smoking not advised.

Avoid use: history of heart disease, infectious hepatitis, sickle cell anaemia, porphyria, liver tumour, undiagnosed vaginal bleeding, pregnancy, hormone-dependent cancer, haemolytic uraemic syndrome (rare kidney disorder), chorea, otosclerosis.

Possible interaction: barbiturates, tetracyclines, griseofulvin, rifampicin, primidone, phenytoin, chloral hydrate, ethosuximide, carbamazepine, glutethimide, dichloralphenazone.

Side effects: fluid retention and bloating, leg cramps/pains, breast enlargement, depression, headaches, nausea, loss of libido, weight gain, vaginal discharge, cervical erosion (alteration of epithelial cells), chloasma (pigmentation of nose, cheeks or forehead), breakthrough bleeding (bleeding between periods).

Manufacturer: Syntex.

NORINYL-1

Description: a combined oestrogen/progestogen contraceptive containing 50μg mestranol and 1mg norethisterone in a white tablet marked NORINYL and SYNTEX.

Used for: oral contraception.

Special care: hypertension, Raynaud's disease (reduced blood supply to an organ of the body's extremities), asthma, severe depression, diabetes, varicose veins, multiple sclerosis, chronic kidney disease, kidney dialysis. Blood pressure, breasts and pelvic organs to be checked regularly; smoking not advised.

Avoid use: history of heart disease, infectious hepatitis, sickle cell anaemia, porphyria, liver tumour, undiagnosed vaginal bleeding, pregnancy, hormone-dependent cancer, haemolytic uraemic syndrome (rare kidney disorder), chorea, otosclerosis.

Possible interaction: barbiturates, tetracyclines, griseofulvin, rifampicin, primidone, phenytoin, chloral hydrate, ethosuximide, carbamazepine, glutethimide, dichloralphenazone.

Side effects: fluid retention and bloating, leg cramps/pains, breast enlargement, depression, headaches, nausea, loss of libido, weight gain, vaginal discharge, cervical erosion (alteration of epithelial cells), chloasma (pigmentation of nose, cheeks or forehead), breakthrough bleeding (bleeding between periods).

Manufacturer: Syntex.

NORISTERAT

Description: a depot progestogen contraceptive, norethisterone oenanthate, available as an oily solution in ampoules containing 200mg/ml

Used for: short-term highly effective contraception irrespective of errors by patient.

Dosage: 200mg by deep intramuscular injection (in gluteal muscle) administered within the first 5 days of the cycle. May be repeated once after 8 weeks.

Special care: liver disorder or diseases that are likely to worsen in pregnancy, severe depression.

Avoid use: acute and severe chronic liver disease, pregnancy, history of thromboembolism, history during pregnancy of itching, idiopathic jaundice or pemphigoid gestationis (skin disorder with large blisters).

Side effects: weight changes, breast discomfort, headache, dizziness, nausea, menstrual changes.

Manufacturer: Schering H.C.

NORMAX

Description: a laxative and faecal softener containing danthron (50mg) and docusate sodium (60mg) in brown capsules marked NORMAX.

Used for: constipation in the elderly, for those with heart failure, coronary thrombosis and constipation induced by analgesics.

Dosage: 1 to 3 tablets at night. Children over 6 years, 1 at night. Not for children under 6 years.

Special care: lactation.

Avoid use: obstruction of the bowel.

Manufacturer: Evans.

NORMEGON

Description: Human menopausal gonadotrophin.
Used for: female or male infertility due to understimulation of the gonads by gonadotrophin. Superovulation for in-vitro fertilization.
Dosage: by intramuscular injection, but see literature.
Special care: exclude other possible causes including gonad abnormalities. Check oestrogen levels and size of ovaries regularly.
Avoid use: ovarian, pituitary or testicular tumours.
Side effects: risk of multiple pregnancy, miscarriage, rash.
Manufacturer: Organon.

NORMISON

Description: an intermediate-acting benzodiazepine, temazepam, available as yellow capsules marked N10 (10mg) and N20 (20mg).
Used for: premedication, short-term treatment of insomnia when sedation during the day is not required.
Dosage: 20–40mg half to 1 hour before surgery (premedication). 10–30mg at bedtime (elderly 10mg), maximum 60mg for severe cases. Not for children.
Special care: chronic liver or kidney disease, chronic lung disease, pregnancy, labour, lactation, elderly. May impair judgement. Withdraw gradually and avoid prolonged use.
Avoid use: depression of respiration, acute lung disease; psychotic, phobic or obsessional states.
Possible interaction: anticonvulsants, depressants of the CNS, alcohol.
Side effects: ataxia, confusion, light-headedness, drowsiness, hypotension, gastro-intestinal upsets, disturbances in vision and libido, skin rashes, retention of urine, vertigo. Sometimes jaundice or blood disorders.
Manufacturer: Wyeth.

NOROXIN

Description: an anti-infective for the eye and a 4-quinolone, norfloxacin, available as 0.3% drops.
Used for: bacterial infections.
Dosage: 1 or 2 drops 4 times per day.
Special care: pregnancy.
Side effects: localized irritation, bitter taste.
Manufacturer: M.S.D.

NORPLANT

Description: a progestogen depot contraceptive, levonorgestrel, available as an implant (228mg) beneath the skin.
Used for: long-term contraception that is reversible.
Dosage: subdermal implant, for those aged 18–40, to be removed within 5 years.
Special care: risk of arterial disease, hypertension, benign intracranial hypertension, migraine. Check blood pressure, breasts and pelvic organs before and during treatment.
Avoid use: thromboembolic disorders, heart disease, liver disease, history of severe arterial disease, pregnancy, undiagnosed vaginal bleeding, hormone-dependent cancer, recent cancer of the uterus.
Possible interaction: phenytoin, primidone, rifampicin, griseofulvin, barbiturates, carbamazepine, phenylbuta-zone, chronic use of tetracyclines.
Side effects: amenorrhoea, ovarian cysts, irregular or extended menstrual bleeding, headache, nausea, weight gain, hirsutism, hair loss, enlargement of related organs.
Manufacturer: Roussel.

NORVAL

Description: a TCAD, mianserin hydrochloride, available as orange tablets in 10, 20 and 30mg strengths, marked with NORVAL and tablet strength.
Used for: depression.
Dosage: 30–40mg per day as 1 dose at night or in divided doses. Increase after

a few days to maintenance levels of 30–90mg per day. Elderly, start no higher than 30mg per day, increase gradually. Not for children.

Special care: elderly, pregnancy, heart block, myocardial infarction, epilepsy, glaucoma, enlarged prostate.

Avoid use: lactation, severe liver disease, mania.

Possible interaction: alcohol, anticoagulants, MAOIs.

Side effects: drowsiness, blood changes. Blood tests advisable monthly for first 3 months. Withdraw if there develops infection, jaundice, convulsions or hypomania.

Manufacturer: Bencard.

NOVA-T

Description: an IUD comprising copper wire with a silver core on a plastic T-shaped carrier.

Used for: contraception.

Special care: diabetes, anaemia, history of endocarditis or pelvic inflammatory disease, epilepsy, hypermenorrhoea (or menorrhagia, long or heavy menstrual periods). Examine after 3 months, then annually

Avoid use: pregnancy, past ectopic pregnancy, uterus disorders, infection of vagina or cervix, acute pelvic inflammatory diseases, cervical cancer, abnormal vaginal bleeding, endometrial disease, immunosuppressive therapy, copper allergy, cancer of the genitalia.

Possible interaction: anticoagulants.

Side effects: pain, pelvic infection, perforation of the uterus, abnormal bleeding. On insertion there may be attack of asthma or epilepsy, bradycardia. Remove if persistent bleeding or cramps, perforation of cervix or uterus, pregnancy, persistent pelvic infection.

Manufacturer: Schering H.C.

NOVAGARD

Description: an IUD comprising copper wire with a silver core on a plastic T-shaped carrier.

Used for: contraception.

Special care: diabetes, anaemia, history of endocarditis or pelvic inflammatory disease, epilepsy, hypermenorrhoea (or menorrhagia, long or heavy menstrual periods). Examine after 3 months, then annually.

Avoid use: pregnancy, past ectopic pregnancy, uterus disorders, infection of vagina or cervix, acute pelvic inflammatory diseases, cervical cancer, abnormal vaginal bleeding, endometrial disease, immunosuppressive therapy, copper allergy, cancer of the genitalia.

Possible interaction: anticoagulants.

Side effects: pain, pelvic infection, perforation of the uterus, abnormal bleeding. *On insertion* there may be attack of asthma or epilepsy, bradycardia. Remove if persistent bleeding or cramps, perforation of cervix or uterus, pregnancy, persistent pelvic infection.

Manufacturer: Kabi Pharmacia

NOVANTRONE

Description: a cytotoxic antibiotic, mitozantrone hydrochloride, available as a solution in vials (2mg/ml).

Used for: treatment of tumours (leukaemia, lymphoma, breast cancer, and solid tumours).

Dosage: by intravenous infusion, see literature.

Special care: check heart after total dose of 160mg/m³ to avoid dose-related cardiotoxicity.

Side effects: suppression of bone marrow, see literature.

Manufacturer: Lederle.

NOXYFLEX

Description: a combined antibacterial and antifungal compound, noxythiolin, available as powder (2.5g) in vials.

Used for: solution to be instilled into bladder or other body cavities.

Dosage: see literature.

Special care: the solution must be freshly prepared and used within 7 days.

Manufacturer: Geistlich.

NOZINAN

Description: a group 1 phenothiazine and antipsychotic, methotrimeprazine, available as white tablets (25mg) marked NOZINAN 25.

Used for: schizophrenia, mental disorders where sedation is needed, control of terminal pain and accompanying vomiting or distress.

Dosage: mental disorders, 25–50mg per day for patients who can walk about, 100–200mg for those who cannot. For pain, 12.5–50mg every 4 to 8 hours. Not for children.

Also, **NOZINAN INJECTION**, 2.5% isotonic solution in ampoules.

Dosage: for pain, 12.5–25mg by intramuscular injection or, after dilution, by intravenous injection, every 6 to 8 hours, up to 50mg for severe cases. Or 25–200mg per day diluted with saline, by continuous subcutaneous infusion. Not for children.

Special care: liver disease, Parkinsonism, epilepsy, cardiovascular disease, pregnancy, lactation.

Avoid use: bone marrow depression (unless terminal), coma.

Possible interaction: alcohol, depressants of the CNS, antihypertensives, antidepressants, analgesics, antidiabetics, levodopa, anticonvulsants.

Side effects: rigidity, tremor, dry mouth, muscle spasms in eye, neck, face and back, tardive dyskinesia (involuntary, repetitive muscle movements in the limbs, face and trunk), tachycardia, constipation, blocked nose, difficulty in urinating, hypotension, weight gain, impotence, galactorrhoea, gynaecomastia, blood changes, jaundice, dermatitis, ECG changes, fatigue, drowsiness, seizures.

Manufacturer: R.P.R.

NUBAIN

Description: an analgesic and opiate, nalbuphine hydrochloride, available as 10mg/ml in ampoules.

Used for: moderate to severe pain. Pain associated with suspected myocardial infarction, pre and post-operative pain.

Dosage: pain, 10–20mg by intravenous, intramuscular or subcutaneous injection. Myocardial infarction, 10–30mg by slow intravenous injection, followed within 30 minutes by 20mg if necessary. Children, starting with up to 0.3mg/kg by intravenous, intramuscular or subcutaneous injection, repeated up to twice if required.

Special care: liver or kidney disease, head injury, pregnancy, labour, respiratory depression, history of opioid abuse.

Possible interaction: depressants of the CNS.

Side effects: sweating, dizziness, dry mouth, nausea, sedation.

Manufacturer: DuPont.

NUELIN SA

Description: a xanthine and bronchodilator, theophylline, available as white sustained-release tablets (175mg) marked NLS175 and 3M.

Used for: bronchitis, emphysema, narrowing of airways in asthma.

Dosage: 1 to 2 tablets twice per day after food. Children over 6 years, 1 tablet twice per day. Not for children under 6.

Also, **NUELIN SA-250**, containing 250mg and marked NLS 250 and 3M.

Dosage: 1 to 2 tablets twice per day after food. Children over 6 years, half the adult dose. Not recommended for children under 6.

Also, **NUELIN** containing 125mg, marked NL over 125 and 3M.

Dosage: 1 to 2 tablets, 3 or 4 times per day, after food. Children aged 7 to 12, half the adult dose. Not for children under 7 years.

Also, **NUELIN LIQUID**, containing 60mg theophylline hydrate (as sodium glycinate) per 5ml.

Dosage: 10–20ml 3 or 4 times per day after food. Children aged 7 to 12, 10ml; aged 2 to 6, 5ml 3 or 4 times per day after food. Not for children under 2 years.

Special care: pregnancy, breastfeeding, heart or liver disease, peptic ulcer.

Possible interaction: B$_2$-agonists, steroids, interferon, erythromycin, diuretics, ciprafloxacin, cimetidine.
Side effects: nausea, gastro-intestinal upset, headache, tachycardia, arrhythmias, insomnia.
Manufacturer: 3M Health Care.

NUVELLE

Description: an oestrogen/progestogen compound available as 16 white tablets containing 2mg oestradiol valerate and 12 pink tablets containing in addition 75µg levonorgestrel.
Used for: post-menopausal osteoporosis, hormone replacement therapy for climacteric syndrome (symptoms associated with the menopause).
Dosage: 1 white tablet per day for 16 days then 12 days of taking 1 pink tablet. Start on fifth day of menses (discharge).
Special care: those at risk of thrombosis or with liver disease. Women with any of the following disorders should be monitored: fibroids in the womb, multiple sclerosis, diabetes, tetany, porphyria, epilepsy, liver disease, hypertension, migraine, otsclerosis, gallstones. Breasts, pelvic organs and blood pressure should be checked at regular intervals during course of treatment.
Avoid use: pregnant women, breastfeeding mothers, women with conditions which might lead to thrombosis, thrombophlebitis, serious heart, kidney or liver disease, breast cancer, oestrogen-dependent cancers including those of reproductive system, endometriosis, vaginal bleeding which is undiagnosed.
Possible interaction: drugs which induce liver enzymes.
Side effects: tenderness and enlargement of breasts, weight gain, breakthrough bleeding, giddiness, vomiting and nausea, gastro-intestinal upset. Treatment should be halted immediately if severe headaches occur, disturbance of vision, hypertension or any indications of thrombosis, jaundice. Also, in the event of pregnancy and 6 weeks before planned surgery.
Manufacturer: Schering H.C.

NYCOPREN

Description: a propionic acid and NSAID, naproxen, available as white, oblong tablets (250 or 500mg strength).
Used for: osteoarthrosis, rheumatoid arthritis, acute gout, ankylosing spondylitis, inflammatory musculoskeletal disorders, juvenile rheumatoid arthritis (JRA).
Dosage: 250–500mg twice per day. Gout, start with 750mg followed by 250mg 8-hourly. Musculoskeletal, 500mg then 250mg 8-hourly. For JRA, over 50kg, 250–500mg twice per day, not recommended for under 50kg.
Special care: elderly, kidney or liver disease, heart failure, history of gastro-intestinal lesions, pregnancy, asthma. Check kidney and liver for long-term treatment.
Avoid use: lactation, allergy to aspirin or anti-inflammatory drugs, active peptic ulcer.
Possible interaction: sulphonamides, sulphonylureas, anticoagulants, quinolones, ß-blockers, lithium, hydantoins, frusemide, methotrexate, probenecid.
Side effects: headache, vertigo, blood changes, tinnitus, rash, gastro-intestinal intolerance.
Manufacturer: Nycomed.

NYSTADERMAL

Description: an antibacterial and potent steroid, nystatin (100,000 units/g) and triamcinolone acetonide (0.1%) available as a cream.
Used for: pruritus and eczema, skin infection and inflammation.
Dosage: apply 2 to 4 times per day.
Special care: thrombophlebitis, psychoses, recent intestinal anastomoses, chronic nephritis, certain cancers, osteoporosis, peptic ulcer, skin eruption/rash related to a disease, viral, fungal or active infections, tuberculosis. Hypertension, glaucoma, epilepsy, acute glomerulonephritis (inflammation of kidney glomerulus), diabetes, cirrhosis, hypo-thyroidism, pregnancy, stress. To be withdrawn gradually.

Possible interaction: NSAIDs, oral anticoagulants, phenytoin, ephedrine, phenobarbitone, rifampicin, diuretics, cardiac glycosides, anticholinesterases, hypoglycaemics.
Side effects: osteoporosis, depression, euphoria, hyperglycaemia, peptic ulcers, Cushingoid changes.
Manufacturer: Squibb.

NYSTAFORM

Description: an antifungal and antibac-terial cream containing 100,000 units of nystatin per gram and 1% chlorhexidine.
Used for: skin infections.
Dosage: apply liberally 2 to 3 times per day until 1 week after healing.
Manufacturer: Bayer.

NYSTAFORM-HC

Description: an antifungal and mildly potent steroid containing 100,000 units of nystatin per gram, 1% chlorhexidine, and 0.5% hydrocortisone available as a cream. Also, **NYSTAFORM-HC OINTMENT** containing 100,000 units of nystatin, 1% chlorhexidine and 1% hydrocortisone.
Used for: skin disorders where there is infection.
Dosage: apply 2 or 3 times per day until 1 week after healing.
Special care: thrombophlebitis, psychoses, recent intestinal anastomoses, chronic nephritis, certain cancers, osteoporosis, peptic ulcer, skin eruption/rash related to a disease, viral, fungal or active infections, tuberculosis. Hypertension, glaucoma, epilepsy, acute glomerulonephritis (inflam-mation of kidney glomerulus), diabetes, cirrhosis, hypothyroidism, pregnancy, stress. To be withdrawn gradually.
Possible interaction: NSAIDs, oral anticoagulants, phenytoin, ephedrine, phenobarbitone, rifampicin, diuretics, anticholinesterases, cardiac glycosides, hypoglycaemics.
Side effects: osteoporosis, depression, euphoria, hyperglycaemia, peptic ulcers, Cushingoid changes.
Manufacturer: Bayer.

NYSTAN

Description: an antibiotic containing 500,000 units of nystatin, available as brown tablets.
Used for: intestinal infection with *Candida*.
Dosage: 1 to 2 tablets 4 times per day. Children should take the suspension. Also, **NYSTAN ORAL SUSPENSION** containing 100,000 units nystatin/ml in a ready-mixed suspension. Also, **NYSTAN FOR SUSPENSION** which in addition is free of lactose, sugar and corn starch.
Used for: infections (candidiasis) of the mouth, oesophagus and intestines.
Dosage: 1ml 4 times per day for oral infections, 5ml 4 times per day for infection of the intestines. Children, 1ml 4 times per day. Prevention in infants under 1 month, 1ml per day. For oral infections the suspension should be retained in the mouth. Continue for 2 days after cure. Also, **NYSTAN PASTILLES** containing 100,000 units nystatin per pastille.
Used for: oral infections.
Dosage: 1 pastille sucked slowly 4 times per day for 7 to 14 days.
Side effects: nausea, vomiting and diarrhoea with high doses.
Also, **NYSTAN** as 100,000 units of nystatin in yellow, diamond-shaped pessaries, marked SQUIBB 457; **NYSTAN VAGINAL CREAM** (100,000 units/4g); **NYSTAN GEL** (100,000 units/ g); and **NYSTAN ORAL TABLETS** (500,000 units in brown tablets).
Used for: candidal vaginitis (vaginal infection caused by *Candida*, thrush).
Dosage: 1 to 2 pessaries or 1 to 2 applications of cream for 14 or more consecutive nights; irrespective of menstruation. Gel; applied topically to anogenital region 2 to 4 times per day for 14 days. Oral treatment, 1 tablet 4 times per day during vaginal treatment. Children use vaginal cream with oral treatment.
Side effects: temporary burning and irritation.

Also **NYSTAN** as cream, ointment and gel (100,000 units nystatin per gram).
Used for: thrush of the skin and mucous membranes.
Dosage: apply 2 to 4 times per day.
Manufacturer: Squibb.

OCUFEN

Description: an NSAID which is a proprionic acid available in the form of eyedrops containing 0.03% flubiprofen sodium.
Used for: to inhibit inflammation and constriction of the pupil (miosis) during operations of the eye.
Dosage: as directed by physician.
Manufacturer: Allergan.

OCUSERT PILO

Description: a cholinergic eye preparation containing pilocarpine 20 available as elliptical-shaped sustained-release inserts delivering 40 micrograms/hour for a 1 week period.
Used for: glaucoma.
Dosage: place 1 insert under eyelid and replace each week.
Avoid use: patients with severe inflammation or infecion.
Side effects: eye irritation, loss of sharpness of vision.
Manufacturer: Cusi.

ODRIK

Description: an ACE inhibitor available as capsules of 3 strengths all containing randolapril. Yellow/red capsules contain 0.5mg; orange/red contain 1mg; red/red contain 2mg.
Used for: hypertension.
Dosage: 0.5mg once each day at first increasing every 2 to 4 weeks to a maximum 4mg as a single daily dose. Maintenance dose is in the order of 1–2mg

once each day. Any diuretics being taken should be discontinued 2 or 3 days before treatment starts.
Special care: liver or kidney disease, receiving kidney dialysis, undergoing anaesthesia or surgery, congestive heart failure. Also, patients with low fluid and salt levels.
Avoid use: pregnancy, breastfeeding, obstruction of blood outflow from heart or aortic stenosis (narrowing of aorta). Also, angioneurotic oedema due to previous treatment with an ACE inhibitor.
Possible interaction: NSAIDs, potassium-sparing diuretics.
Side effects: rash, cough, muscular weakness, headache, dizziness, palpitations, hypotension. Rarely, agranulocytosis (a blood disorder characterized by abnormal reduction in number of white blood cells (granulocytes), angioneurotic oedema, depression of bone marrow.
Manufacturer: Roussel.

OLBETAM

Description: a lipid-lowering nicotinic acid derivative available as pink/red-brown capsules containing 250mg acipimox marked with name.
Used for: raised protein-bound lipid levels in blood (hyperlipoproteinaemia) of type IIa, IIb and IV.
Dosage: adults, 2 or 3 tablets each day taken as divided doses with meals. Maximum dosage is 1200mg each day.
Avoid use: pregnancy, breastfeeding, children, patients with peptic ulcer.
Side effects: gastro-intestinal upset, flushing, headache, inflammation of skin and mucous membranes (erythema), malaise, skin rash.
Manufacturer: Pharmacia.

OMNOPON^{CD}

Description: an analgesic, opiate available as a solution in ampoules for injection containing 15.4mg papaveretum/ml.
Used for: severe pain.
Dosage: adults, 0.5–1ml given by sub-cutaneous, intravenous or intramuscular

injection. Dose may be repeated after 4 hours. Children, under 1 year, 0.0075–0.01ml/kg body weight each day. Over 1 year, 0.01–0.015ml/kg. All given by subcutaneous, intravenous or intramuscular injection as a maximum single dose. Elderly, 0.5ml at first by same route.

Special care: pregnancy, breastfeeding, elderly persons, newborn babies, patients with enlarged prostate gland, underactive thyroid gland, serious liver or kidney disease, having head injury.

Possible interaction: alcohol, phenothiazines, MAOIs, CNS depressants.

Side effects: drug dependence and tolerance, constipation, nausea, constipation.

Manufacturer: Roche.

ONCOVIN

Description: a cytotoxic vinca alkaloid drug produced as a solution in vials for injection containing 1mg vincristine sulphate/ml.

Used for: lymphomas, leukaemia, some solid tumours (e.g. lung and breast cancer).

Dosage: by intravenous injection as directed by physician skilled in cancer chemotherapy.

Special care: care in handling, contact with eyes must be avoided, tissue irritant.

Avoid use: must not be given by intrathecal injection (i.e. into meninges (membrane linings) of the spinal cord).

Side effects: damage to peripheral and autonomic nervous system characterized by muscle weakness and abdominal bloating. Hair loss, vomiting, nausea.

Manufacturer: Lilly.

ONE-ALPHA

Description: a vitamin D analogue, alfacalcidol, available as capsules in 2 strengths; white capsules contain 0.25μg and brown capsules contain 1μg.

ALPHA SOLUTION containing 0.2μg/ml and also **ONE-ALPHA INJECTION** in ampoules containing 2μg/ml.

Used for: bone disorders due to kidney disease or loss of function, bone disease

associated with under or overactivity of parathyroid glands, low calcium levels in newborn babies. Also, rickets and osteomalacia (bone softening).

Dosage: 1μg at first adjusted according to response; children, under 20kg, 0.05μg/kg body weight each day at first; over 20kg, 1μg daily. Injection is given intravenously.

Special care: pregnancy, breastfeeding, kidney failure. Levels of blood calcium must be checked at regular intervals during the course of treatment.

Possible interaction: thiazide diuretics, colestipol, digitalis, barbiturates, antacids, cholestyramine, anticonvulsants, sucralfate, danazol, mineral oils, antacids.

Manufacturer: Leo.

OPERIDINE^{CD}

Description: a narcotic analgesic which is a controlled drug available as a solution in ampoules for injection containing 1mg phenoperidine hydrochloride/ml.

Used for: enhancement of anaesthetics and analgesia during surgery; as a depressant of respiration (especially doses above 1mg) in patients receiving long-term assisted ventilation.

Dosage: up to 1mg by intravenous injection then 500 μg every 40 to 60 minutes as needed. With assisted ventilation, 2–5mg then 1mg as needed. Children, 30–50μg/kg body weight. With assisted ventilation, 100–150μg/kg. Elderly persons receive lower doses.

Special care: myasthenia gravis, serious respiratory or liver disease, underactive thyroid. If used in obstetrics, may cause depression of respiration in baby.

Avoid use: obstructive airways disease or depression of respiration (unless being mechanically ventilated).

Possible interaction: MAOIs, cimetidine.

Side effects: convulsions with high doses, respiratory depression, nausea, vomiting, bradycardia, hypotension which is short-lived.

Manufacturer: Janssen.

OPTHAINE

Description: local anaesthetic eyedrops containing 0.5% proxymetacaine hydrochloride.

Used for: as local anaesthetic during ophthalmic procedures.

Dosage: usual dose, 1 or 2 drops before procedure begins. Protect eye.

Side effects: irritation of eye and, rarely, hypersensitive allergic reactions.

Manufacturer: Squibb.

OPILON

Description: a selective alpha₁-blocker available as film-coated, pale yellow tablets containing 40mg thymoxamine as hydrochloride.

Used for: short-term treatment of Raynaud's disease (a disease affecting the arteries of the fingers which makes them liable to spasm when the hands are cold).

Dosage: 1 tablet 4 times each day increasing to 2 tablets 4 times each day if condition does not respond. If no significant improvement after 2 weeks, drug should be withdrawn.

Special care: angina, recent heart attack, diabetes.

Avoid use: pregnancy, breastfeeding, known hypersensitivity to thymoxamine.

Possible interaction: diarrhoea, nausea, headache, vertigo. Drug should be withdrawn if liver function is affected.

Manufacturer: Parke-Davis.

OPTICROM

Description: an NSAID preparation available in the form of eyedrops containing 2% sodium cromoglycate. Also, OPTICROM EYE OINTMENT containing 4% sodium cromoglycate.

Used for: allergic conjunctivitis.

Dosage: 1 or 2 drops in both eyes 4 times each day, or ointment 3 times daily.

Avoid use: drops, patients wearing soft contact lenses; ointment, all types of contact lenses.

Side effects: burning, stinging sensation in eye which is of short-lived duration.

Manufacturer: Fisons.

ORAMORPH

Description: an analgesic opiate preparation available in a variety of different forms, all containing morphine sulphate. ORAMORPH SR are sustained-release, film-coated tablets of different strengths: 10mg buff tablets; 30mg purple tablets; 60mg orange tablets; 100mg grey tablets. All are marked with strength. ORAMORPH SOLUTION contains 10mg morphine sulphate/5ml in a sugar-containing solution. ORAMORPH UNIT DOSE is a sugar-free solution in single dose vials containing 10mg, 30mg or 100mg morphine sulphate/5ml. ORAMORPH CONCENTRATE is a sugar-free solution containing 100mg morphine sulphate/5ml.

Used for: severe pain.

Dosage: Oramorph SR, 10–20mg every 12 hours at first, increasing as needed. Other preparations, 10–20mg at 4 hourly intervals. Children, all preparations except Oramorph SR, age 1 to 5 years, up to 5mg; 6 to 12 years, 5–10mg, both every 4 hours.

Special care: elderly, breastfeeding, underactivity of thyroid gland, reduced function of adrenal glands, enlarged prostate gland, liver or kidney disease, shock, after surgery.

Avoid use: pregnancy, children under 1 year, obstructive airways disease, disorders characterized by convulsions, depressed respiration, head injuries, coma, severe liver disease, severe alcoholism, raised intracranial pressure.

Possible interaction: central nervous system depressants, MAOIs.

Side effects: vomiting and nausea, constipation, sedation, drug dependence and tolerance.

Manufacturer: Boehringer Ingelheim.

ORAP

Description: an antipsychotic drug, pimozide, which is a diphenylbutylpipe-ridine available as tablets in 3 strengths: scored, white tablets contain 2mg, marked on 1 side with O/2; scored green

tablets contain 4mg, marked on 1 side with O/4. Scored, white tablets contain 10mg, marked 1 side with O/10. On the other side all are marked JANSSEN.
Used for: schizophrenia.
Dosage: adults, 10mg each day at first increasing by 2–4mg daily at weekly intervals. Maximum daily dose is 20mg. To prevent a relapse, 2mg each day. Usual daily dose is in the order of 2–20mg.
Special care: pregnancy, imbalance in electrolyte (salts) levels, liver or kidney disorder, epilepsy, Parkinsonism, endogenous depression (resulting from factors within the body). ECG should be carried out before and during the course of treatment. Patients require careful monitoring.
Avoid use: children, breastfeeding, patients with a very long QT interval (part of the ECG) which can result in a potentially fatal type of tachycardia, history of heart arrhythmias.
Possible interaction: analgesics, levodopa, CNS depressants, antidiabetic drugs, alcohol, antidepressants, antihypertensives, anticonvulsants, some heart drugs and antipsychotics.
Side effects: extrapyramidal effects (characterized by involuntary and reflex muscle movements), apathy, sleepiness, disturbance of sleep, depression. Blocked nose, dry mouth, constipation, blurring of vision, tachycardia, heart arrhythmias, hypotension, changes in EEG and ECG. Changes in breasts and menstrual cycle, weight gain, impotence. Blood and liver changes, jaundice, rash, pigmentation of skin and eyes, sensitivity to light, haemolytic anaemia, difficulty in urination.
Manufacturer: Janssen.

ORBENIN

Description: an antibiotic penicillin which is penicillinase-resistant (i.e. resistant to the penicillinase enzymes produced by certain bacteria). Available as orange/black capsules containing 250mg or 500mg cloxacillin (as sodium salt) and marked with strength and name. Also

ORBENIN INJECTION, available in vials containing 250mg and 500mg cloxacillin.
Used for: infections caused by Gram-positive bacteria including resistant staphylococci.
Dosage: tablets, 500mg every 6 hours taken half an hour to an hour before meals; injection, 250mg intramuscularly or 500mg intravenously every 4 to 6 hours. Children, over 2 years, half adult dose.
Avoid use: children under 2 years.
Side effects: gastro-intestinal upset, allergic responses, rash.
Manufacturer: Forley.

ORELOX

Description: a cephalosporin antibiotic available as film-coated white tablets containing 100mg cefpodoxime (as proxetil) marked 208A.
Used for: bronchitis, tonsilitis, pharyngitis, pneumonia, sinusitis.
Dosage: adults, 1 or 2 tablets (depending upon infection) twice each day taken with a meal in the morning and evening.
Special care: pregnancy, sensitivity to beta-lactam antibiotics, kidney disorders.
Avoid use: children.
Possible interaction: H_2 antagonists, antacids.
Side effects: headache, gastro-intestinal upset, allergic responses, raised liver enzymes, colitis.
Manufacturer: Roussel.

ORGARAN

Description: an antithrombotic heparinoid preparation produced as a solution in ampoules for injection, containing 1250 units danaparoid sodium antifactor Xa activity/ml.
Used for: prevention of deep vein thrombosis in patients undergoing surgery.
Dosage: adults, 0.6ml by subcutaneous injection twice each day for 7 to 10 days before operation. The last dose should be given not less than 1 hour before surgery.
Special care: patients with ulcer, liver or kidney disorder, asthma, history of

heparin-induced thrombocytopenia who test positive to danaparoid.
Avoid use: pregnancy, breastfeeding, children, bleeding disorders, stroke with haemorrhage, peptic ulcer, serious liver or kidney disease, bacterial endocarditis, serious hypertension, retinopathy (disorder of the blood vessels of the retina of the eye) associated with diabetes.
Side effects: risk of haemorrhage, skin rash, haematoma, bruising. Also, changes in liver enzymes, thrombocytopenia.
Manufacturer: Organon Teknika.

ORIMETEN

Description: an anti-cancer drug which inhibits steroid synthesis produced in the form of scored, off-white tablets containing 250mg aminoglutethimide marked GG and CG.
Used for: advanced breast cancer in post-menopausal women or those whose ovaries have been removed. Also, advanced prostate cancer and Cushing's syndrome resulting from malignancy.
Dosage: cancer, 1 tablet each day increasing by 1 tablet daily each week. Maximum daily dose is 4 tablets for breast cancer and 3 for prostate cancer. Cushing's syndrome, 1 each day slowly increasing if required to 4 daily in divided doses. Maximum dose is 8 tablets daily.
Special care: regular monitoring of electrolytes and blood counts is required. Patients with breast or prostate cancer require glucocorticoids (adrenal gland hormones) and these may also be needed by those with Cushing's syndrome. Also, mineralocorticoids (adrenal gland hormones) may be needeed.
Avoid use: pregnancy, breastfeeding.
Possible interaction: synthetic glucocorticoids, anticoagulants, hypoglycaemics taken orally.
Side effects: gastro-intestinal upset, blood changes, effects on CNS, rash, thyroid disorders. If allergic alveolitis (inflammation of the air sacs, alveoli, of the lungs) occurs, the drug should be withdrawn.
Manufacturer: Ciba.

ORTHO DIENOESTROL

Description: an hormonal oestrogen preparation available in the form of a vaginal cream with applicator containing 0.01% dienoestrol.
Used for: inflammaion and irritation of the vagina and vulva, atrophic vaginitis.
Dosage: 1 or 2 applicator doses into the vagina each day for 1 to 2 weeks, then reducing to half the initial dose for a further 1 or 2 weeks. Maintenance is 1 applicator dose 1, 2 or 3 times each week.
Special care: patients considered at risk of thromboembolism, porphyria, multiple sclerosis, epilepsy, fibroids in the womb, migraine, tetany. Also, patients with otosclerosis, gallstones, liver disease. Pelvic organs, breasts and blood pressure should be checked regularly during treatment.
Avoid use: pregnancy, breastfeeding, breast or other cancer of reproductive tract or one which is hormone-dependent. Also, thromboembolism-type disorders, undiagnosed vaginal bleeding or endometriosis, thrombophlebitis, heart, liver or kidney disease. Rotor or Dublin-Johnson syndrome.
Possible interaction: drugs which induce liver enzymes.
Side effects: enlargement and soreness of breasts, gastro-intestinal upset, dizziness, breakthrough bleeding, headache, vomiting and nausea, weight gain.
Manufacturer: Ortho.

ORTHO-GYNEST

Description: an hormonal oestrogen preparation available as vaginal pessaries containing 0.5mg oestriol. Also, **ORTHO-GYNEST CREAM** containing 0.01% oestriol, with applicator.
Used for: vaginal, vulval and cervical inflammation and disorders in post-menopausal women; atrophic vaginitis.
Dosage: 1 pessary or applicator dose inserted high up into the vagina at night. Maintenance is 1 pessary or applicator dose each week.
Special care: patients considered at risk

of thromboembolism, porphyria, multiple sclerosis, epilepsy, fibroids in the womb, migraine, tetany. Also, otosclerosis, gallstones, liver disease. Pelvic organs, breasts and blood pressure should be checked regularly during course of treatment.

Avoid use: pregnancy, breastfeeding, breast or other cancer of reproductive tract or one which is hormone-dependent. Also, patients with thromboembolism-type disorders, undiagnosed vaginal bleeding or endometriosis, thrombophlebitis, heart, liver or kidney disease. Rotor or Dublin-Johnson syndrome.

Possible interaction: drugs which induce liver enzymes.

Side effects: enlargement and soreness of breasts, gastro-intestinal upset, dizziness, breakthrough bleeding, headache, vomiting and nausea, weight gain.

Manufacturer: Ortho.

ORTHO-NAVIN 1/50

Description: an hormonal combined oestrogen/progestogen preparation available as white tablets containing 50µg mestranol and 1mg norethisterone marked C over 50.

Used for: oral contraception.

Dosage: 1 tablet each day for 21 days starting on the fifth day of period followed by 7 tablet-free days.

Special care: patients with multiple sclerosis, serious kidney disease or kidney dialysis, asthma, Raynaud's disease, abnormally high levels of prolactin in the blood (hyperprolactinae-mia), varicose veins, hypertension. Also, patients suffering from severe depression. Thrombosis risk increases with smoking, age and obesity. During the course of treatment, regular checks on blood pressure, pelvic organs and breasts should be carried out.

Avoid use: pregnancy, patients considered to be at risk of thrombosis, suffering from heart disease, pulmonary hypertension, angina, sickle cell

anaemia. Also, undiagnosed vaginal bleeding, history of cholestatic jaundice during pregnancy, cancers which are hormone-dependent, infectious hepatitis, liver disorders. Also, porphyria, Dublin-Johnson and Rotor syndrome, otosclerosis, chorea, haemolytic uraemic syndrome, recent trophoblastic disease.

Possible interaction: barbiturates, ethosuximide, glutethimide, rifampicin, phenytoin, tetracyclines, carbamazepine, chloral hydrate, griseofulvin, dichloral-phenazone, primidone.

Side effects: weight gain, breast enlargement, pains in legs and cramps, headaches, loss of sexual desire, depression, nausea, breakthrough bleeding, cervical erosion, brownish patches on skin (chloasma), vaginal discharge, oedema and bloatedness.

Manufacturer: Ortho.

ORUDIS

Description: an NSAID which is a propionic acid available as capsules in 2 strengths both containing ketoprofen. Purple/green capsules and pink capsules contain 50mg and 100mg respectively, both marked with strength and name. Also, **ORUDIS SUPPOSITORIES** containing 100mg.

Used for: musculo-skeletal disorders, including osteoarthritis, rheumatoid arthritis, joint disorders, ankylosing spondylitis, gout, pain following orthopaedic surgery, dysmenorrhoea (period pain).

Dosage: adults, capsules, 50–100mg twice daily with meals; suppositories, 1 at night with capsules taken during the day, if needed.

Special care: pregnancy, elderly, heart failure, liver or kidney disorders. Patients taking the drug long-term should receive careful monitoring.

Avoid use: children, patients with known allergy to aspirin or NSAID, history of or active stomach ulcer, asthma, serious kidney disease, recent proctitis (inflammation of rectum and anus).

Possible interaction: hydantoins, anticoagulants, sulphonamides, high doses of methotrexate, quinolones.
Side effects: rash, gastro-intestinal upset.
Manufacturer: R.P.R.

ORUVAIL

Description: an NSAID which is a propionic acid available as capsules in 3 strengths all containing ketoprofen. Purple/pink, pink/pink and pink/white capsules contain 100mg, 150mg and 200mg respectively. All are continuous-release and marked with strength and name. Also, **ORUVAIL INJECTION** available as a solution in ampoules containing 50mg/ml.
Used for: musculo-skeletal disorders including osteoarthritis, rheumatoid arthritis, joint disorders, ankylosing spondylitis, gout, pain following orthopaedic surgery, dysmenorrhoea (period pain).
Dosage: capsules, 100–200mg once each day with meal; injection, 50–100mg every 4 hours by deep intramuscular injection. Maximum dose is 200mg each day for 3 days.
Special care: pregnancy, elderly, liver or kidney disease, heart failure.
Avoid use: children, known allergy to NSAID or aspirin, history of or active stomach ulcer, asthma, serious kidney disease.
Possible interaction: hydantoins, anticoagulants, quinolones, high doses methotrexate, sulphonamides.
Side effects: rash, gastro-intestinal upset.
Manufacturer: R.P.R.

ORUVAIL GEL

Description: an NSAID which is a propionic acid available in the form of a gel containing 2.5% ketoprofen.
Used for: sports injuries, strains, sprains, bruises, etc.
Dosage: adults, 15g each day in 2 to 4 divided doses for up to 1 week; massage affected area after applying gel.
Special care: pregnancy, avoid mucous membranes, eyes and broken skin.

Avoid use: breastfeeding, patients with known allergy to NSAID or aspirin, history of asthma.
Side effects: slight local irritation of skin.
Manufacturer: R.P.R.

OTOMIZE

Description: a combined antibiotic and corticosteroid preparation available in the form of a suspension for use with a pump action spray. The solution contains 0.1% dexamethasone, 2% acetic acid and 3250 units neomycin/ml.
Used for: inflammation of external ear.
Dosage: 1 metered dose 3 times each day continuing for 2 days after condition has cleared.
Special care: pregnant women, patients with perforated ear drum.
Side effects: stinging or burning which is short-lived.
Manufacturer: Stafford-Miller.

OTOSPORIN

Description: a combined antibiotic and corticosteroid preparation available in the form of ear drops containing 10,000 units polymixin B sulphate, 3400 units neomycin sulphate and 1% hydrocortisone.
Used for: inflammation and bacterial infections of outer ear.
Dosage: 3 drops 3 or 4 times each day or insert wick soaked in solution which is kept wet.
Special care: avoid long-term use in infants.
Avoid use: perforated eardrum.
Side effects: superinfection.
Manufacturer: Wellcome.

OVESTIN

Description: an hormonal oestrogen preparation available as white tablets containing 1.0mg oestriol coded DG7, ORGANON and with *. Also, **OVESTIN CREAM** with applicator containing 0.1% oestriol.
Used for: tablets, disorders of genital and urinary tract arising from infections when oestrogen is deficient. Cream,

atrophic vaginitis, itching, dryness and atrophy of vulva in elderly women. Treatment of this area before vaginal operations.
Dosage: tablets, 0.5–3mg each day for 4 weeks then 0.5–1mg daily. Cream, 1 applicator dose into vagina each day for 3 weeks with a maintenance dose of 1 applicatorful twice weekly.
Special care: patients considered at risk of thromboembolism, porphyria, multiple sclerosis, epilepsy, fibroids in the womb, migraine, tetany. Also, patients with otosclerosis, gallstones, liver disease. Pelvic organs, breasts and blood pressure should be checked regularly during the course of treatment.
Avoid use: pregnancy, breastfeeding, patients with breast or other cancer of reproductive tract or one which is hormone-dependent. Also, patients with thromboembolism-type disorders, undiagnosed vaginal bleeding or endometriosis, thrombophlebitis, heart, liver or kidney disease. Rotor or Dublin-Johnson syndrome.
Possible interaction: drugs which induce liver enzymes.
Side effects: enlargement and soreness of breasts, gastro-intestinal upset, dizziness, breakthrough bleeding, headache, vomiting and nausea, weight gain.
Manufacturer: Organon.

OVRAN

Description: an hormonal combined oestrogen/progestogen preparation available as white tablets containing 50µg ethinyloestradiol and 250µg levonorgestrel. Also, **OVRAN 30**, white tablets containing 30µg ethinyloestradiol and 250µg levonorgestrel. Both are marked WYETH.
Used for: oral contraception.
Dosage: 1 tablet each day for 21 days starting on first day of period followed by 7 tablet-free days.
Special care: patients with multiple sclerosis, serious kidney disease or kidney dialysis, asthma, Raynaud's disease,

abnormally high levels of prolactin in the blood (hyperprolactinaemia), varicose veins, hypertension. Also, patients suffering from severe depression. Thrombosis risk increases with smoking, age and obesity. During the course of treatment, regular checks on blood pressure, pelvic organs and breasts should be carried out.
Avoid use: pregnancy, patients considered to be at risk of thrombosis, suffering from heart disease, pulmonary hypertension, angina, sickle cell anaemia. Also, undiagnosed vaginal bleeding, history of cholestatic jaundice during pregnancy, cancers which are hormone-dependent, infectious hepatitis, liver disorders. Also, porphyria, Dublin-Johnson and Rotor syndrome, otosclerosis, chorea, haemolytic uraemic syndrome, recent trophoblastic disease.
Possible interaction: barbiturates, ethosuximide, glutethimide, rifampicin, phenytoin, tetracyclines, carbamazepine, chloral hydrate, griseofulvin, dichloral-phenazone, primidone.
Side effects: weight gain, breast enlargement, pains in legs and cramps, headaches, loss of sexual desire, depression, nausea, breakthrough bleeding, cervical erosion, brownish patches on skin (chloasma), vaginal discharge, oedema and bloatedness.
Manufacturer: Wyeth.

OVRANETTE

Description: an hormonal combined oestrogen/progestogen preparation, available as white tablets containing 30µg ethinyloestradiol and 150µg levonorgestrel, marked WYETH and 30.
Used for: oral contraception.
Dosage: 1 tablet each day for 21 days starting on first day of period followed by 7 tablet-free days.
Special care: patients with multiple sclerosis, serious kidney disease or kidney dialysis, asthma, Raynaud's disease, abnormally high levels of prolactin in the blood (hyperprolactinaemia),

varicose veins, hypertension. Also, patients suffering from severe depression. Thrombosis risk increases with smoking, age and obesity. During the course of treatment, regular checks on blood pressure, pelvic organs and breasts should be carried out.

Avoid use: pregnancy, patients considered to be at risk of thrombosis, suffering from heart disease, pulmonary hypertension, angina, sickle cell anaemia. Also, undiagnosed vaginal bleeding, history of cholestatic jaundice during pregnancy, cancers which are hormone-dependent, infectious hepatitis, liver disorders. Also, porphyria, Dublin-Johnson and Rotor syndrome, otosclerosis, chorea, haemolytic uraemic syndrome, recent trophoblastic disease.

Possible interaction: barbiturates, ethosuximide, glutethimide, rifampicin, phenytoin, tetracyclines, carbamazepine, chloral hydrate, griseofulvin, dichloralphenazone, primidone.

Side effects: weight gain, breast enlargement, pains in legs and cramps, headaches, loss of sexual desire, depression, nausea, breakthrough bleeding, cervical erosion, brownish patches on skin (chloasma), vaginal discharge, oedema and bloatedness.

Manufacturer: Wyeth.

OVYSMEN

Description: an hormonal combined oestrogen/progestogen preparation available as white tablets containing 35µg ethinyloestradiol and 500µg norethisterone marked C over 535.

Used for: oral contraception.

Dosage: 1 tablet each day for 21 days starting on fifth day of period followed by 7 tablet-free days.

Special care: patients with multiple sclerosis, serious kidney disease or kidney dialysis, asthma, Raynaud's disease, abnormally high levels of prolactin in the blood (hyperprolactinaemia), varicose veins, hypertension. Also, patients suffering from severe depression.

Thrombosis risk increases with smoking, age and obesity. During the course of treatment, regular checks on blood pressure, pelvic organs and breasts should be carried out.

Avoid use: pregnancy, patients considered to be at risk of thrombosis, suffering from heart disease, pulmonary hypertension, angina, sickle cell anaemia. Also, undiagnosed vaginal bleeding, history of cholestatic jaundice during pregnancy, cancers which are hormone-dependent, infectious hepatitis, liver disorders. Also, porphyria, Dublin-Johnson and Rotor syndrome, otosclerosis, chorea, haemolytic uraemic syndrome, recent trophoblastic disease.

Possible interaction: barbiturates, ethosuximide, glutethimide, rifampicin, phenytoin, tetracyclines, carbamazepine, chloral hydrate, griseofulvin, dichloralphenazone, primidone.

Side effects: weight gain, breast enlargement, pains in legs and cramps, headaches, loss of sexual desire, depression, nausea, breakthrough bleeding, cervical erosion, brownish patches on skin (chloasma), vaginal discharge, oedema and bloatedness.

Manufacturer: Ortho.

OXAZEPAM

Description: an anxiolytic drug and intermediate-acting benzodiazepine available as tablets in 3 strengths containing 10mg, 15mg and 30mg oxazepam.

Used for: anxiety.

Dosage: 15–30mg 3 or 4 times each day increasing to 60mg 3 times daily if exceptionally severe. Elderly persons take reduced dose of 10–20mg 3 to 4 times each day.

Special care: chronic liver or kidney disease, chronic lung disease, pregnancy, labour, lactation, elderly. May impair judgement. Withdraw gradually and avoid prolonged use.

Avoid use: depression of respiration, acute lung disease; psychotic, phobic or obsessional states.

Possible interaction: anticonvulsants, depressants of the CNS, alcohol.
Side effects: ataxia, confusion, light-headedness, drowsiness, hypotension, gastro-intestinal upsets, disturbances in vision and libido, skin rashes, retention of urine, vertigo. Sometimes jaundice or blood disorders.
Manufacturer: non-proprietary but available from APS, Berk, Cox, Kerfoot, Norton, Wyeth.

OXIVENT

Description: an anticholinergic broncho-dilator delivering 100μg oxitropium bromide per dose by metered dose inhaler. Also, **OXIVENT AUTOHALER** delivering 100μg oxitropium bromide per dose by breath-actuated metered dose aerosol.
Used for: obstructive lung disease, asthma.
Dosage: adults, 2 puffs 2 or 3 times each day.
Special care: avoid eyes, patients with enlarged prostate gland, glaucoma.
Avoid use: pregnancy, breastfeeding, children, allergy to ipratropium bromide or atropine.
Side effects: dry mouth, nausea, irritation of throat, anticholinergic effects. If cough or wheezing develops, drug should be withdrawn.
Manufacturer: Boehringer Ingelheim.

PABRINEX

Description: a combined preparation of vitamins B and C in paired ampoules for both intravenous and intramuscular injection. Pairs of intravenous ampoules contain 250mg thiamine hydrochloride, 4mg riboflavine, 50mg pyridoxine hydrochloride, 160mg nicotinamide, 500mg ascorbic acid and 1g anhydrous dextrose. Pairs of intramuscular

ampoules contain the same but without anhydrous dextrose.
Used for: severe deficiencies in vitamin B and C when oral doses cannot be taken or are not adequate.
Dosage: by intravenous injection (over 10 minutes) or infusion, 2 to 4 pairs of ampoules every 4 to 8 hours for up to 2 days. Then 1 pair of intramuscular ampoules by intramuscular injection or 1 pair of intravenous ampoules by intravenous injection or infusion once each day for 5 to 7 days.
Special care: anaphylaxis may occur hence treatment should only be given when it is essential and facilities for resuscitation must be available.
Possible interaction: levodopa.
Side effects: anaphylaxis.
Manufacturer: Link.

PALFIUM^{CD}

Description: an analgesic opiate preparation which is a controlled drug available as scored, white tablets containing 5mg dextromoramide and scored peach tablets containing 10mg dextromoramide. Also, **PALFIUM SUPPOSITORIES** containinng 10mg dextromoramide astartrate.
Used for: severe, intractable pain.
Dosage: tablets, up to 5mg at first then adjusted according to response. Suppositories, 1 as required. Children, 80 μg/kg body weight.
Special care: pregnancy, elderly, underactive thyroid gland, liver disorders.
Avoid use: women in labour, patients with obstructed airways and depression of respiration.
Possible interaction: CNS depressants, MAOIs.
Side effects: sweating, nausea dependence and tolerance.
Manufacturer: B.M. Pharm.

PAMERGAN P100^{CD}

Description: a narcotic analgesic and sedative available in ampoules for injection containing 100mg pethidine hydrochloride and 50mg promethazine hydrochloride/2ml.

Used for: relief of pain in labour, pain during and after operations, pre-medication enhancement of anaesthesia.

Dosage: labour and severe pain, 1–2ml every 4 hours by intramuscular injection if necessary; pre-medication, 25–200mg by intramuscular injection 1 hour before surgery; enhancement of anaesthesia (with nitrous oxide), 10–25mg by slow intravenous injection. Children, pre-medication, age 8 to 12 years, 0.75ml; 13 to 16 years, 1ml all by intramuscular injection.

Special care: pregnancy, breastfeeding. Elderly and debilitated persons should receive reduced doses. Also, liver disorders, asthma, respiratory depression, hypotension, underactivity of thyroid gland. If patient is terminally ill, the benefits may be considered to outweigh any risk.

Avoid use: patients with serious kidney disorders, head injury or raised intracranial pressure.

Possible interaction: MAOIs, cimetidine, anxiolytics and hypnotics.

Side effects: convulsions with high doses, vomiting, nausea, constipation, drowsiness, difficulty passing urine, depression of respiration, hypotension, sweating, dry mouth, flushing palpitations, bradycardia, urticaria, rash, itching, miosis (constriction of pupil of the eye), vertigo. Hallucinations and mood swings.

Manufacturer: Martindale.

PARAMAX

Description: an NSAID combining an analgesic and anti-emetic preparation available as scored, white tablets containing 500mg paracetamol and 5mg metaclopramide hydrochloride, marked PARAMAX. Also **PARAMAX SACHETS**, effervescent powder.

Used for: migraine.

Dosage: adults over 20 years, 2 tablets when attack starts followed by 2 every 4 hours up to maximum dose of 6 in 24

hours. Age 16 to 19 years and over 60kg body weight, 2 tablets at start of attack and maximum dose of 5 in 24 hours. 30–50kg body weight, 1 tablet at start of attack with a maximum of 3 in 24 hours. Age 12 to 14 years, over 30kg body weight, 1 tablet at start of attack with maximum of 3 in 24 hours.

Special care: pregnancy, breastfeeding, liver or kidney disorder.

Avoid use: children under 12 years, patients with phaeochromocytoma, breast cancer which is prolactin-dependent, recent surgery on gastro-intestinal tract.

Possible interaction: phenothiazines, anticholinergics, butyrophenones.

Side effects: drowsiness, raised blood levels of prolactin, diarrhoea, extrapyramidal reactions (characterized by reflex-type muscle movements and spasms).

Manufacturer: Lorex.

PARAPLATIN

Description: an alkylating cytotoxic drug produced as a solution in vials for injection containing 10mg carboplatin/ml.

Used for: ovarian cancer, small cell lung cancer.

Dosage: as directed by physician skilled in cancer chemotherapy.

Special care: patients with kidney disorders.

Possible interaction: aminoglycosides, capreomycin, anticoagulants taken orally.

Side effects: bone marrow suppression, nausea, vomiting, toxic effects on nerves, kidneys, hearing, hair loss.

Manufacturer: Bristol-Myers.

PARLODEL

Description: a dopamine agonist available as scored white tablets in 2 strengths containing 1mg and 2.5mg bromocriptine (as mesylate) respectively, all marked with strength and name. Also, **PARLODEL CAPSULES** in 2 strengths, white/blue containing 5mg bromocriptine, coded PARLODEL 5 and white containing 10mg, coded PARLODEL 10.

PARNATE

Used for: Parkinsonism, additional therapy in acromegaly (enlarged face, feet and hands due to a pituitary gland tumour producing an excess of growth hormone), tumours which are prolactin-dependent, abnormally high prolactin levels in blood, prevention and suppression of milk production after childbirth. Also, benign breast disorders connected with monthly cycle, breast pain, hormone-based infertility.

Dosage: adults, for Parkinsonism, initial dose, 1–1.25mg taken at night for 1 week increasing gradually to 2.5mg 3 times each day in fourth week. Dose is then gradually increased to 10–40mg 3 times each day in divided doses. Drug should be taken with meals. Acromegaly and tumours dependent upon prolactin, initial dose, 1–1.25mg taken at night gradually increasing to 5mg every 6 hours (with daily meals). Prevention and suppression of lactation; 2.5mg on day of birth then 2.5mg twice each day with meals for 2 weeks. Excess prolactin levels in blood, 1–1.25mg taken at night increasing to 7.5mg each day in divided doses with meals with a maximum of 30mg daily. Benign breast disease and pain, 1–1.25mg taken at night increasing gradually to 2.5mg twice each day with meals. Infertility, 1–1.25mg taken at bedtime at first gradually increasing to 7.5mg each day in divided doses with meals, the maximum being 30mg daily.

Special care: history of heart and circulatory disorders or psychoses. Regular gynaecological monitoring necessary for women and non-hormonal methods of contraception should be used for those not wishing to conceive as may cause ovulation.

Avoid use: high blood pressure at time of childbirth, hypersensitivity to ergot alkaloids, toxaemia of pregnancy. Withdraw if conception occurs.

Possible interaction: drugs affecting blood pressure, alcohol, metoclopramide, erythromycin.

Side effects: vomiting, nausea, leg pains, slight constipation, dry mouth, vasospasm. Rarely, heart attack, stroke, headache, hypertension, convulsions, dizziness, confusion. Drug should be withdrawn if peritoneal fibrosis occurs.

Manufacturer: Sandoz.

PARNATE

Description: an MAOI available as sugar-coated red tablets containing 100mg tranylcypromine (as sulphate), marked SKF.

Used for: depression.

Dosage: 1 tablet twice daily increasing to 1 tablet 3 times daily after 1 week. Maintenance dose is 1 tablet daily.

Special care: elderly, epilepsy.

Avoid use: children, patients with phaeochromocytoma, congestive heart failure, heart and circulatory diseases, blood changes, hyperthyroidism, liver disease, disease of cerebral arteries.

Possible interaction: ephedrine, TCADs, narcotic analgesics and pethidine, amphetamine, levodopa, methylphenidate, phenylpropanolamine, fenfluramine. Alcohol, barbiturates, hypnotics, hypoglycaemics, insulin, reserpine, anticholinergics, methyldopa, guanethidine. Many foods should be avoided including yeast extracts, Marmite, meat extracts, Oxo and Bovril, alcoholic drinks, broad bean pods, banana skins, flavoured textured soya protein, pickled herrings. Also any foods that are not completely fresh.

Side effects: severe hypertensive responses with certain foods, constipation, blurred vision, difficulty passing urine, gastro-intestinal upset. Low blood pressure on rising, skin rash, swelling of ankles, fatigue, weariness, dizziness, jaundice, blood disorders, weight gain, changes in libido. Occasionally, confusion and mania.

Manufacturer: S.K. & F.

PARSTELIN

Description: an MAOI available as sugar-coated green tablets containing 10mg tranylcypromine as sulphate and 1mg trifluoperazine as hydrochloride, marked SKF.

Used for: depression.

Dosage: 1 tablet twice each day at first increasing to 1 tablet 3 times each day after 1 week. Maintenance dose is normally 1 daily tablet.

Special care: elderly, epilepsy.

Avoid use: children, phaeochromocytoma, congestive heart failure, heart and circulatory diseases, blood changes, hyperthyroidism, liver disease, disease of cerebral arteries.

Possible interaction: ephedrine, TCADs, narcotic analgesics and pethidine, amphetamine, levodopa, methylphenidate, phenylpropanolamine, fenfluramine. Alcohol, barbiturates, hypnotics, hypoglycaemics, insulin, reserpine, anticholinergics, methyldopa, guanethidine. Many foods should be avoided including yeast extracts, Marmite, meat extracts, Oxo and Bovril, alcoholic drinks, broad bean pods, banana skins, flavoured textured soya protein, pickled herrings. Also any foods that are not completely fresh.

Side effects: severe hypertensive responses with certain foods, constipation, blurred vision, difficulty passing urine, gastrointestinal upset. Low blood pressure on rising, skin rash, swelling of ankles, fatigue, weariness, dizziness, jaundice, blood disorders, weight gain, changes in libido. Occasionally, confusion and mania.

Manufacturer: S.K. & F.

PARTOBULIN

Description: a preparation of human anti-D immunoglobulin available as a solution in ampoules for injection containing 1250 units/ml.

Used for: rhesus (D) incompatibility.

Dosage: antenatal prevention, 1250 units by intramuscular injection in weeks 28 and 34 of pregnancy and a further dose within 72 hours of birth. Following abortion or miscarriage or possible sensitising procedure, e.g. amniocentesis, 1250 units within 72 hours by intramuscular injection. Following transplacental bleeding where more than 25ml of foetal blood has been

transferred (1% of foetal red blood cells), 5000 units or 50 units/ml of foetal blood, by intramuscular injection.

Special care: patients who have IGA antibodies or with known history of unusual reactions to transfused blood or blood products.

Possible interaction: live vaccines.

Manufacturer: Immuno.

PARVOLEX

Description: an amino acid preparation used to treat drug overdose and available as a solution in ampoules for injection containing 200mg acetylcysteine/ml. Acetylcysteine acts to protect the liver from damage.

Used for: paracetamol overdose.

Dosage: by intravenous infusion in glucose intravenous infusion; 150mg/kg body weight in 200ml over 15 minutes at first. Then 50mg/kg body weight in 500ml over 4 hours followed by 100mg/kg body weight in 1000ml over 16 hours.

Special care: history of asthma. Vomiting should be induced if patient is treated within 4 hours of overdose. Plasma concentrations of paracetamol require monitoring. Patients who have taken alcohol, phenobarbitone, rifampicin, carbamazepine or phenytoin may be at risk of live toxicity at lower plasma-paracetamol concentrations.

Possible interaction: metals and rubber.

Side effects: rash, anaphylaxis.

Manufacturer: Evans.

PAVULON

Description: a non-depolarising muscle relaxant available as a solution in ampoules for injection containing 4mg pancuronium bromide/2ml.

Used for: muscle relaxation for intubation of patients undergoing anaesthesia and mechanical ventilation in intensive care.

Dosage: adults, 50–100 µg/kg body weight at first (for intubation) then 10–20 µg/kg body weight as needed to maintain relaxation. Children, 60–100 µg/kg body weight at first then 10–20 µg/kg. Newborn baby, 30–40 µg/kg body weight at first followed by 10–20 µg/kg. Intensive care patients, 60 µg/kg body weight every hour to hour and a half.

Special care: patients with liver and kidney disorders (reduced dose).

Possible interaction: procainamide, quinidine, aminoglycosides, clindamycin, azloallin, colistin, propanolol, verapamil, nifedipine, ecothiopate, demacarium, pyridostigmine, neostigmine, magnesium salts.

Manufacturer: Organon Teknika.

PENBRITIN

Description: an antibiotic broad-spectrum penicillin preparation available as black/red capsules in 2 strengths containing 250mg and 500mg ampicillin, marked with strength and name. Also, **PENBRITIN SYRUP** available as powder for reconstitution with water, then containing 125mg/5ml. **PENBRITIN SYRUP FORTE** contains 250mg/5ml (available as powder for reconstitution). **PENBRITIN PAEDIATRIC SUSPENSION** contains 125mg/1.25ml when reconstituted (available as powder). **PENBRITIN INJECTION** available as powder in vials containing 250mg and 500mg ampicillin sodium.

Used for: ear, nose, throat and respiratory infections, soft tissue infections. Infections of urinary tract and gonorrhoea.

Dosage: adults, oral preparations, 250mg–1g every 6 hours; injection, 250–500mg by intravenous or intramuscular injection, 4, 5 or 6 times each day. Children, oral preparations, 125–250mg every 6 hours; injection, half adult dose.

Special care: patients with glandular fever.

Side effects: gastro-intestinal upset, hypersensitivity reactions.

Manufacturer: Beecham.

PENDRAMINE

Description: a penicillin derivative available as film-coated, scored, oblong white tablets containing 125mg and

250mg penicillamine respectively; the 250mg tablets are marked HB.

Used for: severe rheumatoid arthritis.

Dosage: 125–250mg each day for first 4 to 8 weeks, then increase every 4 weeks by 125–250mg to a maximum dose of 2g each day, if needed. Children, usual dose, 15–20mg/kg body weight each day. Start with lower dose then gradually increase every 4 weeks over period of 3 to 6 months.

Special care: patients sensitive to penicillin checks on blood, urine and kidney function are required regularly during the course of treatment.

Avoid use: pregnancy, breastfeeding, patients with kidney disorders, thrombocytopenia, SLE, agranulocytosis (serious reduction in number of white blood cells [granulocytes]).

Possible interaction: phenylbutazone, zinc or iron salts, cytotoxic drugs, antimalarial drugs, gold salts, antacids.

Side effects: blood changes, myasthenia gravis, anorexia, rash, fever, nausea, protein in urine, blood in urine, SLE, nephrotic syndrome (a kidney abnormality resulting from a number of diseases and conditions).

Manufacturer: Asta Medica.

PENTACARINAT

Description: an antiprotozal preparation available as a powder in vials for reconstitution and injection containing 300mg pentamidine isethionate. Also, **PENTACARINAT SOLUTION** containing 300mg pentamidine isethionate/5ml for nebulization.

Used for: pneumocystis carinii pneumonia, kala-azar, cutaneous leishmaniasis.

Dosage: adults and children, pneumocystis carinii pneumonia, 4mg/kg body weight each day for 14 days; nebulized solution, 600mg each day for 3 weeks; prevention of secondary infection, 300mg every 4 weeks or 150mg every 2 weeks. Kala-azar, 3–4mg/kg body weight each day on alternate days up to a maximum of 10 deep intramuscular injections. May

be repeated, if needed. Cutaneous leishmaniasis, 3–4mg/kg body weight by deep intramuscular injection once or twice each week until condition improves. Trypanosomiasis, 4mg/kg body weight by deep intramuscular injection or intravenous infusion each day on alternate days to a maximum of 7 to 10 injections. *Special care*: must only be given by specialist physician under close medical supervision. Risk of serious hypotension once dose has been given; patient must be lying down and blood pressure monitored. Patients with liver or kidney disorder (reduced dose), hyper or hypotension, anaemia, leucopenia, thrombocytopenia, hypo or hyperglycaemia. *Side effects*: severe and occasionally fatal reactions due to hypotension, pancreatitis, hypoglycaemia, cardiac arrhythmias. Also, leucopenia, thrombocytopenia, hypocalcaemia, serious kidney failure. Vomiting, dizziness, nausea, fainting, rash, flushing, constriction of airways on inhalation, pain, disturbance of sense of taste. Tissue and muscle damage, abscess and pain at injection site.
Manufacturer: Theraplix.

PENTASA

Description: a colorectal salicylate preparation available as an enema containing 1g mesalazine. Also, PENTASA SUPPOSITORY, suppositories containing 1g mesalazine; PENTASA SR sustained-release scored tablets which are light grey and contain 250mg and 500mg mesalazine respectively, marked with strength and PENTASA.
Used for: ulcerative colitis (inflammation and ulceration of the colon and rectum).
Dosage: adults, 1 enema or suppository at night; tablets, 2 500mg tablets 3 times each day increasing to 8 500mg tablets (maximum dose), if needed. Maintenance dose is 500mg 3 times each day.
Special care: pregnancy, breastfeeding, elderly, protein in urine or raised levels of blood urea.
Avoid use: children.

Side effects: headache, abdominal pain, nausea.
Manufacturer: Yamanouchi.

PEPCID

Description: an H_2 blocker available as square, beige tablets and square, brown tablets containing 20mg and 40mg famotidine respectively, both marked with strength and name.
Used for: treatment of stomach and duodenal ulcers, prevention of relapse of duodenal ulcers. Prevention and treatment of reflux disease of stomach and oesophagus, treatment of Zollinger-Ellison syndrome.
Dosage: treatment of ulcers, 40mg taken at night for 4 to 8 weeks; prevention of relapse of duodenal ucer, 20mg taken at night. Gastro-oesophageal reflux disease, 20mg twice each day for 6 weeks to 3 months (or 40mg, if damage or ulceration is present). Prevention, 20mg twice each day. Zollinger-Ellison syndrome, 20mg 6 hours at first adjusted according to response to a maximum dose of 800mg each day.
Special care: pregnancy, breastfeeding, stomach cancer or kidney disease.
Avoid use: children.
Side effects: nausea, diarrhoea, constipation, rash, gastro-intestinal upset, dry mouth, headache, anorexia, dizziness, weariness. Rarely there may be enlargement of breasts in males (reversible).
Manufacturer: Morson.

PERFAN

Description: a phosphodiesterase inhibitor available in ampoules for injection containing 5mg enoximone/ml.
Used for: congestive heart failure where filling pressures are increased and cardiac output reduced.
Dosage: adults, by slow intravenous injection, 0.5–1mg/kg body weight at first then 500 µg/kg every half hour until condition improves or 3mg/kg may be given every 3 to 6 hours, as needed. By intravenous infusion, 90 µg/kg body

weight/ minute at first over 10 to 30 minutes. Then intermittent or continuous infusion of 20 µg/kg body weight. Total maximum dose should not be greater than 24mg/kg body weight in 24 hours. Plastic apparatus must be used as crystals form in glass.
Side effects: tachycardia, heart arrhythmias, unusual heartbeats, nausea, vomiting, headache, diarrhoea, hypotension, insom-nia, fever, chills, urine retention, reduced ability to produce and pass urine, pains in limbs.
Manufacturer: Merrell Dow.

PERGONAL

Description: an hormonal gonadotrophin preparation available as a powder in ampoules for reconstitution and injection containing menotrophin (equivalent to 75 units of both follicle-stimulating hormone and luteinizing hormone, with solvent).
Used for: underactivity (infertility) of testes due to lack of gonadotrophin. Female infertility due to lack of ovulation. Superovulation for in vitro fertilization.
Dosage: male adults, 1 ampoule 3 times each week along with 2000 units chorionic gonadotrophin twice each week for at least 4 months. Female infertility, by intramuscular injection according to levels of oestrogen. Superovulation, 2 or 3 ampoules each day.
Special care: patients with hormonal disorders or intracranial lesions must have these corrected before therapy begins.
Avoid use: pregnancy.
Side effects: overstimulation of ovaries may lead to enlargement and rupture, allergic responses, multiple pregnancy.
Manufacturer: Serono.

PERINAL

Description: a colorectal preparation combining a steroid and local anaesthetic available in the form of a metered dose spray containing 0.2% hydrocortisone and 1% lignocaine hydrochloride.

Used for: pain in anal area.
Dosage: 2 sprays up to 3 times each day.
Special care: short-term use only, pregnancy.
Avoid use: patients with infections of fungal, viral and bacterial origin.
Side effects: systemic corticosteroid effects, e.g. changes as in Cushing's syndrome.
Manufacturer: Dermal.

PERSANTIN

Description: an anti-platelet drug available as sugar-coated orange and white tablets containing 25mg and 100mg dipyridamole, marked with strength and name.
Used for: additional therapy along with oral anticoagulants to prevent thrombosis of artificial heart valves.
Dosage: 300–600mg each day in 3 or 4 doses taken before meals. Children, 5mg/ kg body weight as divided dose each day.
Special care: recent heart attack, worsening angina, narrowing of aorta below valves.
Possible interaction: antacids.
Side effects: gastro-intestinal upset, giddiness, headache.
Manufacturer: Boehringer Ingelheim.

PERTOFRAN

Description: a TCAD available as sugar-coated pink tablets containing 25mg desipramine hydrochloride, marked EW and CG.
Used for: depression.
Dosage: 1 tablet 3 times each day at first increasing to 2, 3 or 4 times daily if needed. Elderly, start with 1 tablet daily.
Special care: elderly, epilepsy.
Avoid use: children, phaeochromocytoma, congestive heart failure, heart and circulatory diseases, blood changes, hyperthyroidism, liver disease, disease of cerebral arteries.
Possible interaction: ephedrine, TCADs, narcotic analgesics and pethidine, amphetamine, levodopa, methylphenidate, phenylpropanolamine, fenfluramine.

Alcohol, barbiturates, hypnotics, hypoglycaemics, insulin, reserpine, anticholinergics, methyldopa, guanethidine. Many foods should be avoided including yeast extracts, Marmite, meat extracts, Oxo and Bovril, alcoholic drinks, broad bean pods, banana skins, flavoured textured soya protein, pickled herrings. Also any foods that are not completely fresh.
Side effects: severe hypertensive responses with certain foods, constipation, blurred vision, difficulty passing urine, gastro-intestinal upset. Low blood pressure on rising, skin rash, swelling of ankles, fatigue, weariness, dizziness, jaundice, blood disorders, weight gain, changes in libido. Occasionally, confusion and mania.
Manufacturer: Geigy.

PEVARYL TC

Description: a preparation in the form of a cream which combines an antifungal and potent steroid, containing 1% econazole nitrate and 0.1% triamcinolone acetonide.
Used for: inflammatory skin conditions where fungal infection is present..
Dosage: rub into affected area twice each day for 14 days.
Special care: short-term use only.
Avoid use: children, long-term or extensive use especially in pregnancy, patients with untreated bacterial or fungal infections or skin infections of tuberculous or viral origin or due to ringworm. Also, dermatitis in area of mouth, acne, leg ulcers or scabies.
Side effects: suppression of adrenal glands, skin thinning, abnormal hair growth, changes as in Cushing's syndrome.
Manufacturer: Cilag.

PHARMORUBICIN

Description: a cytotoxic antibiotic preparation available as a powder in vials for reconstitution and injection containing 10mg, 20mg or 50mg epirubicin hydrochloride. Also, **PHARMORU-BICIN SOLUTION** containing 2mg/ml.

Used for: breast cancer, papillary tumours of bladder.
Dosage: adults, breast cancer, by intravenous injection as directed by physician. Papillary tumours, solution of 50mg in 50ml sterile water is instilled each week for 8 weeks. Prevention, once each week for 4 weeks then once each month for 11 months.
Special care: care in handling, irritant to tissues. Patients with liver disease (reduced doses).
Side effects: bone marrow suppression, nausea, vomiting, hair loss, effects on fertility.
Manufacturer: Pharmacia.

PHYSEPTONE^{CD}

Description: an opiate analgesic preparation which is a controlled drug available as scored, white tablets containing 5mg methadone hydrochloride marked WELLCOME L4A. Also, **PHYSEPTONE INJECTION**, containing 10mg/ml in ampoules for injection.
Used for: severe pain.
Dosage: tablets, 5–10mg every 6 to 8 hours or same dose by subcutaneous or intramuscular injection.
Special care: pregnancy, underactive thyroid gland or serious liver disease.
Avoid use: children, depression of respiration, obstructive airways disease, obstetric patients, those who are not confined to bed.
Possible interaction: central nervous system depressants, MAOIs.
Side effects: dizziness, nausea, sedation, euphoria, drug tolerance and dependence.
Manufacturer: Wellcome.

PIPORTIL DEPOT

Description: a phenothiazine group II available as a depot oily injection in ampoules containing 50mg pipothiazine palmitate/ml.
Used for: ongoing treatment of certain psychiatric disorders particularly schizophrenia.

Dosage: a test dose at first of 25mg by deep intramuscular injection into the gluteal muscle (buttock), then adjusted by 25mg or 50mg increments until best response is achieved. The usual maintenance dose is in the order of 50–100mg every 4 weeks with a maximum of 200mg.
Special care: pregnancy, breastfeeding, history of convulsions, severe extrapyramidal responses to phenothiazines taken orally.
Avoid use: children, severe heart disorder, liver or kidney failure, phaeochromocytoma, depression of bone marrow function, severe hardening of cerebral arteries.
Possible interaction: alcohol, anaesthetics, antacids, antimuscarines, anxiolytics, hypnotics, calcium channel blockers, lithium.
Side effects: extrapyramidal symptoms, changes in ECG and EEG, tachycardia and heart arrhythmias, apathy, drowsiness, insomnia, depression. Dry mouth, blocked nose, difficulty passing urine, constipation, hypotension, blurred vision. Changes in breasts and menstrual cycle, weight gain, impotence, blood changes, effects on liver, jaundice, rash, pigmentation of skin and eyes (especially higher doses).
Manufacturer: Theraplix.

PIPRIL

Description: an antibiotic broad-spectrum penicillin available as powder in vials in strengths of 1g, 2g and 4g piperacillin (as sodium salt), with diluent, for injection (1g and 2g) and infusion (4g).
Used for: local and systemic infections; prevention of infection during operations.
Dosage: adults, by intramuscular or slow intravenous injection or by intravenous infusion. 100–150mg/kg body weight in divided doses each day at first. Severe infections may require up to 200–300mg/kg with 16g or more daily if life is threatened. Single doses over 2g must be given by intravenous injection or infusion. Children may require lesser doses.

Special care: pregnancy, kidney disorder.
Side effects: gastro-intestinal upset, hypersensitive allergic reactions.
Manufacturer: Lederle.

PIPTALIN

Description: an anti-spasmodic used for digestive disorders, combining an anti-cholinergic and deflatulent drug, available as a sugar-free elixir containing 4mg pipenzolate bromide and 40mg activated dimethicone/5ml.
Used for: flatulence, pain due to spasm and overactivity of gastro-intestinal tract, abdominal extension due to gas build-up.
Dosage: 10ml 3 or 4 times each day taken 15 minutes before meal. Children, up to 10kg body weight, 2.5ml; 10–20kg, 2.5–5ml; 20–40kg, 5ml. All taken 15 minutes before meals 3 or 4 times each day.
Special care: urine retention, enlarged prostate gland, glaucoma.
Avoid use: pregnancy, breastfeeding, myasthenia gravis, various disorders of gastro-intestinal tract including obstruction, paralytic ileus, pyloric stenosis, ulcerative colitis. Also, liver or kidney disorders, tachycardia, unstable angina.
Possible interaction: benzodiazepines, TCADs, antihistamines.
Side effects: constipation, urine retention, vomiting and nausea, dry mouth, visual disorder, weakness, tachycardia, blushing, palpitations, insomnia.
Manufacturer: B.M. Pharmaceuticals.

PITRESSIN

Description: A preparation of antidiuretic hormone available as a solution in ampoules for injection containing 20 units agipressin (synthetic vasopressin)/ml.
Used for: pituitary diabetes insipidus.
Dosage: by intramuscular or subcutaneous injection, 5–20 units every 4 hours. By intravenous infusion, 20 units over 15 minutes.
Special care: pregnancy, conditions which might be made worse by water retention,

asthma, heart failure, migraine, epilepsy, kidney disorders. Careful checks on amount of water retention required.
Avoid use: disease of arteries especially coronary arteries, severe nephritis.
Side effects: constriction of coronary arteries possibly leading to angina and reduction in blood flow to heart, hyper-sensitive allergic reactions, feeling of needing to defecate, belching, abdominal pains, nausea, pallor.
Manufacturer: Parke-Davis.

PLAQUENIL

Description: an NSAID which is a 4-aminoquinolone available as sugar-coated orange tablets containing 200mg hydroxychloroquine sulphate.
Used for: rheumatoid arthritis and juvenile rheumatoid arthritis, lupus erythematosus (a severe inflammatory disease affecting internal organs and skin).
Dosage: 2 tablets each day with meals at first, with a maintenance dose of 1 or 2 tablets daily. The maximum dose is 6.5mg/kg body weight each day. If no improvement is seen after 6 months, drug should be withdrawn. Children, 6.5mg/kg body weight each day.
Special care: breastfeeding, porphyria, liver or kidney disease, a history of blood, gastro-intestinal or neurological disorders. Patients on long-term therapy should receive regular eye tests.
Avoid use: pregnancy, patients with maculopathy (a disorder of the eye spot of the retina).
Possible interaction: antacids, drugs which may damage the eyes, aminoglycosides.
Side effects: opacity of the cornea and changes in the retina of the eye, reduced eye accommodation (discontinue if this occurs). Also, gastro-intestinal intolerance, baldness, skin responses, bleaching of hair.
Manufacturer: Sanofi Winthrop.

PLENDIL

Description: an antihypertensive class II calcium antagonist available as film-coated sustained-release tablets containing 5mg and 10mg felodipine.
Used for: hypertension.
Dosage: 5mg once each day increasing if necessary to a usual maintenance dose of 5–10mg. The maximum daily dose is 20mg.
Special care: recent problems of poor blood circulation to the heart or serious liver disease.
Avoid use: pregnancy, breastfeeding.
Possible interaction: phenytoin, pheno-barbitone, cimetidine, carbamazepine.
Side effects: flushing, swelling of ankles, weariness, giddiness, headache, slight swelling of gums, palpitations.
Manufacturer: Schwarz.

PNEUMOVAX II

Description: a preparation of pneumo-coccal vaccine, available as a solution for injection, containing 25 µg of 23 types of pneumococcus/0.5ml as a purified mixture of capsular polysaccharides.
Used for: immunisation against pneumococcal disease.
Dosage: adults and children age 2 years and over, 0.5ml by intramuscular or subcutaneous injection.
Special care: patients with weak hearts or lungs, respiratory diseases or feverish illnesses, revaccination of high risk children.
Avoid use: pregnancy, breastfeeding, children under 2 years, patients with Hodgkin's disease who have had chemo-therapy or radiation treatment. Patients who have recently received immunosup-pressive treatment, revaccination of adults.
Side effects: fever, local skin reactions, relapse of patients with stabilized thrombocytopenic purpura (a bleeding disorder characterized by haemorrhage beneath the skin and mucous membranes).
Manufacturer: Morson.

POLYFAX

Description: a preparation of peptide anti-biotics available as an ointment containing 10,000 units polymyxin B sulphate and 500 units bacitracin zinc per gram.

Used for: eye infections including conjunctivitis, keratitis, styes, blepharitis. Prevent infection after removal of foreign objects from the eye or surgery. Also, impetigo, infected burns and skin infections.
Dosage: apply thinly at least twice per day.
Special care: patients with extensive, open wounds.
Side effects: skin sensitization, toxic effects on kidneys.
Manufacturer: Cusi.

POLYTRIM

Description: A combined antibacterial preparation available in the form of eyedrops containing 1mg trimethoprim and 10,000 units polymyxin B sulphate/ml. Also, POLYTRIM OINTMENT containing 5mg trimethoprim and 10,000 units polymyxin B sulphate/gram.
Used for: bacterial eye infections.
Dosage: apply 3 or 4 times each day continuing for 2 days after symptoms have cleared.
Manufacturer: Cusi.

PONDERAX PACAPS

Description: an anti-obesity serotoninergic drug available as blue/clear sustained-release capsules, with white pellets containing 60mg fenfluramine hydrochloride marked P and PA60.
Used for: severe obesity.
Dosage: adults 1 tablet daily half an hour before a meal for a maximum period of 3 months.
Special care: therapy should last for up to 3 months and drug gradually withdrawn over last 1 or 2 weeks.
Avoid use: patients suffering from depression, epilepsy, psychiatric disorder or drug or alcohol abuse.
Possible interaction: antidiabetics, MAOIs, alcohol, antihypertensives, sedatives, anti-anoretics.
Side effects: dry mouth, nervousness, sedation, hallucinations, frequency of urination, depression (especially if drug abruptly stopped), diarrhoea.
Manufacturer: Pacaps Servier.

PONDOCILLIN

Description: an antibiotic preparation which is a broad-spectrum penicillin available as film-coated, oval, white tablets containing 500mg pivampicillin coded with symbol and 128. Also, PONDOCILLIN SUSPENSION containing 175mg pivampicillin/5ml available as granules for reconstitution.
Used for: skin, soft tissue infections, bronchitis, pneumonia, gonorrhoea and urinary tract infections.
Dosage: adults, 1 tablet or 15ml suspension twice each day with drink or food. Children, under 1 year, 40–60mg/kg; 1 to 5 years, 10–15ml; 6 to 10 years, 15–20ml. All as daily divided doses with food or drink.
Special care: kidney disease.
Avoid use: patients with glandular fever.
Side effects: gastro-intestinal upset, hypersensitive allergic reactions.
Manufacturer: Leo.

PONSTAN FORTE

Description: an NSAID available as blue/ivory capsules containing 250mg mefenamic acid marked PONSTAN 250. Also, PONSTAN FORTE film-coated, yellow tablets containing 500mg marked with name. PONSTAN PAEDIATRIC SUSPENSION containing 50mg/5ml.
Used for: pain, period pain, headache, rheumatoid pain (Stills disease), osteoarthritis, heavy menstrual bleeding.
Dosage: adults, 500mg 3 times each day (on first day of period in patients with heavy menstrual bleeding). Children, use paediatric suspension, aged 6 months to 1 year, 5ml; 2 to 4 years, 10ml; 5 to 8 years, 15ml; 9 to 12 years, 20ml. All doses at 8 hour intervals for no more than 1 week.
Special care: pregnancy, breastfeeding, elderly, allergies, asthma, heart failure, epilepsy.
Avoid use: known allergy to NSAID or aspirin, ulcer, liver or kidney disorder, inflammatory bowel disease.

Possible interaction: sulphonylureas, anticoagulants, hydantoins, quinolones.
Side effects: kidney disorder, gastro-intestinal intolerance, raised level of liver enzymes. Rarely, blood changes. Withdraw drug if skin rash occurs.
Manufacturer: Parke-Davis.

POTABA

Description: an antifibrotic preparation which dissolves fibrous tissue, available as powder in sachets containing 3g potassium p-aminobenzoate. Also, **POTABA TABLETS** white, containing 500mg. **POTABA CAPSULES**, red/white, containing 500mg.
Used for: scleroderma (thickened skin), Peyronie's disease (fibrous hardening of the penis).
Dosage: adults, 12g each day in 4 divided doses with meals.
Special care: kidney disease.
Possible interaction: sulphonamides.
Side effects: anorexia, nausea (discontinue if these occur).
Manufacturer: Glenwood.

PRAXILENE

Description: a preparation that is a peripheral and cerebral activator which improves the use of glucose and oxygen by the tissues, increasing the level of ATP (the energy molecules of cells) and decreasing lactic acid levels. It is available as pink capsules containing 100mg naftidrofuryl oxalate. Also, **PRAXILENE FORTE** available in ampoules for injection containing 20mg naftidrofuryl oxalate/ml.
Used for: disorders of cerebral and peripheral arteries.
Dosage: 1 or 2 tablets 3 times each day.
Special care: use of Praxilene Forte in patients with very weak heart or conduction disorders.
Avoid use: children. Use of Forte in patients with heart block.
Side effects: nausea, stomach ache.
Manufacturer: Lipha.

PRECORTISYL

Description: a glucocorticoid corticosteroid preparation available as white tablets containing 1mg prednisolone and scored, white tablets containing 5mg prednisolone. Also, **PRECORTISYL FORTE** scored, white tablets containing 25mg prednisolone.
Used for: Precortisyl, allergic and rheumatic disorders; Forte, rheumatic fever, systemic lupus erythematosus (severe inflammatory disorder affecting many parts of the body), blood disorders.
Dosage: Precortisyl, 20–40mg each day in divided doses at first, then reducing by 2.5–5mg every third or fourth day until a maintenance dose, in the order of 5–20mg daily, is achieved. Forte, 75mg in 3 divided doses. Children, Precortisyl, age 1 to 7 years, quarter to half adult dose; 7 to 12 years, half to three-quarters adult dose.
Special care: pregnancy, diabetes, kidney inflammation, hypertension, thrombophlebitis, epilepsy, secondary cancer, underactive thyroid, peptic ulcer, glaucoma, recent surgical anastomoses of intestine. Also, patients suffering from stress, psychoses, liver cirrhosis, infections of fungal or viral origin, tuberculosis, other infections. Also avoid contact with chicken pox or *Herpes zoster* and seek medical advice if this occurs or if infected.
Avoid use: children under 1 year.
Possible interaction: diuretics, hypoglycaemics, phenytoin, NSAIDs, rifampicin, anticholinesterases, ephedrine, anticoagulants taken orally, phenobarbitone, cardiac glycosides, diuretics.
Side effects: mood changes, depression and euphoria, changes as in Cushing's syndrome, osteoporosis, peptic ulcer, hyperglycaemia.
Manufacturer: Roussel.

PRED FORTE

Description: a corticosteroid preparation available as eyedrops containing 1% prednisolone acetate.
Used for: inflammation of eyes where no infection is present.

Dosage: 1 or 2 drops 2, 3 or 4 times each day. 2 drops every hour may be needed during the first 48 hours.
Special care: pregnancy, babies.
Avoid use: fungal, viral or tuberculous eye infections or those producing pus. Also, glaucoma, dendritic ulcer, those wearing soft contact lenses.
Side effects: formation of cataracts, thinning of cornea, rise in pressure within eye, secondary fungal or viral infections.
Manufacturer: Allergan.

PREDENEMA

Description: a steroid colorectal agent available as an enema containing 20mg prednisolone (as metasulphobenzoate sodium).
Used for: ulcerative colitis.
Dosage: adults, 1 enema at night for 2, 3 or 4 weeks.
Special care: pregnancy, avoid long-term use.
Avoid use: children. Patients with perforated bowel, infections, fistulae, obstruction of the bowel, peritonitis.
Manufacturer: Pharmax.

PREDFOAM

Description: a steroid colorectal agent available as a white aerosol foam containing 20mg prednisolone (as meta-sulphobenzoate sodium) per metered dose.
Used for: ulcerative colitis, proctitis (inflammation of the rectum).
Dosage: adults, 1 metered dose into rectum twice each day for 2 weeks continuing for another 2 weeks if condition improves.
Special care: pregnancy, short-term use only.
Avoid use: children, patients with perforated bowel, infections, fistulae, obstruction of the bowel, peritonitis.
Manufacturer: Pharmax.

PREDNESOL

Description: a glucocorticoid corticosteroid preparation available as scored, pink tablets containing 5mg prednisolone (as disodium phosphate) marked with name and GLAXO.
Used for: rheumatic, allergic and inflammatory disorders responsive to steroids.
Dosage: adults, 10–100mg in water each day at first, in divided doses, then reducing to lowest dose which is effective. Children, age 1 to 7, quarter to half adult dose; 7 to 12, half to three-quarters adult dose.
Special care: thrombophlebitis, psychoses, recent intestinal anastomoses, chronic nephritis, certain cancers, osteoporosis, peptic ulcer, skin eruption/rash related to a disease, viral, fungal or active infections, tuberculosis. Hypertension, glaucoma, epilepsy, acute glomerulonephritis (inflammation of kidney glomerulus), diabetes, cirrhosis, hypothyroidism, pregnancy, stress. To be withdrawn gradually.
Possible interaction: NSAIDs, oral anticoagulants, phenytoin, ephedrine, phenobarbitone, rifampicin, diuretics, cardiac glycosides, anticholinesterases, hypoglycaemics.
Side effects: osteoporosis, depression, euphoria, hyperglycaemia, peptic ulcers, Cushingoid changes.
Manufacturer: Glaxo.

PREDSOL

Description: a steroid colorectal agent available as an enema containing 20mg prednisolone as disodium phosphate.
Also, **PREDSOL SUPPOSITORIES** containing 5mg prednisolone (as disodium phosphate).
Used for: enema, ulcerative colitis; suppositories, proctitis (inflammation of rectum) and anal disorders resulting from Crohn's disease (a disorder of the intestine or part of digestive tract in which there is inflammation and ulceration).
Dosage: adults, enema, 1 at night for 2, 3 or 4 weeks; suppositories, 1 every night and morning after passing stool.
Special care: pregnancy, short-term use only.
Avoid use: children, bacterial, fungal, tuberculous or viral infections.

Side effects: systemic glucocorticoid effects, e.g. mood swings, euphoria and depression, changes as in Cushing's syndrome, peptic ulcer, hyperglycaemia, osteoporosis.
Manufacturer: Evans.

PREFERID

Description: a potent topical steroid preparation available as cream and ointment containing 0.025% budesonide.
Used for: psoriasis, all types of dermatitis, eczema.
Dosage: apply thinly 2 or 3 times each day.
Special care: thrombophlebitis, psychoses, recent intestinal anastomoses, chronic nephritis, certain cancers, osteoporosis, peptic ulcer, skin eruption/ rash related to a disease, viral, fungal or active infections, tuberculosis. Hypertension, glaucoma, epilepsy, acute glomerulonephritis (inflammation of kidney glomerulus), diabetes, cirrhosis, hypothyroidism, pregnancy, stress. To be withdrawn gradually.
Possible interaction: NSAIDs, oral anticoagulants, phenytoin, ephedrine, phenobarbitone, rifampicin, diuretics, cardiac glycosides, anticholinesterases, hypoglycaemics.
Side effects: osteoporosis, depression, euphoria, hyperglycaemia, peptic ulcers, Cushingoid changes.
Manufacturer: Yamanouchi.

PREGNYL

Description: a preparation of human chorionic gonadotrophin available as powder in ampoules, with solvent for reconstitution and injection, at strengths of 500, 1500 and 5000 units.
Used for: underdevelopment of male sexual organs, deficient production of sperm, delayed puberty in males; infertility due to lack of maturing of follicles and ovulation in females. Along with human menopausal gonadotrophin to produce superovulation for in vitro fertilization treatment.

Dosage: male adults, hypogonadism, 500– 1000 units 2 or 3 times each week by intramuscular injection. Delayed puberty, 1500 units twice each week by intramuscular injection for at least 6 months. Females, infertility, following treatment with human menopausal gonadotrophin, 5000– 10000 units by intra-muscular injection. Then 3 further injections of 5000 units during the next 9 days. Superovulation, 30 to 40 hours after injection with human menopausal gonadotrophin, 5000–10000 units by intramuscular injection.
Special care: patients with heart or kidney disorders, epilepsy, hypertension, migraine, hormone levels should be monitored in female patients.
Avoid use: children, patients with androgen-dependent cancers.
Side effects: skin rashes, salt and water retention.
Manufacturer: Organon.

PREMARIN

Description: an oestrogen preparation available as sugar-coated, oval, maroon tablets and sugar-coated, oval, yellow tablets containing 0.625mg and 1.25mg conjugated oestrogens. Also, **PRE-MARIN VAGINAL CREAM** containing 0.625mg/g conjugated oestrogens.
Used for: tablets, hormone replacement therapy for menopausal women who have had a hysterectomy. Prevention of osteoporosis following menopause. Relief of symptoms of some breast cancers in postmenopausal women. Cream, atrophic vaginitis and urethritis (inflammation due to atrophy of the tissues of the vagina and urethra), Kraurosis vulvae (a disease of the external genital area, characterized by degeneration of tissues and itching, affecting elderly women).
Dosage: tablets, for hormone replacement therapy, 0.625mg–1.25mg each day for 12 to 18 months. Prevention of osteoporosis, same dose for 5 to 10 years. Breast cancer, up to 10mg 3 times each day for at least 9 months. Cream, 1–2g applied daily to

affected area or intra-vaginally (using applicator) for 3 weeks followed by 1 week without treatment.

Special care: those at risk of thromboembolism or with history of disorders relating to this, those with porphyria, gallstones, diabetes, otosclerosis, fibroids in the uterus, tetany, epilepsy, mild liver disease. Blood pressure, breasts and pelvic organs should be checked regularly during the course of treatment.

Avoid use: thromboembolism, thrombophlebitis, vaginal bleeding which is not diagnosed, or endometriosis, genital tract cancer or other oestrogen-dependent cancers. Serious kidney, liver, heart disease, Dublin-Johnson or Rotor syndrome.

Possible interaction: drugs which induce liver enzymes.

Manufacturer: Wyeth.

PREMPAK-C

Description: an oestrogen and progestogen preparation available in the form of sugar-coated oval tablets in 2 strengths, 28 maroon or 28 yellow containing 0.625mg or 1.25mg conjugated oestrogens respectively. Also, 12 sugar-coated brown tablets containing 0.15mg norgestrel in same pack.

Used for: hormone replacement therapy in women who have not had a hysterectomy, for menopausal symptoms, prevention of osteoporosis following menopause.

Dosage: 1 maroon or yellow tablet for 16 days then 1 maroon or yellow tablet and 1 brown tablet for 12 days, starting on first day of period if present.

Special care: patients with history of, or considered to be at risk of thrombosis. Women with any of the following should receive careful monitoring: epilepsy, gallstones, porphyria, multiple sclerosis, otosclerosis, diabetes, migraine, hypertension, tetany, fibroids in the uterus. Blood pressure, breasts and pelvic organs should be examined regularly during the treatment especially in women who may be at risk of breast cancer.

Avoid use: pregnancy, breastfeeding, with breast cancer, cancer of reproductive system or other hormonally dependent cancer, inflammation of veins or other thromboembolic conditions, endometriosis, undiagnosed vaginal bleeding, serious liver, kidney or heart disease, Dublin-Johnson or Rotor syndrome.

Possible interaction: drugs which induce liver enzymes.

Side effects: soreness and enlargement of breasts, breakthrough bleeding, weight gain, gastro-intestinal upset, dizziness, nausea, headache, vomiting. If frequent, severe, migraine-like headaches, disturbance of vision, rise in blood pressure, jaundice or indications of thrombosis occur, drug should immediately be withdrawn, and also in the event of pregnancy. Drug should be stopped 6 weeks before planned major surgery.

Manufacturer: Wyeth.

PREPIDIL

Description: a prostaglandin preparation available as a sterile cervical gel in single use syringes containing 500μg dinoprostone/3g gel.

Used for: induction of labour, softening and dilation of cervix.

Dosage: 1 dose into cervical canal, repeated as directed by physician.

Special care: glaucoma, asthma, raised pressure within eye; high doses may cause rupture of uterus. Should not be given continuously for more than 2 days

Avoid use: patients at risk of rupture of uterus, those in whom delivery is complicated, e.g. placenta praevia, those with serious toxaemia, untreated pelvic infection, multiple pregnancy, previous history of difficult delivery, inflammation of vagina or cervix.

Side effects: chills, shivering, flushing, headache, nausea, vomiting, diarrhoea, raised level of white blood cells, short-lived fever, abnormal increase in muscle tone of uterus, severe contractions.

Manufacturer: Upjohn.

PREPULSID

Description: a prokinetic drug acting on the gastro-intestinal tract, which promotes the movement of food through the oesophagus and stomach. It is available as scored, white tablets containing 10mg cisapride (as monohydrate). Also, **PREPULSID SUSPENSION**, cherry-flavoured solution containing 5mg cisapride/5ml.
Used for: gastro-oesophageal reflux, maintenance treatment of reflux oesophagitis, dyspepsia, relief of symptoms when gastric emptying is delayed as in systemic sclerosis, diabetes, autonomic neuropathy.
Dosage: gastro-oesophageal reflux, 20mg before breakfast and at night time or 10mg 3 times each day for 12 weeks. Then a maintenance dose of 20mg once each day at bedtime or 10mg twice each day before breakfast and at night. Dyspepsia, 10mg 3 times each day for 4 weeks. Delayed gastric emptying, 10mg 3 or 4 times each day, for 6 weeks.
Special care: breastfeeding, elderly, kidney or liver disorders.
Avoid use: pregnancy, children, patients with gastro-intestinal obstruction, haemorrhage or perforation.
Possible interaction: anticholinergics, anticoagulants taken orally, central nervous system depressants.
Side effects: abdominal rumbling and pain, diarrhoea; rarely, extrapyramidal effects, headache, convulsions.
Manufacturer: Janssen.

PRESCAL

Description: an antihypertensive preparation which is a class II calcium antagonist, available as scored yellow tablets containing 2.5mg isradipine marked NM and CIBA.
Used for: hypertension.
Dosage: 1 tablet in the morning and at night, increasing after 3 or 4 weeks to 2 twice each day if needed. Maximum dose is 4 twice daily. Elderly, half a tablet twice each day at first.

Special care: pregnancy, breastfeeding, narrowing of aorta (aortic stenosis), sick sinus syndrome.
Avoid use: children.
Possible interaction: anticonvulsants.
Side effects: tachycardia, palpitations, headache, giddiness, flushing, fluid retention in hands and feet, pain in abdomen, gain in weight, tiredness, skin rashes. Rise in level of transaminase enzymes in blood.
Manufacturer: Ciba.

PRESTIM

Description: an antihypertensive preparation which combines a non-cardioselective ß-blocker and thiazide diuretic available as white, scored tablets containing 10mg timolol maleate and 2.5mg bendrofluazide, marked with a lion and 132.
Also, **PRESTIM FORTE** scored, white tablets containing 20mg timolol maleate and 5mg bendrofluazide, marked with a lion and 146.
Used for: hypertension.
Dosage: Prestim, 1 to 4 tablets each day. Prestim Forte, half dose.
Special care: pregnancy, breastfeeding, patients with weak hearts may require diuretics and digitalis, those with diabetes, undergoing general anaesthesia, kidney or liver disorders, gout. Electrolyte (salts) levels may need to be monitored.
Avoid use: history of bronchospasm or obstructive airways disease, heart block, heart shock, uncompensated heart failure, disease of peripheral arteries, bradycardia. Serious or worsening kidney failure or anuria.
Possible interaction: sympathomimetics, class I antiarrhythmics, central nervous system depressants, clonidine withdrawal, ergot alkaloids, cardiac depressant anaesthetics, verapamil, reserpine, indomethacin, hypoglycaemics, cimetidine, other antihypertensives. Digitalis, potassium supplements, potassium-sparing diuretics, lithium.

Side effects: cold hands and feet, disturbance of sleep, fatigue on exercise, bronchospasm, bradycardia, gastro-intestinal disturbances, heart failure, blood changes, gout, sensitivity to light, muscle weakness. If skin rash or dry eyes occur, withdraw drug gradually.
Manufacturer: Leo.

PRIADEL

Description: an antidepressant preparation which is a lithium salt available as scored, white, continuous-release tablets in 2 strengths. Capsule-shaped tablets contain 200mg lithium carbonate marked P200. Tablets, marked PRIADEL, contain 400mg lithium carbonate. Also, **PRIADEL LIQUID**, a sugar-free solution containing 520mg lithium citrate/5ml.
Used for: tablets, manic depression, mania, aggressive and self-harming behaviour, recurrent bouts of depression.
Dosage: tablets, 400–1200mg as a single dose each day at first; liquid 400–1200mg in 2 divided daily doses at first. Dosage then adjusted to maintain a certain blood level.
Special care: levels in blood must be monitored along with heart, kidney and thyroid function.
Avoid use: children, pregnancy, breast-feeding, hypothyroidism, Addison's disease, heart or kidney disorders, disturbance of salt balance.
Possible interaction: diazepam, metoclopramide, diuretics, flupenthixol, methyldopa, tetracyclines, phenytoin, haloperidol, NSAIDs, carbamazepine.
Side effects: trembling hands, diarrhoea, nausea, disturbance of ECG and central nervous system, gain in weight, hypo and hyperthyroidism, skin rashes, oedema, passing of large quantities of urine, thirstiness, oedema.
Manufacturer: Delandale.

PRIMACOR

Description: a heart drug and phosphodi-esterase inhibitors, which have a mode of action resembling stimulation by the sympathetic nervous system. Primacor is available in ampoules for injection containing 10mg milrinone/ml.
Used for: acute, post-operative heart failure after cardiac surgery; short-term treatment of congestive heart failure which has not responded to other drugs.
Dose: 50µg/kg body weight by slow intravenous injection over 10 minutes. Then by intravenous infusion at a rate of 375–750 nanograms/kg/minute. This is for up to 12 hours in post-operative patients and for 48–72 hours in those with congestive heart failure. The maximum daily dose is 1.13mg/kg.
Special care: certain types of heart failure associated with disease of heart valves and outflow obstruction. Patients with kidney disorder should receive reduced dose. Monitoring of fluid, electrolyte levels, blood pressure, central venous blood pressure, heart rate, ECG, liver enzymes, platelet counts must be carried out.
Side effects: unusual heart beats, hypotension, arrhythmias, vomiting, nausea, insomnia, headache, diarrhoea. Less commonly, chills, pains in limbs, reduced production of urine, urine retention, fever.
Manufacturer: Sanofi Winthrop.

PRIMALAN

Description: an anti-allergic antihista-mine preparation which is a phenothi-azine type drug, available as white tablets containing 5mg mequitazine marked PRIMALAN.
Used for: hay fever, itching, urticaria, inflammation of the nose.
Dosage: 1 tablet twice each day.
Avoid use: pregnancy, liver disease, enlarged prostate gland, epilepsy.
Possible interaction: central nervous system depressants, some sympathomimet-ics (indirect acting), alcohol, MAOIs.
Side effects: sleepiness, impaired reactions, extrapyramidal responses, anticholinergic side effects.
Manufacturer: Theraplix.

PRIMAXIN IV

Description: an antibiotic compound preparation, combining a carbapenem and enzyme inhibitor. It is available as 250mg or 500mg of powder in vials for reconstitution and injection, containing equal parts of imipenem (as monohydrate) and cilastin (as sodium salt). Also, **PRIMAXIN IM**, a preparation containing 500mg cilastin and 500mg imipenem as powder in vials for reconstitution and intramuscular injection.

Used for: septicaemia, bone, skin, joint, soft tissue infections, infections of urinary, genital and lower respiratory tracts, abdominal and gynaecological infections. Also, prevention of infection after surgery.

Dosage: adults, Primaxin IV, 250 mg–1g by intravenous infusion every 6 to 8 hours, depending upon nature and severity of infection. Prevention of infection, 1g when patient is anaesthetized followed by a further 1g dose 3 hours later. Primaxin, depending upon nature and severity of infection, in the order of 500–750mg by deep intramuscular injection. Maximum dose is 1.5g each day. Patients with gonococcal inflam-mation and infection of urethra or cervix receive 500mg as a single dose. Children, Primaxin IV only, age over 3 months, 15mg/kg body weight every 6 hours, the maximum daily dose being 2g.

Special care: pregnancy, breastfeeding, patients with kidney disorders, gastro-intestinal diseases (especially inflammation of bowel), those with known allergy to penicillin.

Avoid use: children under 3 months.

Possible interaction: ganciclovir, probenecid.

Side effects: diarrhoea, colitis (inflammation of the large intestine or bowel), nausea, vomiting, blood changes. Disturbance of central nervous system, convulsions, rise in level of liver enzymes, creatinine and urea in blood.

Manufacturer: M.S.D.

PRIMOLUT N

Description: an hormonal progestogen preparation available as white tablets containing 5mg norethisterone marked AN inside a hexagon shape.

Used for: abnormal menstrual bleeding, other menstrual disorders, postponement of menstruation, endometriosis.

Dosage: adults, heavy menstrual bleeding, 1 tablet twice or 3 times each day from day 19 to day 26 of cycle. Postponement of menstruation, 1 tablet 3 times each day, beginning 3 days before expected start of period. Endometriosis, 2 tablets each day beginning on fifth day of cycle, increasing to 4 or 5 daily if spotting takes place. 2 tablets each day should be taken for at least 4 to 6 months.

Special care: migraine or epilepsy.

Avoid use: pregnancy, history of itching or idiopathic jaundice during pregnancy, serious liver disorders, Dublin-Johnson and Rotor syndromes..

Side effects: disturbance of liver function, masculinization.

Manufacturer: Schering H.C.

PRIMOTESTON DEPOT

Description: an hormonal preparation of a depot androgen available as a solution in ampoules for injection containing 250mg testosterone oenanthate/ml.

Used for: underactivity of testes, breast cancer.

Dosage: underactivity of testes, 250mg by intramuscular injection every 2 or 3 weeks. Same for maintenance once every 2 or 3 weeks. Female breast cancer, 200mg by intramuscular injection every 2 weeks.

Special care: epilepsy, migraine, hyper-tension heart, kidney or liver disease.

Avoid use: liver or prostate cancer, untreated heart failure, heart disease due to insufficient blood supply.

Possible interaction: drugs that induce liver enzymnes.

Side effects: weight gain, oedema, liver tumours. Males, decrease in fertility, premature closure of epiphyses, priapism (abnormal, prolonged and painful erection

of penis, not associated with sexual arousal but with underlying disorder or caused by a drug). Females, masculinization, withdraw drug if hypercalcaemia occurs.
Manufacturer: Schering H.C.

PRO-BANTHINE

Description: an anticholinergic preparation available as sugar-coated, peach-coloured tablets containing 15mg propantheline bromide.
Used for: peptic ulcer, irritable bowel syndrome, enuresis (incontinence of urine).
Dosage: ulcer, 1 tablet 3 times each day taken before meals, and 2 at bedtime; irritable bowel syndrome, up to 8 tablets each day in divided doses. Enuresis, 1 to 2 tablets 3 times each day, with a daily maximum of 8 in divided doses.
Special care: elderly, liver or kidney disease, ulcerative colitis, serious heart disease, degenerative disease of autonomic nervous system.
Avoid use: children, patients with glaucoma, obstruction of gastro-intestinal or urinary tracts.
Possible interaction: digoxin.
Side effects: anticholinergic side effects.
Manufacturer: Baker Norton.

PRO-VIRON

Description: an hormonal androgen preparation available as white, scored tablets containing 25mg mesterolone.
Used for: androgen deficiency, male infertility.
Dosage: 25mg 3 or 4 times each day redcued to 50–70mg in divided doses as a daily maintenance dose.
Special care: elderly patients with kidney or liver disorders, epilepsy, secondary bone cancers (risk of hypercalcaemia, hypertension, ischaemic heart diesease). Boys before age of puberty.
Avoid use: kidney disorder, hypercalcae-mia, breast cancer in men, prostate cancer.
Possible interaction: liver-inducing enzymes.

Side effects: premature closure of epiphyses in boys before puberty, precocious sexual development in boys, suppression of sperm production in men, hypercalcaemia. Increase in bone growth, priapism (prolonged, painful erection of penis not associated with sexual arousal but symptom of underlying disorder or drug), oedema with salt retention.
Manufacturer: Schering Health.

PROCAINAMIDE DURULES

Description: a class I antiarrhythmic drug available as pale yellow, sustained-release tablets containing 500mg procainamide hydrochloride.
Used for: heart arrhythmias, some disorders of muscles.
Dosage: usually 2 to thee tablets 3 times each day.
Special care: heart, liver or kidney failure. Regular blood tests required.
Avoid use: patients with myasthenia gravis, SLE, heart block, asthma.
Side effects: effects on CNS, blood changes, SLE, gastro-intestinal upset.
Manufacturer: Astra.

PROCTOFOAM H.C.

Description: a colorectal preparation combining a steroid and local anaesthetic available as an aerosol foam containing 1% hydrocortisone acetate and 1% pramoxine hydrochloride with applicator.
Used for: haemorrhoids, anal fissures, proctitis (inflammation of rectum and anus), cryptitis (inflammation of a crypt—a blind pit or small sac in the anal region).
Dosage: 1 applicator dose into the rectum 2 or 3 times each day and after passing stool. Apply to external anal area as needed.
Special care: pregnancy, short-term use only.
Avoid use: children, patients with fungal, viral or tuberculous infections.
Side effects: systemic corticosteroid side effects.
Manufacturer: Stafford-Miller.

PROCTOSEDYL

Description: a colorectal preparation combining a steroid and local anaesthetic available as suppositories containing hydrochloride. Also,

PROCTOSEDYL OINTMENT containing 0.5% hydrocortisone and 0.5% cinchocaine hydrochloride.

Used for: haemorrhoids, anal itching, inflammation.

Dosage: 1 suppository and/or 1 application of ointment in the morning and at night, and after passing motion.

Special care: pregnancy, short-term use only.

Avoid use: patients with fungal, viral or tuberculous infections.

Side effects: systemic corticosteroid side effects.

Manufacturer: Schering H.C.

PROFASI

Description: a gonadotrophin preparation available as powder in ampoules along with solvent for reconstitution and injection in different strengths containing 500 units, 1000 units, 2000 units, 5000 units and 10,000 units chorionic gonadotrophin.

Used for: underactivity of testes (infertility), undescended testicles, female infertility due to lack of ovulation, superovulation for in vitro fertilization treatment.

Dosage: underactive testes, 2000 units twice each week; undescended testicles, 500–1000 units every other day. Females, lack of ovulation, up to 10,000 units in middle of monthly cycle; superovulation, up to 10,000 units. All doses in males given intramuscularly, in females by intramuscular or subcutaneous injection.

Special care: any other hormonal disorders should be corrected before treatment starts. Hormone levels in females require monitoring.

Side effects: oedema, allergic reactions, over-stimulation of ovaries.

Manufacturer: Serono.

PROGESIC

Description: an NSAID available as yellow tablets containing 200mg fenprofen (as calcium salt) marked LILLY 4015.

Used for: pain, rheumatic and arthritic disorders including osteoarthritis, rheumatoid arthritis, ankylosing spondylitis.

Dosage: 200–600mg 3 or 4 times each day with a maximum of 3g daily.

Special care: pregnancy, breastfeeding, elderly, history of gastro-intestinal bleeding or peptic ulcer, liver or kidney disease, heart failure, asthma.

Avoid use: children, allergy to aspirin or antiinflammatory drug, severe kidney disease.

Possible interaction: aspirin, loop diuretics, anticoagulants, sulphonylureas, hydantoins, phenobarbitone, quinolones.

Side effects: liver and kidney disorders, allergic reactions, gastro-intestinal bleeding and intolerance.

Manufacturer: Lilly.

PROGYNOVA

Description: an hormonal oestrogen preparation available in the form of beige, sugar-coated tablets, containing 1mg and blue, containing 2mg oestradiol valerate respectively.

Used for: short-term treatment of menopausal symptoms.

Dosage: 1mg each day for 21 days then 7 tablet-free days, 2mg tablets should only be used when needed.

Special care: those at risk of thromboembolism, porphyria, multiple sclerosis, epilepsy, fibroids in the womb, migraine, tetany. Also, otosclerosis, gall-stones, liver disease. Pelvic organs, breasts and blood pressure should be checked regularly during course of treatment.

Avoid use: pregnancy, breastfeeding, breast or other cancer of reproductive tract or 1 which is hormone-dependent. Also, thromboembolism-type disorders, undiagnosed vaginal bleeding or endometriosis, thrombophlebitis, heart, liver or kidney disease, Rotor or Dublin-Johnson syndrome.

Possible interaction: drugs which induce liver enzymes.
Side effects: enlargement and soreness of breasts, gastro-intestinal upset, dizziness, breakthrough bleeding, headache, vomiting and nausea, weight gain.
Manufacturer: Schering H.C.

PROLEUKIN

Description: a highly toxic drug which is a recombinant interleukin-2 available as a powder in vials for reconstitution and injection containing 18 million units aldesleukin.
Used for: secondary cancer of kidney cells in some patients.
Dosage: as individually directed by physician; by intravenous infusion.
Special care: for use in specialist cancer units only.
Possible interaction: antihypertensives.
Side effects: pulmonary oedema, hypotension, serious toxic effects on liver, kidneys, bone marrow, thyroid and central nervous system.
Manufacturer: EuroCetus.

PROLUTON DEPOT

Description: a depot hormonal preparation of a progestogen containing 250mg hydroxyprogesterone hexanoate/ml in ampoules for oily injection.
Used for: habitual abortion.
Dosage: 250–500mg by intramuscular injection each week during the first 5 months of pregnancy.
Special care: hypertension, kidney or heart disease.
Avoid use: pregnancy, liver disease, cancer of breast or reproductive tract, undiagnosed vaginal bleeding, porphyria, serious disease of the arteries.
Side effects: weight changes, oedema, disturbance of menstrual cycle and pre-menstrual symptoms, depression, discomfort in breasts, change in libido, urticaria, acne, baldness, unusual hair growth, anaphylactoid-type reactions. Sleepiness, insomnia; rarely, jaundice.
Manufacturer: Schering H.C.

PROMINAL^{CD}

Description: an anticonvulsant preparation and barbiturate available as white tablets containing 30mg, 60mg and 200mg methylphenobarbitone, marked P30, P60 and P200 respectively.
Used for: focal and grand mal epilepsy.
Dosage: 100–600mg each day, children 5–15mg/kg body weight each day.
Special care: kidney and liver disorders, serious lung insufficiency.
Avoid use: pregnancy, breastfeeding, elderly, patients who are debilitated, suffering from porphyria, pain which is not controlled, history of drug or alcohol abuse.
Possible interaction: CNS depressants, griseofulvin, alcohol, phenytoin, systemic steroids, chloramphenicol, rifampicin, metronidazole, anticoagulants of the coumarin type.
Side effects: headache, respiratory depression, dizziness, unsteadiness, sleepiness, confusion, agitation, allergic responses. Drug tolerance and dependence may occur. Drug is metabolized to phenobarbitone.
Manufacturer: Sanofi Winthrop.

PRONDOL

Description: a TCAD available as yellow tablets containing 15mg iprindole (as hydrochloride) marked WYETH.
Used for: depression.
Dosage: 15–30mg 3 times daily at first with a maximum of 60mg 3 times daily. Elderly start with 15mg 3 times daily.
Special care: liver disorders, hyperthyroidism, glaucoma, lactation, epilepsy, diabetes, adrenal tumour, heart disease, urine retention. Psychotic or suicidal patients.
Avoid use: children, heart block, heart attacks, severe liver disease, pregnancy.
Possible interaction: MAOIs (or within 14 days of their use), alcohol, antidepressants, barbiturates, anticholinergics, local anaesthetics that contain adrenaline or noradrenaline, oestrogens, cimetidine, antihypertensives.

Side effects: constipation, urine retention, dry mouth, blurred vision, palpitations, tachycardia, nervousness, drowsiness, insomnia. Changes in weight, blood and blood sugar, jaundice, skin reactions, weakness, ataxia, hypotension, sweating, altered libido, gynaecomastia, galactorrhoea.
Manufacturer: Wyeth.

PRONESTYL

Description: a class I antiarrhythmic preparation available as scored, white tablets containing 250mg procainamide hydrochloride marked SQUIBB 754. Also, **PRONESTYL INJECTION**, a solution in vials containing 100mg procainamide hydrochloride/ml.
Used for: heart arrhythmias.
Dosage: tablets, up to 50mg/kg body weight each day as divided doses every 3 to 6 hours. Injection, for acute condition, rate not greater than 50mg/minute by slow intravenous injection (or 100mg with monitoring of ECG). This is repeated every 5 minutes until arrhythmia is controlled. Maximum dose 1g. By intravenous infusion, 500–600mg over 25 to 30 minutes while ECG is monitored. Then a maintenance dose of 2–6mg/minute followed by tablets, if needed, 3 to 4 hours after infusion has been given.
Special care: elderly persons, pregnant women, patients with heart or liver failure, myasthenia gravis, regular blood tests should be carried out during the course of treatment.
Avoid use: children, SLE or heart block.
Possible interaction: other antiarrhythmics, terfenadine, astemizole, phenothiazines, cimetidine, neostigmine, pyridostigmine.
Side effects: SLE, blood changes (leucopenia and agranulocytosis—severe reduction in some white blood cells due to chemicals or drugs), gastro-intestinal upset.
Manufacturer: Squibb.

PROPADERM

Description: a potent topical steroid preparation available as cream or ointment containing 0.025% beclomethasone dipropionate.
Used for: inflammatory skin conditions responsive to steroids.
Dosage: apply thinly to affected area twice each day.
Special care: thrombophlebitis, psychoses, recent intestinal anastomoses, chronic nephritis, certain cancers, osteoporosis, peptic ulcer, skin eruption/rash related to a disease, viral, fungal or active infections, tuberculosis. Hypertension, glaucoma, epilepsy, acute glomerulonephritis (inflammation of kidney glomerulus), diabetes, cirrhosis, hypothyroidism, pregnancy, stress.
To be withdrawn gradually.
Possible interaction: NSAIDs, oral anticoagulants, phenytoin, ephedrine, phenobarbitone, rifampicin, diuretics, cardiac glycosides, anticholinesterases, hypoglycaemics.
Side effects: osteoporosis, depression, euphoria, hyperglycaemia, peptic ulcers, Cushingoid changes.
Manufacturer: Yamanouchi.

PROPINE

Description: a sympathomimetic preparation available as eyedrops containing 0.1% dipivefrin hydrochloride.
Used for: hypotension in eye, open angle glaucoma.
Dosage: adults, 1 drop into eye every 12 hours.
Special care: patients without whole or part of lens (aphakia) e.g. as in surgical removal of cataracts, narrow angle between iris and cornea of eye.
Avoid use: children, patients with closed angle glaucoma, wearing soft contact lenses.
Side effects: short-lived stinging, allergic responses, increased blood flow; rarely, raised blood pressure.
Manufacturer: Allergan.

PROSCAR

Description: a preparation which is a selective 5-alpha reductase inhibitor available as film-coated, apple-shaped blue tablets containing 5mg finasteride marked with name and MSD.
Used for: benign enlargement of the prostate gland.
Dosage: 1 tablet each day for at least 6 months, then continuing long-term if condition is responding.
Special care: obstruction or disease of genital tract. Women may absorb drug via semen through sexual intercourse or by handling tablets—risk in pregnancy.
Avoid use: patients with prostate cancer.
Side effects: decreased libido, impotence, reduced volume of ejaculation possibly affecting fertility.
Manufacturer: M.S.D.

PROSTAP SR

Description: a gonadotrophin-releasing hormone analogue available as powder in microcapsule in vial with diluent for depot injection containing 3.75mg leuprorelin acetate.
Used for: advanced cancer of the prostate gland.
Dosage: 3.75mg as a single dose by subcutaneous or intramuscular injection each month.
Special care: patients may require additional treatment with an anti-androgen starting 2 or 3 days before Prostap is given and continuing for 2 to 3 weeks.
Special care: in patients at risk of compression of spinal cord or obstruction of ureter.
Side effects: short-lived bone pain and obstruction of urine, decreased libido, impotence; rarely, swelling of hand and feet due to oedema, decreased libido, nausea, fatigue.
Manufacturer: Lederle.

PROSTIGMIN

Description: an anticholinesterase preparation available as scored, white tablets containing 15mg neostigmine

bromide marked PROSTIGMIN. Also, **PROSTIGMIN INJECTION** available in ampoules containing 2.5mg neostigmin methylsulphate.
Used for: myasthenia gravis, urine retention following surgery, paralytic ileus (decrease or absence of movement—peristalsis—along the intestine due to injury or surgery).
Dosage: urine retention, paralytic ileus, 1 to 2 tablets as needed; myasthenia gravis, 5 to 20 tablets in divided doses each day. Injection, urine retention, paralytic ileus 0.5–2.5mg by subcutaneous or intramuscular injection; myasthenia gravis, 1.0–2.5mg by subcutaneous or intramuscular injection. Children, urine retention, paralytic ileus, 2.5–15mg as required; myasthenia gravis, newborn babies, 1–5mg every 4 hours, other ages 15–90mg in divided doses each day. Injection, urine retention, paralytic ileus, 0.125–1mg by intramuscular or subcutaneous injection; myasthenia gravis, newborn babies, 50–250μg every 4 hours, 30 minutes before feeds. Other ages, 200–500μg as needed.
Special care: Parkinsonism, asthma, heart disease, epilepsy, vagotonia (increased activity of and effects resulting from stimulation of vagus nerve).
Avoid use: patients with obstruction of intestine or urinary tract.
Possible interaction: cyclopropane, halothane, depolarising muscle relaxants.
Side effects: vomiting, nausea, diarrhoea, pains in abdomen, over-production of saliva.
Manufacturer: Roche.

PROSTIN E₂ ORAL

Description: a prostaglandin preparation available as rectangular, white tablets containing 500μg dinoprostone marked 76 on one side and U on the other. Also, **PROSTIN E₂ VAGINAL TABLETS**, white tablets containing 3mg, marked 715 and UPJOHN. **PROSTIN E₂ SOLUTIONS**, alcoholic solution in ampoules in 2 strengths containing 1mg and 10mg/ml. **PROSTIN E$_2$ VAGINAL GEL**, in 2 strengths containing 1mg and 2mg/3g gel.

Used for: induction of labour.

Dosage: tablets, 500µg then 0.5–1mg hourly, the maximum dose being 1.5mg. Vaginal tablets, 3mg inserted high into vagina followed by further 3mg 6 to 8 hours later if labour has not begun. Maximum dose is 6mg. Vaginal gel,1mg intravaginally at first followed by further 1–2mg after 6 hours if labour has not begun. Maximum dose is 3mg; (exceptionally, 4mg maximum dose may be needed).

Special care: higher doses may cause rupture of uterus, should not be given for more than 2 days. Glaucoma, raised pressure within eye, asthma.

Avoid use: previous history of difficult or traumatic birth, multiple pregnancy, risk of uterine rupture, obstruction or failure of uterine contractions, untreated pelvic infections, foetal distress, serious toxaemia.

Side effects: vomiting, diarrhoea, nausea, dizziness, headache, shivering, flushing, temporary fever, raised white blood cell count, exceptionally high muscle tone of uterus, very severe contractions.

Manufacturer: Upjohn.

PROSTIN F$_2$

Description: a prostaglandin available as a solution in ampoules for injection into amniotic fluid containing 5mg dinoprost (as tromethamine salt)/ml.

Used for: induction of labour—rarely used.

Special care: higher doses may cause rupture of uterus, should not be given for more than 2 days. Patients with vaginitis or cervicitis (inflammation of vagina or cervix), glaucoma, raised pressure within eye, asthma.

Avoid use: previous history of difficult or traumatic birth, multiple pregnancy, risk of uterine rupture, obstruction or failure of uterine contractions, untreated pelvic infections, foetal distress, serious toxaemia.

Side effects: vomiting, diarrhoea, nausea, dizziness, headache, shivering, flushing, temporary fever, raised white blood cell count, exceptionally high muscle tone of uterus, very severe contractions.

Manufacturer: Upjohn.

PROSTIN VR

Description: a prostaglandin preparation available as an alcoholic solution in ampoules for infusion containing 0.5mg alprostadil/ml.

Used for: newborn babies with congenital heart defects, before corrective surgery.

Dosage: 50–100 nanograms/kg body weight/minute at first then lowest effective dose.

Special care: risk of haemorrhage, arterial blood pressure must be monitored.

Avoid use: newborn babies with hyaline membrane disease (respiratory distress syndrome) in which lungs are not properly expanded, (usually premature infants between 32 and 37 weeks of gestation).

Side effects: apnoea (especially babies less than 2kg body weight), hypotension, oedema, fever, diarrhoea, tachycardia and bradycardia, flushing, convulsions, cardiac arrest. Effects on blood, weakening of walls of pulmonary artery and ductus arteriosus.

Manufacturer: Upjohn.

PROTHIADEN

Description: a TCAD preparation available as brown/red capsules containing 25mg dothiepin hydrochloride marked P25. Also, **PROTHIADEN TABLETS**, sugar-coated red tablets containing 75mg dothiepin hydrochloride marked P75.

Used for: depression and anxiety.

Dosage: adults, 75–150mg each day either as divided doses or taken as single dose at night.

Special care: liver disorders, hyperthyroidism, glaucoma, lactation, epilepsy, diabetes, adrenal tumour, heart disease, urine retention. Psychotic or suicidal patients.

Avoid use: children, heart block, heart attacks, severe liver disease, pregnancy.
Possible interaction: MAOIs (or within 14 days of their use), alcohol, antidepressants, barbiturates, anticholinergics, local anaesthetics that contain adrenaline or noradrenaline, oestrogens, cimetidine, antihypertensives.
Side effects: constipation, urine retention, dry mouth, blurred vision, palpitations, tachycardia, nervousness, drowsiness, insomnia. Changes in weight, blood and blood sugar, jaundice, skin reactions, weakness, ataxia, hypotension, sweating, altered libido, gynaecomastia, galactorrhoea.
Manufacturer: Boots.

PROVERA

Description: an hormonal progestogen preparation available as scored tablets in 3 strengths all containing medroxyprogesterone acetate. Orange, 2.5mg, marked U64; blue, 5mg, marked 286; white, 10mg, marked Upjohn 50.
Used for: abnormal uterine bleeding, endometriosis, secondary ammenorrhoea (situation where menstrual periods stop due to underlying physical, psychiatric or environmental factors). Breast cancer in women after menopause, renal cell and endometrial cancer.
Dosage: abnormal uterine bleeding 2.5–10mg each day for 5 to 10 days, repeated for 2 or 3 monthly cycles. Endometriosis, 10mg 3 times each day starting on first day of cycle and and continuing for 90 days without a break. Ammenorrhoea, 2.5–10mg each day for 5 to 10 days beginning on what is thought to be 16th continuing to 21st day of cycle. Repeat for 3 monthly cycles without break. Breast cancer, 400–800mg each day, renal cell and endometrial cancer, 200–400 mg daily.
Special care: diabetes, asthma, heart or kidney disorders, migraine, history of depression.
Avoid use: pregnancy, cancer of genital tract, liver disease, history of or present thromboembolic conditions.

Side effects: gain in weight, abnormal production of breast milk, slight oedema, breast pain. Gastro-intestinal upset, central nervous system effects, skin and mucous membrane reactions.
Manufacturer: Upjohn.

PROZAC

Description: an antidepressant preparation which is a 5HT reuptake inhibitor, promoting the availability of this neurotransmitter. It is available as white/green capsules containing 20mg fluoxetine hydrochloride marked DISTA 3105. Also, **PROZAC LIQUID**, a syrup containing 20mg/5ml.
Used for: depression especially when sedation is not needed. Obsessive-compulsive disorders, bulimia nervosa (over-eating phase of anorexia nervosa).
Dosage: depression, usual dose in the order of 20mg each day; obsessive compulsive disorder, 20–60mg each day; bulimia nervosa, 60mg each day.
Special care: pregnancy, heart disease, epilepsy, diabetes, kidney disorder, liver failure, heart disease.
Avoid use: children, breastfeeding, severe kidney failure, unstable epilepsy.
Possible interaction: vinblastine, MAOIs, lithium, carbamazepine, TCADs, flecainide, encainide, tryptophan.
Side effects: diarrhoea, vomiting, nausea, insomnia, headache, dizziness, drowsiness, anxiety, weakness, fever, hypomania, convulsions, mania. Withdraw drug if allergic reactions or rash occur.
Manufacturer: Dista.

PULMADIL

Description: a broncho-dilator which is a selective beta$_2$-agonist available as a metered dose aerosol delivering 0.2mg rimiterol hydrobromide per dose.
Used for: bronchospasm resulting from chronic bronchitis and bronchial asthma.
Dosage: 1 to 3 doses which can be repeated after half an hour, if needed. Maximum of 24 doses in 24 hours.

Special care: pregnancy, weak heart, arrhythmias, angina, hyperthyroidism, hypertension.
Possible interaction: sympathomimetics.
Side effects: dilation of peripheral blood vessels, headache.
Manufacturer: 3M Health Care.

PULMICORT

Description: a bronchodilator corticosteroid preparation delivering 200µg budesonide per metered dose aerosol, suitable for use with a standard inhaler, nebuhaler or collapsible space delivery unit. Also, **PULMICORT LS** delivering 50µg per dose. **PULMICORT TURBOHALER** for use with a powder inhaler delivering 100, 200 or 400µg budesonide per metered dose. **PULMICORT RESPULES** available at strengths of 0.25mg and 0.5mg per ml available in ampoules for nebulisation.
Used for: bronchial asthma.
Dosage: Pulmicort, 1 puff twice daily up to 8 puffs daily in severe attack. Pulmicort turbohaler 200–1600µg in divided doses daily. Pulmicort respules, in the order of 1–2mg twice each day with a maintenance dose of 0.5–1mg twice daily. Children, Pulmicort, 1 to 2 puffs twice each day. Pulmicort LS (children only), 1 to 8 puffs each day. Pulmicort turbo-haler, 200–800µg in divided doses daily. Pulmicort respules, age 3 months to 12 years, 0.5–1mg twice each day with a maintenance dose of 0.25–0.5mg twice daily.
Special care: pregnancy, pulmonary tuberculosis either active or statis, those transferring from other (systemic) steroids.
Side effects: candidiasis of throat and mouth, dryness and hoarseness.
Manufacturer: Astra.

PUMP-HEP

Description: an anticoagulant preparation of sodium heparin available in single dose ampoules for continuous infusion, at a strength of 1000 units/ml.
Used for: pulmonary embolism and deep vein thrombosis.

Dosage: 15,000 units; children 250 units/kg body weight, both 12 hourly. Both following on from first doses given by intravenous infusion or injection.
Special care: pregnancy, kidney or liver disease. Drug should be withdrawn gradually if taken for more than 5 days. Platelet counts are required if taken for more than 5 days.
Avoid use: patients with bleeding disorders, haemophilia, serious hypertension, recent operation on eye or nervous system, cerebral aneurysm, serious liver disease, peptic ulcer, allergy to heparin, thrombocytopenia.
Possible interaction: aspirin, dipyridamole, glyceryl trinitrate infusion.
Side effects: allergic reactions, skin necrosis, osteoporosis (if taken longterm). Stop drug immediately if thrombocytopenia occurs.
Manufacturer: Leo.

PURI-NETHOL

Description: a cytotoxic drug available as scored, fawn-coloured tablets containing 50mg mercaptopurine coded WELLCOME 04A.
Used for: leukaemia, especially in children.
Dosage: adults and children, 2.5mg/kg bod yweight each day at first, used for maintenance treatment.
Special care: pregnancy, kidney disorder. Dosage should be reduced if allopurinol is also being received.
Possible interaction: allopurinol, warfarin.
Side effects: vomiting, nausea, bone marrow suppression, anorexia, toxic effects on liver.
Manufacturer: Wellcome.

PYOPEN

Description: an antibiotic preparation of penicillin available as powder in vials for reconstitution and injection containing 1g and 5g carbenicillin sodium.
Used for: endocarditis, meningitis, septicaemia, infected burns and wounds, urinary and respiratory tract infections,

sepsis within abdomen, infections following operations.
Dosage: by rapid infusion, 5g every 4 to 6 hours; children, 250–400mg/kg body weight in divided doses each day.
Special care: kidney disorders.
Side effects: gastro-intestinal upset, allergic hypersensitivity reactions, hypokalaemia, change in function of blood platelets.
Manufacturer: Link.

PYROGASTRONE

Description: a compound preparation combining an antacid and cytoprotectant available as off-white tablets containing 20mg carbenoxolone sodium, 60mg magnesium trisilicate, 600mg alginic acid, 240mg dried aluminium hydroxide, 210mg sodium bicarbonate marked PG and with symbol. Also, **PYROGAS-TRONE LIQUID** containing 10mg carbenoxolone sodium, 150mg dried aluminium hydroxide/5ml.
Used for: gastro-oesophageal reflux, oesophagitis.
Dosage: 1 tablet or 10ml suspension 3 times each day after meals plus 2 tablets or 20ml suspension at bedtime.
Special care: patients with fluid and salt retention.
Avoid use: pregnancy, children, elderly, hypokalaemia, liver or kidney failure.
Possible interaction: diuretics, digoxin.
Side effects: hypertension, heart failure, hypokalaemia, retention of water and salt.
Manufacturer: Sanofi Winthrop.

QUESTRAN A

Description: a bile acid sequestrant available as a low sugar powder in sachets containing 4g cholestyramine. Also, **QUESTRAN**, powder in sachets containing 4g cholestyramine.
Used for: diarrhoea resulting from

surgery, radiation, Crohn's disease, damage or disease of vagus nerve, itching resulting from liver disease. Also, prevention of coronary heart disease in men with very high lipid/cholesterol levels in the blood who are aged between 35 and 59. Treatment of type II hyperlipoproteinaemias (high levels of lipid-bound proteins).
Dosage: diarrhoea and elevated lipid and lipid/protein levels, 1 sachet each day at first gradually increasing to 3 to 6 each day after 3 or 4 weeks, taken as single or divided doses; daily maximum is 9 sachets. Itching, 1 or 2 sachets daily; children over 6 years of age, dose in proportion to that of adult weighing 70kg.
Special care: pregnancy, breastfeeding, dietary supplements of vitamins A, D amd K may be needed with high doses taken long term, patients with phenylke-tonuria (abnormal presence of phenylketones in urine) taking Questran A. Any other drugs should be taken 1 hour before Questran A or 4 hours afterwards.
Avoid use: children under 6 years of age, total obstruction of bile duct.
Possible interaction: antibiotics, digitalis, diuretics.
Side effects: increased tendency for bleeding in patients taking drug long-term due to deficiency in vitamin K, constipation.
Manufacturer: Bristol-Myers.

QUINOCORT

Description: a topical preparation combining a mildly potent steroid and antifungal, antibacterial agent available as a cream containing 0.5% potassium hydroxyquinolone sulphate and 1% hydrocortisone.
Used for: inflammatory, infected skin conditions responsive to steroids.
Dosage: apply thinly 2 or 3 times each day.
Special care: thrombophlebitis, psychoses, recent intestinal anastomoses, chronic nephritis, certain cancers, osteoporosis, peptic ulcer, skin eruption/

rash related to a disease, viral, fungal or active infections, tuberculosis. Hypertension, glaucoma, epilepsy, acute glomerulonephritis (inflammation of kidney glomerulus), diabetes, cirrhosis, hypothyroidism, pregnancy, stress. To be withdrawn gradually.
Possible interaction: NSAIDs, oral anticoagulants, phenytoin, ephedrine, phenobarbitone, rifampicin, diuretics, cardiac glycosides, anticholinesterases, hypoglycaemics.
Side effects: osteoporosis, depression, euphoria, hyperglycaemia, peptic ulcers, Cushingoid changes.
Manufacturer: Quinoderm.

RAPIFEN^{CD}

Description: a narcotic analgesic and controlled drug, alfentanil hydrochloride, available in ampoules containing 500μg/ml. Also **RAPIFEN INTENSIVE CARE** (5mg/ml).
Used for: analgesia during short operations, enhancement of anaesthesia, suppression of respiration for patients in intensive care receiving assistance with ventilation.
Dosage: 500μg over 30 seconds to start then 250μg; with assisted ventilation (for adult and child) 30–50μg/kg then 15μg/kg, all by intravenous injection. 50–100μg/kg over 10 minutes by intravenous infusion for adult or child with assisted ventilation. For analgesia and respiratory suppression, 2mg/hour adjusted according to response.
Special care: myasthenia gravis, elderly, liver disease, pregnancy, respiratory disease.
Avoid use: respiratory depression, diseases causing obstruction of the airways.
Possible interaction: erythromycin, anxiolytics and hypnotics, cimetidine, cisapride, antidepressants.

Side effects: respiratory depression, temporary hypotension, nausea, vomiting, bradycardia.
Manufacturer: Janssen.

RASTINON

Description: a sulphonylurea, tolbutamide, available as white tablets (500mg) marked with symbol and RASTINON 0.5.
Used for: maturity-onset diabetes.
Dosage: 2 per day at the start, adjusted depending upon response. Maintenance dose of 1 to 3 per day as a single or divided dose. Not for children.
Special care: the elderly or patients with kidney failure.
Avoid use: during pregnancy or lactation; juvenile, growth-onset or unstable brittle diabetes (insulin-dependent diabetes mellitus); ketoacidosis; severe kidney or liver disorders; stress, infections or surgery; endocrine disorders.
Possible interaction: MAOIs, corticosteroids, ß-blockers, diuretics, corticotrophin (ACTH), oral contraceptives, alcohol. Also aspirin, oral anticoagulants, and the generic drugs bezafibrate, clofibrate, phenylbutazone, cyclophosphamide, rifampicin, sulphonamides and chloramphenicol. Also glucagon.
Side effects: skin rash and other sensitivity reactions. Other conditions tend to be rare, e.g. hyponatraemia (low blood sodium concentration) or aplastic anaemia.
Manufacturer: Hoechst.

RAZOXIN

Description: a cytotoxic and antineoplastic drug, razoxone, available as white tablets (125mg), marked ICI.
Used for: leukaemias.
Dosage: 150–500mg/m² per day for 3 to 5 days.
Side effects: nausea, vomiting, bone marrow suppression, hair loss, suppression of the immune system, teratogenic.
Manufacturer: Zeneca.

RECORMON

Description: recombinant human erythro-poietin (hormone-regulating red blood cell production) available as powder in vials (1000, 2000, 5000 units epoetin beta).
Used for: anaemia in patients with chronic kidney failure and on dialysis.
Dosage: 20 units/kg 3 times per week for 4 weeks, by subcutaneous injection, or 40 units/kg by intravenous injection with the same frequency. Dose may be doubled depending upon haemoglobin response. May be increased by 20 units/kg at monthly intervals to a maximum of 720 units/kg per week. For maintenance, reduce the dosage to half and adjust weekly. Children over 2 as per adults; not recommended for children under 2.
Special care: history of epilepsy, thrombocytosis (increase in blood platelet count giving an increased tendency to blood clots), hypertension, chronic liver failure, pregnancy, lactation. May need iron supplements, check haemoglobin, blood pressure, platelet count and serum electrolytes.
Side effects: symptoms resembling flu, hypertension, clotting in atrio-ventricular fistula.
Manufacturer: B.M. Pharm.

REDEPTIN

Description: an antipsychotic and diphe-nylbutylpiperidine, fluspirilene, available as 2mg/ml in ampoules and 6ml vials.
Used for: schizophrenia.
Dosage: starting with 2mg per week by intramuscular injection increasing as necessary by 2mg per week to a maximum of 20mg. Dose for maintenance, 2–8mg per week. Elderly, start with 0.5mg per week and adjust depending upon response. Not for children.
Special care: lactation, epilepsy, liver or kidney disease, Parkinsonism.
Avoid use: pregnancy.
Possible interaction: alcohol, depres-sants of the CNS, antihypertensives, antidepressants, analgesics, antidiabet-ics, levodopa, anticonvulsants.

Side effects: rigidity, tremor, dry mouth, muscle spasms in eye, neck, face and back, tardive dyskinesia (involuntary, repetitive muscle movements in the limbs, face and trunk), tachycardia, constipation, blocked nose, difficulty in urinating, hypotension, weight gain, impotence, galactorrhoea, gynaecomastia, blood changes, jaundice, dermatitis, ECG changes, fatigue, drowsiness, seizures.
Manufacturer: S.H. & F.

REFOLINON

Description: Folinic acid (as a calcium salt) available as pale yellow tablets (15mg) marked F and CF.
Used for: megaloblastic anaemia, antidote or rescue after treatment with methotrexate.
Dosage: 1 tablet daily for anaemia, see literature for antidote use.
Also, **REFOLINON INJECTION**, containing 3mg/ml.
Avoid use: vitamin B_{12} deficiency anaemia.
Manufacturer: Farmitalia.

REGAINE

Description: a hair restorer, minoxidil, available as a liquid containing 20mg/ml.
Used for: alopecia.
Dosage: 1ml applied to the scalp 2 times per day for at least 4 months. Hair loss will recur if treatment ceases.
Special care: hypotension, broken skin, check blood pressure in susceptible patients.
Side effects: dermatitis.
Manufacturer: Upjohn.

RELIFEX

Description: an NSAID and naphthylal-kanone, nabumetone, available as red tablets (500mg) marked RELIFEX 500.
Also, **RELIFEX SUSPENSION** (500mg/5ml).
Used for: rheumatoid arthritis and osteoarthritis.
Dosage: 2 tablets or 10ml as 1 dose at bedtime. An extra 1 to 2 tablets or 5–10ml may be taken in the morning for severe

cases. Elderly, 1 to 2 tablets or 5–10ml per day. Not for children.
Special care: elderly, allergy-induced by aspirin or anti-inflammatory drugs, liver or kidney disease, history of peptic ulcer.
Avoid use: active peptic ulcer, pregnancy, breastfeeding, severe liver disease.
Possible interaction: sulphonylurea, hypoglycaemics, hydantoin, oral anticoagulants, anticonvulsants.
Side effects: nausea, diarrhoea, abdominal pain, dyspepsia, constipation, headache, dizziness, rashes, sedation.
Manufacturer: Bencard.

REMEDEINE

Description: an analgesic containing 500mg paracetamol, 20mg dihydrocodeine tartrate in white tablets marked PD/20. Also, **REMEDEINE FORTE** containing 500mg paracetamol and 30mg dihydrocodeine tartrate in white tablets marked PD/30.
Used for: severe pain.
Dosage: 1 to 2 tablets 4 to 6 hourly up to a daily maximum of 8 tablets. Not for children.
Special care: chronic liver disease, hypothyroidism, allergies, kidney disease.
Avoid use: raised intracranial pressure, depression of respiration, diseases causing obstruction of the respiratory tract.
Possible interaction: alcohol, MAOIs.
Side effects: nausea, vomiting, drowsiness, headache, vertigo, constipation, retention of urine.
Manufacturer: Napp.

RESPACAL

Description: a β_2-agonist and bronchodilator, tulobuterol hydrochloride, available as white tablets (2mg) marked ucb.
Used for: prevention and control of bronchospasm in asthma.
Dosage: 1 tablet twice per day increasing to 3 times per day if required. Children over 10 years, $^1/_2$ to 1 tablet twice per day. Not for children under 10.
Also, **RESPACAL SYRUP**, 1mg per 5ml.
Dosage: 10ml 2 or 3 times per day.

Children over 10 years, 5–10ml; 6 to 10 years, 2.5–5ml both twice per day. Not for children under 6.
Special care: epilepsy, hypertension, hyperthyroidism, diabetes, disease of the heart and blood vessels.
Avoid use: acute liver failure or chronic liver disease, kidney failure.
Side effects: tremor, palpitations, tachycardia, possible serious hypokalaemia.
Manufacturer: UCB.

RESTANDOL

Description: an androgen, testosterone undecanoate, available as brown, oval gelatin capsules (40mg strength), marked ORG and DV3.
Used for: osteoporosis caused by androgen deficiency, deficiency in the male of the secretory activity of the testis whether due to castration or other disorder.
Dosage: starting with 3 to 4 capsules per day for 2 to 3 weeks, adjusting to 1 to 3 depending upon response.
Special care: epilepsy, hypertension, heart, liver or kidney disease, migraine.
Avoid use: untreated heart failure, cancer of the liver or prostate, abnormal condition of the kidney (nephrosis/nephrotic syndrome), ischaemic heart disease.
Possible interaction: drugs that induce liver enzymes.
Side effects: oedema, weight increase, tumours of the liver, lower fertility, premature epiphyseal closure, extended erection of the penis not associated with sexual arousal.
Manufacturer: Organon.

RETIN-A

Description: a vitamin A derivative, tretinoin available as a 0.025% lotion. Also, **RETIN-A GEL** (0.01% and 0.025%), **RETIN-A CREAM** (0.025% and 0.05%).
Used for: acne vulgaris (common in adolescents) where there are pustules, papules (solid, raised lesion less than 1cm across) and comedones (blackheads).
Dosage: apply once or twice per day for at least 8 weeks. Not for children.

Special care: pregnancy, avoid UV light.
Avoid use: eczema, abrasions, cuts. Do not get on eyes or mucous membranes.
Possible interaction: keratolytics.
Side effects: irritation, erythema, alteration to skin pigmentation.
Manufacturer: Cilag.

RETROVIR

Description: an antiviral compound, zidovudine, available as white capsules (100mg) marked 100 and Y9C and white/blue capsules (250mg) marked 250 and H2F. Both bear the company logo and a blue securiband. Also, **RETROVIR SYRUP**, 50mg/5ml, a pale-yellow strawberry-flavoured solution.
Used for: HIV disease.
Dosage: adults (asymptomatic) 500–1500mg per day in 4 or 5 divided doses; 6 200mg per day if tolerable for symptomatic HIV. Children over 3 months, 180mg/m^2 4 times per day. Not for children under 3 months.
Special care: blood tests every 2 weeks for the first 3 months, then monthly. Alter dose should there be anaemia or bone marrow suppression. Kidney or liver disease, elderly, pregnancy.
Avoid use: low neutrophil (white blood cell) counts or low levels of haemoglobin, lactation.
Possible interaction: analgesics (paracetamol particularly), potentially nephroptoxics or bone marrow suppressives, probenecid, methadone, drugs affecting liver activity. Warn patients about accompanying use of self-administered drugs.
Side effects: neutropenia, leucopenia, nausea, anaemia, abdominal pain, fever, rash, headache, muscle pain, insomnia, numbness or tingling sensations.
Manufacturer: Wellcome.

REVANIL

Description: a dopamine agonist, lysuride maleate, available as white tablets (200µg) marked CM in a hexagon.
Used for: Parkinsonism.

Dosage: start with 1 tablet at bedtime with food increasing weekly by 1 tablet daily to a maximum of 25 daily. Not for children.
Special care: pregnancy, tumour of the pituitary.
Avoid use: weak heart, disturbance of peripheral circulation.
Possible interaction: dopamine antagonists, psychotropics (affecting behaviour and psychic functions).
Side effects: nausea, vomiting, hypotension, headache, dizziness, lethargy, drowsiness, abdominal pain, constipation, psychiatric reactions.
Manufacturer: Roche.

RHEUMOX

Description: a benzotriazine and NSAID, azapropazone dihydrate, available as orange capsules (300mg) marked RHEUMOX and AHR. Also, **RHEUMOX TABLETS** containing 600mg in orange, oblong tablets marked RHEUMOX 600.
Used for: gout, hyperuricaemia (high blood uric acid), rheumatoid arthritis, osteoarthritis, ankylosing spondylitis.
Dosage: acute gout, 2.4g in divided doses over 24 hours then 1.8g per day and 1.2g per day; 600mg morning and night for chronic gout. For other conditions, 1.2g per day in 2 or 4 divided doses. Elderly, 300mg morning and night up to a maximum of 900mg per day if kidneys function normally. Not for children.
Special care: pregnancy, heart failure, elderly, liver or kidney disease (monitor if on long-term treatment), past peptic ulcer.
Avoid use: kidney disorder, past blood changes, peptic ulcer.
Possible interaction: sulphonamides, hypoglycaemics, anticoagulants, methotrexate, phenytoin.
Side effects: oedema, gastro-intestinal bleeding, sensitivity to light, alveolitis (allergic lung reaction to substances inhaled). Discontinue upon a positive Coomb's test (antiglobulin test—an antibody against globulin).
Manufacturer: Wyeth.

RHINOCORT

Description: a corticosteroid, budesonide, available as a metered dose (50µg) nasal aerosol.
Used for: rhinitis.
Dosage: apply twice to each nostril twice per day, reducing to 1 application twice daily. Not recommended for long-term continuous treatment for children. Also, **RHINOCORT AQUA**, a 100µg metered pump nasal spray.
Dosage: start with 2 applications in each nostril every morning; 1 application for maintenance. Not for children.
Special care: pregnancy, infections of a fungal, viral or tuberculous nature.
Side effects: sneezing
Manufacturer: Astra.

RHINOLAST

Description: an antihistamine, azelastine hydrochloride, available as a 0.1% metered dose nasal spray.
Used for: rhinitis.
Dosage: 1 application per nostril twice per day. Not for children.
Special care: pregnancy, breastfeeding.
Side effects: nasal irritation, effect on taste.
Manufacturer: Asta Medica.

RIDAURA

Description: a gold salt, auranofin, available as pale yellow square tablets (3mg).
Used for: progressive rheumatoid arthritis not controlled by NSAIDs.
Dosage: start with 6mg per day and continue for 3 to 6 months minimum. Dosage can be increased to 3mg 3 times per day if response is inadequate. Cease after a further 3 months if response still inadequate. Not for children.
Special care: kidney and liver disorders, rash, past bone marrow depression, bowel inflammation. Blood and urinary protein should be monitored before and during treatment. Women should use effective contraception during and 6 months after treatment.
Avoid use: past necrotising enterocolitis (an acute inflammatory bowel disorder affecting large and small intestines), exfoliative dermatitis, severe blood disorders, kidney disease, severe liver disease, SLE, pregnancy, breastfeeding, pulmonary fibrosis.
Side effects: nausea, abdominal pain, diarrhoea, rashes, itching, hair loss, ulcerative enterocolitis, inflammation of the mouth (stomatitis), conjunctivitis, nephrotic syndrome (oedema, low protein in the urine and low blood albumin levels), upset to taste.
Manufacturer: Bencard.

RIFADIN

Description: an antibiotic and antimalarial, rifampicin, available as blue/red capsules (150mg) and red capsules (300mg), marked LEPETIT. Also, **RIFADIN SYRUP** (100mg/5ml) and **RIFADIN INFUSION** as 600mg powder in a vial with 10ml solvent in an ampoule.
Used for: prevention of meningococcal meningitis, treatment of carriers of *Haemophilus influenzae*, additional therapy for brucellosis, Legionnaire's disease and serious staphylococcal infections, tuberculosis and mycobacterial infections, leprosy.
Dosage: meningitis—600g twice per day for 2 days; influenza—20mg/kg per day for 4 days; brucellosis—600–1200mg per day as 2 to 4 doses; tuberculosis—8–12mg/kg per day thirty minutes before or 2 hours after a meal; leprosy—600mg once per month or 10mg/kg per day. Children: meningitis—1 to 12 years, 10mg/kg twice per day for 2 days; 3 months to 1 year, 5mg/kg, not for children under 3 months; influenza—20mg/kg daily for 4 days, infants up to 1 month 10mg/kg daily for 4 days; tuberculosis—10–30mg/kg per day to a daily maximum of 600mg; leprosy—as adult dose.
Special care: pregnancy, breastfeeding, liver disease, elderly, poorly nourished or the very young.
Avoid use: jaundice.

Possible interaction: digitalis, hypoglycae-mics, cyclosporin, corticosteroids, anticoagulants, oral contraceptives, dapsone, quinidine, phenytoin, narcotics.
Side effects: rashes, gastro-intestinal upset, flu-like symptoms, upset liver function, orange discolouration of urine and secretions.
Manufacturer: Merrell Dow.

RIFATER

Description: a compound drug containing 50mg isoniazid, 300mg pyrazinamide and 120mg rifampicin in pink-beige tablets.
Used for: pulmonary tuberculosis in the initial intensive phase.
Dosage: a single dose thirty minutes before or 2 hours after a meal—over 65kg, 6 tablets per day; 50–64kg, 5 tablets; 40–49kg, 4 tablets; under 40 kg, 3 tablets per day, to continue for 2 months followed by rifampicin/isoniazid compound. For the initial period, the additional use of ethambutol or streptomycin is advised. For children contact the manufacturer.
Special care: history of epilepsy, gout, liver disease, haemoptysis (coughing up blood).
Avoid use: jaundice.
Possible interaction: digitalis, hypo-glycaemics, cyclosporin, corticosteroids, anticoagulants, oral contraceptives, dapsone, quinidine, phenytoin, narcotics.
Side effects: rashes, gastro-intestinal upset, flu-like symptoms, upset liver function, orange discolouration of urine and secretions.
Manufacturer: Merrell Dow.

RIFINAH

Description: a combination of rifampicin (150mg) and isoniazid (100mg) in pink tablets marked RH150 and also orange tablets, coded RH300 containing 300mg rifampicin and 150mg isoniazid.
Used for: tuberculosis.
Dosage: 2 Rifinah 300 daily if over 50kg; 3 Rifinah 150 daily if under 50kg,

as a single dose thirty minutes before or 2 hours after a meal. Not for children.
Special care: pregnancy, lactation, under-nourished, elderly, liver disease (monitor).
Avoid use: jaundice.
Possible interaction: digitalis, hypoglycae-mics, cyclosporin, corticosteroids, anticoagulants, oral contraceptives, dapsone, quinidine, phenytoin, narcotics.
Side effects: rashes, gastro-intestinal upset, flu-like symptoms, upset liver function, orange discolouration of urine and secretions.
Manufacturer: Merrell Dow.

RIMACTANE

Description: a rifamycin, rifampicin, available in red capsules coded JZ 150 (150mg) and red/brown capsules coded C3 300 (300mg), both also marked CG. Also, **RIMACTANE SYRUP** (100mg/5ml).
Used for: prevention of meningococcal meningitis, additional treatment in tuberculosis and certain mycobacterial infections.
Dosage: (meningitis) 600mg twice per day for 2 days; children 1 to 12 years 10mg/kg; up to 1 year, 5mg/kg both twice per day for 2 days. For tuberculo-sis etc., 450–600mg thirty minutes before breakfast; children up to 20mg/k per day to a maximum single dose of 600mg.
Also, **RIMACTANE INFUSION** as 300mg rifampicin powder in a vial.
Special care: porphyria, pregnancy, breastfeeding, liver disease (monitor), elderly, poorly-nourished or the very young.
Avoid use: jaundice.
Possible interaction: corticosteroids, digitalis, anticoagulants, hypoglycae-mics, cyclosporin, oral contraceptives, phenytoin, quinidine, antacids, dapsone anticholinergics, opiates.
Side effects: rashes, gastro-intestinal upse flu-like symptoms, upset liver function, discolouration of urine and secretions.
Manufacturer: Ciba.

RIMACTAZID

Description: a combination of rifampicin and isoniazid in pink tablets '150' marked El and CG (150mg/100mg respectively) and orange oblong tablets '300' marked OH and CG (300mg/150mg respectively).
Used for: tuberculosis.
Dosage: 2 300 tablets per day before breakfast (for over 50kg) or 3 150 tablets per day (for under 50kg). Not for children.
Special care: porphyria, elderly, epilepsy, pregnancy, lactation, liver disease (monitor).
Avoid use: acute liver disease, neuritis (peripheral), past drug-induced hepatitis.
Possible interaction: anticoagulants, anticholinergics, corticosteroids, antacids, digitalis, hypoglycaemics, cyclosporin, oral contraceptives, phenytoin, dapsone, narcotics, quinidine, disulfiram
Side effects: rashes, gastro-intestinal upset, flu-like symptoms, upset liver function, discolouration of urine and secretions.
Manufacturer: Ciba.

RIMSO-50

Description: a bladder irrigator, dimethyl sulphoxide (50%, sterile solution).
Used for: relief of interstitial cystitis.
Dosage: see literature.
Special care: malignancy of the urinary tract. Check liver and kidney function and eyes regularly.
Side effects: hypersensitivity reactions because of histamine release.
Manufacturer: Britannia.

RINATEC

Description: an anticholinergic nasal spray, ipratropium bromide, in 20µg metered dose spray.
Used for: rhinorrhoea (runny nose) associated with perennial rhinitis.
Dosage: 1 or 2 sprays in the nostrils up to 4 times per day. Not for children.
Special care: enlarged prostate, glaucoma.
Side effects: irritation, nasal dryness.
Manufacturer: Boehringer Ingelheim.

RISPERDAL

Description: an antipsychotic and benzisoxazole derivative, risperidone available as 1mg white (Ris/1), 2mg orange (Ris/2), 3mg yellow (Ris/3) and 4mg green oblong tablets (Ris/4), all marked Janssen.
Used for: schizophrenia and other psychoses.
Dosage: (over 15 years) 1mg on first day, 2mg on second day, 3mg on third day , all twice per day. Maximum 8mg twice per day. Elderly, start with 0.5mg, increasing by 0.5mg to 1-2mg twice daily. Not for children.
Special care: epilepsy, elderly, disease of kidney, liver or heart and blood vessels, Parkinsonism, pregnancy, breastfeeding. If driving or operating machine. Cease if signs of tardive dyskinesia.
Possible interaction: levodopa, dopamine agonists, drugs acting centrally.
Side effects: hypotension when standing, tachycardia, galactorrhoea, sexual disorders, extrapyramidal symptoms, anxiety, insomnia, headache, fatigue, dizziness, weight gain, gastro-intestinal upset, rash, rhinitis, blurred vision, poor concentration.
Manufacturer: Janssen/Organon.

RIVOTRIL

Description: an anticonvulsant and benzodiazepine, clonazepam, available as beige tablets (0.5mg) and white tablets (2mg) marked RIV and with tablet strength.
Used for: epilepsy.
Dosage: start with maximum daily dose of 1mg increasing to maintenance of 4–8mg per day. Elderly, 0.5mg daily maximum initially. Children: 5 to 12 years, 0.5mg maximum per day initially rising to maintenance of 3–6mg per day; 1 to 5 years, 0.25mg, and 1–3mg (same criteria); up to 1 year, 0.25mg and 0.5–1mg (same criteria). Gradually increase all to maintenance dose.
Also, **RIVOTRIL INJECTION**, 1mg in solvent in ampoules (with diluent).

Used for: status epilepticus (continual seizures producing brain damage unless halted).
Dosage: 1mg by slow intravenous injection. Children, 0.5mg by same means, but see literature.
Special care: chronic lung insufficiency, chronic liver or kidney disease, the elderly, pregnant, during labour or lactation. Judgement and dexterity may be affected, long-term use is to be avoided. To be withdrawn gradually.
Avoid use: acute lung insufficiency, depression of respiration (except in cases of acute muscle spasms). Also when treating anxiety, obsessional states or chronic psychosis.
Possible interaction: alcohol and other depressants of the central nervous system, anticonvulsants.
Side effects: vertigo, gastro-intestinal upsets, confusion, ataxia, drowsiness, light-headedness, hypotension, disturbance of vision, skin rashes. Also urine retention, changes in libido. Dependence a potential problem.
Manufacturer: Roche.

RO-A-VIT

Description: Vitamin A as 50,000 units per ml in an aqueous solution (in ampoules).
Used for: vitamin A deficiency.
Dosage: 1/2 to 1 ampoule by deep intra-muscular injection, weekly or monthly.
Special care: do not mix with other vitamin injections, liver disease. Monitor.
Side effects: possible hypervitaminosis (toxic effects of excessive doses) in children and infants.
Manufacturer: Cambridge.

ROACCUTANE

Description: a vitamin A derivative, isotretinoin, available in red/white gelatin capsules (5 and 20mg) marked with R and strength.
Used for: acne, especially severe forms unresponsive to antibiotics.
Dosage: start with 0.5mg/kg with food

for 4 weeks adjusting depending upon response within the range 0.1–1.0mg/kg for an additional 8 to 12 weeks. Not normally repeated. Not for children.
Special care: (hospital use only) exclude pregnancy, effective contraception necessary 1 month before and up to 4 weeks after treatment. Check liver function and blood lipids regularly.
Avoid use: pregnancy, breastfeeding, liver or kidney disease.
Possible interaction: high doses of vitamin A.
Side effects: hair loss, dryness, mucosal erosion, nausea, headache, drowsiness, sweating, seizures, menstrual disorders, mood changes, rise in liver enzymes; sometimes hearing loss, thrombo-cytopenia.
Manufacturer: Roche.

ROBAXIN

Description: a carbamate and muscle relaxant, methocarbamol, available as white, oblong tablets marked AHR (750mg strength).
Used for: skeletal muscle spasm.
Dosage: 2 tablets 4 times per day.
Elderly—1 tablet 4 times per day. Not for children.
Also, **ROBAXIN INJECTABLE** (100mg/ml in ampoules).
Special care: liver or kidney disease, pregnancy, breastfeeding.
Avoid use: coma, brain damage, myasthenia gravis, epilepsy.
Possible interaction: depressants and stimulants of the CNS, alcohol, anticholinergics.
Side effects: allergies, drowsiness.
Manufacturer: Shire.

ROBAXISAL FORTE

Description: a carbamate and salicylate and muscle relaxant comprising 400mg methocarbamol and 325g aspirin in pink/white, two-layered tablets marked AHR.
Used for: skeletal muscle spasms.
Dosage: 2 tablets (elderly 1) 4 times daily. Not for children.

Special care: pregnancy, breastfeeding, liver or kidney disease, past bronchospasm, allergy to anti-inflammatory drugs.
Avoid use: brain damage, coma, myasthenia gravis, peptic ulcer, epilepsy, haemophilia.
Possible interaction: anticholinergics, alcohol, stimulants and depressants of the CNS, hypoglycaemics, hydantoins, anticoagulants.
Side effects: gastro-intestinal bleeding, allergies, drowsiness.
Manufacturer: Shire.

ROBINUL

Description: an anticholinergic, glycopyrronium bromide, available as ampoules containing 0.2mg/ml. Also, **ROBINUL NEOSTIGMINE** which contains 0.5mg glycopyrronium bromide and 2.5mg/ml neostigmine methysulphate in ampoules.
Used for: reduction of secretions during anaesthesia.
Dosage: for premedication 200–400μg Robinul by intramuscular or intravenous injection (child: 4–8μg/kg to a maximum of 200μg). Robinul neostigmine: 1–2ml (child 0.02ml) by intravenous injection over 10 to thirty seconds.
Special care: cardiovascular disease, atropine should be given, asthma, epilepsy, peptic ulcer, pregnancy, breast-feeding, hypotension, Parkinsonism, bradycardia, recent myocardial infarction.
Possible interaction: cisapride, antihistamines, nefopam, disopyramide, TCADs, MAOIs, phenothiazines, amantadine.
Side effects: nausea, vomiting, diarrhoea, abdominal cramps, tachycardia.
Manufacturer: Wyeth.

ROCALTROL

Description: a vitamin D analogue, calcitriol, available as capsules containing 0.25μg (red/white) and 0.5μg (red).
Used for: in cases of renal osteodystrophy (bone development defect due to kidney disorder affecting calcium and phosphorus metabolism).

Dosage: 1–2μg per day increasing if required to 2–3μg by 0.25–0.5μg increments. Not for children.
Special care: pregnancy, do not use other vitamin D preparations. Check serum calcium levels.
Avoid use: hypercalcaemia metastatic calcification (due to spread of malignancy).
Side effects: hypercalciuria (calcium in urine), hypercalcaemia.
Manufacturer: Roche.

ROCEPHIN

Description: a cephalosporin, ceftriaxone, available as a powder in vials (250mg, 1g and 2g).
Used for: meningitis, pneumonia, septicaemia. Infections of bone, skin and soft tissue. Gonorrhoea, preventitive for operations, infections in patients with neutropenia.
Dosage: 1g per day by deep intramuscular injection, slow intravenous injection or infusion. 2–4g as 1 dose, per day, for severe infections. Gonorrhoea—250mg intramuscularly; preventitive—1g intramuscularly or slow intravenous injection; also colorectal surgery—2g intramuscularly or by slow intravenous injection or infusion. Children (over 6 weeks only): 20–50mg/kg daily by the same means, up to 80mg/kg for severe infections.
Special care: severe liver or kidney disease, hypersensitivity to β-lactam.
Avoid use: pregnancy.
Side effects: primarily skin infections, blood changes, gastro-intestinal upset.
Manufacturer: Roche.

ROFERON-A

Description: an interferon, interferon alfa-2a, available in vials of 3, 4.5 and 18 million units, with syringe, needles and water for injection.
Used for: AIDS-related Kaposi's sarcoma, some leukaemias, T-cell lymphoma, hepatitis B, renal cell carcinoma.
Dosage: by subcutaneous and intramuscular injection. See literature.

Avoid use: pregnancy.
Possible interaction: theophylline.
Side effects: (dose-related) depression,
flu-like symptoms, bone marrow
suppression, hypo-and hypertension,
arrhythmia, rash, seizures; rarely, coma.
Manufacturer: Roche.

ROGITINE

Description: an alpha-blocker and
antihypertensive, phentolamine
mesylate, in ampoules of 10mg/ml.
Used for: hypertension associated with
phaeochromocytoma.
Dosage: 2–5mg by intravenous injection,
repeated if required. Children: 1mg.
Special care: asthma, gastritis, kidney
disorder, peptic ulcer. Elderly,
pregnancy, lactation. Monitor blood.
Avoid use: hypotension, weak heart,
myocardial infarction, hypersensitivity
to sulphites, disease of coronary arteries.
Possible interaction: antihypertensives,
antipsychotics.
Side effects: weakness, dizziness,
tachycardia, hypotension, flushes,
blocked nose, gastro-intestinal upset.
Manufacturer: Ciba.

ROHYPNOL

Description: an hypnotic and intermediate-acting benzodiazepine, fluni-
trazepam, in diamond-shaped purple
tablets (1mg) marked ROHYPNOL.
Used for: short-term treatment of severe
or disabling insomnia, to induce sleep at
unusual times.
Dosage: ¹/₂ to 1 tablet at bedtime
(elderly, ¹/₂ tablet). Not for children.
Special care: chronic liver or kidney
disease, chronic lung disease, pregnancy,
labour, lactation, elderly. May impair
judgement. Withdraw gradually and
avoid prolonged use.
Avoid use: depression of respiration,
acute lung disease; psychotic, phobic or
obsessional states.
Possible interaction: anticonvulsants,
depressants of the CNS, alcohol.
Side effects: ataxia, confusion, light-

headedness, drowsiness, hypotension,
gastro intestinal upsets, disturbances in
vision and libido, skin rashes, retention
of urine, vertigo. Sometimes jaundice or
blood disorders.
Manufacturer: Wyeth.

ROWACHOL

Description: Essential oils comprising
32mg menthol, 17mg a and ß-pinenes,
6mg menthone, 5mg camphene, 5mg
borneol and 2mg cineole in green,
spherical, soft, gelatin capsules.
Used for: additional treatment for
disposal of stones in the common bile
duct (with chenodeoxycholic acid).
Dosage: start with 1 capsule 3 times per
day, increasing to 1 to 2 capsules 3 times
per day, before meals. Not for children.
Possible interaction: oral contraceptives,
oral anticoagulants.
Manufacturer: Monmouth.

ROWATINEX

Description: Essential oils comprising
31mg a and ß pinenes, 15mg camphene,
10mg borneol, 4mg anethol, 4mg
fenchone, 3mg cineole in yellow,
spherical, soft, gelatin capsules.
Used for: stones in the urinary tract or
kidney, mild urinary tract infections.
Dosage: 1 capsule 3 or 4 times per day
before meals. Not for children.
Possible interaction: oral contraceptives,
oral anticoagulants.
Manufacturer: Monmouth.

RUBAVAX

Description: a live attenuated virus,
Rubella vaccine, with 25μg neomycin
per dose, as powder in vial with syringe
of diluent (0.5ml).
Used for: immunisation of girls aged 10
to 14 and women (not pregnant) who are
seronegative.
Dosage: 0.5ml by deep subcutaneous or
intramuscular injection. Not for children
under 10.
Avoid use: pregnancy, or pregnancy within
3 months of injection, acute infections.

Possible interaction: live vaccines, immunoglobulin, transfusions of blood or plasma.
Side effects: rash, joint pain, sore throat, fever, malaise, disorder of the lymph system.
Manufacturer: Merieux.

RYTHMODAN

Description: a class I antiarrhythmic, disopyramide, available as green/beige capsules (100mg) marked RY RL.
Used for: disturbance in heart beat.
Dosage: 300–800mg per day in divided doses. Not for children. Also, **RYTHMODAN RETARD**, 250mg disopyramide phosphate in white, sustained-release tablets marked RY and R with symbol.
Dosage: 1–1¹/₂ tablets twice per day. Not for children. Also, **RYTHMODAN INJECTION**, 10mg/ml in ampoules.
Special care: 1st degree atrioventricular block (slowed conduction or stopped heart impulse), heart, liver or kidney failure, enlarged prostate, urine retention, hyperkalaemia, glaucoma.
Avoid use: 2nd or 3rd degree atrioventricular block, severe heart failure.
Possible interaction: ß-blockers, anticholinergics, diuretics, other class I antiarrhythmics, erythromycin.
Side effects: anticholinergic effects, sometimes jaundice, hypoglycaemia, psychosis.
Manufacturer: Roussel.

SABRIL

Description: an anticonvulsant preparation which is an analogue of a gamma-aminobutyric acid available as oval, white, scored tablets containing 500mg vigabatrin. Also, **SABRIL SACHET** containing 500mg vigabatrin as powder.
Used for: control of epilepsy which has not responded to other drugs.

Dosage: 2g each day as single or divided doses, at first along with any other drug being taken. Then dose altered according to response with a maximum of 4g daily. Children, 40mg/kg body weight each day at first increasing, if needed, to a maximum of 80–100mg/kg.
Special care: elderly, kidney disorders, history of psychiatric illness or behavioural problems. Neurological function should be monitored during the course of treatment. Withdraw drug gradually.
Avoid use: pregnancy, breastfeeding.
Possible interaction: other anti-epileptic drugs.
Side effects: behavioural disturbances, irritability, aggression, dizziness, sleepiness, fatigue, disturbance of vision and memory, nervousness. Children may show agitated behaviour. Patients with a certain type of convulsion (myoclonic) may experience an increase in frequency.
Manufacturer: Merrell Dow.

SAIZEN

Description: a preparation of growth hormone as powder in vials containing 4 units and 10 units somatropin for reconstitution and injection.
Used for: failure of growth in children due to deficiency in growth hormone. Turner syndrome.
Dosage: children, deficiency of growth hormone, 0.07–0.08 units/kg body weight each day by intramuscular or subcutaneous injection. Or, 0.2 units/kg 3 times each week. Turner syndrome, 0.09–0.1 units/kg each day at first then 0.11–0.14 units/kg if needed.
Special care: diabetes, lesion on the brain, deficiency in ACTH (adrenocorticotrophic hormone). Thyroid function should be monitored.
Avoid use: Girls who are pregnant or breastfeeding, children with fusion of epiphyses or tumour.
Side effects: pain at site of injection, breakdown of fat beneath skin at injection site, oedema, hypothyroidism.
Manufacturer: Serono.

SALAMOL

Description: a preparation which is a bronchodilator and selective ß₂-agonist available as a metered dose aerosol delivering 100µg salbutamol per dose. Also, **SALAMOL STERI-NEB** available as a preservative-free solution for nebulization containing 2.5mg and 5mg salbutamol as sulphate/2.5ml, as single dose units.

Used for: Salamol, bronchospasm as in bronchitis, emphysema and asthma. Salamol Steri-Neb, severe bronchospasm and acute severe asthma which has failed to respond to other drugs.

Dosage: Salamol, adults, for attack, 1 or 2 puffs; prevention, 2 puffs 3 to 4 times each day. Salamol Steri-Neb, 2.5mg nebulized 3 or 4 times each day increasing to 5mg if needed. Children, Salamol, half adult dose.

Special care: pregnancy, weak heart, heart arrhythmias, angina, hypertension, hyperthyroidism.

Possible interaction: ß-blockers, sympathomimetics.

Side effects: headache, dilation of peripheral blood vessels, tremor, hypokalaemia.

Manufacturer: Baker Norton.

SALAZOPYRIN

Description: a colorectal NSAID which is a salicylate and sulphonamide, available as scored, yellow tablets containing 500mg sulphasalazine marked with logo. Also, **SALAZOPYRIN EN-TABS**, enteric-coated yellow tablets (500mg) marked with logo. **SALAZOPYRIN SUSPEN-SION**, fruit-flavoured containing 250mg/5ml. **SALAZOPYRIN ENEMA** containing 3g; **SALAZOPYRIN SUPPOSITORIES** containing 500mg.

Used for: ulcerative colitis (inflammation of colon), Crohn's disease. Salazopyrin En-Tabs, rheumatoid arthritis which has not responded to other NSAIDs.

Dosage: oral preparations, for ulcerative colitis and Crohn's disease, 2 to 4 tablets or 20–40ml 4 times each day with a maintenance dose of 4 tablets or 40ml in divided doses daily. Enema, 1 at night; suppositories, 2 in the morning and after passing stool in addition to oral dose. Rheumatoid arthritis, 1 En-Tab daily for 1 week increasing over 6 weeks to 6 each day in divided doses. Children, over 2 years of age, oral preparations, 40–60mg/kg body weight each day with a maintenance dose of 20–30mg/kg daily. Suppositories, a reduced dose in proportion to that for 70kg adult.

Special care: patients with allergies, liver or kidney disorders. Any ill effects should be reported and patients should receive regular checks of liver function and blood.

Avoid use: children under 2 years.

Possible interaction: rash, nausea, fever, headache, appetite loss, gastro-intestinal disturbance. Effects on CNS and kidneys, blood changes, allergic hypersensitivity reactions. Reduced production of, and presence of abnormal spermatozoa in males.

Manufacturer: Pharmacia.

SALBULIN

Description: a bronchodilator which is a selective ß₂-agonist available as a metered dose aerosol delivering 100µg salbutamol/dose.

Used for: bronchospasm in bronchitis, emphysema, asthma.

Dosage: adults, attack, 1 or 2 puffs; prevention, 2 puffs 3 or 4 times each day. Children, half adult dose.

Special care: pregnancy, hyperthyroidism.

Possible interaction: ß-blockers, sympathomimetics.

Side effects: headache, dilation of peripheral blood vessels, nervousness, tremor.

Manufacturer: 3M Health Care.

SALOFALK

Description: a colorectal preparation and salicylate available as oval, yellow, enteric-coated tablets containing 250mg mesalazine.

Used for: ulcerative colitis, maintenance treatment.
Dosage: adults, for active condition, 6 tablets each day in 3 divided doses. Maintenance treatment, 3 to 6 tablets each day in divided doses.
Special care: pregnancy, kidney disorder.
Avoid use: children, blood clotting disorders, serious liver or kidney disease, allergy to salicylates, peptic ulcer.
Possible interaction: preparations that make the stools more acid, lactulose.
Side effects: allergic hypersensitivity responses, increased haemoglobin levels.
Manufacturer: Thames.

SALURIC

Description: a thiazide diuretic available as scored, white tablets containing 500mg chlorothiazide marked MSD 432.
Used for: hypertension, oedema.
Dosage: hypertension, half to 1 tablet in single or divided doses each day with a maximum of 2 tablets. Oedema, $^1/_2$ to 2 tablets once or twice each day or on days when required, with a maximum of 4 daily. Children, age under 6 months, 35mg/kg body weight each day; 6 months to 2 years, 125–375mg each day. 2 to 12 years, 375mg–1g each day. All in 2 divided doses.
Special care: elderly, pregnancy, breastfeeding, gout, liver or kidney disorders, SLE, liver cirrhosis, diabetes. Glucose, electrolyte and fluid levels should be monitored during the course of treatment.
Avoid use: hypercalcaemia, allergy to sulphonamides, serious liver or kidney failure. Addison's disease.
Possible interaction: NSAIDs, lithium opioids, corticosteroids, alcohol cardiac glycosides, barbiturates, tubocurarine, carbenoxolone, antidiabetic drugs.
Side effects: gastro-intestinal upset, dizziness, disturbance of metabolism and electrolyte balance, blood changes, pancreatitis, impotence, anorexia.
Manufacturer: M.S.D.

SANDIMMUN

Description: a fungal metabolite immunosuppressant available as a yellow, sugar-free, oily solution containing 100mg cyclosporin/ml. Also, **SANDIMMUN CAPSULES** available in 3 strengths, oval, light pink 25mg; oblong, yellow, 50mg; and oblong, deep pink, 100mg all containing cyclosporin. **SANDIMMUN INTRAVENOUS INFUSION** available in ampoules containing 50mg/ml.
Used for: serious rheumatoid arthritis which has not responded to other drugs, suppression of immune system in patients undergoing bone marrow or organ transplants, prevention and treatment of graft-versus-host disease. Serious atopic dermatitis and psoriasis which has not responded to other drugs or where these are not considered to be suitable.
Dosage: 1.25–5mg/kg body weight per day depending upon condition. See literature.
Special care: pregnancy, breastfeeding, hyperkalaemia, herpes, hyperuricaemia (raised levels of uric acid in blood). Treatment must be given in specialist unit and close monitoring of blood potassium levels, blood pressure, liver and kidney function is required before and during treatment. Avoid sunbathing.
Avoid use: malignant diseases (except of skin), kidney disorders, uncontrolled infections or hypertension.
Possible interaction: barbiturates, systemic antibiotics, rifampicin, live vaccines, ketoconazole, erythromycin, phenytoin, carbamazepine, itraconazole, fluconazole, ACE inhibitors, oral contraceptives, calcium antagonists, certain enzyme inhibitors, colchicine, drugs with toxic effects on kidneys. Potassium supplements and potassium-sparing diuretics, prednisolone, lipid solutions, methyl prednisolone, NSAIDs, propafenone.
Side effects: weakness, tiredness, muscle cramps, burning sensation in feet and

hands, tremor, gastro-intestinal upset. Rarely, other blood changes, headache, weight gain, oedema, rash, fits, colitis, pancreatitis. Also, hyperkalaemia, rise in uric acid levels in blood, damage to nerves, effects on menstruation, enlargement of breasts. If uncontrolled hypertension or liver and kidney disorders occur, drug should be withdrawn.
Manufacturer: Sandoz.

SANDOGLOBULIN

Description: a freeze-dried preparation of human normal immunoglobulin available with diluent for intravenous infusion.
Used for: globulin deficiencies in newborn babies, thrombocytopenic purpura (a bleeding disorder).
Dosage: deficiency, 0.1–0.3g/kg body weight every 2 to 4 weeks. Thrombocytopenic purpura, 0.4g/kg each day for 5 days. Then maintenance dose of same order when needed.
Special care: during infusion, patients must be monitored for signs of anaphylaxis.
Avoid use: patients with selective immunoglobulin A deficiency who have antibodies to Ig A and who are sensitized.
Possible interaction: live viral vaccines.
Side effects: allergic anaphylactoid-type reactions, inflammatory responses which may be delayed.
Manufacturer: Sandoz.

SANDOSTATIN

Description: a sandostatin analogue available as a solution in ampoules for injection at strengths of 0.05mg, 0.1mg and 0.5mg/ml and 1mg/5ml multi-dose vial, all containing octreotide (as acetate).
Used for: short-term treatment of acromegaly (abnormal enlargement of face, hands and feet due to excess secretion of growth hormone by a pituitary gland tumour), before surgery or X-ray therapy. Relief of symptoms of certain tumours of the gastro-intestinal tract and pancreas, and carcinoid tumours which release hormones.

Dosage: acromegaly, 0.1–0.2mg 3 times each day. Tumours, 0.05mg once or twice each day increasing to 0.2mg 3 times daily if needed. Carcinoid tumours, stop drug if no improvement after 1 week.
Special care: diabetes. Those taking drug long-term require monitoring of thyroid function and for development of gallstones.
Avoid use: pregnancy, breastfeeding.
Possible interaction: cimetidine, cyclosporin.
Side effects: pain, swelling and soreness at injection site, pain in abdomen, vomiting, diarrhoea, steatorrhoea (increased amount of fat in faeces which are pale, frothy and foul-smelling), anorexia, gallstones.
Manufacturer: Sandoz.

SANOMIGRAN

Description: a serotonin antagonist available as sugar-coated, ivory-coloured tablets containing 0.5mg and 1.5mg pizotifen (as hydrogen maleate), marked SMG and SMG 1.5 respectively. Also, **SANOMIGRAN ELIXIR** containing 0.25mg/5ml as a sugar-free solution.
Used for: prevention of migraine.
Dosage: 1.5mg each day in 3 divided doses or 1 dose at night. Dosage may be increased to a maximum of 4.5mg each day if needed with up to 3mg as a maximum single dose. Children, up to 1.5mg each day in divided doses or 1mg as a single night time dose.
Special care: urine retention, glaucoma.
Side effects: gain in weight, sleepiness.
Manufacturer: Sandoz.

SAVENTRINE

Description: a heart stimulant and ß-agonist available as mottled white tablets containing 30mg isoprenaline hydrochloride marked with a P inside a hexagon shape. Also, **SAVENTRINE I.V.** available as a solution in ampoules for injection containing 1mg/ml.
Used for: heart block, severe bradycardia, Stokes Adams attacks.

Dosage: tablets (rarely used) 30mg every 6 hours with usual dose in the order of 90–840mg each day. Infusion, 0.5–10µg/minute.
Special care: diabetes or hypertension.
Avoid use: hyperthyroidism, serious heart disease, tachycardia, ventricular fibrillation, cardiac asthma.
Side effects: headache, tremor, sweating, diarrhoea, palpitations.
Manufacturer: Pharmax.

SCHERING PC4

Description: an oestrogen/progestogen preparation available as sugar-coated white tablets containing 50µg ethinyloestradiol and 0.5mg norgestrel.
Used for: emergency and contraception (the "morning-after" pill) to be taken within 72 hours of unprotected sexual intercourse.
Dosage: 2 tablets taken as soon as possible after intercourse followed, 12 hours later, by another 2 tablets.
Special care: porphyria, gallstones, liver disorders, heart, kidney, circulatory diseases, diabetes, epilepsy, hypertension, history of severe depression. If patient still becomes pregnant, monitoring required to ensure pregnancy is not ectopic. Intercourse should be avoided for the remainder of the cycle.
Avoid use: patients with overdue menstrual period, those not within 72 hours of unprotected intercourse.
Possible interaction: barbiturates, chlorpromazine, rifampicin, chloral hydrate, glutethimide, tetracyclines, dichloralphenazone, griseofulvin, ethosuximide, phenytoin, carbamazepine, primidone.
Side effects: vomiting (reduces drug's effect) and nausea. Period normally starts later than expected, following treatment.
Manufacturer: Schering H.C.

SCHERIPROCT

Description: a combined steroid and local anaesthetic preparation available as

an ointment containing 0.19% prednisolone hexanoate and 0.5% cinchocaine hydrochloride. Also,
SCHERIPROCT SUPPOSITORIES containing 1.3mg prednisolone hexanoate and 1mg cinchocaine hydrochloride.
Used for: anal fissure, haemorrhoids, proctitis (inflammation of rectum), anal itching.
Dosage: apply ointment 2, 3 or 4 times each day; insert 1 suppository 1, 2 or 3 times each day after passing stool.
Special care: pregnant women, short-term use only.
Avoid use: patients with tuberculous, viral or fungal infections.
Side effects: systemic corticosteroid side effects.
Manufacturer: Schering H.C.

SCOLINE

Description: a depolarising muscle relaxant of short-lived duration available as a solution for injection containing 50mg suxamethonium chloride/ml.
Used for: paralysis following induction of anaesthesia usually to allow tracheal tube to be inserted. Has duration of action lasting 5 minutes and repeated doses may be given to allow longer-lasting procedures to be carried out.
Special care: with unusual or low concentration of pseudocholinesterase enzymes in whom more prolonged paralysis may occur. Dual block involving longer-lasting paralysis may develop after repeated doses of suxamethonium.
Avoid use: liver disease or burns.
Possible interaction: digoxin, ecothiopate, demacarium, eyedrops, neostigmine, pyndostigmine, thiotepa, cyclophoshamide, bambuterol.
Side effects: short-lived rise in creatine, phosphokinase (enzyme) and potassium levels in blood plasma, post-operative muscle pains.
Manufacturer: Evans.

SCOPODERM

Description: an anti-emetic, anticholinergic preparation available as a self-adhesive pink patch containing 1.5mg hyoscine.
Used for: motion sickness.
Dosage: adults and children over 10 years, apply patch to clean, dry skin behind ear 5 to 6 hours before travelling. Replace after 72 hours if needed and remove when travelling is finished.
Special care: pregnancy, breastfeeding, liver or kidney disorders, obstruction of intestine, bladder or pyloric stenosis.
Avoid use: children under 10 years, glaucoma. Consumption of alcohol.
Possible interaction: drugs affecting CNS, anticholinergics, alcohol.
Side effects: skin rashes and irritation, urine retention, dry mouth, disturbance of vision, sleepiness, dizziness. Rarely, withdrawal symptoms.
Manufacturer: Ciba.

SECADREX

Description: an antihypertensive preparation combining a cardioselective ß-blocker and thiazide diuretic available as film-coated white tablets containing 200mg acebutolol (as hydrochloride) and 12.5mg hydrochlorothiazide, marked SECADREX.
Used for: hypertension.
Dosage: 1 to 2 tablets as a single dose each day.
Special care: pregnancy, breastfeeding, patients with weak hearts may require diuretics and digitalis, diabetes, undergoing general anaesthesia, kidney or liver disorders, gout. Electrolyte (salts) levels may need to be monitored.
Avoid use: history of bronchospasm or obstructive airways disease, heart block, heart shock, uncompensated heart failure, disease of peripheral arteries, bradycardia. Serious or worsening kidney failure or anuria.
Possible interaction: sympathomimetics, class I antiarrhythmics, CNS depressants, clonidine withdrawal, ergot alkaloids,

cardiac depressant anaesthetics, verapamil, reserpine, indomethacin, hypoglycaemics, cimetidine, other antihypertensives. Digitalis, potassium supplements, potassium-sparing diuretics, lithium.
Side effects: cold hands and feet, disturbance of sleep, fatigue on exercise, bronchospasm, bradycardia, gastrointestinal disturbances, heart failure, blood changes, gout, sensitivity to light, muscle weakness. If skin rash or dry eyes occur, withdraw drug gradually.
Manufacturer: Theraplix.

SECONAL SODIUM^{CD}

Description: a barbiturate preparation available as 50mg and 100mg orange capsules, coded F42 and F40 respectively, both containing quinalbarbitone sodium.
Used for: short-term treatment of serious insomnia.
Dosage: 50–100mg taken at night.
Special care: extremely dangerous, addictive drug with narrow margin of safety. Liable to abuse by overdose leading to coma and death or if combined with alcohol. Easily produces dependence and severe withdrawal symptoms. Drowsiness may persist next day affecting driving and performance of skilled tasks.
Avoid use: should be avoided if possible in all patients. Not to be used for children, young adults, pregnant and nursing mothers, elderly, those with drug or alcohol related problems, patients with liver, kidney or heart disease or porphyria. Insomnia where the cause is pain.
Possible interaction: alcohol, CNS depressant drugs, Griseofulvin, metronidazone, rifampicin, phenytoin, chloramphenicol. Anticoagulant drugs of the coumarin type, steroid drugs including contraceptive pill.
Side effects: hangover with drowsiness, shakiness, dizziness, headache, anxiety, confusion, excitement, rash and allergic responses, gastro intestinal upsets, urine retention, loss of sexual desire.
Manufacturer: Kite.

SECTRAL

Description: an anti-arrhythmic, anti-anginal preparation which is a cardioselective ß-blocker available as capsules in 2 strengths, both containing acebutolol (as hydrochloride). White/buff, 100mg and pink/buff 200mg both marked with strength and SECTRAL. Also, **SECTRAL TABLETS**, white, film-coated, containing 400mg marked SECTRAL 400.

Used for: heart arrhythmias, angina.

Dosage: adults, arrhythmias, maintenance dose of 400–1200mg in 2 or 3 divided doses each day. Angina, 400mg once each day taken with breakfast or 200mg twice daily. The maximum is 1.2g each day.

Special care: history of bronchospasm and certain ß-blockers, diabetes, liver or kidney disease, pregnancy, lactation, general anaesthesia. Withdraw gradually. Not for children.

Avoid use: heart block or failure, bradycardia, sick sinus syndrome (associated with sinus node disorder), certain ß-blockers, severe peripheral arterial disease.

Possible interaction: verapamil, hypoglycaemics, reserpine, clonidine withdrawal, some antiarrhythmics and anaesthetics, antihypertensives, depressants of the CNS, cimetidine, indomethacin, sympathomimetics.

Side effects: bradycardia, cold hands and feet, disturbance to sleep, heart failure, gastro-intestinal upset, tiredness on exertion, bronchospasm.

Manufacturer: Theraplix.

SECURON SR

Description: a class I calcium antagonist available as film-coated, oblong, scored, green, sustained-release tablets containing 240mg verapamil hydrochloride and marked with logo. Also, **HALF SECURON SR**, white, film-coated, sustained-release tablets containing 120mg marked 120 SR and company name. Also, **SECURON TABLETS** white, film-coated and available in strengths of 40mg, 80mg and 120mg, all marked with strength, name and KNOLL. Also, **SECURON I.V.** available as a solution in pre-filled syringes containing 2.5mg/ml.

Used for: supraventricular tachycardia, angina, hypertension.

Dosage: tachycardias, Securon Tablets, 40–120mg 3 times each day. Angina, Securon SR, Half Securon SR or Securon Tablets, 120mg 3 times each day. Hypertension, Securon SR or Half Securon SR, 240mg once each day with a maximum of 480mg in divided doses daily. Patients who have not taken verapamil before start with lower dose of 120mg once daily. Securon Tablets, 120mg twice each day at first increasing to 160mg twice daily if needed. Maximum dose is 480mg in divided doses daily. Children, for tachycardias, Securon Tablets only, age under 2 years, 20mg; age over 2 years, 20–40mg, both 2 or 3 times each day.

Special care: pregnancy, breastfeeding, patients with liver or kidney disorders, heart conduction disturbances, bradycardia, 1st degree heart block. Patients with weak hearts require digitalis and/or diuretics.

Avoid use: some kinds of heart block, heart shock, sick sinus syndrome, serious bradycardia, heart attack, severe hypotension, uncompensated heart failure, certain types of heart flutter or fibrillation. Patients should not receive intravenous ß-blockers at same time.

Possible interaction: digoxin, ß-blockers, cimetidine, muscle relaxant drugs, inhaled anaesthetics, cyclosporin, rifampicin, antihypertensives, lithium, carbamazepine, theophylline, phenobarbitone, phenytoin.

Side effects: constipation; rarely, nausea, headache, dizziness, allergic reactions, hypotension, enlargement of breasts, increased growth of gum tissues, flushes. (Effects on heart rate, heart muscle and hypotension when given intravenously).

Manufacturer: Knoll.

SECUROPEN

Description: an antibiotic preparation which is an antipseudomonal penicillin

available as powder in vials for reconstitution and injection at strengths of 500mg, 1g, 2g and 5g all containing azlocillin (as monosodium).
Used for: local and systemic infections especially those caused by pseudomonas bacteria.
Dosage: adults, 2g every 8 hours by intravenous injection; serious infections, 5g every 8 hours by intravenous infusion. Children, premature baby, 50mg/kg body weight every 12 hours; newborn baby, 100mg/kg every 12 hours; aged 1 week to 1 year, 100mg/kg every 8 hours; 1 to 14 years, 75mg/kg every 8 hours.
Special care: pregnancy, kidney disorders.
Possible interaction: tubocurarine and other non-depolarising muscle relaxants, methotrexate.
Side effects: gastro-intestinal upset, allergic hypersensitive responses.
Manufacturer: Bayer.

SEMPREX

Description: an antihistamine preparation of the arylalkylamine type available as white capsules containing 8mg acrivastine marked with symbol, 09C and company name.
Used for: allergic rhinitis, urticaria.
Dosage: adults, 1 tablet 3 times each day.
Special care: pregnancy, breastfeeding.
Avoid use: children, elderly, kidney failure.
Possible interaction: CNS depressants, alcohol.
Side effects: rarely, drowsiness.
Manufacturer: Wellcome.

SEPTRIN

Description: an antibiotic preparation combining a folic acid inhibitor and sulphonamide available as white tablets and orange dissolvable tablets, both containing 80mg trimethoprim and 400mg sulphamethoxazole. Tablets are both marked with maker's name, tablet name and coded Y2B. **SEPTRIN ADULT SUSPENSION** same components/5ml. **SEPTRIN PAEDIAT-RIC SUSPENSION**, sugar-free,

containing 40mg trimethoprim and 200mg sulphamethoxazole/5ml. Also, **SEPTRIN FOR INFUSION** available in ampoules containing 80mg trimethoprim and 400mg sulphamethoxazole/5ml.
Used for: infections of skin, gastro-intestinal, respiratory and urinary tracts.
Dosage: tablets, 1 to 3 twice each day; suspension, 5–15ml twice daily; Septrin Forte, 1 to 1 $1/2$ tablets twice each day. Infusion, 960mg every 12 hours increasing to 1.44g if infection is extremely severe, given intravenously. Children, Paediatric Suspension, 6 weeks to 6 months, 2.5ml; 6 months to 6 years, 5ml; over 6 years, 10ml, all twice each day. Tablets, children over 6 years, 1 tablet or 5ml adult suspension. Infusion, 36mg/kg body weight each day in 2 divided doses increasing to 54mg/kg in the case of severe infections.
Special care: breastfeeding, elderly, patients with kidney disorders (require reduced or less frequent doses). Regular blood tests should be carried out in patients taking the drug long-term.
Avoid use: pregnancy, newborn babies, severe liver or kidney disorders, blood changes.
Possible interaction: anticonvulsants, folate inhibitors, hypoglycaemics, anticoagulants.
Side effects: vomiting, nausea, inflammation of tongue, blood changes, skin rashes, folate deficiency; rarely erythema multiformae (allergic disorder affecting skin and mucous membranes), Lyell syndrome.
Manufacturer: Wellcome.

SERC

Description: an anti-emetic preparation which is a histamine analogue available as white tablets in 2 strengths containing 8mg and 16mg betahistine, dihydrochloride, marked Duphar 256 or 267 respectively.
Used for: symptoms associated with Ménière's syndrome including hearing loss, tinnitus and vertigo.

Dosage: 16mg 3 times each day at first with a maintenance dose of 24–48mg daily.
Special care: patients with peptic ulcer, bronchial asthma.
Avoid use: phaeochromocytoma.
Side effects: gastro-intestinal upset.
Manufacturer: Duphar.

SERENACE

Description: an anti-depressant preparation which is a butyrophenone available as green/light green capsules containing 0.5mg haloperidol marked Norton 500 and SERENACE. Also, SERENACE TABLETS in 4 strengths all containing haloperidol; white, 1.5mg; pink, 5mg; 10mg and 20mg all marked with strength on one side and SERENACE on other, and coded NORTON. SERENACE LIQUID, containing 2mg/ml; SERENACE INJECTION available as a solution in ampoules for injection in strengths of 5mg and 10mg/ml.
Used for: capsules, additional treatment for anxiety; tablets and liquid, manic states, psychoses, schizophrenia, behaviour disorders in children.
Dosage: capsules, 1 twice each day; tablets or liquid, 1.5–20mg each day at first increasing as needed to control disorder. Then decreasing to a maintenance dose in the order of 3–10mg each day. The maximum daily dose is 200mg. Injection, for emergency treatment, 5–30mg by intravenous or intramuscular injection every 6 hours, then preparations taken by mouth. Children, tablets or liquid only, 0.025–0.05mg/kg body weight each day at first. Usual daily maximum is 10mg.
Special care: pregnancy, tardive dyskinesia disorder characterized by repeated involuntary muscle movements), hyperthyroidism, kidney or liver failure, serious heart or circulatory disorders, epilepsy.
Avoid use: breastfeeding, parkinsonism, coma.
Possible interaction: rifampicin, fluoxetine, carbamazepine, anxiolytics, hypnotics.

Side effects: extrapyramidal side effects, drowsiness, hypothermia, insomnia, pallor, nightmares, depression, constipation, dry mouth, blocked nose, difficulty in urination. Changes in ECG and EEG, effects on heart, e.g. tachycardia, arrhythmias, blood changes, changes in endocrine system, e.g. effects on menstruation, breasts, impotence, weight gain. Effects on liver, jaundice, sensitivity to light, purple pigmentation of skin and eyes.
Manufacturer: Baker Norton.

SEREVENT

Description: a bronchodilator and selective β_2-agonist available as a metered dose aerosol delivering 25µg salmeterol (as xinafoate) per dose. Also, SEREVENT DISKHALER, using disks containing 4 x 50µg blisters salmeterol (as xinafoate) with breath-actuated delivery system.
Used for: various types of asthma along with anti-inflammatory therapy.
Dosage: adults, Serevent, 2 puffs twice each day, 4 puffs if exceptionally severe. Serevent Diskhaler, 1 blister twice each day or 2 if very severe. Children, Serevent, age over 4 years, 2 puffs twice each day. Serevent Diskhaler, 1 blister twice each day.
Special care: pregnancy, breastfeeding, thyrotoxicosis, acute symptoms of asthma or if unstable and severe. Steroid therapy should be continued.
Avoid use: children under 4 years.
Possible interaction: β-blockers.
Side effects: paradoxical bronchospasm, hypokalaemia; rarely, skin eruptions, pain in chest, joints and muscles, headache, palpitations, tremor, irritation of throat.
Manufacturer: A. & H.

SEROPHENE

Description: an antioestrogen preparation available as scored, white tablets containing 50mg clomiphene citrate.
Used for: female infertility caused by disorder of hypothalamus-pituitary gland

function. Also, with gonadotrophins in invitro fertilization treatment.
Dosage: infertility, 1 tablet each day for 5 days, ideally starting within 5 days of menstruation. Superovulation, 2 tablets each day starting on day 2 continuing to day 6 of monthly cycle.
Special care: ensure patient is not pregnant before and during course of treatment.
Avoid use: patients with undiagnosed bleeding from uterus, large cyst on ovary, cancer of endometrium, liver disorder.
Side effects: pain or discomfort in abdomen, enlargement of ovaries, flushes. Withdraw drug if blurring of vision occurs.
Manufacturer: Serono.

SEROXAT

Description: an antidepressant available as film-coated, oval, scored tablets in 2 strengths; containing 20mg (white) and 30mg (blue) paroxetine (as hydrochloride). Both marked with strength and name.
Used for: depression and depressive illness with anxiety.
Dosage: 20mg once each day at first, taken in the morning with breakfast. Then increasing gradually every 2 or 3 weeks by 10mg to a maximum daily dose of 50mg. Elderly persons start with lower dose of 20mg once each day increasing gradually to 40mg daily, if needed.
Special care: pregnancy, breastfeeding, serious liver or kidney disorders, heart disease or disease of arteries of heart, epilepsy, history of mania.
Avoid use: children.
Possible interaction: anticonvulsants, tryptophan, drugs affecting liver enzymes, phenytoin, MAOIs, anticonvulsants.
Side effects: dry mouth, sweating, sleepiness, tremor, nausea, weakness, effects on sexual habits.
Manufacturer: S.K. & F.

SEVREDOL^{CD}

Description: an analgesic opiate available as film-coated, capsule-shaped, scored tablets in 2 strengths, blue

containing 10mg, and pink containing 20mg morphine sulphate. Both are marked with strength and IR.
Used for: severe pain.
Dosage: 10mg every 4 hours at first increasing dose if necessary. Children, age 3 to 5 years, 5mg every 4 hours; 6 to 12 years, 5–10mg every 4 hours.
Special care: elderly, enlarged prostate gland, underactive thyroid, liver or kidney disease, paralytic ileus, respiratory problems, reduced function of adrenal glands, following surgery.
Avoid use: pregnancy, breastfeeding, children under 3 years, obstructive airways disease, serious liver disease, head injuries, raised pressure within brain, coma, depression of respiration, alcoholism.
Possible interaction: CNS depressants, MAOIs.
Side effects: nausea, vomiting, constipation, sedation, drug tolerance and addiction.
Manufacturer: Napp.

SIMPLENE

Description: a sympathomimetic preparation available in the form of eyedrops in 2 strengths containing 0.5% and 1% adrenaline.
Used for: primary open angle and secondary glaucoma.
Dosage: 1 drop twice each day.
Avoid use: patients with narrow angle glaucoma or diabetes.
Possible interaction: MAOIs, ß-blockers, tricyclics.
Side effects: pain or discomfort in eye, headache, skin reactions, pigmentation with melanin. Rarely, systemic side effects.
Manufacturer: Chauvin.

SINEMET

Description: an anti-Parkinsonism preparation combining a dopamine precursor and dopa decarboxylase inhibitor available in the form of tablets "LS" scored, oval, yellow tablets contain

50mg levodopa and 12.5mg carbidopa (as monohydrate), marked with name. "Plus" scored, oval, yellow tablets contain 100mg and 25mg marked with name. "110" scored, oval, blue tablets contain 100mg and 10mg, marked MSD 547. "275" scored, oval, blue tablets contain 250mg and 25mg marked MSD 554. Also, SINEMET CR, oval, mottled, peach-coloured, continuous-release tablets containing 200mg and 50mg marked 521 and DPP. Also, HALF SINEMET CR, oval, pink, continuous-release tablets containing 100mg and 25mg marked 601 and DPP.

Used for: Parkinsonism.

Dosage: adults over 18 years, not receiving levodopa, 1 "LS" or 1 "Plus" tablet 3 times each day at first increasing by 1 tablet every other day to the equivalent of 8 "Plus" tablets each day. Patients who have been taking levodopa should stop this 8 hours before taking Sinemet. Sinemet CR, 1 tablet twice each day in first instance, if not receiving levodopa, then adjusted according to response.

Special care: liver or kidney disease, disease of heart or heart blood vessels, endocrine disorders, peptic ulcer, wide angle glaucoma. Liver, kidney and heart function should be monitored and blood values checked regularly if patients are taking drug long-term.

Avoid use: children, pregnancy, breast-feeding, narrow angle glaucoma, history of malignant melanoma, severe psychoses.

Possible interaction: MAOIs, sympathomimetics, antihypertensives, drug acting on central amines.

Side effects: CNS effects, low blood pressure on rising, discolouration of urine, vomiting, nausea, involuntary muscle movements, anorexia.

Manufacturer: DuPont.

SINEQUAN

Description: a TCAD preparation available as tablets in different strengths, all containing doxepin (as hydrochloride).

Red, 10mg capsules, coded SQN; red/blue 25mg capsules, coded SQN 25; blue, 50mg capsules, coded SQN 50; blue/yellow 75mg capsules coded SQN 75. All are marked PFIZER.

Used for: depression.

Dosage: 10–100mg 3 times each day or a maximum of 100mg as a single night-time dose.

Special care: liver disorders, hyperthyroidism, glaucoma, lactation, epilepsy, diabetes, adrenal tumour, heart disease, urine retention. Psychotic or suicidal patients.

Avoid use: heart block, heart attacks, severe liver disease, pregnancy.

Possible interaction: MAOIs (or within 14 days of their use), alcohol, antidepressants, barbiturates, anticholinergics, local anaesthetics that contain adrenaline or noradrenaline, oestrogens, cimetidine, antihypertensives.

Side effects: constipation, urine retention, dry mouth, blurred vision, palpitations, tachycardia, nervousness, drowsiness, insomnia. Changes in weight, blood and blood sugar, jaundice, skin reactions, weakness, ataxia, hypotension, sweating, altered libido, gynaecomastia, galactorrhoea.

Manufacturer: Pfizer.

SINTHROME

Description: a coumarin anticoagulant preparation available as white tablets containing 1mg nicoumalone, marked CG and AA.

Used for: thromboembolic disorders.

Dosage: 8–12mg on first day, 4–8mg on following day, then according to response.

Special care: breastfeeding, elderly, serious heart failure, liver disorders, hypertension, disorders of absorption from gastro-intestinal tract, reduced protein binding. If intramuscular injections are given there is a risk of haematoma (accumulation of leaked blood which forms a solid mass within tissues).

Avoid use: pregnancy, children, patients who have had surgery or undergone

labour in last 24 hours, those with liver or kidney disorders, serious hypertension, blood changes, inflammation of or leakage of fluid from pericardium, bacterial endocarditis. Patients who are unco-operative.
Possible interaction: quinidine, corticosteroids, NSAIDs, antibiotics, hypoglycaemics taken by mouth, cimetidine, sulphonamides, phenformin. Drugs affecting the halting of bleeding, liver enzymes, vitamin K, absorption.
Side effects: allergic responses, damage to liver, reversible hair loss, haemorrhage. Rarely, headache, nausea, skin necrosis, anorexia.
Manufacturer: Geigy.

SKINOREN

Description: an antibacterial preparation available as a cream containing 20% azelaic acid.
Used for: acne.
Dosage: apply in the morning and evening to affected skin and rub in, maximum dose is 10g daily. Treatment should be continued according to response but for no more than 6 months.
Special care: pregnancy, breastfeeding, avoid eyes.
Side effects: sensitivity to light, local skin irritation.
Manufacturer: Schering H.C.

SLO-PHYLLIN

Description: a xanthine bronchidilator available as sustained-release capsules enclosing white pellets, in 3 strengths, all containing theophylline. White/clear 60mg, brown/clear 125mg and blue/clear 250mg capsules are all marked with strength, SLO-PHYLLIN and LIPHA.
Used for: bronchospasm in asthma, emphysema, bronchitis.
Dosage: 250–500mg twice each day; children, age 2 to 6 years, 60–120mg; 6 to 12 years, 125–250mg; all twice each day.
Special care: pregnancy, breastfeeding, peptic ulcer, liver or heart disease.
Avoid use: children under 2 years.

Possible interaction: interferon, erythromycin, diuretics, ß$_2$-agonists, cimetidine, steroids, ciprofloxacin.
Side effects: gastro-intestinal upset, nausea, heart arrhythmias, tachycardia, headache, insomnia.
Manufacturer: Lipha.

SLOW-FE FOLIC

Description: a haematinic preparation available as film-coated, cream-coloured tablets containing 160mg dried ferrous sulphate and 400µg folic acid, marked TP and CIBA.
Used for: prevention of iron and folic acid deficiencies in pregnant women.
Dosage: 1 to 2 tablets each day.
Possible interaction: anticonvulsants, penicillamine, tetracyclines, antacids, zinc salts.
Side effects: constipation nausea.
Manufacturer: Ciba.

SLO-TRASICOR

Description: an antianginal, antihypertensive preparation available as film-coated, white, sustained-release tablets containing 160mg oxprenolol hydrochloride, marked with name and manufacturer's name.
Used for: angina, hypertension.
Dosage: angina, 1 each morning at first increasing to 2 or 3 if needed. If nocturnal angina is present, an evening dose may be taken. Hypertension, 1 tablet each morning.
Special care: history of bronchospasm and certain ß-blockers, diabetes, liver or kidney disease, pregnancy, lactation, general anaesthesia. Withdraw gradually. Not for children.
Avoid use: heart block or failure, bradycardia, sick sinus syndrome (associated with sinus node disorder), certain ß-blockers, severe peripheral arterial disease.
Possible interaction: verapamil, hypoglycaemics, reserpine, clonidine withdrawal, some antiarrhythmics and anaesthetics, antihypertensives,

depressants of the CNS, cimetidine, indomethacin, sympathomimetics.
Side effects: bradycardia, cold hands and feet, disturbance to sleep, heart failure, gastro-intestinal upset, tiredness on exertion, bronchospasm.
Manufacturer: Ciba.

SNO-PHENICOL

Description: a broad-spectrum antibiotic preparation available as eyedrops containing 0.5% chloramphenicol.
Used for: bacterial Infections of the eye.
Dosage: 1 or more drops into eye, as needed. Children, 1 drop as needed.
Side effects: local allergic hypersensitive responses (stop immediately). Rarely, aplastic anaemia.
Manufacturer: Chauvin.

SNO-PILO

Description: a cholinergic eye preparation available in the form of drops in different strengths containing 1%, 2% and 4% pilocarpine.
Used for: glaucoma.
Dosage: 1 or 2 drops 4 times each day.
Avoid use: severe inflammation of iris, wearing soft contact lenses.
Side effects: short-lived loss of visual sharpness.
Manufacturer: Chauvin.

SODIUM AMYTAL^{CD}

Description: an hypnotic barbiturate preparation, available as blue capsules in 2 strengths containing 60mg and 200mg amylobarbitone sodium, coded LILLY F23 or F33 respectively.
Used for: insomnia, which has not responded to other drugs.
Dosage: tablets, 60–200mg taken at night.
Special care: extremely dangerous, addictive drug with narrow margin of safety. Liable to abuse by overdose leading to coma and death or if combined with alcohol. Easily produces dependence and severe withdrawal symptoms. Drowsiness may persist next day affecting driving and performance of skilled tasks.

Avoid use: should be avoided if possible in all patients. Not to be used for children, young adults, pregnant and nursing mothers, elderly pesons, those with drug or alcohol related problems, patients with liver, kidney or heart disease, porphyria. Insomnia where the cause is pain.
Possible interaction: alcohol, CNS depressant drugs, Griseofulvin, metronidazole, rifampicin, phenytoin, chloramphenicol. Anticoagulant drugs of the coumarin type, steroid drugs including contraceptive pill.
Side effects: hangover with drowsiness, shakiness, dizziness, headache, anxiety, confusion, excitement, rash and allergic responses, gastro intestinal upsets, urine retention, loss of sexual desire.
Manufacturer: Kite.

SODIUM AMYTAL INJECTION^{CD}

Description: a barbiturate preparation, available as a powder in vials for reconstitution and injection containing 500mg amylobarbitone sodium.
Used for: status epilepticus (but not grand mal epilepsy).
Dosage: 250 mg–1g by slow intravenous or intramuscular injection. Children, age over 6 years, 65–500mg by slow intravenous or intramuscular injection.
Special care: kidney and liver disorders, serious lung insufficiency.
Avoid use: pregnancy, breastfeeding, elderly, patients who are debilitated, porphyria, pain which is not controlled, history of drug or alcohol abuse.
Possible interaction: CNS depressants, griseofulvin, alcohol, phenytoin, systemic steroids, chloramphenicol, rifampicin, metronidazole, anticoagulants of the coumarin type.
Side effects: headache, respiratory depression, dizziness, unsteadiness, sleepiness, confusion, agitation, allergic responses. Drug tolerance and dependence may occur.
Manufacturer: Kite.

SOFRA-TULLE

Description: a gauze dressing for
wounds impregnated with 1%
framycetin sulphate available in
individual foil sachets.
Used for: burns, wounds, ulcers,
infected areas.
Dosage: apply to affected area.
Avoid use: large open wounds—danger
of ototoxicity (damage to organs of
balance and hearing), especially in
children, elderly and patients with
kidney disorders.
Manufacturer: Roussel.

SOFRADEX

Description: a compound preparation
combining a corticosteroid,
aminoglycoside and antibiotic available
in the form of drops containing 0.05%
dexamethasone, 0.5% framycetin
sulphate and 0.005% gramicidin.
Also, **SOFRADEX OINTMENT**
containing 0.05% dexamethasone, 0.5%
framycetin sulphate and 0.005%
gramicidin.
Used for: inflammation and infection of
outer ear. Inflammation of eye and
prevention of infection, short term only,
blepharitis (inflammation of hair
follicles of eye lashes which may be
caused by infection.
Dosage: drops, ear, apply 2 to 3 drops 3
or 4 times each day; ointment, ear, apply
once or twice daily. Drops, eye, 1 or 2
drops up to 6 times each day or more
frequently if necessary. Ointment, eye,
apply 2 or 3 times each day or at night if
drops are being used.
Special care: pregnant women.
Avoid use: long-term use in babies or by
pregnant women, perforated eardrum (if
for ear infections), eye infections
producing pus or those with tuberculous,
fungal or viral origin.
Side effects: superinfection, use in eyes
may lead to thinning of cornea, fungal
infection, cataract, rise in pressure
within eye.
Manufacturer: Roussel.

SOFRAMYCIN

Description: an antibiotic aminoglycoside preparation available in the form of
drops containing 0.5% framycetin
sulphate. Also, **SOFRAMYCIN
OINTMENT** containing 0.5%
framycetin sulphate.
Used for: eye infections, styes,
blepharitis (inflammation and infection
of hair follicles of eye lashes),
conjunctivitis. Ointment also used for
bacterial infections of skin.
Dosage: eyes, apply 1 or 2 drops 3 or 4
times each day; apply ointment 2 or 3
times each day or at night if drops are
being used. Skin, apply to affected area
up to 3 times each day.
Special care: use on more extensive
areas of skin.
Side effects: sensitization, ototoxicity
(damage to organs of balance and hearing).
Manufacturer: Roussel.

SOLPADOL

Description: a compound analgesic
preparation available as scored, white,
effervescent tablets containing 500mg
paracetamol and 30mg codeine
phosphate. Also, **SOLPADOL
CAPLETS**, capsule-shaped, white
tablets containing the same.
Used for: severe pain.
Dosage: 2 tablets every 4 hours with a
maximum of 8 in any 24 hour period.
Special care: labour, pregnancy,
breastfeeding, elderly, liver or kidney
disorders, underactive thyroid gland,
obstruction or inflammation of the
bowel.
Avoid use: children, depression of
respiration, obstruction of airways, head
injury, raised pressure within brain,
alcoholism, surgery to the biliary tract
(bile duct, gall bladder).
Possible interaction: CNS depressants,
MAOIs.
Side effects: constipation, blurred vision,
dizziness, dry mouth, nausea, sedation,
drug dependence and tolerance.
Manufacturer: Sanofi Winthrop.

SOLU-CORTEF

Description: a glucocorticoid-mineralocorticoid (corticosteroid) preparation available in vials with diluent for reconstitution and injection, containing 100mg hydrocortisone (as sodium succinate).

Used for: medical emergencies requiring rapid corticosteroid dose, e.g. anaphylaxis, asthma.

Dosage: 100–500mg by slow intravenous injection. Children, may require reduced doses but not less than 25mg each day.

Special care: thrombophlebitis, psychoses, recent intestinal anastomoses, chronic nephritis, certain cancers, osteo-porosis, peptic ulcer, skin eruption/rash related to a disease, viral, fungal or active infections, tuberculosis. Hypertension, glaucoma, epilepsy, acute glomerulonephritis (inflammation of kidney glomerulus), diabetes, cirrhosis, hypothyroidism, pregnancy, stress. To be withdrawn gradually.

Possible interaction: NSAIDs, oral anticoagulants, phenytoin, ephedrine, phenobarbitone, rifampicin, diuretics, cardiac glycosides, anticholinesterases, hypoglycaemics.

Side effects: osteoporosis, depression, euphoria, hyperglycaemia, peptic ulcers, Cushingoid changes.

Manufacturer: Upjohn.

SOLU-MEDRONE

Description: a glucocorticoid corticosteroid preparation available as powder in vials for reconstitution and injection, in strengths of 40mg, 125mg, 500mg and g all containing methylprednisolone (as sodium succinate). Also, **SOLU-MEDRONE 2G** available in vials with diluent, containing 2g methylprednisolone as sodium succinate).

Used for: Solu-Medrone, allergic conditions, ulcerative colitis, Crohn's disease, Stevens-Johnson syndrome, removal of stomach contents by aspiration, cerebral oedema resulting from tumour, transplant operations. Solu-Medrone 2G, serious spinal cord injuries.

Dosage: Solu-Medrone, transplants, up to 1g each day; other conditions, 10–500mg by slow intravenous or intramuscular injection over 30 minutes or longer. Solu-Medrone 2G, 30mg/kg body weight by intravenous injection over 15 minutes starting within 8 hours of injury. Then, further dose after 45 minutes at rate of 5.4mg/kg/hour for 23 hours, by intravenous infusion. Children, Solu-Medrone only, up to 30mg/kg each day depending upon condition; status asthmaticus (severe, prolonged asthma attack), 1–4mg/kg each day for 1 to 3 days.

Special care: thrombophlebitis, psychoses, recent intestinal anastomoses, chronic nephritis, certain cancers, osteoporosis, peptic ulcer, skin eruption/rash related to a disease, viral, fungal or active infections, tuberculosis. Hypertension, glaucoma, epilepsy, acute glomerulonephritis (inflammation of kidney glomerulus), diabetes, cirrhosis, hypothyroidism, pregnancy, stress. To be withdrawn gradually.

Possible interaction: NSAIDs, oral anticoagulants, phenytoin, ephedrine, phenobarbitone, rifampicin, diuretics, cardiac glycosides, anticholinesterases, hypoglycaemics.

Side effects: osteoporosis, depression, euphoria, hyperglycaemia, peptic ulcers, Cushingoid changes.

Manufacturer: Upjohn.

SONERYL^{CD}

Description: an hypnotic barbiturate available as pink, scored tablets containing 100mg butobarbitone marked SONERYL.

Used for: insomnia which has not responded to other drugs.

Dosage: 1–2 tablets taken at bedtime.

Special care: extremely dangerous, addictive drug with narrow margin of safety. Liable to abuse by overdose leading to coma and death or if combined with alcohol. Easily produces dependence and severe withdrawal symptoms. Drowsiness may persist next day affecting driving and performance of skilled tasks.

Avoid use: should be avoided if possible in all patients. Not to be used for children, young adults, pregnant and nursing mothers, elderly pesons, those with drug or alcohol related problems, patients with liver, kidney or heart disease, porphyria. Insomnia where the cause is pain.

Possible interaction: alcohol, CNS depressants, griseofulvin, metronidazone, rifampicin, phenytoin, chloramphenicol. Anticoagulant drugs of the coumarin type, steroid drugs including contraceptive pill.

Side effects: hangover with drowsiness, shakiness, dizziness, headache, anxiety, confusion, excitement, rash and allergic responses, gastro intestinal upsets, urine retention, loss of sexual desire.

Manufacturer: Theraplix.

SOTACOR

Description: a non-cardioselective ß-blocker available as white tablets in 2 strengths of 80mg and 160mg containing solatol hydrochloride, both marked with strength and name. Also, **SOTACOR INJECTION** available as a solution in ampoules for injection containing 10mg/ml.

Used for: prevention of second heart attack, arrhythmias, angina, hypertension.

Dosage: prevention of heart attack, 320mg once each day starting 5 to 14 days after first attack. Arrhythmias, 160–240mg each day in divided or single doses. Angina, 160mg each day in single or divided doses; hypertension, 160mg each day at first increasing to 320mg daily if needed.

Special care: history of bronchospasm and certain ß-blockers, diabetes, liver or kidney disease, pregnancy, lactation, general anaesthesia. Withdraw gradually. Not for children.

Avoid use: heart block or failure, bradycardia, sick sinus syndrome (associated with sinus node disorder), certain ß-blockers, severe peripheral arterial disease.

Possible interaction: verapamil, hypoglycaemics, reserpine, clonidine withdrawal, some antiarrhythmics and anaesthetics, antihypertensives, depressants of the CNS, cimetidine, indomethacin, sympathomimetics.

Side effects: bradycardia, cold hands and feet, disturbance to sleep, heart failure, gastro-intestinal upset, tiredness on exertion, bronchospasm.

Manufacturer: Bristol-Myers.

SOTAZIDE

Description: an antihypertensive compound which combines a non-cardioselective ß-blocker and thiazide diuretic, available as oblong, scored, blue tablets containing 160mg solatol hydrochloride and 25mg hydrochlorothiazide.

Used for: hypertension.

Dosage: 1 tablet each day increasing to 2 if needed.

Special care: pregnancy, breastfeeding, patients with weak hearts may require diuretics and digitalis, those with diabetes, undergoing general anaesthesia, kidney or liver disorders, gout. Electrolyte (salts) levels may need to be monitored.

Avoid use: history of bronchospasm or obstructive airways disease, heart block, heart shock, uncompensated heart failure, disease of peripheral arteries, bradycardia. Serious or worsening kidney failure or anuria.

Possible interaction: sympathomimetics, class I antiarrhythmics, CNS depressants, clonidine withdrawal, ergot alkaloids, cardiac depressant anaesthetics, verapamil, reserpine, indomethacin, hypoglycaemics, cimetidine, other antihypertensives. Digitalis, potassium supplements, potassium-sparing diuretics, lithium.

Side effects: cold hands and feet, disturbance of sleep, fatigue on exercise, bronchospasm, bradycardia, gastrointestinal disturbances, heart failure, blood changes, gout, sensitivity to light, muscle weakness. If skin rash or dry eyes occur, withdraw drug gradually.

Manufacturer: Bristol-Myers.

SPARINE

Description: an antipsychotic and group I phenothiazine available as a yellow suspension containing promazine embonate equivalent to 50mg hydrochloride/5ml. Also, **SPARINE INJECTION** containing 50mg promazine hydrochloride/ml as a solution in ampoules.

Used for: additional therapy in treatment of agitation, restlessness and agitation in elderly people, prolonged hiccough. Injection additionally used for vomiting and nausea, EEG and cardiac investigative proceudres in children.

Dosage: 100–200mg 4 times each day; elderly, half adult dose or 25–50mg for agitation and restlessness. Injection, 50mg every 6 to 8 hours by intramuscular injection; elderly, half adult dose. Children, injection only, 0.7mg/kg body weight given intramuscularly.

Special care: pregnancy, breastfeeding, Parkinsonism, liver disorders, disease of heart or arteries of heart.

Avoid use: depresssed bone marrow function or in coma.

Possible interaction: alcohol, anaesthetics, anticonvulsants, levodopa, analgesics, antidiabetic drugs, antihypertensives, antidepressants, tranquillizers.

Side effects: extrapyramidal side effects, drowsiness, hypothermia, insomnia, pallor, nightmares, depression, constipation, dry mouth, blocked nose, difficulty in urination. Changes in ECG and EEG, effects on heart, e.g. tachycardia, arrhythmias, blood changes, changes in endocrine system, e.g. effects on menstruation, breasts, impotence, weight gain. Effects on liver, jaundice, sensitivity to light, purple pigmentation of skin and eyes.

Manufacturer: Wyeth.

SPIROCTAN

Description: a potassium-sparing diuretic, available in the form of blue tablets containing 25mg and green tablets containing 50mg spironolacetone, coded BM B2 and BM A8 respectively. Also, **SPIROCTAN CAPSULES**, green, containing 100mg, coded BM A7. Also, **SPIROCTAN-M**, available as a solution in ampoules containing 20mg canrenoate potassium/ml.

Used for: congestive heart failure, cirrhosis of the liver, nephrotic syndrome (a kidney abnormality), primary aldosteronism (a disease of the adrenal glands in which an excess of aldosterone, the hormone which regulates blood levels of sodium and potassium, is produced). Also, ascites (a collection of fluid in the peritoneal cavity of the abdomen, resulting from various diseases or disorders).

Dosage: tablets and capsules, 50–200mg each day which may be increased, if needed, to a maximum of 400mg. The maximum single dose is 100mg. Spiroctan-M, 200–400mg, maximum 800mg, each day. Children, tablets or capsules, 1.5–3mg/kg body weight each day.

Special care: liver or kidney disorders, long-term use in young people. Fluid, electrolyte and levels of blood urea nitrogen should be monitored.

Avoid use: pregnancy, breastfeeding, Addison's disease, serious kidney disorders, hyperkalaemia.

Possible interaction: potassium-sparing diuretics, potassium supplements, carbenoxolone, ACE inhibitors, NSAIDs, cardiac glycosides.

Side effects: disturbance of metabolism and electrolyte levels, menstrual changes, gastro-intestinal upset, enlargement of breasts, deepening of voice, rash, loss of co-ordination, confusion.

Manufacturer: B.M. Pharm.

SPORANOX

Description: a triazole antifungal drug available as pink/blue capsules enclosing coated pellets containing 100mg itraconazole.

Used for: candidiasis (fungal infections)

of vagina, oropharynx (the part of the pharynx containing the tonsils), skin disorders.
Dosage: vulvo-vaginal infections, 2 tablets twice for 1 day; infections of oropharynx, 1 tablet each day for 15 days (2 tablets daily in patients with AIDS or who are neutropenic). Skin disorders, 1 tablet each day for 15 days or 30 days or 2 for 7 days, depending upon condition.
Special care: liver disease or those who have suffered toxic effects to the liver from taking other drugs.
Avoid use: elderly, children, pregnancy, breastfeeding. Contraception must be used during treatment and for 1 month following taking Sporanox.
Possible interaction: antacids, astemizole, rifampicin, terfenadine, cyclosporin, H_2 antagonists.
Side effects: pain in abdomen, indigestion, nausea, headache.
Manufacturer: Janssen.

STAFOXIL

Description: a penicillinase-resistant penicillin (i.e. resistant to the enzymes produced by some bacteria), available as brown/cream capsules in 2 strengths, containing 250mg and 500mg flucloxacillin (as sodium salt).
Used for: soft tissue, skin, ear, nose and throat infections caused by Gram-positive bacteria.
Dosage: 250mg 4 times each day taken 1 hour before meals. Children, over 2 years, half adult dose.
Avoid use: children under 2 years.
Side effects: gastro-intestinal upset, allergic hypersensitive reactions; rarely, cholestatic jaundice.
Manufacturer: Yamanouchi.

STARIL

Description: an antihypertensive and ACE inhibitor available as diamond-shaped, white tablets containing 10mg fosinopril sodium marked with star, 158 and SQUIBB. Also, white 20mg tablets, marked with star, 609 and SQUIBB.

Used for: hypertension which has not responded to other drugs or where these are not appropriate.
Dosage: 10mg once each day at first with a maintenance dose in the order of 10–20mg daily. The maximum daily dose is 40mg. Any diuretic being taken should be stopped a few days before treatment starts but can be resumed after 4 weeks, if needed.
Special care: congestive heart failure, kidney or liver disorders, receiving dialysis, depletion of fluid or salts.
Avoid use: pregnancy, breastfeeding, children.
Possible interaction: antacids, potassium-sparing diuretics, potassium supplements, lithium, NSAIDs, antihypertensives.
Side effects: chest and muscle pains, rash, gastro-intestinal upset, fatigue, dizziness, palpitations, cough, disturbance of sense of taste; rarely, pancreatitis. If angioneurotic oedema occurs, withdraw drug.
Manufacturer: Squibb.

STD INJECTION

Description: a sclerosant drug available as a solution in ampoules for injection at strengths of 0.5%, 1% and 3% all containing sodium tetradecyl sulphate.
Used for: varicose veins in the leg by compression sclerotherapy.
Dosage: for large veins, 0.25–1ml of 3% solution into section of vein by intravenous injection followed immediately by compression applied continuously. Maximum treatment of 4 sites in any 1 session of treatment. Small veins, 0.25–1ml of 1% solution in same way as for large veins. Maximum treatment of 10 sites in any 1 session. Very small veins or venules, 0.1–1ml of 0.5% solution as above. Maximum treatment of 10 sites in any 1 session.
Special care: pregnancy, breastfeeding, disease of the arteries, history of allergy. Treatment must be carried out by specialist with emergency equipment available in the event of anaphylaxis.

Avoid use: thrombophlebitis, infections, varicose veins caused by tumours, diabetes which is not controlled. Patients who are obese or immobile, taking oral contraceptives.
Manufacturer: STD.

STELAZINE
Description: an anxiolytic, antidepressant and anticonvulsant preparation which is a phenothiazine group II drug. It is available as sugar-coated, blue tablets in 2 strengths containing 1mg and 5mg trifluoperazine (as hydrochloride), and marked SKF. Also, **STELAZINE SYRUP** containing 1mg/5ml; **STELAZINE SPANSULES,** yellow/clear, sustained-release capsules containing 2mg, 10mg and 15mg as white and blue pellets, marked 2. **STELAZINE CONCENTRATE,** containing 10mg/ml; **STELAZINE INJECTION** available as a solution in ampoules containing 1mg/ml.
Used for: anxiety and agitation which may be accompanied by depression, psychosis, schizophrenia, disturbed behaviour; vomiting and nausea.
Dosage: anxiety, Stelazine tablets, syrup, spansules, 2–4mg each day with a maximum of 6mg. Schizophrenia, psychosis, disturbed behaviour, tablets or syrup, 5mg twice each day at first increasing to 15mg after 7 days. If needed, dosage may be further increased every 3 days by 5mg until condition is controlled and then reduced again for maintenance. Spansules, 1 10mg strength each day at first, increasing to 1 15mg spansule daily after 7 days. Injection, 1–3mg each day in divided doses, by intramuscular injection. Nausea and vomiting, tablets, syrup, spansules, 2–6mg each day. Elderly persons, tablets or syrup, all disorders, 1mg each day at first which may require gradual increase according to response. Children, usually use syrup, all disorders, age 3 to 5 years, up to 1mg; 6 to 12 years, up to 4mg, all as daily divided doses.

Special care: pregnancy, breastfeeding, elderly, heart disease or disease of heart blood vessels, epilepsy, Parkinsonism, vomiting which is undiagnosed.
Avoid use: children under 3 years, depressed bone marrow function, liver damage, coma.
Possible interaction: analgesics, alcohol, CNS depressants, antihypertensives.
Side effects: dry mouth, blurring of vision, disturbance of CNS, changes to ECG, hormonal changes. Rarely, extrapyramidal side effects and allergic responses with low doses. Judgement and performance of skilled tasks may be impaired.
Manufacturer: S.K. & F.

STEMETIL
Description: an antipsychotic and anticonvulsant and phenothiazine group III drug, available as cream tablets 5mg and 25mg (scored) both containing prochlorperazine maleate and marked with strength and name. Also, **STEMETIL SYRUP** containing 5mg prochlorperazine mesylate/5ml. **STEMETIL EFF,** effervescent granules in sachets for reconstitution in water containing 5mg prochlorperazine mesylate. Also, **STEMETIL SUPPOSITORIES,** available in strengths of 5mg and 25mg containing prochlorperazine. **STEMETIL INJECTION** available as a solution in ampoules for injection containing 1 25% prochlorperazine mesylate.
Used for: psychoses, schizophrenia, minor psychiatric and emotional disorders, severe vomiting and nausea, migraine, vertigo resulting from Ménière's disease (an inner ear disorder accompanied by ringing in the ears and progressive deafness).
Dosage: psychiatric disorders, oral preparations, 15–25mg each day, maximum 40mg for minor illnesses; 75–100mg daily for schizophrenia, all in divided doses. Suppositories, 25mg 2 or 3 times each day, then oral preparations. Injection, 12.5–25mg 2 or 3 times each

day by deep intramuscular injection then oral preparations. Vertigo, oral preparations, 5mg 3 times each day with a maximum of 30mg. Nausea, vomiting, 20mg as single dose then 10mg after 2 hours if needed. Prevention, 5–10mg 2 or 3 times each day. Suppositories, for vertigo, nausea and vomiting, 25mg as single dose then oral preparations after 6 hours, if needed. Injection, 12.5mg by deep intramuscular injection, then oral preparations if needed. Children, use syrup for nausea, vomiting only, over 10kg in weight, 0.25mg/kg body weight 2 or 3 times each day.

Special care: breastfeeding, heart disease or disease of heart blood vessels, Parkinsonism, prolonged vomiting which is not diagnosed.

Avoid use: pregnancy, children under 10kg body weight, epilepsy, depressed bone marrow function, liver or kidney disorders, coma.

Possible interaction: alcohol, antidiabetics, CNS depressants, antihypertensives, anticholinergics, analgesics, anticonvulsants.

Side effects: anticholinergic side effects and disturbance of CNS, hypotension on rising (following injection), blood disorders, jaundice. At low doses there may rarely be endocrine changes, extrapyramidal side effects and allergic responses. Judgement and performance of skilled tasks may be impaired.

Manufacturer: Theraplix.

STER-ZAC DC

Description: a disinfectant preparation available as a cream containing 3% hexachlophane.

Used for: disinfection of hands prior to surgery.

Dosage: wash hands with 3–5ml used as soap.

Special care: children under 2 years.

Manufacturer: Hough, Hoseason.

STESOLID

Description: a preparation for use rectally, with applicator, which is a long-acting benzodiazepine, available as a solution in single doses containing 5mg or 10mg diazepam.

Used for: agitation, acute anxiety, convulsions, status epilepticus in which rapid treatment is necessary but injection intravenously is not desirable. Also, muscle spasm and pre-medication.

Dosage: for all conditions, 10mg via rectum, elderly persons, 5mg. Children, age 1 to 3 years, 5mg; over 3 years, 10mg.

Special care: chronic liver or kidney disease, chronic lung disease, pregnancy, labour, lactation, elderly. May impair judgement. Withdraw gradually and avoid prolonged use.

Avoid use: children under 1 year, depression of respiration, acute lung disease; psychotic, phobic or obsessional states.

Possible interaction: anticonvulsants, depressants of the CNS, alcohol.

Side effects: ataxia, confusion, light-headedness, drowsiness, hypotension, gastro-intestinal upsets, disturbances in vision and libido, skin rashes, retention of urine, vertigo. Sometimes jaundice or blood disorders.

Manufacturer: Durmex.

STIEDEX

Description: a topical potent steroid preparation available as an oily cream containing 0.25% desoxymethasone. STIEDEX LP, a moderatly potent steroid preparation available as an oily cream containing 0.05%. Also, STIEDEX LOTION, combining a potent steroid and keratolytic agent in a lotion containing 0.25% desoxymethasone and 1% salicylic acid.

Used for: Stiedex cream and LP cream, skin inflammations responsive to steroids. Lotion, psoriasis, especially of scalp and various other skin conditions.

Dosage: creams, apply thinly 2 or 3 times each day and rub in. Lotion, apply once or twice each day in morning and/or evening and rub in. When condition improves, use once each day.

Special care: thrombophlebitis,

psychoses, recent intestinal anastomoses, chronic nephritis, certain cancers, osteoporosis, peptic ulcer, skin eruption/rash related to a disease, viral, fungal or active infections, tuberculosis. Hypertension, glaucoma, epilepsy, acute glomerulonephritis (inflammation of kidney glomerulus), diabetes, cirrhosis, hypothyroidism, pregnancy, stress. To be withdrawn gradually.
Avoid use: children (Stiedex).
Possible interaction: NSAIDs, oral anticoagulants, phenytoin, ephedrine, phenobarbitone, rifampicin, diuretics, cardiac glycosides, anticholinesterases, hypoglycaemics.
Side effects: osteoporosis, depression, euphoria, hyperglycaemia, peptic ulcers, Cushingoid changes.
Manufacturer: Stiefel.

STIEMYCIN

Description: an antibiotic solution containing 2% erythromycin.
Used for: acne.
Dosage: adults, apply twice each day in the morning and evening after washing.
Side effects: possible slight irritation and dryness of skin at site of application.
Manufacturer: Stiefel.

STREPTASE

Description: a fibrinolytic preparation available as powder in vials for reconstitution and injection containing 250,000 units or 750,000 units streptokinase. Also, **STREPTASE 1.5 MEGA UNITS**, as powder in vials for reconstitution and injection containing 1,500,000 units streptokinase.
Used for: Streptase, pulmonary embolism, deep vein thrombosis, blockage of peripheral arteries, thrombosis of retinal blood vessels. Streptase 1.5 Mega Units, acute heart attack.
Dosage: Streptase, initial dose of 250,000 units by intravenous infusion, then 100,000 units by infusion/hour for 24–72 hours depending upon response. Streptase 1.5 Mega Units, single dose over 1 hour by intravenous infusion of 1.5 million units, accompanied by oral doses of 150mg aspirin each day for at least 4 weeks. Children, Streptase only, initial dose adjusted according to condition, body weight then 20 units/ml of blood volume.
Special care: heart disorders; blood tests and anticoagulant therapy are also required.
Avoid use: pregnancy, patients who have received streptokinase treatment in last 5 days to 12 months, those with known allergy to streptokinase. Patients with recent bleeding disorders, clotting disorders, liver or kidney damage, brain growth, lung disease, inflammation and bacterial infection of endocardium, serious bronchitis, pancreatitis, diabetes. Having recently had surgery or with history of bleeding.
Possible interaction: drugs affecting blood platelets, anticoagulants.
Side effects: feverish reactions, heart arrhythmias, hypotension, pulmonary oedema, haemorrhage, embolism caused by cholesterol. Rarely, anaphylaxis.
Manufacturer: Hoechst.

STROMBA

Description: an anabolic steroid available as white, scored tablets containing 5mg stanozolol marked STROMBA.
Used for: Behcet's disease, (a rare disease affecting the blood vessels of the eye), prevention of angio-oedema which is hereditary.
Dosage: Behcet's disease, 10mg each day; angio-oedema, 2.5–10mg each day at first then reduce dose as condition responds. Children, angio-oedema, aged 1 to 6 years, 2.5mg each day at first; 6 to 12 years, 2.5–5mg daily in first instance. Dose is then adjusted according to response.
Special care: use for long periods in children, women past menopause, patients with kidney or heart disorders. Monitoring of liver function is required if patient has history of jaundice.

Avoid use: pregnancy, porphyria, cancer of prostate gland, liver disease, type 1 diabetes.
Possible interaction: oral anticoagulants.
Side effects: indigestion, headache, skin rash, pains and cramps; toxic effects on liver, masculinizing effects on women and children before puberty.
Manufacturer: Sanofi Winthrop.

SUBLIMAZE^{CD}

Description: a narocotic analgesic available as a solution in ampoules containing 50µg fentanyl/ml.
Used for: analgesia during operations, enhancement of analgesic, respiratory depression in patients receiving artificial ventilation.
Dosage: adults breathing unaided, 50–200µg at first then 50µg as needed. Adults being ventilated, 0.3–3.5mg at first then 100–200µg as needed. Children, 3 to 5 µg/kg body weight then 1µg/kg as needed. Child being ventilated, 15µg/kg then 1–3 µg/kg as needed.
Special care: liver disease, underactive thyroid, respiratory disorders, myasthenia gravis. If used in obstetric patients, may cause depression of respiration in baby.
Avoid use: obstructive airways disease or depression of respiration unless being artificially ventilated.
Possible interaction: MAOIs, anxiolytics, hypnotics, cimetidine.
Side effects: depression of respiration, bradycardia, vomiting, nausea, short-lived hypotension.
Manufacturer: Janssen.

SULPITIL

Description: an antipsychotic preparation and substituted benzamide available as scored, white tablets containing 200mg sulpiride marked L113.
Used for: schizophrenia.
Dosage: adults and young persons over 14 years, 200–400mg twice each day with a maximum of 1800mg daily. Elderly, 50–100mg twice each day at first increasing slowly to normal adult dose.

Special care: pregnancy, epilepsy, kidney disorders, hypertension, hypomania.
Avoid use: breastfeeding, phaeochromocytoma, porphyria.
Possible interaction: alcohol, anxiolytics, hypnotics, tetrabenazine, calcium channel blockers, cimetidine.
Side effects: extrapyramidal side effects, ECG and EEG changes. Effects on heart rhythm, blocked nose, dry mouth, constipation, blurring of vision, difficulty passing urine, drowsiness, apathy, depression, insomnia. Blood changes involving white blood cells, hormonal changes, e.g. enlargement of breasts, change in libido, impotence, sensitivity to light, effects on liver, changes in weight.
Manufacturer: Pharmacia.

SUTTRIN

Description: a compound sulphonamide antibacterial preparation available as lozenge-shaped, white, vaginal tablets (with applicator) containing 172.5mg sulphathiazole, 143.75mg sulphacetamide and 184mg sulphabenzamide marked with C and symbol. Also, **SULTRIN CREAM** containing 3.42% sulphathiazole, 2.86% sulphacetamide, 3.7% sulphabenzamide, with applicator.
Used for: inflammation and infection of vagina and cervix caused by bacteria, post-cervical cautery, post-operative treatment.
Dosage: tablets, 1 intravaginally twice each day for 10 days. Cream, 1 applicator dose intravaginally twice each day for 10 days which may need to be reduced to 1 dose daily, depending upon response.
Avoid use: children, kidney disorders.
Side effects: allergic reactions.
Manufacturer: Cilag.

SUPRAX

Description: an antibiotic cephalosporin available as film-coated, scored white tablets containing 200mg cefixime marked LL200 and SUPRAX. Also, **SUPRAX PAEDIATRIC SUSPENSION**

containing 100mg/5ml solution.
Used for: infections of urinary and respiratory tract.
Dosage: 200–400mg as single or 2 divided doses for 7 to 14 days. Children, age 6 to 12 months, 3.75ml; 1 to 4 years, 5ml; 5 to 10 years, 10ml; 11 to 12 years, 15ml. All as daily doses of paediatric suspension.
Special care: pregnancy, breastfeeding, allergy to ß-lactams, serious kidney disorders.
Avoid use: children under 6 months.
Side effects: rashes, gastro-intestinal upset, headache, dizziness. Rarely, pseudomembranous colitis.
Manufacturer: Lederle.

SUPRECUR

Description: a preparation which is a GnRH (gonadotrophin-releasing hormone) analogue that acts on the pituitary gland inhibiting the release of gonadotrophin, resulting in a lowering of the levels of oestrogen produced by the ovaries. It is available in the form of a nasal spray, with pump, delivering a metered dose of 150μg buserelin (as acetate) per application.
Used for: endometriosis, pituitary desensitization prior to controlled stimulation of the ovaries (with gonadotrophins) as a part of infertility treatment.
Dosage: for endometriosis, 1 spray into each nostril in the morning, middle of the day and evening for a maximum period of 6 months. Treatment should begin on first or second day of monthly cycle. Infertility, 1 spray in 1 nostril 4 times each day, as directed by specialist, usually for 2 to 3 weeks.
Special care: patients subject to depression or at risk of osteoporosis. Barrier methods of contraception must be used.
Avoid use: pregnancy, breastfeeding, hormone-dependent tumours, undiagnosed vaginal bleeding.
Possible interaction: nasal decongestants.
Side effects: local irritation of nose, menopausal symptoms, e.g. hot flushes,

change in libido, vaginal dryness, sweating, nausea, headache, changes in breasts and tenderness, cysts on ovaries, backache, dry skin, acne, rash, palpitations, changes in density of bones.
Manufacturer: Hoechst.

SUPREFACT

Description: a gonadotrophin-releasing hormone analogue, acting on pituitary gland receptors resulting in the inhibition of the release of luteinizing hormone and lower levels of testosterone in the blood. Suprefact is available in vials for injection containing 1mg buserelin (as acetate)/ml. Also, **SUPREFACT NASAL SPRAY** containing 100 μg per dose.
Used for: Stage C or D cancer of the prostate gland in which it is desirable for levels of testosterone to be reduced.
Dosage: 0.5ml every 8 hours by subcutaneous injection for 1 week. Then 1 spray in each nostril 6 times each day as maintenance dose.
Special care: anti-androgens may be needed.
Avoid use: patients with tumours that are not responsive to hormones; those who have had 1 or both testes surgically removed (orchidectomy).
Side effects: short-lived irritation of nostrils, loss of libido, hot flushes.
Manufacturer: Hoechst.

SURGAM SA

Description: an NSAID which is a propionic acid available as sustained-release maroon/pink capsules enclosing white pellets containing 300mg tiaprofenic acid, marked SURGAM SA. Also, **SURGAM TABLETS**, white, in strengths of 200mg and 300mg, marked with symbol on one side and name and strength on the reverse.
Used for: disorders of joints, skeleton and muscles including osteoarthritis, rheumatoid arthritis, lumbago, ankylosing spondylitis, injuries.
Dosage: capsules, 2 as a single daily

dose; tablets, 600mg as divided doses each day.

Special care: pregnancy, breastfeeding, elderly, heart failure, liver or kidney disorders, known allergy to aspirin or NSAID.

Avoid use: children, history of or active peptic ulcer.

Possible interaction: sulphonamides, hypoglycaemics, diuretics, anticoagulants, hydantoins.

Side effects: headache, gastro-intestinal upset, sleepiness, rash. Withdraw if cystitis and haematuria (blood in urine) occur (rare).

Manufacturer: Roussel.

SURMONTIL

Description: a TCAD preparation available as white tablets in strengths of 10mg and 25mg containing trimipramine (as maleate), both marked with strength and SURMONTIL. Also, **SURMONTIL CAPSULES**, white/green containing 50mg marked SU50.

Used for: depression and/or anxiety, agitation, disturbance of sleep.

Dosage: mild or moderate symptoms, 50–75mg as single dose, 2 hours before going to bed. Continue for a minimum of 3 weeks. Moderate to severe symptoms, 75mg each day under specialist supervision gradually increasing according to condition. Usual dose is in the order of 150–300mg each day then reducing for maintenance once condition improves. Elderly, 10–25mg 3 times each day.

Special care: liver disorders, hyperthyroidism, glaucoma, lactation, epilepsy, diabetes, adrenal tumour, heart disease, urine retention. Psychotic or suicidal patients.

Avoid use: heart block, heart attacks, severe liver disease, pregnancy.

Possible interaction: MAOIs (or within 14 days of their use), alcohol, antidepressants, barbiturates, anticholinergics, local anaesthetics that contain adrenaline or noradrenaline, oestrogens, cimetidine, antihypertensives.

Side effects: constipation, urine retention, dry mouth, blurred vision, palpitations, tachycardia, nervousness, drowsiness, insomnia. Changes in weight, blood and blood sugar, jaundice, skin reactions, weakness, ataxia, hypotension, sweating, altered libido, gynaecomastia, galactorrhoea.

Manufacturer: Theraplix.

SURVANTA

Description: a lung surfactant available as a solution in single dose vials containing 25mg beractant (a natural lung extract)/ml.

Used for: newborn babies with respiratory distress undergoing mechanical ventilation whose birthweight exceeds 700g and who are receiving continuous monitoring.

Dosage: 100mg/kg body weight in volume not greater than 4ml/kg by endotracheal tube. Best given within 8 hours of birth and a maximum of 4 further doses at a minimum of 6 hourly intervals, may be given within 48 hours.

Special care: continuous monitoring of oxygen level in arterial blood required.

Side effects: endotracheal tube may become blocked by mucous, possible haemorrhage in lung.

Manufacturer: Abbott.

SUSTAMYCIN

Description: a tetracycline antibiotic preparation available as sustained-release capsules in light and darker blue containing 250mg tetracycline hydrochloride.

Used for: infections responsive to tetracyclines, severe acne.

Dosage: infections, 2 capsules twice each day at first reducing to 1 as condition improves. Acne, 4 tablets each day for first 2 to 3 weeks then 1 for 3 to 4 months.

Special care: liver or kidney disorders.

Avoid use: pregnancy, breastfeeding, children.

Possible interaction: mineral supplements, milk, antacids, oral contraceptives.

Side effects: allergic responses, superinfections, gastro-intestinal upset.
Manufacturer: B.M. Pharmaceuticals.

SUSTANON 100

Description: an hormonal depot androgen preparation available in ampoules for injection containing 20mg testosterone propionate, 40mg testosterone phenylpropionate, 40mg testosterone isocaproate/ml. Also, **SUSTANON 250** available in ampoules for injection containing 30mg testosterone propionate, 60mg testosterone phenylpropionate, 60mg testosterone isocaproate and 100mg testosterone decanoate/ml.
Used for: androgen deficiency in males, osteoporosis resulting from androgen deficiency.
Dosage: 1ml by deep intramuscular injection every 2 weeks; Sustanon 250, 1ml by deep intramuscular injection every 3 weeks.
Special care: heart, liver or kidney disorders, migraine, hypertension, epilepsy.
Avoid use: heart disease, heart failure which is untreated, cancer of prostate gland or liver, nephrotic syndrome (a kidney abnormality resulting from various diseases and disorders).
Possible interaction: drugs which induce liver enzymes.
Side effects: weight gain, liver tumours, oedema, reduced fertility, premature closure of epiphyses, priapism (painful and prolonged erection of penis not connected with sexual arousal but caused by drug treatment or sickle-cell trait. Causes tissue damage if not relieved by decompression).
Manufacturer: Organon.

SYMMETRAL

Description: a dopaminergic, tricyclic amine preparation available as reddish-brown capsules containing 100mg amantadine hydrochloride marked GEIGY. Also, **SYMMETRAL SYRUP** containing 50mg amantadine hydrochloride/ml.
Used for: Parkinsonism, prevention and treatment of patients with certain strains of influenza (A$_2$, A/New Jersey) who are at risk from complications. *Herpes zoster* infections.
Dosage: Parkinsonism, 100mg capsules of syrup each day for 7 days at first then same dose twice daily. Influenza, treatment, 1 capsule twice each day for 5 to 7 days; prevention, 1 capsule twice each day for 7 to 10 days. *Herpes zoster*, 1 capsule or 10ml syrup twice each day for 14 to 28 days. Children, for influenza age over 10 years, treatment and prevention, 1 capsule in morning for 7 to 10 days.
Special care: pregnancy, congestive heart failure, liver or kidney disorders, suffering from confusion.
Avoid use: children under 10 years, serious kidney disease, history of or active stomach ulcer, history of convulsions.
Possible interaction: anticholinergics, levodopa, CNS stimulants.
Side effects: livedo reticularis (a disorder of the veins resulting in a mottled "fish-net" appearance of legs and occasionally arms), oedema in hands and feet, skin rash, gastro-intestinal upset, disturbance of vision, effects on central nervous system.
Manufacturer: Geigy.

SYNACTHEN DEPOT

Description: a depot preparation of adrenal stimulating hormone available in ampoules for injection containing 1mg tetracosactrin acetate and zinc complex/ml.
Used for: collagen and rheumatic disorders, Crohn's disease, ulcerative colitis.
Dosage: acute treatment, 1–2g by intramuscular injection each day with reduced doses for maintenance. Children, age 1 month to 2 years, 0.25mg by intramuscular injection each day at first; 2 to 5 years, 0.25–0.5mg by intramuscular injection each day at first; 5 to 12 years, 0.25–1mg by intramuscular injection each day at first. For maintenance, these doses are repeated every 2 to 8 days.

Special care: thrombophlebitis, psychoses, recent intestinal anastomoses, chronic nephritis, certain cancers, osteoporosis, peptic ulcer, skin eruption/ rash related to a disease, viral, fungal or active infections, tuberculosis. Hypertension, glaucoma, epilepsy, acute glomerulonephritis (inflammation of kidney glomerulus), diabetes, cirrhosis, hypothyroidism, pregnancy, stress. To be withdrawn gradually.
Avoid use: allergic conditions, asthma.
Possible interaction: NSAIDs, oral anticoagulants, phenytoin, ephedrine, phenobarbitone, rifampicin, diuretics, cardiac glycosides, anticholinesterases, hypoglycaemics.
Side effects: osteoporosis, depression, euphoria, hyperglycaemia, peptic ulcers, Cushingoid changes.
Manufacturer: Ciba.

SYNALAR

Description: a potent topical steroid preparation available as cream and ointment containing 0.025% fluocinolone acetonide. **SYNALAR 1:4**, a moderately potent steroid cream and ointment containing 0.00625%. **SYNALAR CREAM 1:10**, a mildly potent steroid cream containing 0.0025%. **SYNALAR C** a combined potent steroid, antibacterial, antifungal cream and ointment containing 0.025% fluocinolone acetonide and 3% clioquinol. **SYNALAR N**, a potent steroid and antibacterial cream and ointment containing 0.025% fluocinolone acetonide and 0.5% neomycin sulphate. Also, **SYNALAR GEL** containing 0.025% fluocinolone acetate.
Used for: Synalar steroid preparations, skin conditions responsive to steroid treatment; Synalar combined preparations, infected skin conditions responsive to steroid treatment. Synalar Gel, skin conditions of the scalp responsive to steroid treatment.
Dosage: apply thinly 2 or 3 times each day and rub in. Synalar Gel, rub into scalp in the morning and at night at first and then once or twice each week for maintenance.
Special care: thrombophlebitis, psychoses, recent intestinal anastomoses, chronic nephritis, certain cancers, osteoporosis, peptic ulcer, skin eruption/ rash related to a disease, viral, fungal or active infections, tuberculosis. Hypertension, glaucoma, epilepsy, acute glomerulonephritis (inflammation of kidney glomerulus), diabetes, cirrhosis, hypothyroidism, pregnancy, stress. To be withdrawn gradually.
Avoid use: use only mild steroid preparations in children.
Possible interaction: NSAIDs, oral anticoagulants, phenytoin, ephedrine, phenobarbitone, rifampicin, diuretics, cardiac glycosides, anticholinesterases, hypoglycaemics.
Side effects: osteoporosis, depression, euphoria, hyperglycaemia, peptic ulcers, Cushingoid changes.
Manufacturer: Zeneca.

SYNARD

Description: a gonadotrophin-releasing hormone analogue available as a nasal spray delivering 200µg nafarelin (as acetate) per metered dose. It acts on the pituitary gland to lower the levels of oestrogen produced by the ovaries and endometrial growth.
Used for: endometriosis.
Dosage: 1 spray into 1 nostril in the morning and then a second spray into th other nostril in the evening. Treatment should continue for a maximum period of 6 months and start between day 2 and 4 of monthly cycle.
Special care: patients at risk of osteoporosis. Barrier methods of contraception should be used.
Avoid use: pregnancy, breastfeeding, undiagnosed vaginal bleeding. Treatmer should not be repeated.
Possible interaction: nasal decongestants.
Side effects: changes in libido and bone density, changes in breast size and

enderness. Menopausal symptoms, e.g. ot flushes, sweating, vaginal dryness, nood changes, depression, aches and ramps. Migraine, palpitations, cysts on varies, allergic hypersensitive esponses, hair loss, blurring of vision. *Manufacturer*: Syntex.

YNFLEX

Description: an NSAID available as lm-coated orange tablets containing 75mg napoxen sodium marked YNTEX.

Used for: period pain, pain following perations, migraine, muscle and bone ains, strains and sprains.

Dosage: age over 16 years, usual dose, 2 ablets as 1 dose then 1 tablet 6 to 8-ourly as required. Maximum dose is 4 ablets daily. Migraine, 3 tablets as first ose then 1 or 2 tablets 6 to 8-hourly ith a daily maximum of 5.

Special care: pregnancy, breastfeeding, lderly, liver or kidney disorders, history f lesions in gastro-intestinal tract, heart ailure, asthma. Patients taking drug ong-term require careful monitoring.

Avoid use: children under 16 years, nown allergy to NSAID or aspirin, eptic ulcer.

Possible interaction: sulphonylureas, nticoagulants, frusemide, ß-blockers, uinolones, ACE inhibitors, hydantoins, thium probenecid, methotrexate.

Side effects: blood changes, gastrointestinal intolerance, vertigo, rash, nnitus.

Manufacturer: Syntex.

YNPHASE

Description: a combined oestrogen/ rogestogen oral contraceptive eparation available as: 7 white tablets ntaining 35µg ethinyloestradiol, 5mg norethisterone; 9 yellow tablets ntaining 35µg and 1mg norethisterone; 5 hite tablets containing 35µg and 0.5mg spectively. All are marked SYNTEX d the white tablets also with a B.

Used for: oral contraception.

Dosage: 1 tablet each day starting on fifth day of period then 7 tablet-free days.

Special care: multiple sclerosis, serious kidney disease or kidney dialysis, asthma, Raynaud's disease, abnormally high levels of prolactin in the blood (hyperprolactinaemia), varicose veins, hypertension, severe depression. Thrombosis risk increases with smoking, age and obesity. During the course of treatment, regular checks on blood pressure, pelvic organs and breasts should be carried out.

Avoid use: pregnancy, patients at risk of thrombosis, suffering from heart disease, pulmonary hypertension, angina, sickle cell anaemia. Also, undiagnosed vaginal bleeding, history of cholestatic jaundice during pregnancy, cancers which are hormone-dependent, infectious hepatitis, liver disorders. Also, porphyria, Dublin-Johnson and Rotor syndrome, otosclerosis, chorea, haemolytic uraemic syndrome, recent trophoblastic disease.

Possible interaction: barbiturates, ethosuximide, glutethimide, rifampicin, phenytoin, tetracyclines, carbamazepine, chloral hydrate, griseofulvin, dichloralphenazone, primidone.

Side effects: weight gain, breast enlargement, pains in legs and cramps, headaches, loss of sexual desire, depression, nausea, breakthrough bleeding, cervical erosion, brownish patches on skin (chloasma), vaginal discharge, oedema and bloatedness.

Manufacturer: Syntex.

SYNTARIS

Description: a corticosteroid preparation available as a nasal spray delivering 25µg flunisolide per metered dose.

Used for: allergic and inflammatory conditions affecting the nose, e.g. hay fever.

Dosage: 2 sprays into each nostril 2, or maximum of 3, times each day reducing to a minimum effective dose for control. Treatment should continue long-term. Children, age 5 to 12 years, 1 spray in each nostril 3 times each day.

Special care: pregnancy, patients who have had recent trauma or surgery, ulcers of the nose. Also, special care in patients changing from other steroid drugs.
Avoid use: children under 5, untreated infections of nose or eyes.
Side effects: short-lived irritation of nose.
Manufacturer: Syntex.

SYNTOCINON

Description: a uterotropic hormonal preparation containing synthetic oxytocin used in obstetrics, and available as a solution in ampoules for injection at strengths of 2 units/2ml, 5 units/ml, 10 units/ml, 50 units/5ml.
Used for: to induce and augment labour, missed abortion.
Dosage: by slow intravenous infusion as a solution containing 1 unit per litre, adjusted as needed.
Special care: disorders of heart and heart circulation, hypertension, previous Caesarian section, abnormal presentation of baby, multiple birth.
Avoid use: placental praevia, serious toxaemia, obstruction of delivery, distress in baby, hypertonic (very active) activity of uterus, tendency to amniotic fluid embolism.
Side effects: danger of severe uterine contractions leading to rupture (with higher doses), hypertension and subarachnoid haemorrhage in mother, heart arrhythmias, water intoxication and lung oedema (infusion volume must remain low).
Manufacturer: Sandoz.

SYNTOMETRINE

Description: a uterotropic hormonal preparation used in obstetrics available as a solution in ampoules for injection containing 0.5mg ergometrine maleate and 5 units synthetic oxytocin/ml.
Used for: bleeding due to incomplete abortion (before surgery to remove contents of uterus), during delivery (third stage of labour) after or when baby's shoulders have emerged.

Dosage: 1ml by intramuscular injection.
Special care: porphyria, multiple birth, hypertension, heart disease, liver or kidney disease.
Avoid use: serious heart, liver, kidney or lung disease, severe hypertension, sepsis, circulatory disease, toxaemia, in first or second stage of labour.
Side effects: vomiting and nausea, short-lived hypertension, constriction of blood vessels, heart attack, stroke, lung oedema.
Manufacturer: Sandoz.

SYNTOPRESSIN

Description: a vasopressin analogue available as a solution for use with a nasal spray delivering 50 units lypressin/ml.
Used for: diabetes insipidus.
Dosage: 1 or 2 sprays into one or both nostrils 3 to 7 times a day.
Special care: pregnancy, patients with epilepsy, hypertension, disease of peripheral blood vessels, hypertension, advanced arteriosclerosis, heart failure.
Avoid use: coronary heart disease, undergoing anaesthesia with cyclopropane or halothane.
Possible interaction: chlorpropamide, lithium, carbamazepine, clofibrate.
Side effects: blocked nose and ulceration of lining of nose, nausea, pain in abdomen, feeling of needing to defecate.
Manufacturer: Sandoz.

TAGAMET

Description: an H_2 blocker cimetidine for treatment of ulcers, available in green tablets (200mg) and green oblong tablets (400mg) marked TAGAMET, SK & F and strength, and green oval tablets (800mg) marked SK & F and T 800. Also, **TAGAMET EFFERVESCENT**, 400mg white effervescent tablet and **TAGAMET SYRUP** (200mg/5ml).

Used for: ulcers—duodenal. benign gastric, recurrent and stomach. Dyspepsia, oesophageal reflux and where gastric acid has to be reduced.

Dosage: for duodenal ulcer, 800mg at bedtime or 400mg twice daily for 4 weeks, then half dose for maintenance. See literature for other conditions. Children over 1 year, 25–30mmg/kg per day in divided doses. Also, **TAGAMET INJECTION** (200mg/2ml) and **TAGAMET INFUSION** (400mg in 100ml).

Special care: eliminate malignancy first; kidney disorder, pregnancy, breastfeeding.

Possible interaction: theophylline, oral anticoagulants, phenytoin.

Side effects: rash, dizziness, tiredness, diarrhoea, confusion, gynaecomastia; rarely pancreatitis, thrombocytopenia, muscle and joint pain.

Manufacturer: S.K. & F.

TAMBOCOR

Description: a class I antiarrhythmic, flecainide acetate, available as white tablets marked 3M TR 50 (50mg) or 3M TR 100 (100mg).

Used for: tachycardia, arrhythmias.

Dosage: 50–100mg twice per day to a maximum of 400mg daily, depending upon condition, reduced after 3 to 5 days to the lowest possible maintenance dose. Not for children.

Also, **TAMBOCOR INJECTION**, 10mg/ml in ampoules.

Dosage: see literature. Not for children.

Special care: start therapy in hospital. Pacemakers, weak liver or kidneys, heart disease, pregnancy. Monitor plasma levels.

Avoid use: heart failure, past myocardial infarction, 2nd or 3rd degree atrioventricular block, sinus node disease, atrial fibrillation.

Possible interaction: digoxin, other class I antiarrhythmics, cardiac depressants.

Side effects: nausea, dizziness, vomiting, sight disturbances, sensitivity to light, jaundice, upset to liver enzymes, ataxia, tingling sensations.

Manufacturer: 3m Health Care.

TAMOFEN

Description: an antioestrogen, tamoxifen citrate, available as white tablets with 10mg (marked T10), 20mg (T20) and 40mg (T40).

Used for: infertility, breast cancer.

Dosage: 20mg per day for 4 days starting on second day on menstruation increasing to 40g and then 80mg for later treatments if required. For breast cancer 20mg per day increasing to 40mg if required.

Avoid use: pregnancy.

Possible interaction: warfarin.

Side effects: gastro-intestinal upset, hot flushes, vaginal bleeding, dizziness, disturbance to sight.

Manufacturer: Tillotts.

TAMPOVAGAN

Description: an oestrogen, stilboestrol, available as a pessary with 5% lactic acid.

Used for: vaginitis after the menopause.

Dosage: 2, high in the vagina at night for 2 to 3 weeks. Not for children.

Special care: patients considered to be at risk of thrombosis or with liver disease. Women with any of the following disorders should be carefully monitored: fibroids in the womb, multiple sclerosis, diabetes, tetany, porphyria, epilepsy, liver disease, hypertension, migraine, otosclerosis, gallstones. Breasts, pelvic organs and blood pressure should be checked at regular intervals during the course of treatment.

Avoid use: pregnancy, breastfeeding, conditions which might lead to thrombosis, thrombophlebitis, serious heart, kidney or liver disease, breast cancer, oestrogen-dependent cancers including those of reproductive system, endometriosis, vaginal bleeding which is undiagnosed.

Possible interaction: drugs which induce liver enzymes.

Side effects: tenderness and enlargement of breasts, weight gain, breakthrough bleeding, giddiness, vomiting and nausea, gastro-intestinal upset. Treatment should be halted immediately

if severe headaches occur, disturbance of vision, hypertension or any indications of thrombosis, jaundice. Also, in the event of pregnancy and 6 weeks before planned surgery.
Manufacturer: Norgine.

TARCORTIN

Description: a mild steroid and antipsoriatic, comprising 0.5% hydrocortisone and 5% coal tar extract in a cream.
Used for: eczema, psoriasis and other skin disorders.
Dosage: apply twice or more per day.
Special care: thrombophlebitis, psychoses, recent intestinal anastomoses, chronic nephritis, certain cancers, osteoporosis, peptic ulcer, skin eruption/rash related to a disease, viral, fungal or active infections, tuberculosis. Hypertension, glaucoma, epilepsy, acute glomerulonephritis (inflammation of kidney glomerulus), diabetes, cirrhosis, hypothyroidism, pregnancy, stress. To be withdrawn gradually.
Possible interaction: NSAIDs, oral anticoagulants, phenytoin, ephedrine, phenobarbitone, rifampicin, diuretics, cardiac glycosides, anticholinesterases, hypoglycaemics.
Side effects: osteoporosis, depression, euphoria, hyperglycaemia, peptic ulcers, Cushingoid changes.
Manufacturer: Stafford-Miller.

TARGOCID

Description: a glycopeptide and antibiotic, teicoplanin, available as powder in vials (200 and 400mg).
Used for: serious Gram-positive infections or staphylococcal infections where there is no response or a sensitivity to penicillins or cephalosporins.
Dosage: 400mg intravenously on first day, then 200mg per day. For severe infections, 400mg intravenously every 12 hours for 3 doses then 400mg daily. Over 85kg, 3–6mg/kg but see literature. If kidney disease, reduce dose from day 4. Children, up to 2 months, 16mg/kg on first day, then 8mg/kg per day; over 2 months, 10mg/kg every 12 hours for 3 doses then 6mg/kg per day. For severe infections 10mg/kg every 12 hours for 3 doses then same dose daily.
Special care: check blood, liver and kidneys regularly.
Avoid use: pregnancy, lactation.
Side effects: thrombophlebitis, rash, fever, reaction at site of injection, bronchospasm, nausea, vomiting, dizziness, diarrhoea, blood changes.
Manufacturer: Merrell Dow.

TARIVID

Description: a 4-quinolone antibiotic, ofloxacin, available as white, oblong tablets (200mg) and yellow, oblong tablets (400mg).
Used for: infections of the urinary tract, respiratory tract. Sexually transmitted diseases.
Dosage: 200–400mg per day depending upon the infection and its severity. Doses over 400mg to be given as 2 divided doses. Not for children.
Also, **TARIVID INFUSION**, 2mg/ml ofloxacin hydrochloride.
Used for: infections of the respiratory tract, upper and lower urinary tract, septicaemia.
Dosage: 200–800mg per day for 7 to 10 days, varying according to infection and its severity. Not for children.
Special care: kidney damage, psychiatric disorders, exposure to UV light or strong sunlight, when driving or operating machinery.
Avoid use: pregnancy, breastfeeding, history of epilepsy, growing adolescents.
Possible interaction: NSAIDs, anticoagulants, iron, antacids with aluminium or magnesium. Hypotensives, barbiturate anaesthetics (for injection).
Side effects: skin reactions, convulsions, disturbances to CNS, gastro-intestinal upset, hypersensitivity reactions, colitis. For injection—thrombophlebitis, pain at the site of injection, hypotension.
Manufacturer: Hoechst.

TAXOL

Description: a taxane, paclitaxel, available as a solution (6mg/ml) in vials.
Used for: ovarian cancer (metastatic) resistant to treatment with platinum.
Dosage: 175mg/m^2 by intravenous infusion over 3 hours, repeated 3-weekly. Additional, preliminary treatment necessary with antihistamines, H$_2$-antagonists and corticosteroids.
Special care: abnormalities in heart conduction, disease of peripheral nerves, liver or kidney failure. Check blood. Have resuscitation equipment available.
Avoid use: if neutrophils are low, pregnancy, lactation, severe liver damage.
Side effects: peripheral nerve disease, suppression of bone marrow, joint and muscle pain, hair loss, hypotension, gastro-intestinal upset, bradycardia, oedema.
Manufacturer: BMS.

TAZOCIN

Description: a ß-lactamase inhibitor (active against ß-lactamase-producing bacteria) and broad spectrum penicillin comprising piperacillin (2g) with tazobactam (250mg) both as sodium salts also as 4g/500mg both as powder in vials.
Used for: infections of the lower respiratory tract, urinary tract, of the skin, abdominal. Septicaemia and infections caused by more than 1 organism.
Dosage: 4.5g every 8 hours by slow intravenous infusion or injection. Not for children.
Special care: pregnancy, breastfeeding, kidney failure, low potassium levels.
Possible interaction: drugs that affect blood coagulation or platelet function, probenecid.
Side effects: allergic reactions, superinfection, gastro-intestinal upset, skin reactions.
Manufacturer: Lederle.

TEGRETOL

Description: an iminostilbene and diben-zazepine, carbamazepine, available as white tablets (100 and 200mg) marked with name and strength, and white oblong tablets (400mg) marked with name and strength. Also, **TEGRETOL CHEWTABS**, 100 and 200mg as square, pale orange chewable tablets marked T, tablet strength and name. **TEGRETOL RETARD**, 200mg in continuous-release, orange, oblong tablets marked CG and HC and 400mg tablets coloured brown and marked CG and ENE. Also, **TEGRETOL LIQUID**, a sugar-free liquid containing 100mg/5ml.
Used for: prevention of manic depressive psychosis which does not respond to therapy with lithium, epilepsy, trigeminal neuralgia.
Dosage: manic depression—start with 400mg per day in divided doses and increase until the symptoms are controlled (to a maximum of 1.6g per day), usually 400–600mg. Epilepsy, start with 100–200mg once or twice per day increasing to 800mg–1.2g and a maximum of 1.6g. Children, 10 to 15 years, 600mg–1g; 5 to 10 years, 400–600mg; 1 to 5 years, 200–400mg; up to 1 year, 100–200mg. All per day, in divided doses. Neuralgia, start with 100mg once or twice per day increasing to gain control, usually 600–800mg per day in divided doses (daily maximum 1.6g).
Special care: pregnancy, breastfeeding, liver and kidney disease, elderly, severe cardiovascular disease. Check blood and liver function.
Avoid use: abnormalities in atrioventricular conduction (heart conduction block).
Possible interaction: MAOIs, combined oral contraceptives, oral anticoagulants, steroids, lithium, phenytoin, cimetidine, dextropropoxyphene, doxycycline, isoniazid, erythromycin, diltiazem, verapamil, viloxazine.
Side effects: double vision, dry mouth, dizziness, drowsiness, gastric upset, oedema, rashes, blood changes, hair loss, toxic epidermal necrolysis (a rare skin disease producing exfoliation), kidney failure, hepatitis, enlargement of lymph nodes, changes in heart conduction, jaundice.
Manufacturer: Geigy.

TEMAZEPAM

Description: an intermediate benzodiazepine and hypnotic, temazepam, available as a solution (10mg/5ml). Also, **TEMAZEPAM TABLETS** (10 and 20mg) and **TEMAZEPAM GEL FILLED**, 10, 15, 20 and 30mg gel-filled capsules.
Used for: insomnia.
Dosage: 10–30mg at bedtime (elderly, 5–15mg). For severe cases, up to 60mg maximum. Not for children.
Special care: chronic liver or kidney disease, chronic lung disease, pregnancy, labour, lactation, elderly. May impair judgement. Withdraw gradually and avoid prolonged use.
Avoid use: depression of respiration, acute lung disease; psychotic, phobic or obsessional states.
Possible interaction: anticonvulsants, depressants of the CNS, alcohol.
Side effects: ataxia, confusion, lightheadedness, drowsiness, hypotension, gastro-intestinal upsets, disturbances in vision and libido, skin rashes, retention of urine, vertigo. Sometimes jaundice or blood disorders.
Manufacturer: non-proprietary.

TEMGESIC^{CD}

Description: an opiate and analgesic, buprenorphine hydrochloride, available as white, sublingual tablets (200 and 400µg) marked with 2 or 4 and symbol.
Used for: moderate to severe pain.
Dosage: 200–400µg sublingually every 6 to 8 hours or as required. Children, not for under 16kg; 16–25kg, 100µg; 25–37.5kg, 100–200µg; 37.5–50kg, 200–300µg, taken sublingually every 6 to 8 hours. Also, **TEMGESIC INJECTION** (300µg/ml in ampoules).
Dosage: 300–600µg every 6 to 8 hours, by intramuscular or slow, intravenous injection. Children, not for under 6 months; over 6 months, 3–6µg/kg every 6 to 8 hours to a maximum of 9µg/kg.
Special care: pregnancy, labour, reduced breathing or liver functions, dependence on narcotics or large doses previously.
Possible interaction: depressants of the CNS, MAOIs.
Side effects: nausea, dizziness, drowsiness, sweating.
Manufacturer: Reckitt & Colman.

TEMOPEN

Description: a penicillin, temocillin (as sodium) that is resistant to penicillinase, available as powder (1g) in vials.
Used for: septicaemia, infections of the urinary and lower respiratory tracts caused by Gram-negative bacilli which are susceptible to temocillin.
Dosage: 1–2g every 12 hours intramuscularly or intravenously. For urinary tract infection, 1g per day. Contact manufacturer re dosage for children.
Special care: pregnancy, breastfeeding, kidney disease.
Side effects: pain at the point of injection, diarrhoea. Discontinue if rash occurs.
Manufacturer: Bencard.

TENIF

Description: a cardioselective ß-blocker and class II calcium antagonist, atenolol (50mg) with nifedipine (20mg) available in red-brown capsules marked with TENIF and logo.
Used for: angina, hypotension.
Dosage: 1 capsule twice per day (angina); 1 per day increasing to 2 per day if necessary (elderly, 1) for hypertension. Not for children.
Special care: anaesthesia, diabetes, liver or kidney disease, weak heart or heart conduction defect.
Avoid use: heart failure, heart block, cardiagenic shock, pregnancy, breastfeeding.
Possible interaction: heart depressants, quinidine, cimetidine.
Side effects: oedema, headache, dizziness, flushes, rash, dry eyes, jaundice, hyperplasia of the gums.
Manufacturer: Stuart.

TENORET 50

Description: a cardioselective ß-blocker and thiazide diuretic comprising 50mg atenolol and 12.5mg chlorthalidone in brown tablets marked TENORET 50 and logo.

Used for: hypertension, especially in the elderly.

Dosage: 1 tablet per day. Not for children.

Special care: history of bronchospasm and certain ß-blockers, diabetes, liver or kidney disease, pregnancy, lactation, general anaesthesia, gout, check electrolyte levels, K⁺ supplements may be required depending on the case. Withdraw gradually. Not for children.

Avoid use: heart block or failure, slow heart rate (bradycardia), sick sinus syndrome (associated with sinus node disorder), certain ß-blockers, severe peripheral arterial disease, pregnancy, lactation, severe kidney failure, anuria, hepatic cornea.

Possible interaction: verapamil, hypoglycaemics, reserpine, clonidine withdrawal, some antiarrhythmics and anaesthetics, antihypertensives, depressants of the CNS, cimetidine, indomethacin, sympathomimetics, lithium, potassium supplements with potassium-sparing diuretics, digitalis.

Side effects: bradycardia, cold hands and feet, disturbance to sleep, heart failure, gastro-intestinal upset, tiredness on exertion, bronchospasm, gout, weakness, blood disorders, sensitivity to light.

Manufacturer: Stuart.

TENORETIC

Description: a cardioselective ß-blocker and thiazide diuretic containing 100mg atenolol, 25mg chlorthalidone in brown tablets marked with logo and TENORETIC.

Used for: hypertension.

Dosage: 1 tablet per day. Not for children.

Special care: history of bronchospasm and certain ß-blockers, diabetes, liver or kidney disease, pregnancy, lactation, general anaesthesia, gout, check

electrolyte levels, K⁺ supplements may be required depending on the case. Withdraw gradually. Not for children.

Avoid use: heart block or failure, slow heart rate (bradycardia), sick sinus syndrome (associated with sinus node disorder), certain ß-blockers, severe peripheral arterial disease, pregnancy, lactation, severe kidney failure, anuria, hepatic cornea.

Possible interaction: verapamil, hypoglycaemics, reserpine, clonidine withdrawal, some antiarrhythmics and anaesthetics, antihypertensives, depressants of the CNS, cimetidine, indomethacin, sympathomimetics, lithium, potassium supplements with potassium-sparing diuretics, digitalis.

Side effects: bradycardia, cold hands and feet, disturbance to sleep, heart failure, gastro-intestinal upset, tiredness on exertion, bronchospasm, gout, weakness, blood disorders, sensitivity to light.

Manufacturer: Stuart.

TENORMIN

Description: a cardioselective ß-blocker, atenolol, available in white tablets (25mg, marked with TENORMIN, 25 and logo) and orange tablets (100mg, marked with TENORMIN and logo). Also, **TENORMIN LS**, 50mg orange tablets marked 9 with name and **TENORMIN SYRUP**, a lemon-lime sugar-free syrup containing 25mg/ml. Also available as **TENORMIN INJEC-TION** (0.5mg/ml in 10ml ampoule).

Used for: cardiac arrhythmias, early treatment of acute myocardial infarction, angina, hypertension.

Dosage: 50–100mg per day, reduced for the elderly or where there is kidney disorder. Not for children.

Special care: history of bronchospasm and certain ß-blockers, diabetes, liver or kidney disease, pregnancy, lactation, general anaesthesia. Withdraw gradually. Not for children.

Avoid use: heart block or failure, slow heart rate (bradycardia), sick sinus syndrome (associated with sinus node disorder), certain ß-blockers, severe peripheral arterial disease.

Possible interaction: verapamil, hypoglycaemics, reserpine, clonidine withdrawal, some antiarrhythmics and anaesthetics, antihypertensives, depressants of the CNS, cimetidine, indomethacin, sympathomimetics.

Side effects: bradycardia, cold hands and feet, disturbance to sleep, heart failure, gastro-intestinal upset, tiredness on exertion, bronchospasm.

Manufacturer: Stuart.

TENUATE DOSPAN^{CD}

Description: a CNS stimulant, diethylpropion hydrochloride, available as sustained-release, white, oblong tablets marked MERRELL.

Used for: obesity.

Dosage: 1 tablet mid-morning. Not for children.

Special care: angina, peptic ulcer, hypertension, arrhythmias.

Avoid use: severe hypertension, arteriosclerosis, hyperthyroidism, glaucoma, pregnancy, breastfeeding, past drug or alcohol abuse or psychiatric illness.

Possible interaction: other anoretics, antihypertensives, antidiabetics, guanethidine, methyldopas, MAOIs, sympathomimetics, psychotropics.

Side effects: dependence, tolerance, psychoses, agitation, sleeplessness. Do not use over long period.

Manufacturer: Merrell Dow.

TEOPTIC

Description: a ß-blocker, carteolol hydrochloride, available as 1% and 2% drops.

Used for: hypertension in the eye, certain glaucomas.

Dosage: start with 1 drop of 1% solution in affected eye twice per day. Use 2% solution if 1% is ineffective. Not for children.

Special care: heart block, cardiogenic shock, diabetes.

Avoid use: heart failure, asthma, serious lung disease, pregnancy, soft or gas-permeable contact lenses.

Possible interaction: other ß-blockers.

Side effects: blurred vision, burning sensation, pain, irritation of the eye, hyperaemia (greater than normal amount of blood in the vessels).

Manufacturer: Ciba Vision.

TERRA-CORTRIL

Description: an antibiotic 0.5% oxytetracycline hydrochloride, with a mild steroid, 0.17% hydrocortisone, in a spray.

Used for: infected eczema, infected intertrigo (dermatitis of skin surfaces in contact), insect bites.

Dosage: spray 2 to 4 times per day. Not for children.

Also **TERRA-CORTRIL OINTMENT**, 3% oxytetracycline hydrochloride with 1% hydrocortisone.

Dosage: use 2 to 4 times per day. Not for children.

Also, **TERRA-CORTRIL NYSTATIN**, as for the ointment but with 100,000 units nystatin (an antifungal).

Used for: infected skin conditions.

Dosage: apply 2 to 4 times per day. Not for children.

Special care: thrombophlebitis, psychoses, recent intestinal anastomoses, chronic nephritis, certain cancers, osteoporosis, peptic ulcer, skin eruption/rash related to a disease, viral, fungal or active infections, tuberculosis. Hypertension, glaucoma, epilepsy, acute glomerulonephritis (inflammation of kidney glomerulus), diabetes, cirrhosis, hypothyroidism, pregnancy, stress. To be withdrawn gradually.

Possible interaction: NSAIDs, oral anticoagulants, phenytoin, ephedrine, phenobarbitone, rifampicin, diuretics, cardiac glycosides, anticholinesterases, hypoglycaemics.

Side effects: osteoporosis, depression, euphoria, hyperglycaemia, peptic ulcers, Cushingoid changes.

Also, an antibiotic/corticosteroid combination with 5mg oxytetracycline hydrochloride, 15mg hydrocortisone

acetate and 10,000 units/ml polymyxin in B sulphate, in drop form.
Used for: external ear infections.
Dosage: 2 to 4 drops 3 times per day for up to 7 days. Not for children.
Avoid use: pregnancy, perforated ear drum, infections of a viral, fungal or tuberculous nature or those containing pus.
Side effects: superinfection, allergy.
Manufacturer: Pfizer.

TERRAMYCIN

Description: a tetracycline, oxytetracycline, available as yellow tablets (250mg) marked Pfizer. Also, **TERRAMYCIN CAPSULES**, 250mg in yellow capsules marked TER 250 and Pfizer.
Used for: infections sensitive to Terramycin; severe acne.
Dosage: 250–500mg 4 times per day. Not for children.
Special care: liver or kidney disease.
Avoid use: pregnancy, breastfeeding.
Possible interaction: antacids, mineral supplements, milk, oral contraceptives.
Side effects: superinfections, allergic reactions, gastro-intestinal upsets.
Manufacturer: Pfizer.

TERTROXIN

Description: a thyroid hormone, liothyronine sodium (20µg), in white tablets marked with EVANS and name.
Used for: severe thyroid deficiency, myxoedema coma.
Dosage: start with 10–20µg 8-hourly increasing after 7 days if required to 60µg per day in divided doses. For elderly and children, start with 5µg per day in divided doses.
Special care: diabetes, breastfeeding.
Avoid use: angina caused by effort, cardiovascular problems.
Possible interaction: phenytoin, anticoagulants, tricyclics, cholestyramine.
Side effects: tachycardia, arrhythmias, muscle cramps or weakness, anginal pain, flushes, headache, sweating, diarrhoea, weight loss, excitability.
Manufacturer: Link.

TETAVAX

Description: a purified tetanus toxoid vaccine containing 40 units/0.5ml on aluminium hydroxide in syringes, ampoules and vials.
Used for: immunisation and booster doses.
Dosage: first immunisation: 0.5ml, then 0.5ml after 1 month and 0.5ml after 1 more month. Reinforcing (booster) doses: 0.5ml 10 years after first immunisation. When required after injuries, 0.5ml single dose unless a booster has been administered in previous 12 months. All given by deep subcutaneous or intramuscular injection.
Special care: hypersensitivity may occur if a dose is given within 12 months of a booster.
Avoid use: acute infectious disease unless in a wound susceptible to tetanus.
Side effects: malaise, fever.
Manufacturer: Merieux.

TETRABID

Description: 250mg tetracycline hydrochloride in purple/yellow sustained-release capsules.
Used for: acne, infections sensitive to this drug such as bronchitis.
Dosage: 1 capsule per day for at least 3 months (acne). For infections, start with 2 capsules then 1 every 12 hours. Not for children.
Special care: liver or kidney disorder.
Avoid use: pregnancy, breastfeeding.
Possible interaction: antacids, mineral supplements, milk, digoxin, oral anticoagulants, oral contraceptives.
Side effects: superinfections, allergic reactions, gastro-intestinal upset. Cease use if there is intracranial hypertension.
Manufacturer: Organon.

TETRALYSAL

Description: a tetracycline, lymecycline (408mg), in white capsules marked Farmitalia.
Used for: acne; infections of the skin and

soft tissue; ear, nose and throat or the respiratory tract.
Dosage: 1 twice per day (for at least 8 weeks in the case of acne). Not for children.
Special care: liver and kidney disorders.
Avoid use: pregnancy, breastfeeding.
Possible interaction: mineral supplements, antacids, oral contraceptives.
Side effects: superinfections, allergic reactions, gastro-intestinal upset.
Manufacturer: Farmitalia.

TICAR

Description: a penicillin, ticarcillin sodium, available as a 5g infusion bottle and powder in vials.
Used for: septicaemia, peritonitis, infections of the urinary or respiratory tract, infected wounds, endocarditis and post-operative infections especially those caused by *Pseudomonas aeruginosa*.
Dosage: up to 20g by slow intravenous injection or rapid infusion (children 300mg/kg) or up to 4g per day intramuscularly and in divided doses (children 100mg/kg).
Special care: kidney disease.
Side effects: gastro-intestinal upset, hypersensitivity reactions.
Manufacturer: Link.

TILADE MINT SYNCRONER

Description: an anti-inflammatory and non-steroid, nedocromil sodium, available as a mint-flavoured suspension delivered by aerosol with spacer device (2mg). Also, **TILADE MINT**, utilising a metered dose aerosol
Used for: bronchial asthma where anti-inflammatory control is required.
Dosage: start with 2 puffs 4 times per day (2 puffs twice per day for maintenance). Not for children.
Special care: pregnancy.
Side effects: cough, passing headache, gastro-intestinal upset.
Manufacturer: Fisons.

TILDIEM

Description: a class III calcium antagonist, diltiazem hydrochloride, available as off-white tablets (60mg) marked TILDIEM 60.
Used for: angina.
Dosage: 60mg 3 times per day to a maximum of 480mg per day in divided doses. Not for children.
Also, **TILDIEM RETARD**, white, sustained-release tablets (90 and 120mg).
Dosage: start with 90mg or 120mg twice per day increasing if required to a maximum of 2 120mg tablets twice per day. Elderly; 60mg twice per day, increasing to 90 or 120mg. Not for children.
Also, **TILDIEM LA**, white/yellow, sustained-release capsules containing 300mg.
Used for: hypertension.
Dosage: 1 at the same time every day. For the elderly, start with Retard 120mg each day. Using Retard–120mg twice per day increasing if required to 180mg twice daily. Elderly, 120mg daily to a maximum of 120mg twice per day. Not for children.
Special care: check heart rate in elderly or cases of liver and kidney disorder. Monitor patients with mild bradycardia.
Avoid use: pregnancy, bradycadia, heart block, sick sinus syndrome.
Possible interaction: other antihypertensives, ß-blockers, heart depressants, digoxin, dantrolene infusion, cyclosporin, diazepam, lithium cimetidine, theophylline, carbamazepine.
Manufacturer: Lorex.

TIMECEF

Description: a cephalosporin antibiotic, cefodizime (as sodium salt) available in vials (1g).
Used for: infections of the urinary and lower respiratory tracts.
Dosage: 1g twice per day (respiratory tract), 2g per day as 1 or divided doses (urinary tract) by intravenous injection, infusion or intramuscular injection. Not for children.

Special care: sensitivity to penicillin, severe kidney disorder, pregnancy, breastfeeding, colitis.
Possible interaction: aminoglycosides, loop diuretics.
Side effects: gastro-intestinal upset, passing rise in liver enzymes, hypersensitivity reactions, eosinophilia (increase of eosinophils, a type of white blood cell, in the blood).
Manufacturer: Roussel.

TIMENTIN

Description: a ß-lactamase inhibitor with penicillin, comprising clavulanic acid (as potassium salt) with ticarcillin (as sodium salt) available as powder in vials (1.6 or 3.2g containing 100mg/1.5g and 200mg/3g).
Used for: severe infections in patients in hospital with poor host defence to infection.
Dosage: 3.2g every 6 to 8 hours by intermittent intravenous infusion to a maximum frequency of 4-hourly. Children up to 1 month, 80mg/kg every 12 hours, increasing to 8-hourly; others 80mg/kg every 6 to 8 hours.
Special care: kidney disorder, severe liver disorder.
Side effects: gastro-intestinal upset, hypersensitivity reactions, hepatitis.
Manufacturer: Beecham.

TIMODINE

Description: a combined antifungal, mild steroid and disinfectant comprising 100,000 units/g nystatin, 0.5% hydrocortisone, 0.2% benzalkonium chloride solution with 10% dimethicone.
Used for: skin disorders, severe nappy rash infected with *Candida*.
Dosage: apply sparingly 3 times per day or at nappy change.
Special care: thrombophlebitis, psychoses, recent intestinal anastomoses, chronic nephritis, certain cancers, osteoporosis, peptic ulcer, skin eruption/ rash related to a disease, viral, fungal or active infections, tuberculosis.

Hypertension, glaucoma, epilepsy, acute glomerulonephritis (inflammation of kidney glomerulus), diabetes, cirrhosis, hypothyroidism, pregnancy, stress. To be withdrawn gradually.
Possible interaction: NSAIDs, oral anticoagulants, phenytoin, ephedrine, phenobarbitone, rifampicin, diuretics, cardiac glycosides, anticholinesterases, hypoglycaemics.
Side effects: osteoporosis, depression, euphoria, hyperglycaemia, peptic ulcers, Cushingoid changes.
Manufacturer: Reckitt & Colman.

TIMOPTIL

Description: a ß-blocker, timolol maleate, available as metered dose drops (0.25% and 0.5%).
Used for: ocular hypertension, certain glaucomas.
Dosage: 1 drop of 0.25% solution twice per day increasing to 0.5% solution if required. Not for children.
Special care: pregnancy, breastfeeding, withdraw gradually.
Avoid use: heart failure, heart block, asthma, sinus bradycardia, past obstructive lung disease, soft lenses.
Possible interaction: adrenaline, antihypertensives, verapamil.
Side effects: irritation, systemic ß-blocker effects (e.g. cold hands and feet, tiredness, stomach upset, rash).
Manufacturer: M.S.D.

TINSET

Description: an antihistamine and mast cell stabiliser, oxatomide, available as white tablets (30mg) marked JANSSEN and Ox over 30.
Used for: allergic rhinitis, urticaria, other allergic conditions.
Dosage: 1 to 2 tablets twice per day; children over 5 up to 1 tablet twice per day. Not for children under 5.
Possible interaction: depressants of the CNS, alcohol.
Side effects: drowsiness, slowed reactions.
Manufacturer: Janssen.

TOBRALEX

Description: an aminoglycoside, tobramycin, available as 0.3% drops.
Used for: bacterial infections of the eye.
Dosage: 1 or 2 drops every 4 hours, up to 2 drops every hour for severe cases. Reduce dose before ceasing treatment.
Side effects: passing irritation.
Manufacturer: Alcon.

TOFRANIL

Description: a TCAD, imipramine hydrochloride, available as red-brown triangular (10mg) and round (25mg) tablets, both marked GEIGY.
Also, **TOFRANIL SYRUP** (25mg/5ml).
Used for: depression; bed-wetting in children.
Dosage: 25mg 3 times per day, up to 150–200mg per day after 7 days. Maintenance dose, 50–100mg per day. Elderly, 10mg per day increasing to 30–50mg. Children: over 11 years, 10–15ml; 8 to 11 years, 5–10ml; 6 to 7 years, 5ml; at bedtime for 3 months maximum (withdraw gradually). Not for children under 6 years.
Special care: liver disorders, hyperthyroidism, glaucoma, lactation, epilepsy, diabetes, adrenal tumour, heart disease, urine retention. Psychotic or suicidal patients.
Avoid use: heart block, heart attacks, severe liver disease, pregnancy.
Possible interaction: MAOIs (or within 14 days of their use), alcohol, antidepressants, barbiturates, anticholinergics, local anaesthetics that contain adrenaline or noradrenaline, oestrogens, cimetidine, antihypertensives.
Side effects: constipation, urine retention, dry mouth, blurred vision, palpitations, tachycardia, nervousness, drowsiness, insomnia. Changes in weight, blood and blood sugar, jaundice, skin reactions, weakness, ataxia, hypotension, sweating, altered libido, gynaecomastia, galactorrhoea.
Manufacturer: Geigy.

TOLANASE

Description: a sulphonylurea, tolazamide, available as white tablets marked UPJOHN 70 (100mg) or UPJOHN 114 (250mg).
Used for: maturity-onset diabetes.
Dosage: 100–250mg per day to a maximum of 1g if necessary (in divided doses). Not for children.
Special care: elderly, kidney failure.
Avoid use: during pregnancy or lactation; juvenile, growth-onset or unstable brittle diabetes (insulin-dependent diabetes mellitus); ketoacidosis; severe kidney or liver disorders; stress, infections or surgery; endocrine disorders.
Possible interaction: MAOIs, corticosteroids, ß-blockers, diuretics, corticotrophin (ACTH), oral contraceptives, alcohol. Also aspirin, oral anticoagulants, and the generic drugs bezafibrate, clofibrate, phenylbutazone, cyclophosphamide, rifampicin, sulphonamides and chloramphenicol. Also glucagon.
Side effects: skin rash and other sensitivity reactions. Other conditions tend to be rare, e.g. hyponatraemia (low blood sodium concentration) or aplastic anaemia.
Manufacturer: Upjohn.

TOLECTIN

Description: a derivative of acetic acid, tolmetin (as sodium salt), available as orange/ivory capsules marked T200 (200mg) or orange capsules marked T400 (400mg).
Used for: osteoarthritis, rheumatoid arthritis, ankylosing spondylitis, juvenile rheumatoid arthritis, joint disorders.
Dosage: 600–1800mg per day in 2 to 4 divided doses. Children, 20–25mg/kg per day in 3 or 4 divided doses.
Special care: liver or kidney disease (check on long-term treatment), heart failure, past gastro-intestinal disease, pregnancy, breastfeeding, elderly.
Avoid use: allergy to aspirin or anti-inflammatory drugs, active peptic ulcer.
Side effects: oedema, rash, epigastric pain.
Manufacturer: Cilag.

TOLERZIDE

Description: a non-cardioselective ß-blocker and thiazide diuretic comprising 80mg sotalol hydrochloride and 12.5mg hydrochlorothiazide in a lilac tablet marked TOLERZIDE.
Used for: hypertension.
Dosage: 1 tablet per day. Not for children.
Special care: history of bronchospasm and certain ß-blockers, diabetes, liver or kidney disease, pregnancy, lactation, general anaesthesia, gout, check electrolyte levels, K⁺ supplements may be required depending on the case. Withdraw gradually.
Avoid use: heart block or failure, slow heart rate (bradycardia), sick sinus syndrome (associated with sinus node disorder), certain ß-blockers, severe peripheral arterial disease, pregnancy, lactation, severe kidney failure, anuria, hepatic cornea.
Possible interaction: verapamil, hypoglycaemics, reserpine, clonidine withdrawal, some antiarrhythmics and anaesthetics, antihypertensives, depressants of the CNS, cimetidine, indomethacin, sympathomimetics, lithium, potassium supplements with potassium-sparing diuretics, digitalis.
Side effects: bradycardia, cold hands and feet, disturbance to sleep, heart failure, gastro-intestinal upset, tiredness on exertion, bronchospasm, gout, weakness, blood disorders, sensitivity to light.
Manufacturer: Bristol-Myers.

TONOCARD

Description: a class I antiarrhythmic, tocainide hydrochloride, available as yellow tablets marked A/TT (400mg).
Used for: life-threatening ventricular arrhythmias.
Dosage: 1.2g per day in 2 or 3 divided doses, to a maximum of 1.8–2.4g. Not for children.
Special care: severe liver or kidney disease, elderly, heart failure, pregnancy.

Avoid use: heart block in the absence of a pacemaker.
Possible interaction: other anti-arrhythmics.
Side effects: leucopenia, agranulocytosis, tremor, SLE, dizziness, gastro-intestinal upset.
Manufacturer: Astra.

TOPICYCLINE

Description: an antibiotic, tetracycline hydrochloride, available as a 0.22% solution.
Used for: acne.
Dosage: apply liberally twice per day until the skin is wet. Not for children.
Special care: kidney disease, pregnancy, breastfeeding. Avoid mouth, eyes and mucous membranes.
Side effects: stinging.
Manufacturer: P. & G.P.

TOPILAR

Description: a potent steroid, fluclorolone acetonide, available as a cream (0.025%). Also **TOPILAR OINTMENT** (0.025%).
Used for: skin disorders that respond to steroids, plaque psoriasis of soles and palms.
Dosage: apply 2 times per day.
Special care: thrombophlebitis, psychoses, recent intestinal anastomoses, chronic nephritis, certain cancers, osteoporosis, peptic ulcer, skin eruption/rash related to a disease, viral, fungal or active infections, tuberculosis. Hypertension, glaucoma, epilepsy, acute glomerulonephritis (inflammation of kidney glomerulus), diabetes, cirrhosis, hypothyroidism, pregnancy, stress. To be withdrawn gradually.
Possible interaction: NSAIDs, oral anticoagulants, phenytoin, ephedrine, phenobarbitone, rifampicin, diuretics, cardiac glycosides, anticholinesterases, hypoglycaemics.
Side effects: osteoporosis, depression, euphoria, hyperglycaemia, peptic ulcers, Cushingoid changes.
Manufacturer: Bioglan.

TORADOL

Description: an NSAID, ketorolac trometamol, available as solutions (10mg/ml and 30mg/ml) in ampoules.
Used for: short-term control of moderate or severe post-operative pain.
Dosage: start with 10mg intravenously or intramuscularly then 10–30mg 4 to 6 hourly. Maximum 90mg daily for 2 days. Elderly, maximum 60mg daily for 2 days. Not for children under 16. Also, TORADOL TABLETS, 10mg in white tablets marked TORADOL 10 and SYNTEX.
Dosage: 1 tablet 4 to 6 hourly, maximum 4 per day, for up to 7 days. If following injections, 90mg maximum dose on day 1 and 40mg thereafter. Elderly, 1 tablet 6 to 8-hourly for up to 7 days. Maximum dose after injections 60mg on day 1 and then 40mg. Not for children under 16.
Special care: elderly; heart, liver kidney or allergic disease, gastro-intestinal disease.
Avoid use: allergy to aspirin or anti-inflammatory drugs, pregnancy, breast-feeding, peptic ulcer, angioneurotic oedema, asthma, blood coagulation disorders, kidney disease, gastro-intestinal or cerebrovascular bleeding, low volume of circulating blood, dehydration, high risk of haemorrhage induced by surgery.
Possible interaction: NSAIDs, anticoagulants, lithium, methotrexate, probenecid, frusemide, oxypentifylline.
Side effects: ulcers, wound haemorrhage, gastro-intestinal upsets, drowsiness, oedema, kidney failure, bronchospasm, anaphylaxis, pain at site of injection, abnormal liver functions.
Manufacturer: Syntex.

TOTAMOL

Description: a cardioselective ß-blocker, atenolol, available as orange tablets (25, 50 and 100mg) each marked ATL, CP and with tablet strength.
Used for: cardiac arrhythmias, early treatment of acute myocardial infarction; angina; hypertension.

Dosage: 50–100mg per day, less for the elderly or where there is impaired kidney function. Not for children.
Special care: history of bronchospasm and certain ß-blockers, diabetes, liver or kidney disease, pregnancy, lactation, general anaesthesia. Withdraw gradually. Not for children.
Avoid use: heart block or failure, brady-cardia, sick sinus syndrome (associated with sinus node disorder), certain ß-blockers, severe peripheral arterial disease.
Possible interaction: verapamil, hypoglycaemics, reserpine, clonidine withdrawal, some antiarrhythmics and anaesthetics, antihypertensives, depressants of the CNS, cimetidine, indomethacin, sympathomimetics.
Side effects: bradycardia, cold hands and feet, disturbance to sleep, heart failure, gastro-intestinal upset, tiredness on exertion, bronchospasm.
Manufacturer: C.P. Pharm.

TRACRIUM

Description: a muscle relaxant, atracurium besylate, available in ampoules (10mg/ml).
Used for: surgery, long-term ventilation.
Dosage: start with 300–600µg/kg, then 100–200µg/kg as required, by intravenous injection; 5–10µg/kg/minute by intravenous infusion.
Special care: respiration should be assisted until drug is inactivated or antagonised.
Avoid use: myasthenia gravis.
Possible interaction: lithium, nifedipine, verapamil.
Manufacturer: Wellcome.

TRANCOPAL

Description: a muscle relaxant and tranquilliser, chlormezanone, available in yellow tablets (200mg) marked TR.
Used for: short-term treatment of insomnia, and anxiety where there is muscle tension; painful muscle spasms.
Dosage: 200mg up to 4 times per day or 1 400mg dose at night. Half doses for the elderly. Not for children.

Special care: liver or kidney disease, pregnancy. Judgement and dexterity may be impaired.
Avoid use: porphyria.
Possible interaction: alcohol, MAOIs, CNS depressants.
Side effects: headache, dry mouth, nausea, lethargy, dizziness, rashes, jaundice.
Manufacturer: Sanofi Winthrop.

TRANDATE

Description: an a/ß-blocker, labetolol hydrochloride, available as orange tablets (50, 100, 200 and 400mg) marked with name and strength.
Used for: angina, hypertension.
Dosage: start with 100mg twice per day with food, increasing at intervals of 14 days to a maximum of 2.4g per day in divided doses. Elderly start with 50mg twice per day. Not for children.
Also, TRANDATE INJECTION, ampoules containing 5mg/ml.
Special care: history of bronchospasm and certain ß-blockers, diabetes, liver or kidney disease, pregnancy, lactation, general anaesthesia. Withdraw gradually. Not for children.
Avoid use: heart block or failure, slow heart rate, sick sinus syndrome (associated with sinus node disorder), certain ß-blockers, severe peripheral arterial disease.
Possible interaction: verapamil, hypoglycaemics, reserpine, clonidine withdrawal, some antiarrhythmics and anaesthetics, antihypertensives, depressants of the CNS, cimetidine, indomethacin, sympathomimetics.
Side effects: bradycardia, cold hands and feet, disturbance to sleep, heart failure, gastro-intestinal upset, tiredness on exertion, bronchospasm. Withdraw if liver reaction (rare).
Manufacturer: D.F.

TRANXENE

Description: a long-acting benzodi-azepine, clorazepate potassium available in capsules containing 15mg (pink/grey) and 7.5mg (maroon/grey), marked with

TRANXENE, capsule strength and symbol.
Used for: anxiety whether or not depression is present.
Dosage: 7.5–22.5mg per day, elderly 7.5mg. Not for children under 16.
Special care: chronic liver or kidney disease, chronic lung disease, pregnancy, labour, lactation, elderly. May impair judgement. Withdraw gradually and avoid prolonged use.
Avoid use: depression of respiration, acute lung disease; psychotic, phobic or obsessional states.
Possible interaction: anticonvulsants, depressants of the CNS, alcohol.
Side effects: ataxia, confusion, light-headedness, drowsiness, hypotension, gastro-intestinal upsets, disturbances in vision and libido, skin rashes, retention of urine, vertigo. Sometimes jaundice or blood disorders.
Manufacturer: Boehringer Ingelheim.

TRASICOR

Description: a non-cardioselective ß-blocker, oxprenolol hydrochloride, available as tablets containing 20 or 40mg (white), 80mg (beige) and 160mg (orange) all marked with strength, CIBA and TRASICOR.
Used for: cardiac arrhythmias, angina, hypertension, anxiety.
Dosage: from 20–160mg 2 or 3 times per day, depending upon condition being treated. Maximum daily dose 480mg. Not for children.
Special care: history of bronchospasm and certain ß-blockers, diabetes, liver or kidney disease, pregnancy, lactation, general anaesthesia. Withdraw gradually. Not for children.
Avoid use: heart block or failure, bradycardia, sick sinus syndrome (associated with sinus node disorder), certain ß-blockers, severe peripheral arterial disease.
Possible interaction: verapamil, hypoglycaemics, reserpine, clonidine withdrawal, some antiarrhythmics and

anaesthetics, antihypertensives, depressants of the CNS, cimetidine, indomethacin, sympathomimetics.
Side effects: bradycardia, cold hands and feet, disturbance to sleep, heart failure, gastro-intestinal upset, tiredness on exertion, bronchospasm.
Manufacturer: Ciba.

TRASIDREX

Description: a non-cardioselective ß-blocker and thiazide, comprising 160mg oxprenolol hydrochloride in a sustained-release core and 0.25mg cyclopenthiazide in a red outer coat. The tablet is marked with Ciba and TRASIDREX.
Used for: hypertension.
Dosage: start with 1 tablet each morning increasing to 3 per day if required. Not for children.
Special care: history of bronchospasm and certain ß-blockers, diabetes, liver or kidney disease, pregnancy, lactation, general anaesthesia, gout, check electrolyte levels, K⁺ supplements may be required depending on the case. Withdraw gradually. Not for children.
Avoid use: heart block or failure, bradycardia, sick sinus syndrome (associated with sinus node disorder), certain ß-blockers, severe peripheral arterial disease, pregnancy, lactation, severe kidney failure, anuria, hepatic cornea.
Possible interaction: verapamil, hypoglycaemics, reserpine, clonidine withdrawal, some antiarrhythmics and anaesthetics, antihypertensives, depressants of the CNS, cimetidine, indomethacin, sympathomimetics, lithium, potassium supplements with potassium-sparing diuretics, digitalis.
Side effects: bradycardia, cold hands and feet, disturbance to sleep, heart failure, gastro-intestinal upset, tiredness on exertion, bronchospasm, gout, weakness, blood disorders, sensitivity to light.
Manufacturer: Ciba.

TRASYLOL

Description: a haemostatic and antifibrinolytic, aprotinin, available as vials containing 500,000 units per 50ml.
Used for: where there is risk of major blood loss during open heart surgery, or where blood conservation is vital, haemorrhage.
Dosage: by slow intravenous injection or infusion, up to 2 or 3 million units.
Side effects: localized thrombophlebitis, sometimes hypersensitivity reactions.
Manufacturer: Bayer.

TRAVOGYN

Description: an antifungal drug, isoconazole nitrate, available as white, almond-shaped vaginal tablets (300mg) marked with CT in a hexagon.
Used for: vaginal infections from *Candida* or mixed fungal and Gram-positive bacteria.
Dosage: 2 tablets inserted in 1 dose. Not for children.
Side effects: passing irritation and burning sensation.
Manufacturer: Schering H.C.

TRAXAM

Description: an NSAID, felbinac, available as a 3% gel. Also, **TRAXAM FOAM** (3.17%).
Used for: strains, sprains and injury to soft tissue.
Dosage: 1g rubbed into the area 2 to 4 times per day initially for 14 days. Maximum daily usage 25g. Not for children.
Special care: pregnancy, breastfeeding.
Avoid use: allergy to aspirin or anti-inflammatory drugs.
Side effects: dermatitis, itching, erythema.
Manufacturer: Lederle.

TRENTAL

Description: a peripheral vasodilator and xanthine, oxpentifylline, available in pink, oblong, sustained-release tablets (400mg).
Used for: disorders of the peripheral vascular system.

Dosage: 400mg 2 or 3 times per day.
Not for children.
Special care: coronary artery disease,
hypotension, kidney disease.
Avoid use: porphyria.
Possible interaction: antihypertensives.
Side effects: flushes, vertigo, gastro-
intestinal upsets.
Manufacturer: Hoechst.

TRI-ADCORTYL

Description: a potent steroid with
antifungal and antibacterial comprising
0.1% triamcinolone acetate, 100,000
units/g nystatin, 0.25% neomycin
sulphate and 0.025% gramicidin, as
cream and ointment.
Used for: inflamed skin disorders with
infection.
Dosage: use 2 to 4 times per day.
Special care: thrombophlebitis,
psychoses, recent intestinal anastomoses,
chronic nephritis, certain cancers,
osteoporosis, peptic ulcer, skin eruption/
rash related to a disease, viral, fungal or
active infections, tuberculosis.
Hypertension, glaucoma, epilepsy, acute
glomerulonephritis (inflammation of
kidney glomerulus), diabetes, cirrhosis,
hypothyroidism, pregnancy, stress. To be
withdrawn gradually.
Possible interaction: NSAIDs, oral
anticoagulants, phenytoin, ephedrine,
phenobarbitone, rifampicin, diuretics,
cardiac glycosides, anticholinesterases,
hypoglycaemics.
Side effects: osteoporosis, depression,
euphoria, hyperglycaemia, peptic ulcers,
Cushingoid changes.
Manufacturer: Squibb.

TRI-ADCORTYL OTIC

Description: a combined preparation of
corticosteroid, antibiotic and antifungal
containing 0.1% triamcinolone acetonide,
0.25% neomycin sulphate, 0.025%
gramicidin and 100,000 units/g nystatin.
Used for: inflammation of the outer ear.
Dosage: use 2 to 4 times per day.
Special care: pregnancy, perforated ear

drum, do not use long-term in infants.
Avoid use: viral and tuberculous lesions.
Manufacturer: Squibb.

TRI-CICATRIN

Description: a topical corticosteroid
containing 1% hydrocortisone, 250
units/g bacitracin zinc, 3400 units/g
neomycin sulphate and 100,000 units/g
nystatin, as an ointment.
Used for: mild inflammatory skin
disorders.
Dosage: use 2 to 3 times per day, less
frequently upon improvement.
Special care: thrombophlebitis,
psychoses, recent intestinal anastomoses,
chronic nephritis, certain cancers,
osteoporosis, peptic ulcer, skin eruption/
rash related to a disease, viral, fungal or
active infections, tuberculosis.
Hypertension, glaucoma, epilepsy, acute
glomerulonephritis (inflammation of
kidney glomerulus), diabetes, cirrhosis,
hypothyroidism, pregnancy, stress. To be
withdrawn gradually.
Possible interaction: NSAIDs, oral
anticoagulants, phenytoin, ephedrine,
phenobarbitone, rifampicin, diuretics,
cardiac glycosides, anticholinesterases,
hypoglycaemics.
Side effects: osteoporosis, depression,
euphoria, hyperglycaemia, peptic ulcers,
Cushingoid changes
Manufacturer: Wellcome.

TRI-MINULET

Description: an oestrogen/progestogen
compound containing ethinyloestradiol
and gestodene in 6 beige tablets (30/50µg)
5 dark brown tablets (40/70µg) and 10
white tablets (30/100µg respectively).
Used for: oral contraception.
Dosage: 1 tablet daily for 21 days
starting on first day of menstruation,
then 7 days without tablets.
Special care: hypertension, Raynaud's
disease (reduced blood supply to an
organ of the body's extremities), asthma,
severe depression, diabetes, varicose
veins, multiple sclerosis, chronic kidney

disease, kidney dialysis. Blood pressure, breasts and pelvic organs to be checked regularly; smoking not advised.
Avoid use: history of heart disease, infectious hepatitis, sickle cell anaemia, porphyria, liver tumour, undiagnosed vaginal bleeding, pregnancy, hormone-dependent cancer, haemolytic uraemic syndrome (rare kidney disorder), chorea, otosclerosis.
Possible interaction: barbiturates, tetracyclines, griseofulvin, rifampicin, primidone, phenytoin, chloral hydrate, ethosuximide, carbamazepine, glutethimide, dichloralphenazone.
Side effects: fluid retention and bloating, leg cramps/pains, breast enlargement, depression, headaches, nausea, loss of libido, weight gain, vaginal discharge, cervical erosion (alteration of epithelial cells), chloasma (pigmentation of nose, cheeks or forehead), breakthrough bleeding (bleeding between periods).
Manufacturer: Wyeth.

TRIADENE

Description: an oestrogen/progestogen compound containing ethinyloestradiol and gestodene in 6 beige tablets (30/50µg) 5 dark brown tablets (40/70µg) and 10 white tablets (30/100µg respectively).
Used for: oral contraception.
Dosage: 1 tablet daily for 21 days starting on first day of menstruation, then 7 days without tablets.
Special care: hypertension, Raynaud's disease (reduced blood supply to an organ of the body's extremities), asthma, severe depression, diabetes, varicose veins, multiple sclerosis, chronic kidney disease, kidney dialysis. Blood pressure, breasts and pelvic organs to be checked regularly; smoking not advised.
Avoid use: history of heart disease, infectious hepatitis, sickle cell anaemia, porphyria, liver tumour, undiagnosed vaginal bleeding, pregnancy, hormone-dependent cancer, haemolytic uraemic syndrome (rare kidney disorder), chorea, otosclerosis.

Possible interaction: barbiturates, tetracyclines, griseofulvin, rifampicin, primidone, phenytoin, chloral hydrate, ethosuximide, carbamazepine, glutethimide, dichloralphenazone.
Side effects: fluid retention and bloating, leg cramps/pains, breast enlargement, depression, headaches, nausea, loss of libido, weight gain, vaginal discharge, cervical erosion (alteration of epithelial cells), chloasma (pigmentation of nose, cheeks or forehead), breakthrough bleeding (bleeding between periods).
Manufacturer: Schering H.C.

TRIAM-CO

Description: a potassium-sparing diuretic and thiazide, triamterene (50mg) and hydro-chlorothiazide (25mg) in peach tablets marked with logo and TTRIAM-CO.
Used for: oedema, hypertension.
Dosage: start with 1 per day for hypertension; 1 twice per day after meals for oedema, reducing to 1 daily or 2 on alternate days. Maximum 4 per day. Not for children.
Special care: diabetes, gout, pancreatitis, acidosis, liver or kidney disease, pregnancy, breastfeeding.
Avoid use: severe kidney failure, hyperkalaemia, hypercalcaemia, Addison's disease, diabetic ketoacidosis, liver disorder.
Possible interaction: potassium supplements, potassium-sparing diuretics, digitalis, lithium, NSAIDs, ACE inhibitors, antihypertensives.
Side effects: headache, cramps, weakness, diarrhoea, nausea, vomiting, dry mouth, rash, hypotension, hypercalcaemia, hyperglycaemia, SLE, reversible kidney failure.
Manufacturer: Baker Norton.

TRIBIOTIC

Description: an aminoglycoside and antibiotic in aerosol form containing 500,000 units neomycin sulphate, 10,000 units bacitracin zinc and 150,000 units/110g polymyxin B sulphate.
Used for: prevention and control of infection during surgery.

Dosage: apply 1 aerosol sparingly for a maximum of 7 days;
(children 1 second/kg/day).
Special care: pregnancy, breastfeeding, loss of hearing, large areas of damaged skin.
Avoid use: burns.
Possible interaction: other aminoglycoside antibiotics.
Side effects: sensitization, toxicity of the kidney or organs of hearing and balance.
Manufacturer: 3M Health Care.

TRIDIL

Description: an antiarrhythmic and anti-anginal, glyceryl nitrate available in ampoules containing 0.5mg/ml.
Used for: angina, arrhythmias.
Dosage: see literature.
Special care: hypotension, tolerance.
Avoid use: anaemia, cerebral haemorrhage, certain glaucomas, head trauma.
Possible interaction: anticoagulants.
Side effects: flushes, headache, dizziness, tachycardia, hypotension on standing.
Manufacturer: DuPont.

TRIMOPAN

Description: a folic acid inhibitor, trimethoprim, available in white tablets marked 2H7 (100mg) and 3H7 (200mg).
Used for: infections sensitive to trimethoprim, urinary tract infections.
Dosage: 200mg twice per day. Children should use the suspension.

Also, **TRIMOPAN SUSPENSION** containing 50mg/5ml
Dosage: children, 6 to 12 years, 10ml; 2 to 6 years, 5ml; 4 months to 2 years, 2.5ml; all twice per day. Not for infants under 4 months.
Special care: kidney disorder, folate deficiency, elderly, breastfeeding. Check blood during long-term treatment.
Avoid use: pregnancy, infants up to 1 month, severe kidney disease where blood levels cannot be monitored.
Side effects: folate deficiency, gastrointestinal and skin reactions.
Manufacturer: Berk.

TRIMOVATE

Description: a moderately potent steroid with antifungal and antibiotic comprising 0.05% clobetasone butyrate, 100,000 units/g nystatin, 3% oxytetracycline, as a cream.
Used for: skin disorders that respond to steroids, especially in moist or covered areas where there may be infection.
Dosage: use up to 4 times per day.
Special care: thrombophlebitis, psychoses, recent intestinal anastomoses, chronic nephritis, certain cancers, osteoporosis, peptic ulcer, skin eruption/rash related to a disease, viral, fungal or active infections, tuberculosis. Hypertension, glaucoma, epilepsy, acute glomerulonephritis (inflammation of kidney glomerulus), diabetes, cirrhosis, hypothyroidism, pregnancy, stress. To be withdrawn gradually.
Possible interaction: NSAIDs, oral anticoagulants, phenytoin, ephedrine, phenobarbitone, rifampicin, diuretics, cardiac glycosides, anticholinesterases, hypoglycaemics.
Side effects: osteoporosis, depression, euphoria, hyperglycaemia, peptic ulcers, Cushingoid changes.
Manufacturer: Glaxo.

TRINORDIOL

Description: an oestrogen/progestogen combined contraceptive containing ethinyloestradiol and levonorgestrel as 6 brown tablets (30/50μg respectively), 5 white tablets (40/75μg) and 10 ochre tablets (30/125μg).
Used for: oral contraception.
Dosage: 1 tablet for 21 days starting on the first day of menstruation, then 7 days without tablets.
Special care: hypertension, Raynaud's disease (reduced blood supply to an organ of the body's extremities), asthma, severe depression, diabetes, varicose veins, multiple sclerosis, chronic kidney disease, kidney dialysis. Blood pressure, breasts and pelvic organs to be checked regularly; smoking not advised.

Avoid use: history of heart disease, infectious hepatitis, sickle cell anaemia, porphyria, liver tumour, undiagnosed vaginal bleeding, pregnancy, hormone-dependent cancer, haemolytic uraemic syndrome (rare kidney disorder), chorea, otosclerosis.

Possible interaction: barbiturates, tetracyclines, griseofulvin, rifampicin, primidone, phenytoin, chloral hydrate, ethosuximide, carbamazepine, glutethimide, dichloralphenazone.

Side effects: fluid retention and bloating, leg cramps/pains, breast enlargement, depression, headaches, nausea, loss of libido, weight gain, vaginal discharge, cervical erosion (alteration of epithelial cells), chloasma (pigmentation of nose, cheeks or forehead), breakthrough bleeding (bleeding between periods).

Manufacturer: Wyeth.

TRINOVUM

Description: a combined oestrogen/progestogen contraceptive containing ethinyloestradiol and norethisterone as 7 white tablets marked C535 (35µg/0.5mg respectively), 7 light peach tablets marked C735 (35µg/0.75mg) and 7 peach tablets marked C135 (35µg/1mg).

Used for: oral contraception.

Dosage: 1 tablet per day for 21 days commencing on first day of menstruation then 7 days without tablets.

Also, **TRINOVUM ED**, as for Trinovum but with 7 light-green inert lactose tablets marked CC.

Dosage: starting on first day of menstruation, 1 tablet per day for 28 days with no break.

Special care: hypertension, Raynaud's disease (reduced blood supply to an organ of the body's extremities), asthma, severe depression, diabetes, varicose veins, multiple sclerosis, chronic kidney disease, kidney dialysis. Blood pressure, breasts and pelvic organs to be checked regularly; smoking not advised.

Avoid use: history of heart disease, infectious hepatitis, sickle cell anaemia,

porphyria, liver tumour, undiagnosed vaginal bleeding, pregnancy, hormone-dependent cancer, haemolytic uraemic syndrome (rare kidney disorder), chorea, otosclerosis.

Possible interaction: barbiturates, tetracyclines, griseofulvin, rifampicin, primidone, phenytoin, chloral hydrate, ethosuximide, carbamazepine, glutethimide, dichloralphenazone.

Side effects: fluid retention and bloating, leg cramps/pains, breast enlargement, depression, headaches, nausea, loss of libido, weight gain, vaginal discharge, cervical erosion (alteration of epithelial cells), chloasma (pigmentation of nose, cheeks or forehead), breakthrough bleeding (bleeding between periods).

Manufacturer: Ortho.

TRIPTAFEN

Description: an anti-depressant combining a TCAD and group III phenothiazine, as 25mg amitryptiline hydrochloride with 2mg perphenazine in pink tablets marked 1D. Also, **TRIPTAFEN-M**, containing 10mg amitriptyline hydrochloride and 2mg perphenazine in pink tablets marked 2D.

Used for: depression with anxiety.

Dosage: 1 tablet 3 times per day plus 1 at bedtime if needed. Assess after 3 months. Not for children.

Special care: pregnancy, breastfeeding, Parkinsonism, liver disorders, hyperthyroidism, epilepsy, diabetes, glaucoma, retention of urine, cardiovascular disease, psychotic patients.

Avoid use: cardiovascular disease, bone marrow depression, heart block, acute myocardial infarction, severe liver disease.

Possible interaction: antidepressants, anticonvulsants, alcohol, within 2 weeks of taking MAOIs, barbiturates, adrenaline, noradrenaline, antihypertensives, anticholinergics, oestrogens, cimetidine.

Side effects: sleepiness, vertigo, lightheadedness, unsteadiness, disturbance of vision, rash, hypotension, gastro-intestinal upset, changes in libido, retention of

urine. Allergic reactions, dry mouth, constipation, sweating, tachycardia, nervousness, heart arrhythmias. Impotence, effects on breasts, weight loss or gain.
Manufacturer: Forley.

TRISEQUENS

Description: an oestrogen/progestogen combination available as 12 blue tablets (marked 270) containing 2mg oestradiol and 1mg oestriol, 10 white tablets (marked 271) containing 2mg oestradiol, 1mg oestriol and 1mg norethisterone acetate and 6 red tablets (marked 272) containing 1mg oestradiol and 0.5mg oestriol.
Also, **TRISEQUENS FORTE**, with the same components as 12 yellow tablets marked 273 (4mg/2mg), 10 white tablets marked 274 (4mg/2mg/1mg) and 6 red tablets marked 272 (1mg/0.5mg).
Used for: symptoms of the menopause, prevention of post-menopausal osteoporosis.
Dosage: 1 tablet per day without a break, starting on fifth day of discharge with a blue tablet (or yellow if Forte).
Special care: patients considered to be at risk of thrombosis or with liver disease. Women with any of the following disorders should be carefully monitored: fibroids in the womb, multiple sclerosis, diabetes, tetany, porphyria, epilepsy, liver disease, hypertension, migraine, otosclerosis, gallstones. Breasts, pelvic organs and blood pressure should be checked at regular intervals during the course of treatment.
Avoid use: pregnancy, breastfeeding, conditions which might lead to thrombosis, thrombophlebitis, serious heart, kidney or liver disease, breast cancer, oestrogen-dependent cancers including those of reproductive system, endometriosis, vaginal bleeding which is undiagnosed.
Possible interaction: drugs which induce liver enzymes.
Side effects: tenderness and enlargement of breasts, weight gain, breakthrough bleeding, giddiness, vomiting and nausea, gastro-intestinal upset.
Treatment should be halted immediately if severe headaches occur, disturbance of vision, hypertension or any indications of thrombosis, jaundice. Also, in the event of pregnancy and 6 weeks before planned surgery.
Manufacturer: Novo Nordisk.

TRITACE

Description: an ACE inhibitor, ramipril, available as yellow/white (1.25mg), orange/white (2.5mg) and crimson/white (5mg) capsules.
Used for: hypertension.
Dosage: start with 1.25mg per day moving to maintenance dose of 2.5–5mg per day; maximum of 10mg per day. Any diuretic should be stopped 2 to 3 days before taking Tritace. Not for children.
Special care: start treatment in hospital for congestive heart failure or liver disease; haemodialysis, kidney disease (reduce dose and monitor during treatment).
Avoid use: pregnancy, breastfeeding, narrowing of the aorta, past angioneurotic oedema, outflow obstruction.
Possible interaction: lithium, potassium supplements, potassium-sparing diuretics, antihypertensives.
Side effects: headache, fatigue, nausea, vomiting, dizziness, abdominal pain, cough, diarrhoea, hypersensitivity reactions.
Manufacturer: Hoechst.

TRIVAX

Description: a vaccine containing the triple antigen for diphtheria, tetanus and whooping cough, available in ampoules.
Also **TRIVAX-AD** which is adsorbed on aluminium hydroxide.
Used for: active immunisation against these diseases.
Dosage: for children under 5, 3 doses of 0.5ml at 4 weekly intervals. Not for children over 5 or adults.
Avoid use: acute fever, past convulsions, cerebral irritation, neurological diseases.

Reaction to a preceding dose. Epilepsy in the family or history of severe allergies.
Side effects: fever, loss of appetite, irritability, crying.
Manufacturer: Evans.

TROBICIN

Description: an antibacterial compound similar to an aminoglycoside, spectinomycin, as powder (as dihydrochloride pentahydrate) in a vial (400mg/ml) with diluent.
Used for: gonorrhoea.
Dosage: 2g by deep intramuscular injection or 4g for severe cases. Children over 2, 40mg/kg.
Special care: pregnancy, liver or kidney disease.
Possible interaction: lithium.
Side effects: fever, urticaria, nausea, dizziness, lower urine output.
Manufacturer: Upjohn.

TROSYL

Description: an imidazole antifungal, tioconazole, available as a solution containing 280mg/ml.
Used for: nail infections caused by *Candida* and fungi.
Dosage: apply 12 hourly for 6 to 12 months.
Avoid use: pregnancy.
Side effects: nail irritation.
Manufacturer: Novex.

TRYPTIZOL

Description: a TCAD, amitriptyline hydro-chloride, available as blue tablets marked MSD 23 (10mg), yellow tablets marked MSD 45 (25mg) and brown tablets marked MSD 102 (50mg). Also, **TRYPTIZOL CAPSULES**, 75mg orange, sustained-release capsules (marked MSD 649) and **TRYPTIZOL SYRUP** 10mg amitriptyli-ne embonate/5ml.
Used for: depression (adults), bedwetting (children).
Dosage: 75mg up to 150mg per day, in divided doses and 50–100mg for maintenance usually as 1 bedtime dose.

Elderly, 50mg per day in divided doses or as 1 bedtime dose. Children; 11 to 16 years, 25–50mg per day; 6 to 10 years, 10–20mg per day. Not for children under 6. Also, **TRYPTIZOL INJECTION** as 10mg/ml.
Dosage: 10–20mg 4 times per day, intravenously or intramuscularly. Not for children.
Special care: liver disorders, hyperthy-roidism, glaucoma, lactation, epilepsy, diabetes, adrenal tumour, heart disease, urine retention. Psychotic or suicidal patients.
Avoid use: children, heart block, heart attacks, severe liver disease, pregnancy.
Possible interaction: MAOIs (or within 14 days of their use), alcohol, antidepressants, barbiturates, anticholin-ergics, local anaesthetics that contain adrenaline or noradrenaline, oestrogens, cimetidine, antihypertensives.
Side effects: constipation, urine retention, dry mouth, blurred vision, palpitations, tachycardia, nervousness, drowsiness, insomnia. Changes in weight, blood and blood sugar, jaundice, skin reactions, weakness, ataxia, hypotension, sweating, altered libido, gynaecomastia, galactorrhoea.
Manufacturer: Morson.

TUINAL^{CD}

Description: a barbiturate, quinal barbitone sodium and amylobarbitone sodium in equal amounts, available as orange/blue capsules (100mg) marked LILLY F65.
Used for: short-term treatment of severe insomnia for those tolerant to barbiturates.
Dosage: 100–200mg at bedtime. Not for children.
Special care: extremely dangerous, addictive drug with narrow margin of safety. Liable to abuse by overdose leading to coma and death or if combined with alcohol. Easily produces dependence and severe withdrawal symptoms. Drowsiness may persist next day affecting driving and performance of skilled tasks.

Avoid use: should be avoided if possible in all patients. Not to be used for children, young adults, pregnancy, nursing mothers, elderly, those with drug or alcohol related problems, patients with liver, kidney or heart disease, porphyria. Insomnia where the cause is pain.
Possible interaction: alcohol, central nervous system depressant drugs, Griseofulvin, metronidazole, rifampicin, phenytoin, chloramphenicol. Anticoagulant drugs of the coumarin type, steroid drugs including contraceptive pill.
Side effects: hangover with drowsiness, shakiness, dizziness, headache, anxiety, confusion, excitement, rash and allergic responses, gastro intestinal upsets, urine retention, loss of sexual desire.
Manufacturer: Lilly.

TYLEX

Description: an analgesic comprising 500mg paracetamol and 30mg codeine phosphate in red and white capsules marked C30.
Used for: severe pain.
Dosage: 1 or 2 capsules 4-hourly to a maximum of 8 per day. Not for children.
Special care: head injury, raised intracranial pressure, bowel disorders, Addison's disease, hypothyroidism, liver or kidney disease, elderly.
Avoid use: pregnancy, breastfeeding, chronic alcoholism, depression of respiration, diseases causing obstruction of airways.
Possible interaction: CNS depressants, MAOIs.
Side effects: nausea, dry mouth, blurred vision, dizziness, sedation, constipation, tolerance, dependence.
Manufacturer: Cilag.

TYPHIM VI

Description: an inactivated surface antigen of *Salmonella typhi* as 25µg/ 0.5ml in pre-filled syringe.
Used for: active immunisation against typhoid.
Dosage: 0.5ml by intramuscular or deep subcutaneous injection. Children over 18 months, as adult dosage; under 18 months, assess risk of exposure.
Special care: pregnancy, breastfeeding.
Avoid use: acute infections.
Side effects: headache, fever, malaise, localized reactions.
Manufacturer: Merieux

UBRETID

Description: an anticholinesterase, distigmine bromide, available as white tablets (5mg) marked UBRETID, and **UBRETID INJECTION** as 1ml ampoules (0.5mg/ml).
Used for: intestinal and ileal weakness after operations, myasthenia gravis, post-operative urine retention, neurogenic bladder (bladder disorder caused by a lesion of the nervous system).
Dosage: 1 tablet daily, 30 minutes before breakfast up to 4 for myasthenia gravis (2 for children). Post-operative conditions, 0.5mg 12 hours intramuscularly after surgery then 24-hourly until normal function restored. Not for children.
Special care: asthma, heart disease, epilepsy, Parkinsonism, peptic ulcer.
Avoid use: pregnancy, post-operative shock, obstruction in intestines or urinary tract, weak circulation.
Possible interaction: depolarising muscle relaxants.
Side effects: nausea, vomiting, colic, diarrhoea, increased salivation.
Manufacturer: R.P.R.

UCERAX

Description: an antihistamine, hydroxyzine hydrochloride, available as white, oblong tablets (25mg). Also, **UCERAX SYRUP** (10mg/5ml).
Used for: anxiety, skin disorders, pruritus (itching) due to urticaria.

Dosage: 50–100mg 4 times per day for anxiety; otherwise 25mg at night up to 25mg 3 or 4 times per day if required. Children: over 6 years start with 15–25mg at night increasing to 50–100mg per day in divided doses; 6 months to 6 years, 5–15mg increasing to 50mg daily maximum in divided doses.
Special care: kidney disease. Judgement and dexterity may be affected.
Avoid use: pregnancy, breastfeeding.
Possible interaction: depressants of the CNS, alcohol.
Side effects: anticholinergic effects, drowsiness.
Manufacturer: U.C.B.

UKIDAN

Description: a fibrinolytic, urokinase, available as powder in vials containing 5000, 25,000 and 100,000 units.
Used for: pulmonary embolism, deep vein thrombosis, bleeding into the eye in front of the lens, clot in haemodialysis shunt, blockage in peripheral vessel.
Dosage: see the literature.
Special care: peptic ulcer.
Avoid use: severe liver or kidney disease, pregnancy, severe hypertension, recent surgery.
Possible interaction: glucose.
Side effects: fever, haemorrhage.
Manufacturer: Serono.

ULTRADIL

Description: a moderately potent steroid containing 0.1% fluocortolone pivalate and 0.1% fluocortolone hexanoate as cream and ointment.
Used for: eczema, skin disorders and skin conditions that respond to steroids.
Dosage: start by applying 3 times per day, reducing to once per day.
Special care: thrombophlebitis, psychoses, recent intestinal anastomoses, chronic nephritis, certain cancers, osteoporosis, peptic ulcer, skin eruption/rash related to a disease, viral, fungal or active infections, tuberculosis. Hypertension, glaucoma, epilepsy, acute glomerulonephritis (inflammation of kidney glomerulus), diabetes, cirrhosis, hypothyroidism, pregnancy, stress. To be withdrawn gradually.
Possible interaction: NSAIDs, oral anticoagulants, phenytoin, ephedrine, phenobarbitone, rifampicin, diuretics, cardiac glycosides, anticholinesterases, hypoglycaemics.
Side effects: osteoporosis, depression, euphoria, hyperglycaemia, peptic ulcers, Cushingoid changes.
Manufacturer: Schering H.C.

ULTRALANUM

Description: a moderately potent steroid containing 0.25% fluocortolone pivalate and 0.25% fluocortolone hexanoate as a cream. Also, **ULTRALANUM OINTMENT** containing 0.25% fluocortolone and 0.25% fluocortolone hexanoate.
Used for: skin conditions responding to steroids.
Dosage: apply 2 or 3 times per day and reduce to once per day.
Special care: thrombophlebitis, psychoses, recent intestinal anastomoses, chronic nephritis, certain cancers, osteoporosis, peptic ulcer, skin eruption/rash related to a disease, viral, fungal or active infections, tuberculosis. Hypertension, glaucoma, epilepsy, acute glomerulonephritis (inflammation of kidney glomerulus), diabetes, cirrhosis, hypothyroidism, pregnancy, stress. To be withdrawn gradually.
Possible interaction: NSAIDs, oral anticoagulants, phenytoin, ephedrine, phenobarbitone, rifampicin, diuretics, cardiac glycosides, anticholinesterases, hypoglycaemics.
Side effects: osteoporosis, depression, euphoria, hyperglycaemia, peptic ulcers, Cushingoid changes.
Manufacturer: Schering H.C.

ULTRAPROCT

Description: a steroid and local anaesthetic containing fluocortolone pivalate (0.61mg), fluocortolone

hexanoate (0.63mg) and cinchocaine hydrochloride (1mg) as suppositories.
Used for: haemorrhoids, anal fissure, itching, proctitis (inflammation of the rectum).
Dosage: 1 to 3 per day, after defaecation. Not for children.
Also, **ULTRAPROCT OINTMENT**, containing 0.092% fluocortolone pivalate, 0.095% fluocortolone hexanoate and 0.5% cinchocaine hydrochloride.
Dosage: use 2 to 4 times per day. Not for children.
Special care: pregnancy. Do not use for a long period.
Avoid use: infections of a viral, fungal or tuberculous nature.
Side effects: corticosteroid effects.
Manufacturer: Schering H.C.

UNIHEP

Description: an anticoagulant, heparin sodium, available as 1000, 5000, 10,000 and 25,000 units in ampoules.
Used for: treatment and prophylaxis of deep vein thrombosis and pulmonary embolism, angina, acute occlusion of peripheral arteries.
Dosage: varies with condition, see literature.
Special care: pregnancy, liver and kidney disease. Monitor platelet count if treatment exceeds 5 days and cease treatment should thrombocytopenia occur.
Avoid use: thrombocytopenia, cerebral aneurysm, severe hypertension, haemophilia, haemorrhagic disorders, severe liver disease, recent eye or nervous system surgery, hypersensitivity to heparin.
Possible interaction: aspirin, ketorolac, dipyridamole, glyceryl trinitrate.
Side effects: thrombocytopenia, skin necrosis, haemorrhage, hypersensitivity reactions, osteoporosis with prolonged use.
Manufacturer: Leo.

UNIPARIN

Description: an anticoagulant, heparin sodium, available as 5000 units/0.2ml in pre-filled syringe. Also, **UNIPARIN**

FORTE (10,000 units/0.4ml) and **UNIPARIN Ca**, heparin calcium as 25,000 units per ml in pre-filled syringes.
Used for: treatment and prophylaxis of deep vein thrombosis and pulmonary embolism, angina, acute occlusion of peripheral arteries.
Dosage: by subcutaneous injection. See literature for dosage.
Special care: pregnancy, liver and kidney disease. Monitor platelet count if treatment exceeds 5 days and cease treatment should thrombocytopenia occur.
Avoid use: thrombocytopenia, cerebral aneurysm, severe hypertension, haemophilia, haemorrhagic disorders, severe liver disease, recent eye or nervous system surgery, hypersensitivity to heparin.
Possible interaction: aspirin, ketorolac, dipyridamole, glyceryl trinitrate.
Side effects: thrombocytopenia, skin necrosis, haemorrhage, hypersensitivity reactions, osteoporosis with prolonged use.
Manufacturer: C.P. Pharm.

UNIROID-HC

Description: a steroid (5mg hydrocortisone) and local anaesthetic (5mg cinchocaine hydrochloride) available as suppositories.
Used for: haemorrhoids, itching around the anus.
Dosage: Insert 1 dose 3 times per day, and after defaecation for up to 7 days. Not for children.
Also, **UNIROID-HC OINTMENT** containing 5mg hydrocortisone and 5mg/g cinchocaine hydrochloride.
Dosage: use 3 times per day and after defaecation, for up to 7 days. Not for children.
Special care: pregnancy. Do not use over a prolonged period.
Avoid use: infections of a viral, fungal or tuberculous nature.
Side effects: corticosteroid effects.
Manufacturer: Unigreg.

UNIVER

Description: a class I calcium antagonist, verapamil hydrochloride, available as sustained-release capsules coloured yellow/dark blue (120mg and 240mg, marked V120 and V240) and yellow (180mg, marked V180).
Used for: angina, hypertension.
Dosage: 360mg once per day to a maximum of 480mg (angina). For hypertension, 240mg once per day, unless new to verapamil in which case start with 120mg per day.
Special care: 1st degree heart block, weak heart, liver or kidney disease, bradycardia, hypotension, disturbance in heart conduction, pregnancy.
Avoid use: 2nd or 3rd degree heart block, heart failure, sick sinus syndrome.
Possible interaction: quinidine, digoxin, ß-blockers.
Side effects: flushes, constipation, occasionally nausea, vomiting, headache, allergy or liver disorder.
Manufacturer: Rorer.

URIBEN

Description: a quinolone, nalidixic acid, available as a suspension (300mg/5ml).
Used for: infections of the gastro-intestinal tract caused by Gram-negative organisms, urinary tract infections.
Dosage: gastro-intestinal tract infections: 10–15ml 4 times per day, children over 3 months 1ml/kg per day. Contact manufacturer regarding children under 3 months. For urinary tract infections: acute cases, 15ml 4 times per day for at least 7 days; chronic cases 10ml. Children's doses as above.
Special care: severe kidney disease, liver disease, avoid excessive sunlight.
Avoid use: past convulsions.
Possible interaction: probenecid, anticoagulants.
Side effects: rashes, blood disorders, seizures, disturbances in sight, gastro-intestinal upset.
Manufacturer: R.P. Drugs.

URISPAS

Description: an antispasmodic drug, flavoxate hydrochloride, available as white tablets containing 100mg and marked URISPAS, and 200mg (marked URISPAS 200).
Used for: incontinence, frequent or urgent urination, painful urination, bedwetting.
Dosage: 200mg 3 times per day. Not for children.
Special care: pregnancy, glaucoma.
Avoid use: conditions causing obstruction in the urinary or gastro-intestinal tracts.
Side effects: diarrhoea, dry mouth, blurred vision, nausea, fatigue, headache.
Manufacturer: Syntex.

UROMITEXAN

Description: a protectant for the urinary tract, mesna, available as solution in ampoules (100mg/ml).
Used for: prevention of toxicity in the urinary tract caused by the metabolite acrolein.
Dosage: orally or intravenously. See literature for details.
Side effects: fatigue, headache, gastro-intestinal upset, depression, irritability, rash, malaise, pain in the limbs.
Manufacturer: ASTA Medica.

URSOFALK

Description: a bile acid, ursodeoxycholic acid, available as white capsules containing 250mg.
Used for: dissolving cholesterol gallstones.
Dosage: 8–12mg/kg/day in 2 divided doses after meals of which one must be the evening meal. Use for 3 to 4 months after the stones have been dissolved. Not for children.
Avoid use: if gall bladder does not function. Women who are not using contraception.
Possible interaction: drugs to lower cholesterol levels, oral contraceptives, oestrogens.
Manufacturer: Thames.

UTINOR

Description: a 4-quinolone compound, norfloxacin, available as white, oval tablets (400mg) marked UTINOR.
Used for: acute and chronic infections of the urinary tract.
Dosage: 1 tablet twice per day. Duration depends upon the condition. Not for children.
Special care: past epilepsy, kidney disorder.
Avoid use: pregnancy, breastfeeding, growing adolescents and children before puberty.
Possible interaction: NSAIDs, antacids, oral anticoagulants, cyclosporin, theophylline, nitrofurantoin, probenecid, sucralfate.
Side effects: diarrhoea, nausea, headache, dizziness, heartburn, rash, abdominal cramp, irritability, convulsions, anorexia, disturbance to sleep.
Manufacturer: M.S.D.

UTOVLAN

Description: a progestogen, norethisterone, available as white tablets (5mg) marked SYNTEX.
Used for: dysmenorrhoea (painful menstruation), menorrhagia (long or heavy menstrual periods), uterine bleeding, metropathia haemorrhagica (endometrial hyperplasia—irregular bleeding due to excess activity of oestrogen).
Dosage: 1 tablet 3 times per day for 10 days then twice per day for days 19–26 of the next 2 cycles.
Used for: postponement of menses (discharge).
Dosage: 1 tablet 3 times per day commencing 3 days before anticipated start.
Used for: endometriosis.
Dosage: 1 tablet 3 times per day for at least 6 months, increasing to 4 or 5 per day if necessary.
Used for: pre-menstrual syndrome.
Dosage: 1 per day from days 16–25 of the cycle.
Used for: breast cancer.

Dosage: start with 8 per day increasing to 12 if required.
Special care: epilepsy, migraine, diabetes.
Avoid use: not for children. Carcinoma of the breast dependent upon progestogen, past thromboembolic disorders, undiagnosed abnormal vaginal bleeding, liver disease, severe itching, pregnancy, jaundice, past herpes.
Side effects: liver or gastro-intestinal upset.
Manufacturer: Syntex.

VAGIFEM

Description: an hormonal oestrogen preparation available as vaginal pessaries with applicator containing 25µg oestradiol.
Used for: atrophic vaginitis.
Dosage: adults, 1 pessary inserted into vagina each day for 2 weeks, then 1 twice each week for 3 months.
Special care: those at risk of thrombosis or with liver disease. Women with any of the following disorders should be carefully monitored: fibroids in the womb, multiple sclerosis, diabetes, tetany, porphyria, epilepsy, liver disease, hypertension, migraine, otosclerosis, gallstones. Breasts, pelvic organs and blood pressure should be checked at regular intervals during the course of treatment.
Avoid use: pregnancy, breastfeeding, women with conditions which might lead to thrombosis, thrombophlebitis, serious heart, kidney or liver disease, breast cancer, oestrogen-dependent cancers including those of reproductive system, endometriosis, vaginal bleeding which is undiagnosed.
Possible interaction: drugs which induce liver enzymes.
Side effects: tenderness and enlargement of breasts, weight gain, breakthrough bleeding, giddiness, vomiting and nausea,

gastro-intestinal upset. Treatment should be halted immediately if severe headaches occur, disturbance of vision, hypertension or any indications of thrombosis, jaundice. Also, in the event of pregnancy and 6 weeks before planned surgery.
Manufacturer: Novo Nordisk.

VALIUM

Description: a long-acting benzodiazepine drug available as white 2mg tablets, yellow 5mg tablets and blue 10mg tablets all containing diazepam. Tablets are scored and marked with ROCHE and strength. Also, **VALIUM SYRUP** containing 2mg diazepam/5ml; **VALIUM INJECTION** available as a solution in ampoules containing 5mg diazepam/ml.
Used for: severe and disabling anxiety, insomnia, severe alcohol withdrawal symptoms, sleep disorders in children. Feverish convulsions, status epilepticus (injection only), spasm of muscles and cerebral spasticity, as a sedative during medical or surgical procedures.
Dosage: oral preparations, 2–60mg in divided doses each day depending upon condition being treated. Injection, 10–20mg, or 0.2mg/kg body weight depending upon condition being treated, by intrav-enous or intramuscular injection every 4 hours. Status epilepticus, this dose may be repeated after half an hour to an hour with a maximum of 3mg/kg by intravenous infusion over 24 hours. Elderly, oral preparations, 1–30mg each day in divided doses; injection 5mg by intravenous or intramuscular injection every 4 hours. Children, oral preparations, 1–40mg each day in divided doses depending upon condition being treated; 1–5mg at bedtime for sleep disorders. Injection, status epilepticus and convulsions, 0.2–0.3mg/kg by intravenous or intramuscular injection.
Special care: elderly, pregnancy, breastfeeding, liver or kidney disorders, lung disease. Drug should be gradually withdrawn.
Avoid use: patients with serious lung disease, depression of respiration, obsessional and phobic disorders, severe psychosis. Avoid long-term use.
Possible interaction: CNS depressants, anticonvulsants, alcohol. Drugs which induce or inhibit liver enzymes.
Side effects: impaired judgement and performance of skilled tasks, confusion, shakiness, sleepiness, vertigo. Gastrointestinal upset, retention of urine, disturbance of vision, changes in libido, skin rashes, hypotension. Thrombophlebitis at site of injection; rarely, jaundice and blood changes. The longer treatment lasts and the higher the dose the greater the risk of drug dependence.
Manufacturer: Roche.

VALLERGAN

Description: an anti-allergic preparation, which is an antihistamine of the phenothiazine type, available as film-coated, blue tablets containing 10mg trimeprazine tartrate marked V10. Also, **VALLERGAN SYRUP** containing 7.5mg/5ml; **VALLERGAN FORTE SYRUP**, containing 30mg/5ml.
Used for: itching, urticaria, premedication before surgery in children.
Dosage: 10mg 2 or 3 times each day with a maximum of 100mg daily. Elderly persons, 10mg once or twice daily. Children, for itching and allergic conditions age over 2 years, 2.5–5mg 3 or 4 times each day. Premedication, age 2 to 7 years, up to 2mg/kg body weight 1 or 2 hours before surgery.
Avoid use: pregnancy, breastfeeding, liver or kidney disorders, Parkinson's disease, epilepsy, phaeochromocytoma, underactive thyroid gland, myasthenia gravis, glaucoma.
Possible interaction: antihypertensives, hypoglycaemics, alcohol, sympathomimetics, anticholinergics, MAOIs, central nervous system depressants.
Side effects: sleepiness, rash, drowsiness, impaired performance and reactions, heart disturbances, hypotension, depression of respiration. Anticholinergic and

extrapyramidal effects, convulsions, raised levels of prolactin in blood, abnormally low level of white blood cells, jaundice, sensitivity to light (with high doses).
Manufacturer: Theraplix.

VANCOCIN CP

Description: an antibiotic glycopeptide preparation available as powder in vials for reconstitution and injection containing 250mg, 500mg and 1g vancomycin (as hydrochloride). Also, **VANCOCIN MATRIGEL** available as peach/blue capsules containing 125mg (coded Lilly 3125); grey/blue capsules containing 250mg (coded Lilly 3126).
Used for: potentially fatal infections caused by staphylococci which are resistant to other antibiotics. Vancocin Matrigel, staphylococcal enterocolitis and pseudo-membraneous colitis.
Dosage: 500mg every 6 hours or 1g every 12 hours given by slow intravenous infusion over 1 hour. Children, 10mg/kg body weight by slow intravenous infusion over 1 hour at 6 hourly intervals. Vancocin Matrigel, 500mg each day for 7 to 10 days in divided doses with a daily maximum of 2g. Children, 40mg/kg for 7 to 10 days in 3 or 4 divided doses with a daily maximum of 2g.
Special care: elderly, pregnancy, patients with existing loss of hearing, kidney disorders. Blood, kidney function and hearing shoudl be carefully monitored during the course of treatment.
Possible interaction: drugs with toxic effects on central nervous system or kidneys, anaesthetics.
Side effects: chills, fever, nausea, phlebitis, reduction in number of some white blood cells and rise in number of eosinophils, toxic effects on kidneys and organs of hearing and balance. Anaphylactoid allergic reactions.
Manufacturer: Lilly.

VARIDASE

Description: a preparation of fibrinolytic and proteolytic enzymes available as powder in vials containing 100,000 units streptokinase and 25,000 units streptodomase.
Used for: cleansing and removal of debris from wounds and ulcers.
Dosage: apply as wet dressing once or twice each day.
Avoid use: patients with active haemorrhage.
Manufacturer: Lederle.

VASCACE

Description: an antihypertensive preparation which is an ACE inhibitor, available in the form of oval, film-coated, scored tablets in various strengths, all containing cilazapril and marked with strength and CIL. Pink, 0.25mg strength; white, 0.5mg strength; yellow, 1mg strength; red, 2.5mg streength and brown 5mg strength.
Used for: hypertension and renovascular hypertension.
Dosage: hypertension, 1mg once each day at first with a maintenance dose in the order of 1–2.5mg daily. Any diuretic being taken should be withdrawn 2 or 3 days before treatment starts. Renovascular hypertension, 0.25–0.5mg once each day then adjusted according to response of condition. Elderly, hypertension, 0.5mg each day at first; renovascular hypertension, 0.25mg once each day at first.
Special care: liver or kidney disease, congestive heart failure, undergoing renal dialysis, anaesthesia or surgery, suffering from lack of fluid or salt.
Avoid use: children, pregnancy, breastfeeding, patients with outflow obstruction of the heart, aortic stenosis, ascites (abnormal collection of fluid in the peritoneal cavity which is a complication of various diseases).
Possible interaction: NSAIDs, potassium-sparing diuretics.
Side effects: nausea, headache, fatigue, rash, indigestion, giddiness. Rarely, pancreatitis, changes in blood count, angioneurotic oedema.
Manufacturer: Roche.

VASOCON-A

Description: an anti-inflammatory compound preparation combining an antihistamine and sympathomimetic, available as eyedrops containing 0.5% antazoline phosphate and 0.05% naphazoline hydrochloride.

Used for: inflammatory eye conditions including allergic conjunctivitis.

Dosage: adults, 1 or 2 drops up to 4 times each day.

Special care: diabetes, hypertension, hyperthyroidism, disease of coronary arteries.

Avoid use: narrow angle glaucoma, wearing soft contact lenses.

Possible interaction: MAOIs.

Side effects: sleepiness, tachycardia, headache, insomnia, short-lived stinging in eye.

Manufacturer: Lolab.

VASOXINE

Description: an antiarrhythmic and a-agonist, available as a solution in ampoules for injection containing 20mg methoxamine hydrochloride.

Used for: hypotension during anaesthesia.

Dosage: adults, 5–10mg by slow intravenous injection or 5–20mg by intramuscular injection.

Special care: pregnancy, patients with hyperthyroidism.

Avoid use: serious disease of the coronary arteries or heart blood vessels.

Possible interaction: anoretic drugs, cough and cold remedies.

Side effects: hypertension, bradycardia, headache.

Manufacturer: Wellcome.

VELBE

Description: a drug which is a vinca alkaloid available as powder in vials with diluent containing 10mg vinblastine sulphate.

Used for: leukaemias, lymphomas, some solid tumours, e.g. of lung and breast.

Dosage: by intravenous injection as directed by specialist physician.

Special care: caution in handling (trained personnel, protective clothing), irritant to tissues.

Avoid use: intrathecal route.

Side effects: bone marrow suppression, toxic effects on peripheral and autonomic nervous system, reversible hair loss, nausea, vomiting, effects on fertility.

Manufacturer: Lilly.

VELOSEF

Description: an antibiotic preparation which is a cephalosporin available as capsules in 2 strengths both containing cephradine. Blue/orange 250mg capsules, coded SQUIBB 113 and blue 500mg capsules coded SQUIBB 114. Also, VELOSEF SYRUP containing 250mg/5ml. VELOSEF INJECTION as powder in vials for reconstitution and injection containing 500mg and 1g cephradine.

Used for: infections of skin, soft tissues, respiratory, gastro-intestinal and urinary tracts, joints and bones. Also, endocarditis and septicaemia and for prevention of infection during surgery.

Dosage: oral preparations, 1–2g each day in 2, 3 or 4 divided doses with a maximum daily dose of 4g. Injection, 2–4g by intramuscular or intravenous injection or intravenous infusion in divided daily doses. Children, oral preparations, 25–50mg/kg body weight in 2, 3 or 4 daily divided doses. For inflammation of middle ear, 75–100mg/kg each day in divided doses. Injection, 50–100mg/kg each day in divided doses. All treatment should continue for 48–72 hours after symptoms have disappeared.

Special care: kidney disorders, known hypersensitivity to penicillins.

Possible interaction: aminoglycosides.

Side effects: gastro-intestinal upset, allergic hypersensitive responses. Rarely, blood changes involving white blood cells, rise in levels of urea and liver enzymes in blood, positive Coomb's test (a test to detect Rhesus antibodies), candidiasis.

Manufacturer: Squibb.

VENTIDE

Description: a bronchodilator, anti-inflammatory preparation which combines a selective ß-agonist and corticosteroid. It is available as an aerosol delivering 100µg salbutamol and 50µg beclomethasone dipropionate per metered dose. Also, **VENTIDE ROTACAPS** available as clear/grey capsules containing 400µg salbutamol as sulphate and 200µg beclomethasone dipropionate, marked VENTIDE, for use with Rotahaler. Also, **VENTIDE PAEDIATRIC ROTACAPS**, clear/light grey capsules containing 200µg salbutamol as sulphate and 100µg beclomethasone dipropionate, for use with Rotahaler.

Used for: long-term treatment of asthma which requires inhaled bronchodilator and corticosteroid therapy.

Dosage: Ventide, 2 puffs 3 to 4 times each day; Ventide Rotacaps, 1 puff 3 to 4 times each day. Children, Ventide, 1 or 2 puffs 2, 3 or 4 times each day. Ventide Paediatric Rotacaps, 1 puff 2, 3 or 4 times each day.

Special care: pregnancy, weak heart, angina, heart arrhythmias, hyperthyroidism, hypertension, tuberculosis. Special care in patients changing from systemic steroids.

Possible interaction: sympathomimetics.

Side effects: dilation of peripheral blood vessels, headache, nervous tension, tremor, fungal infections of throat and mouth and hoarseness.

Manufacturer: A. & H.

VENTODISKS

Description: a bronchodilator, anti-inflammatory preparation, which is a selective ß₂-agonist, available as light blue disks of 200µg strength and dark blue disks of 400µg strength, containing salbutamol as sulphate. Both are marked with strength and name.

Used for: bronchospasm occurring in bronchitis, emphysema and bronchial asthma.

Dosage: acute attack, 200 or 400µg 3 to 4 times each day. Children, acute attack, 200µg as single dose; prevention, half the dose of adult.

Special care: pregnancy, weak heart, angina, heart arrhythmias, hyperthyroidism, hypertension.

Possible interaction: sympathomimetics.

Side effects: headache, dilation of peripheral blood vessels, nervous tension, tremor.

Manufacturer: A. & H.

VENTOLIN

Description: a bronchodilator/anti-inflammatory preparation which is a selective ß₂-agonist, available as pink tablets containing 2mg and 4mg salbutamol as sulphate, marked AH and IK and AH and 2K respectively. Also, **VENTOLIN SYRUP**, sugar and colour-free, containing 2mg/5ml. Also, **VENTOLIN INHALER**, a metered dose aerosol delivering 100µg salbutamol per puff. **VENTOLIN ROTACAPS** available as clear/light blue capsules containing 200µg and clear/dark blue capsules containing 400 µg, both marked with strength and name for use with Rotahaler. **VENTOLIN INJECTION** available as a solution in ampoules containing 50 and 500µg/ml. **VENTOLIN INFUSION**, available as a solution in ampoules containing 1mg/ml. **VENTOLIN RESPIRATOR SOLUTION**, for hospital use only containing 5mg/ml in bottles. **VENTOLIN NEBULES** for use with nebuliser available as single dose units containing 2.5mg and 5mg/2.5ml.

Used for: bronchospasm occurring in bronchitis, emphysema and bronchial asthma. Injection, status asthmaticus and severe bronchospasm.

Dosage: oral preparations, 2–8mg 3 or 4 times each day. Ventolin Inhaler, attack, 1 or 2 puffs; prevention, 2 puffs 3 or 4 times each day. Ventolin Rotacaps, acute attack, 200 or 400µg as 1 dose; prevention, 400µg 3 or 4 times each day. Injection, 8µg/kg body weight by intramuscular or subcutaneous injection. Or, 4 µg/kg by slow intravenous injection. Nebules, 2.5–5mg nebulised up to 4 times each day. Other preparations, see literature. Children, oral preparations, aged 2 to 6 years, 1–2mg; 6 to 12 years, 2mg, all 3 or 4 times each day. Ventolin Inhaler, half adult dose; Rotacaps, acute attack, 200µg as 1 dose; prevention, half adult dose. Nebules, same as adult dose.

Special care: pregnancy, patients with hyperthyroidism, hypertension, weak heart, angina, heart arrhythmias.
Avoid use: children under 2 years (oral preparations).
Possible interaction: sympathomimetics.
Side effects: headache, dilation of peripheral blood vessels, nervous tension, tremor.
Manufacturer: A. & H.

VEPESID

Description: an anti-cancer drug which is a podophyllotoxin available as pink gelatin capsules containing 50mg and 100mg etoposide. Also, **VEPESID INJECTION** available as a solution in vials containing 20mg etoposide/ml.
Used for: lymphomas, cancer of the bronchus, teratoma of the testes.
Dosage: as directed by specialist but in divided doses over 3 to 5 days. Oral doses are double those of inection which is given intravenously.
Special care: care in handling (trained staff, protective clothing), irritant to tissues.
Side effects: hair loss, bone marrow suppression, vomiting, nausea, effects on fertility.
Manufacturer: Bristol-Myers.

VERMOX

Description: an antihelmintic preparation available as a sugar-free suspension containing 100mg mebendazole/5ml. Also, **VERMOX TABLETS**, scored, pink, containing 100mg mebendazole marked Me/100 and JANSSEN.

Used for: infestations of large roundworm, threadworm, common and American hookworm, whipworm.
Dosage: adults and children aged over 2 years; threadworm, 100mg with dose repeated after 2 or 3 weeks if necessary. Other types of worm, 100mg morning and night for 3 days.
Avoid use: pregnancy.
Side effects: gastro-intestinal upset.
Manufacturer: Janssen.

VIBRAMYCIN

Description: a tetracycline antibiotic preparation available as green capsules containing 100mg doxycycline (as hydrochloride), marked VBM 100 and Pfizer. Also, **VIBRAMYCIN-D**, off-white, dissolvable tablets containing 100mg vibramycin marked Pfizer and D-9.
Used for: gastro-intestinal and respiratory tract infections, pneumonia, soft tissue, urinary tract infections, sexually transmitted diseases, eye infections, acne vulgaris.
Dosage: all infections except sexually transmitted diseases, 200mg with food or drink on first day then 100–200mg daily. Acne, 50mg each day with food or drink for 6 to 12 weeks. (Sexually transmitted diseases, as advised in literature).
Special care: patients with liver disease.
Avoid use: pregnancy, breastfeeding, children.
Possible interaction: carbamazepine, antacids, phenytoin, mineral supplements, barbiturates, methoxyflurane.
Side effects: superinfections, gastrointestinal upset, allergic responses. Withdraw if intracranial hypertension occurs.
Manufacturer: Invicta.

VILLESCON

Description: a combined sympathomimetic and vitamin preparation available as a tonic containing 2.5mg prolintane hydrochloride, 1.67mg thiamine-hydrochloride, 1.36mg riboflavine sodium phosphate, 0.5mg pyridoxine hydrochloride, 5mg nicotinamide/5ml.

Used for: a general tonic.
Dosage: 10ml after breakfast with second dose in afternoon for 1 to 2 weeks. Children, age 5 to 12 years, 2.5–10ml twice each day.
Avoid use: children under 5 years, patients with epilepsy or thyrotoxicosis.
Possible interaction: levodopa, MAOIs.
Side effects: nausea, insomnia, tachycardia, colic.
Manufacturer: Boehringer Ingelheim.

VIRAZID

Description: an antiviral preparation available as a powder in vials for nebusation containing 20mg tribavirin/ml.
Used for: serious respiratory syncitial virus bronchiolitis (inflammation and infection of bronchioles).
Dosage: children only, delivery via an oxygen hood, tent or mask for 12 to 18 hours each day for at least 3 days and for maximum of 7 days.
Special care: patient and equipment require careful monitoring.
Avoid use: pregnancy, females of child-caring age.
Side effects: worsening of respiratory condition, reticulocytosis (increase in number of reticulocytes—immature erythrocyte red blood cells), pneumothorax, bacterial pneumonia.
Manufacturer: Britannia.

VIRORMONE

Description: a sex hormone (androgen) preparation available as a solution in ampoules containing 50mg testosterone propionate/ml.
Used for: cryptorchidism (undescended testicle), male hypogonadism (deficiency in secretion of hormones by testes), delayed puberty in males. Breast cancer after menopause in women.
Dosage: for hypogonadism, 50mg 2 or 3 times each week; cryptorchidism or delayed puberty, 50mg each week. Breast cancer in women, 100mg 2 or 3 times each week, all by intramuscular injection.

Special care: liver, kidney, or heart disorders, migraine, epilepsy, hypertension.
Avoid use: cancer of liver or prostate gland, heart disease or heart failure which is untreated, kidney nephrosis (an abnormality resulting from various diseases or conditions). Hypercalcaemia, high levels of calcium in urine.
Possible interaction: drugs that induce liver enzymes.
Side effects: weight gain, reduced fertility, oedema, tumours of liver, priapism (painful and prolonged erection of penis not connected with sexual arousal but resulting from drug treatment or underlying disorder). Also, premature closure of epiphyses, increased bone growth, masculinization (women).
Manufacturer: Paines and Byrne.

VIRUDOX

Description: an antiviral preparation available as a solution with applicator brush containing 5% idoxuridine, dimethyl sulphoxide to 100%.
Used for: skin infections caused by Herpes simplex and Herpes zoster.
Dosage: adults, apply to affected skin 4 times each day for 4 days.
Special care: avoid mucous membranes and eyes. May damage clothing.
Avoid use: pregnancy, breastfeeding, children.
Side effects: stinging when applied, unusual, distinctive taste during treatment. Over-use may cause skin to soften and break down.
Manufacturer: Bioglan.

VISKALDIX

Description: a non-cardioselective ß-blocker and thiazide, pindolol (10mg) with clopamide (5mg) in white tablets marked with name.
Used for: hypertension.
Dosage: start with 1 tablet in the morning increasing if required, after 2 or 3 weeks, to 2 or a maximum of 3 per day. Not for children.

Special care: history of bronchospasm and certain ß-blockers, diabetes, liver or kidney disease, pregnancy, lactation, general anaesthesia, gout, check electrolyte levels, K⁺ supplements may be required depending on the case. Withdraw gradually. Not for children.
Avoid use: heart block or failure, bradycardia, sick sinus syndrome (associated with sinus node disorder), certain ß-blockers, severe peripheral arterial disease, pregnancy, lactation, severe kidney failure, anuria, hepatic cornea.
Possible interaction: verapamil, hypoglycaemics, reserpine, clonidine withdrawal, some antiarrhythmics and anaesthetics, antihypertensives, depressants of the CNS, cimetidine, indomethacin, sympathomimetics, lithium, potassium supplements with potassium-sparing diuretics, digitalis.
Side effects: bradycardia, cold hands and feet, disturbance to sleep, heart failure, gastro-intestinal upset, tiredness on exertion, bronchospasm, gout, weakness, blood disorders, sensitivity to light.
Manufacturer: Stuart.

VISKEN

Description: a non-cardioselective ß-blocker, pindolol, available as white tablets (5 and 15mg) marked with name and strength.
Used for: angina, hypertension.
Dosage: half to 1 tablet 3 times per day (angina); 10–15mg per day increasing weekly to a maximum of 45mg if necessary. Not for children.
Special care: history of bronchospasm and certain ß-blockers, diabetes, liver or kidney disease, pregnancy, lactation, general anaesthesia. Withdraw gradually. Not for children.
Avoid use: heart block or failure, bradycardia, sick sinus syndrome (associated with sinus node disorder), certain ß-blockers, severe peripheral arterial disease.
Possible interaction: verapamil, hypoglycaemics, reserpine, clonidine withdrawal, some antiarrhythmics and

anaesthetics, antihypertensives, depressants of the CNS, cimetidine, indomethacin, sympathomimetics.
Side effects: bradycardia, cold hands and feet, disturbance to sleep, heart failure, gastro-intestinal upset, tiredness on exertion, bronchospasm.
Manufacturer: Sandoz.

VISTA-METHASONE

Description: a corticosteroid, betamethasone sodium phosphate, available as 0.1% drops.
Used for: non-infected inflammatory conditions of the nose, ear and eye.
Also, **VISTA-METHASONE N** (also includes 0.5% neomycin sulphate).
Used for: infected inflammation of the nose, ear and eye.
Dosage: 1 to 3 drops from 2 hourly to twice daily, depending upon condition.
Special care: pregnancy; avoid prolonged use during pregnancy, or with infants.
Avoid use: infections of a viral, fungal o tuberculous nature, perforated eardrum (for ear conditions), glaucoma or soft contact lenses (for eye conditions).
Side effects: superinfection. For eyes—corneal thinning, cataract, fungal infection, rise in pressure within the eye
Manufacturer: Daniels.

VIVALAN

Description: an antidepressant and oxazine, viloxazine hydrochloride, in white tablets (50mg) marked V and ICI.
Used for: depression, particularly where sedation is not required.
Dosage: 300mg per day in divided dose (maximum 400mg/day). Elderly, start with 100mg per day. Not for children.
Special care: heart block, heart failure, ischaemic heart disease, pregnancy, epilepsy, suicidal tendency.
Avoid use: past peptic ulcer, liver disease, mania, recent myocardial infarction, breastfeeding.
Possible interaction: phenytoin, levodopa theophylline, CNS depressants, carbamazepine, clonidine, MAOIs.

ide effects: anticholinergic effects, jaundice, convulsions, vomiting, headache, affected reactions.
Manufacturer: Zeneca.

VIVOTIF

Description: a live attenuated vaccine, *salmonella typhi*, Ty 21a strain in white/pink capsules.
Used for: immunisation against typhoid fever.
Dosage: 1 capsule with cold drink 1 hour before a meal on days 1, 3 and 5. Annual boost of 3 capsules for those regularly at risk. Children over 6 years, adult dose. Not for children under 6.
Special care: pregnancy, breastfeeding.
Avoid use: acute fever or gastro-intestinal illness, immunosuppressed patients.
Possible interaction: antibiotics, cytotoxics, immunosuppressants, sulphonamides, mefloquine.
Side effects: mild gastro-intestinal upset.
Manufacturer: Evans.

VOLITAL

Description: a stimulant of the CNS, pemoline, available as white tablets (20mg) marked P9.
Used for: hyperkinesia (overactive restlessness) in children.
Dosage: aged 6 to 12 years, start with 20mg in the morning increasing weekly by 20mg to 60mg/day, or possible 120mg if no improvement on lower doses. Not for children under 6.
Special care: reduce dose if side effects occur (improvement usually happens within 6 weeks).
Possible interaction: MAOIs.
Side effects: weight loss, anorexia, headache, sweating, palpitations, dizziness, irritability.
Manufacturer: L.A.B.

VOLMAX

Description: a selective ß₂-agonist, salbutamol sulphate, in white hexagonal continuous-release tablets (4 and 9mg) marked with strength.

Used for: chronic bronchitis, emphysema, bronchospasm.
Dosage: 8mg twice per day. Children, aged 3 to 12 years, 4mg twice per day. Not for those under 3 years.
Special care: angina, hypertension, cardiac arrhythmias, pregnancy, hyperthyroidism, weak heart.
Possible interaction: sympathomimetics.
Side effects: headache, dilatation of peripheral vessels, nervousness.
Manufacturer: A. & H.

VOLRAMAN

Description: a phenylacetic acid, diclofenac sodium, in 25 and 50mg orange tablets.
Used for: pain or inflammation associated with rheumatic disease, gout, musculo-skeletal disorders.
Dosage: 75–150mg per day in divided doses after food.
Special care: elderly, kidney, liver or heart disease.
Avoid use: porphyria, hypersensitivity to aspirin or other NSAIDs, pregnancy, peptic ulcer.
Possible interaction: ACE inhibitors, other NSAIDs, quinolones, anticoagulants, antidiabetics, antihypertensives, diuretics, lithium.
Side effects: gastro-intestinal upset, nausea, diarrhoea, hypersensitivity reactions, dizziness, blood disorders, headache.
Manufacturer: Eastern.

VOLTAROL

Description: a phenylacetic acid, diclofenac sodium, available as yellow (25mg) and brown (50mg) tablets marked with name, strength and GEIGY.
Used for: rheumatoid arthritis, osteoarthrosis, ankylosing spondylitis, chronic juvenile arthritis, acute gout.
Dosage: 75–150mg per day in divided doses. Children over 1 year, 1–3mg/kg/day.
Also, **VOLTAROL DISPERSIBLE** as pink, triangular tablets (50mg) marked V and GEIGY.

Dosage: 1 taken 3 times daily in water for a maximum of 3 months. Not for children.

Also, **VOLTAROL SUSTAINED-RELEASE SR**, as pink, triangular tablets (75mg) marked V 75 SR and GEIGY, and **RETARD** as 100mg red tablets marked VOLTAROL R and GEIGY.

Dosage: 1 SR once or twice per day, 1 Retard per day.

Also, **VOLTAROL SUPPOSITORIES** (100mg).

Dosage: 1 at night and **VOLTAROL PAEDIATRIC SUPPOSITORIES** (12.5mg).

Dosage: children, 1–3mg/kg/day in divided doses.

Also, **VOLTAROL INJECTION** (25mg/ml).

Used for: back pain, post-operative pain, pain in trauma or from fractures.

Dosage: 75mg intramuscularly once or twice per day for 2 days maximum. Continue with tablets or suppositories if required.

Special care: monitor long-term treatment. Liver, kidney or heart disease, porphyria, past gastro-intestinal lesions, pregnancy, breastfeeding, elderly, blood disorders.

Avoid use: allergy to aspirin or anti-inflammatory drugs, proctitis (inflammation of anus and rectum), peptic ulcer.

Possible interaction: lithium, diuretics, digoxin, methotrexate, salicylates, cyclosporin, oral hypoglycaemics, NSAIDs, steroids, quinolones.

Side effects: headache, oedema, gastro-intestinal upset.

Manufacturer: Geigy.

VOLTAROL EMULGEL

Description: an NSAID, diclofenac diethyl-lammonium salt as 1.16g in an aqueous gel (equivalent to 1g diclofenac sodium).

Used for: soft tissue rheumatism, strains, sprains, bruises.

Dosage: 2–4g rubbed into area 3 to 4 times per day. Not for children.

Special care: pregnancy, breastfeeding, avoid eyes, mucous membrane, broken skin.

Avoid use: allergy to aspirin or anti-inflammatory drugs.

Side effects: itching, dermatitis, localized erythema, sensitivity to light.

Manufacturer: Geigy.

VOLTAROL OPHTHA

Description: an NSAID, diclofenac sodium, available as 0.1% single dose eyedrops.

Used for: reduction of miosis (excessive constriction of the sphincter muscle of the iris) in cataract surgery, post-operative inflammation.

Dosage: see literature.

Possible interaction: ACE inhibitors, other NSAIDs, quinolones, anticoagulants, antidiabetics, antihypertensives, diuretics, lithium.

Manufacturer: Ciba Vision.

WARTICON

Description: a cytotoxic drug, 0.5% podophyllotoxin, available as a solution with applicator. Also, **WARTICON FEM** including mirror.

Used for: external genital warts.

Dosage: use twice per day over 3 days, repeated weekly for up to 4 weeks if necessary. Not for children.

Avoid use: pregnancy, breastfeeding.

Side effects: localized irritation.

Manufacturer: Perstop.

WELLDORM

Description: a sedative and hypnotic, chloral betaine, available in purple oval tablets (strength 707mg, equivalent to 414mg of chloral hydrate).

Used for: insomnia over the short-term.

Dosage: 1 or 2 tablets at bedtime to a maximum of 2g chloral hydrate equivalent per day.

Also, **WELLDORM ELIXIR**, 143mg
chloral hydrate/5ml.
Dosage: 15–45ml at bedtime to a daily
maximum of 2g. Children: 30–50mg/kg
to a daily maximum of 1g.
Avoid use: severe heart, kidney or liver
disease, porphyria, gastritis, pregnancy,
breastfeeding.
Possible interaction: anticoagulants, anticholinergics, CNS depressants, alcohol.
Side effects: headache, nausea, vomiting,
flatulence, bloating, rashes, blood
disorders, excitability.
Manufacturer: S.N.P.

WELLFERON

Description: an interferon (affects
immunity and cell function) interferon
alfa-N1, available as vials containing 3
million units/ml.
Used for: chronic hepatitis B, hairy-cell
leukaemia.
Dosage: by subcutaneous and intramuscular injection. See literature for dose.
Special care: see literature.
Avoid use: see literature.
Possible interaction: theophylline.
Side effects: lethargy, flu-like symptoms,
depression, bone marrow depression,
hypo- and hypertension, arrhythmias,
rashes, seizures.
Manufacturer: Wellcome.

XANAX

Description: a long-acting benzodiazepine,
alprazolam, available as white, oval tablets
(250µg) marked UPJOHN 29 and pink,
oval tablets (500µg) marked UPJOHN 55.
Used for: short-term treatment of anxiety
and anxiety with depression.
Dosage: 250–500µg 2 or 3 times per
day, elderly, 250µg, to a daily maximum
of 3mg. Not for children.
Special care: chronic liver or kidney

disease, chronic lung disease, pregnancy,
labour, lactation, elderly. May impair
judgement. Withdraw gradually and
avoid prolonged use.
Avoid use: depression of respiration,
acute lung disease; psychotic, phobic or
obsessional states.
Possible interaction: anticonvulsants,
depressants of the CNS, alcohol.
Side effects: ataxia, confusion, light-
headedness, drowsiness, hypotension,
gastro-intestinal upsets, disturbances in
vision and libido, skin rashes, retention
of urine, vertigo. Sometimes jaundice or
blood disorders.
Manufacturer: Upjohn.

XATRAL

Description: a selective a₁-blocker,
alfuzosin hydrochloride, available as white
tablets (2.5mg) marked XATRAL 2.5.
Used for: benign prostatic hypertrophy
(enlargement of prostate gland).
Dosage: 1 tablet 3 times per day to a
maximum of 4. Elderly, 1 at morning
and evening to start, to a maximum of 4.
Special care: weak heart, hypertension.
Monitor blood pressure especially when
starting treatment. Stop 24 hours before
anaesthesia, or if angina worsens.
Avoid use: severe liver disease, past
orthostatic hypotension (low blood
pressure on standing).
Possible interaction: antihypertensives,
calcium antagonists, other a-blockers.
Side effects: gastro-intestinal upset,
headache, dizziness, vertigo, tachycardia, orthostatic hypotension, chest pain,
fatigue, rash, flushing, oedema, itching,
palpitations, fainting.
Manufacturer: Lorex.

XURET

Description: a thiazide-like diuretic,
metolazone, available as white tablets
(0.5mg) marked X and GALEN.
Used for: hypertension.
Dosage: 1 per day each morning
(maximum 2 per day). Not for children.
Special care: diabetes, gout, SLE, elderly,

cirrhosis of the liver, liver or kidney disease, pregnancy, breastfeeding. Check, fluid, glucose and electrolyte levels.
Avoid use: Addison's disease, hypercalcaemia, severe kidney or liver failure, sensitivity to sulphonamides.
Possible interaction: NSAIDs, alcohol, antidiabetics, opioids, barbiturates, corticosteroids, cardiac glycosides, lithium, tubocurarine.
Side effects: gastro-intestinal upset, blood disorders, rash, sensitivity to light, impotence, anorexia, dizziness, pancreatitis, disturbance to metabolism and electrolyte levels.
Manufacturer: Galen.

XYLOCAINE

Description: a local anaesthetic, lignocaine hydrochloride, available as vials of strength 0.5%, 1% and 2% with or without adrenaline.
Used for: local anaesthetics.
Dosage: 200mg maximum (without adrenaline) or 500mg (with). Children: given in proportion to adult dose. See literature.
Also, **XYLOCAINE OINTMENT** (5% lignocaine) in tube or accordion syringe.
Also, **XYLOCAINE GEL**, 2% lignocaine hydrochloride in tube or accordion syringe, and **XYLOCAINE ANTISEPTIC GEL** containing, in addition, 0.25% chlorhexidine gluconate solution.
Used for: anaesthesia of urethra or vagina, surface anaesthesia.
Dosage: women, 3–5ml; men 10ml to start, then 3–5ml. Not for children.
Also, **XYLOCAINE 4% TOPICAL** (4% lignocaine hydrochloride).
Used for: bronchoscopy, dental treatment, reduced sensitivity to pain in oropharyngeal region, surface anaesthesia.
Dosage: up to 5ml but see literature. Children: up to 3mg/kg.
Also, **XYLOCAINE PUMP SPRAY**, 10mg lignocaine per dose.
Used for: dental treatment, ear, nose and throat surgery, surface anaesthesia in obstetrics.

Dosage: a maximum of 20 doses. Children: in proportion.
Special care: epilepsy.
Avoid use: cardiovascular disease if adrenaline is used, any surgery of the extremities, thyrotoxicosis.
Possible interaction: phenothiazines, tricyclics, MAOIs (if adrenaline version).
Manufacturer: Astra.

XYLOCARD

Description: a class I antiarrhythmic, lignocaine hydrochloride, available in preloaded syringes (100mg).
Used for: arrhythmia of the ventricle associated with myocardial infarction.
Dosage: 50–100mg over 2 minutes, by intravenous injection. Repeat once or twice 5 to 10 minutes, if required. Not for children.
Special care: liver or kidney disease.
Avoid use: heart block, heart conduction disorders, heart failure.
Possible interaction: loop diuretics, thiazides, cimetidine, propanolol.
Side effects: nausea, blurred vision, hypotension, agitation, drowsiness, depression of respiration.
Manufacturer: Astra.

XYLOPROCT

Description: a combined local anaesthetic and steroid containing 60mg lignocaine, 50mg aluminium acetate, 400mg zinc oxide, and 5mg hydrocortisone acetate in suppository form.
Used for: haemorrhoids, itching, anal fissure, anal fistula.
Dosage: 1 at night and after defecation.
Also, **XYLOPROCT OINTMENT** containing 5% lignocaine, 18% zinc oxide, 3.5% aluminium acetate and 0.275% hydrocortisone.
Dosage: use several times per day.
Special care: pregnancy. Do not use over a long period.
Avoid use: infections of a viral, fungal or tuberculous nature.
Side effects: corticosteroid effects.
Manufacturer: Astra.

YUTOPAR

Description: a ß-agonist for relaxation of uterine smooth muscle, ritodrine hydrochloride, available in yellow tablets (10mg) marked YUTOPAR.
Used for: premature labour (with no complications), foetal asphyxiation in labour.
Dosage: 1, half an hour before the end of intravenous therapy. For maintenance, 1 every 2 hours for 24 hours, then 1 or 2 every 4 to 6 hours. Also, **YUTOPAR INJECTION** (10mg/ml in ampoules).
Special care: diabetes, thyrotoxicosis or cardiovascular disease of the mother, monitor heart rate of mother and foetus.
Avoid use: if a prolonged pregnancy would be hazardous, toxaemia of pregnancy, cord compression, antepartum haemorrage (bleeding before the birth and after 28th week), threatened abortion.
Possible interactions: ß-agonists, MAOIs.
Side effects: anxiety, tachycardia, tremor, higher blood sugar levels.
Manufacturer: Duphar.

ZADITEN

Description: an anti-allergic agent and antihistamine, ketotifen, as hydrogen fumarate, available as white, scored tablets (1mg) marked ZADITEN 1. Also **ZADITEN CAPSULES** (1mg white capsules marked CS) and **ZADITEN ELIXIR** (1mg/5ml, sugar-free).
Used for: prevention of bronchial asthma, allergic rhinitis and conjunctivitis.

Dosage: 1–2mg twice per day with food. Children over 2 years, 1mg twice per day with food. Not for children under 2 years.
Avoid use: pregnancy, breastfeeding.
Possible interaction: antihistamines, oral hypoglycaemics, alcohol, depressants of the CNS.
Side effects: dry mouth, dizziness, drowsiness, affected reactions.
Manufacturer: Sandoz.

ZADSTAT

Description: a nitro imidazole and antibacterial/amoeboride/antiprotozoal, metronidazole, available as white tablets (200mg) marked LL and M200.
Used for: infections caused by anaerobic bacteria, amoebiasis, trichomonal infections, ulcerative gingivitis.
Dosage: average 600–800mg per day in divided doses, reduced doses for children. See literature for amoebiasis. Partner should also be treated for trichomonal infections when the dose may be up to 2g as a single dose.
Also **ZADSTAT SUPPOSITORIES** (500mg and 1g).
Dosage: see literature.
Special care: pregnancy, breastfeeding (a high dose treatment is not recommended).
Possible interaction: oral anticoagulants, alcohol, phenobarbitone.
Side effects: leucopenia, urticaria, angioneurotic oedema, furred tongue, unpleasant taste, gastro-intestinal upset, dark urine, disturbance to CNS, seizures on prolonged or intensive treatment.
Manufacturer: Lederle.

ZANTAC

Description: an H_2 blocker, ranitidine hydrochloride, available as white, pentagonal tablets (150mg) and white tablets (300mg) both marked with GLAXO, strength and ZANTAC. Also, **ZANTAC EFFERVESCENT**, 150 and 300mg white effervescent tablets, and **ZANTAC SYRUP**, 150mg/10ml with 7.5% ethanol in a sugar-free syrup.
Used for: duodenal, benign gastric and

post-operative ulcers; ulcers due to NSAIDs. Oesophageal reflux, prevention of ulcers induced by NSAIDs, dyspepsia, oesophagitis.
Dosage: 150mg 2 times per day or 300mg at bedtime. 150mg 4 times per day for oesophagitis. Also see literature. Not for children under 8 years. Over 8 years, for peptic ulcer, 2–4mg/kg twice per day. Also, **ZANTAC INJECTION**, 50mg/2ml as a solution in ampoules.
Special care: exclude malignancy first, kidney disease, pregnancy, lactation.
Side effects: dizziness, headache, sometimes hepatitis, leucopenia, thrombocytopenia, hypersensitivity, confusion.
Manufacturer: Glaxo.

ZARONTIN

Description: a succinimide and anticonvulsant, ethosuximide, in amber oblong capsules (250mg), marked P-D. Also, **ZARONTIN SYRUP** (250mg/5ml).
Used for: petit mal.
Dosage: 500mg per day increasing as required by 250mg at 4 to 7 day intervals to a maximum of 2g per day. Children, 6 to 12 years, adult dose, under 6, 250mg per day adjusted according to response.
Special care: pregnancy, breastfeeding, liver or kidney disease. Withdrawal should be gradual.
Side effects: gastric upset, disturbance to CNS, rashes, blood disorders, SLE.
Manufacturer: Parke-Davis.

ZAVEDOS

Description: a cytotoxic antibiotic, idarubicin hydrochloride, as powder in vials (5 and 10mg). Also, **ZAVEDOS CAPSULES**, 5, 10 and 25mg strengths in capsules coloured orange, red/white and orange/white respectively. Also as powder for reconstitution and injection.
Used for: acute leukaemia.
Special care: teratogenic, liver and kidney disease, irritant to skin and tissues (when handling), heart disease, elderly, monitor heart.

Avoid use: of simultaneous radiotherapy, pregnancy.
Side effects: nausea, vomiting, hair loss, bone marrow suppression, tissue necrosis upon extravasation, inflammation of mucous membranes.
Manufacturer: Farmitalia.

ZESTORETIC

Description: an ACE inhibitor and thiazide diuretic containing 20mg lisinopril and 12.5mg hydrochlorothiazide, in white tablets.
Used for: hypertension.
Dosage: 1 tablet per day (maximum of 2). Not for children.
Special care: liver or kidney disease, gout, diabetes, anaesthesia, ischaemic heart or cerebrovascular disease, haemodialysis, imbalance in fluid or electrolyte levels.
Avoid use: pregnancy, breastfeeding, anuria, angioneurotic oedema in conjunction with previous treatment using ACE inhibitor.
Possible interaction: lithium, NSAIDs, hypoglycaemics, potassium supplements, potassium-sparing diuretics, tubocurarine.
Side effects: headache, fatigue, hypotension, cough, dizziness, nausea, impotence, angioneurotic oedema, diarrhoea.
Manufacturer: Zeneca.

ZESTRIL

Description: an ACE inhibitor, lisinopril, available as tablets, marked with heart shape and strength: 2.5mg (white), 5 and 10mg (pink), and 20mg (red). 2.5, 5, 10 and 20mg have company symbol; 10 and 20mg have a trade mark.
Used for: additional therapy (to digitalis and diuretics) in congestive heart failure, hypertension.
Dosage: start with 2.5mg per day, increasing gradually to a maintenance dose of 5–20mg once per day. Cease using diuretic 2 to 3 days before treatment for hypertension. Reduce dose of diuretic in treating heart failure and start treatment in hospital. Not for children.
Special care: renovascular hypertension

(increased pressure in hepatic portal vein), kidney disease, haemodialysis, congestive heart failure, anaesthesia, breastfeeding.
Avoid use: pregnancy, angioneurotic oedema from past treatment with ACE inhibitor, narrowing of aorta, enlargement of right ventricle.
Possible interaction: potassium supplement, potassium-sparing diuretics, lithium, antihypertensives, indomethacin.
Side effects: kidney failure, angioneurotic oedema, hypotension, dizziness, headache, diarrhoea, fatigue, cough, nausea, palpitations, rash, weakness.
Manufacturer: Zeneca.

ZIMOVANE

Description: a cyclopyrrolone and hypnotic, zopiclone, available as white tablets (7.5mg) marked ZM.
Used for: insomnia.
Dosage: 1 tablet at bedtime (2 if required). Elderly , $^1/_2$ tablet. Not for children.
Special care: liver disorder, check for withdrawal symptoms on completing treatment.
Avoid use: pregnancy, breastfeeding.
Possible interaction: trimipramine, alcohol, other depressants of the CNS.
Side effects: gastro-intestinal upset, metallic aftertaste, allergic reactions, drowsiness, minor behavioural changes, judgement and dexterity may be impaired.
Manufacturer: R.P.R.

ZINACEF

Description: a cephalosporin and antibacterial, cefuroxime (as sodium salt) available in 250mg, 750mg and 1.5g vials.
Used for: infections of soft tissue, the respiratory and urinary tracts, meningitis, gonorrhoea, prevention of infection during surgery.
Dosage: see literature.
Possible interaction: aminoglycosides, loop diuretics.
Side effects: gastro-intestinal upset, hypersensitivity reactions. Occasionally leucopenia, neutropenia, candidosis.
Manufacturer: Glaxo.

ZINAMIDE

Description: a derivative of nicotinic acid, pyrazinamide, in white tablets (500mg) marked MSD 504.
Used for: tuberculosis when used with other anti-tuberculous drugs.
Dosage: 20–35mg/kg/day in divided doses, to a maximum of 3g. Not for children.
Special care: past gout or diabetes, check liver function and blood uric acid.
Avoid use: liver disease. Withdraw if there is liver damage or high blood uric acid with gouty arthritis.
Side effects: hepatitis.
Manufacturer: M.S.D.

ZINERYT

Description: an antibiotic containing erythromycin (4%), zinc acetate (1.2%) in an alcoholic solution.
Used for: acne.
Dosage: use twice daily.
Special care: avoid mucous membranes and eyes.
Side effects: passing irritation.
Manufacturer: Brocades.

ZINNAT

Description: a cephalosporin and antibacterial, cefuroxime axetil, in white tables containing 125 or 250mg, marked GLAXO and 125 or 250. Also, **ZINNAT SUSPENSION** (125mg/5ml).
Used for: infections of the ear, nose and thorat, respiratory or urinary tracts, skin and soft tissues.
Dosage: usually 250mg twice per day after food, 500mg for severe infections and a 1g single dose per day for gonorrhoea. Children over 2 years 250mg twice per day; 3 months–2 years, 125mg twice per day. Not for infants under 3 months.
Special care: pregnancy, breastfeeding, hypersensitivity to penicillin.
Side effects: colitis, hypersensitivity reactions, headache, gastro-intestinal upset, candidosis, increase in liver enzymes.
Manufacturer: Glaxo.

ZIRTEK

Description: an antihistamine, cetirizine hydrochloride, in white oblong tablets (10mg) marked Y/Y.
Used for: urticaria, seasonal rhinitis.
Dosage: 1 tablet per day. Not for children under 6 years; over 6 years, adult dose.
Also, **ZIRTEK SOLUTION** (1mg/ml) in banana-flavoured, sugar-free solution.
Dosage: 10ml per day for adults and children over 6 years. Not for children under 6 years.
Special care: pregnancy, kidney disease.
Avoid use: breastfeeding.
Side effects: agitation, gastro-intestinal upset, dizziness, headache, dry mouth, drowsiness.
Manufacturer: UCB.

ZITA

Description: an H$_2$-blocker, cimetidine, in 200, 400 and 800mg tablets.
Used for: ulcer (stomach, benign gastric and duodenal), reflux oesophagitis, Zollinger-Ellison syndrome.
Dosage: usually 400mg twice per day or 800mg at night for 4 to 8 weeks, depending upon condition. Children, 20–30mg/kg per day in divided doses.
Special care: liver or kidney disease, pregnancy, breastfeeding.
Possible interaction: warfarin, phenytoin, theophylline, pethidine, antiarrhythmics, anticoagulants, rifampicin, antidepressants, antidiabetics, ß-blockers, benzodiazepines, some antipsychotics, chloroquine, carbamazepine.
Side effects: rash, dizziness, fatigue. Occasionally liver disorder, muscle or joint pain, bradycardia and heart block, gynaecomastia (with high dosages).
Manufacturer: Eastern.

ZITHROMAX

Description: a macrolide and antibacterial, azithromycin dihydrate, in white capsules (250mg) marked ZTM250 and Pfizer.
Used for: infections of skin, soft tissue, and respiratory tract, otitis media and certain genital infections.
Dosage: 2 per day for 3 days taken 1 hour before or 2 hours after food.
Also, **ZITHROMAX SUSPENSION**, 200mg/5ml.
Dosage: children: 12 to 14 years, 10ml; 8 to 11 years, 7.5ml; 3 to 7 years, 5ml; under 3 years, 10mg/kg.
Special care: pregnancy, breastfeeding, liver or kidney disorder.
Avoid use: liver disease.
Possible interaction: antacids, cyclosporin, warfarin, digoxin, ergot derivatives.
Side effects: allergic reaction, rash, anaphylaxis, gastro-intestinal upset, angioneurotic oedema.
Manufacturer: Richborough.

ZOCOR

Description: an HMG CoA reductase inhibitor, simvastatin, in oval tablets (10mg, peach; 20mg, tan) marked with strength and ZOCOR.
Used for: primary high blood cholesterol levels.
Dosage: start with 10mg at night, altered to match response, within the range 10–40mg. Not for children.
Special care: past liver disease, check liver function.
Avoid use: pregnancy, women should use non-hormonal contraception, breastfeeding, liver disease.
Possible interaction: cyclosporin, digoxin, coumarin anticoagulants, gemfibrozil, nicotinic acid.
Side effects: headache, nausea, dyspepsia, diarrhoea, abdominal pain, constipation, flatulence, weakness, myopathy.
Manufacturer: M.S.D.

ZOFRAN

Description: a 5HT$_3$-antagonist (blocks nausea and vomiting reflexes), ondansetron hydrochloride in yellow, oval tablets (4 and 8mg) marked with GLAXO and strength.

Also, **ZOFRAN INJECTION** (2mg/ml).
Used for: post-operative nausea and
vomiting or that due to chemo- and
radiotherapy.
Dosage: see literature.
Special care: pregnancy.
Avoid use: breastfeeding.
Side effects: flushes, headache,
constipation.
Manufacturer: Glaxo.

ZOLADEX

Description: a gonadotrophin release
hormone analogue, goserelin acetate, as
a biodegradable depot (3.6mg).
Used for: endometriosis, advanced
breast cancer, prostate cancer.
Dosage: 1 depot subcutaneously in
abdominal wall every 28 days for up
to 6 months.
Special care: those at risk of osteoporosis, or males at risk of obstruction of the
ureter or compression of the spinal cord.
Avoid use: pregnancy, breastfeeding.
Non-hormonal contraception should
be used.
Side effects: headaches, hot flushes,
breast swelling or tenderness, rashes,
vaginal dryness, hypercalcaemia.
Manufacturer: Zeneca.

ZOVIRAX

Description: a nucleoside analogue and
antiviral, acyclovir, available in shield-
shaped tablets; 200mg, blue and marked
ZOVIRAX with a triangle; 400mg, pink
and marked ZOVIRAX 400 with a
triangle. Also 800mg in white, elongated
tablet marked ZOVIRAX 800. Also
ZOVIRAX SUSPENSION (200mg/
5ml) and **ZOVIRAX CHICKENPOX
TREATMENT** (400mg/5ml).
Used for: Herpes simplex and Herpes
zoster particularly in immunocompromised patients.
Dosage: from 800mg–4g per day
depending upon condition. Children
from 200mg 4 times per day. See literature.
Also, **ZOVIRAX INFUSION** (250 and
500mg as powder in vials) and

ZOVIRAX CREAM (5%).
Dosage: use 5 times per day at 4-hour
intervals, for 5 days. Also ointment, (3%).
Used for: herpetic keratitis (inflammation of the cornea).
Dosage: insert 1cm into lower conjuctival
sac 5 times per day continuing 3 days
after healing.
Special care: kidney disease, do not use
cream in eyes.
Possible interaction: probenecid.
Side effects: erythema, flaking skin with
topical use, passing irritation, kidney
disorder, stinging (with ointment).,
Manufacturer: Wellcome.

ZUMENON

Description: an oestrogen, oestradiol,
available as blue tablets (2mg) marked
381 and DUPHAR.
Used for: symptoms of the menopause.
Dosage: start with 1 per day, increased
to 2 if necessary, reducing to 1 as soon
as possible. Commence on fifth day of
menstruation (any time if absent).
Special care: patients at risk of
thrombosis or with liver disease. Women
with any of the following disorders
should be carefully monitored: fibroids
in the womb, multiple sclerosis,
diabetes, tetany, porphyria, epilepsy,
liver disease, hypertension, migraine,
otosclerosis, gallstones. Breasts, pelvic
organs and blood pressure should be
checked at regular intervals during the
course of treatment.
Avoid use; pregnancy, breastfeeding,
women with conditions which might
lead to thrombosis, thrombophlebitis,
serious heart, kidney or liver disease,
breast cancer, oestrogen-dependent
cancers including those of reproductive
system, endometriosis, vaginal bleeding
which is undiagnosed.
Possible interaction: drugs which induce
liver enzymes.
Side effects: tenderness and enlargement
of breasts, weight gain, breakthrough
bleeding, giddiness, vomiting and nausea,
gastro-intestinal upset. Treatment should

be halted immediately if severe headaches occur, disturbance of vision, hypertension or any indications of thrombosis, jaundice. Also, in the event of pregnancy and 6 weeks before planned surgery.
Manufacturer: Duphar.

ZYLORIC
Description: an inhibitor of xanthine oxidase which forms uric acid. Allopurinol is available as white tablets coded U4A (100mg) and ZYLORIC 300 with C9B (300mg).
Used for: gout, prevention of stones of uric acid and calcium oxalate.
Dosage: start with 100–300mg per day. Maintenance dose of 200–600mg per day. Not for children.
Special care: pregnancy, liver or kidney disease, elderly. Anti-inflammatory drug to be given for 1 month at start of treatment. Maintain fluid intake.
Avoid use: acute gout.
Possible interaction: anticoagulants, azathioprine, mercaptopurine, chlorpropamide.
Side effects: nausea, acute gout, withdraw if there are skin reactions.
Manufacturer: Wellcome.

MEDICAL TERMS

ABDOMEN the region of the body which lies below the THORAX, being divided from it by the DIAPHRAGM, and above the pelvis. The abdominal cavity contains the DIGESTIVE ORGANS (e.g. the STOMACH and INTESTINES), the EXCRETORY ORGANS (BLADDER and KIDNEYS) and, in females, the REPRODUCTIVE ORGANS (WOMB and OVARIES).

ABLATION the surgical removal (i.e. by cutting) of any part of the body.

ABORTIFACIENT one of a number of drugs used to bring about an induced ABORTION.

ABORTION the removal of an embryo or foetus from the womb, either by natural expulsion or by human intervention, before it is considered to be viable at the 24th week of pregnancy. An abortion may be SPONTANEOUS, and this is commonest during the first three months of pregnancy and is thought to be most often associated with abnormalities in the foetus. Or, an abortion may be INDUCED, when it is also known as THERAPEUTIC, or TERMINATION OF PREGNANCY, and is carried out for medical or social reasons. Unless the mother's life is at risk, UK legislation requires a therapeutic abortion to be carried out before 24 weeks gestation. A THREATENED ABORTION occurs when the foetus is alive but there is bleeding from the UTERUS and/or pain. If the foetus has died the abortion is referred to as INEVITABLE. An INCOMPLETE ABORTION describes the situation where some of the foetal material is left behind in the uterus.

A HABITUAL ABORTION is where a woman loses each foetus in three consecutive pregnancies before the 20th week. The foetus weighs less than 500 grams and an abnormality in the uterus is one of the reasons why this occurs.

ABO SYSTEM a blood group classification, *see* BLOOD GROUPS.

ABRUPTIO PLACENTAE bleeding from the PLACENTA after the 28th week of PREGNANCY which may result in the placenta becoming completely or partially detached from the wall of the UTERUS.

ABSCESS a collection of pus at a localized site anywhere in the body resulting from an infection caused by bacteria. Treatment is by the surgical opening of the abscess and by the administration of ANTIBIOTICS.

ABSCISSION the surgical removal of tissue by cutting.

ACARDIA the condition which describes the congenital absence of the heart. It may arise where there are Siamese twins, in which case one heart is responsible for the circulation of both infants.

ACETONE a chemical substance which is formed in the body when normal metabolism is upset, as during prolonged bouts of vomiting, starvation, DIABETES MELLITUS and sometimes as a result of severe fevers, particularly in children. The acetone is excreted in the urine and in the breath, and in diabetes may be a forewarning of coma.

ACETYLCHOLINE an important organic chemical substance present in the body which is known as a NEURO TRANSMITTER and is involved in the transmission of electrical impulses along nerves.

ACHALASIA means failure to relax and usually refers to a condition called achalasia of the cardia. It describes the situation where the muscle fibres surrounding the opening of the OESOPHAGUS (gullet) into the stomach do not relax properly, and hinder the passage of food.

ACHONDROPLASIA this is the commonest cause of DWARFISM in which the long bones of the limbs are abnormally short. It is inherited as a dominant characteristic which affects both sexes.

ACIDOSIS describes a condition in which the acidity of the blood and body fluids rises to an abnormally high level due to a failure in the mechanisms which regulate the acid/base balance in the body. It is commonly caused by a faulty metabolism of fat, as in DIABETES MELLITUS or during starvation and excessive vomiting. It may also have a respiratory origin e.g. during drowning when a higher than normal level of carbon dioxide is retained in the body. It also occurs as a result of kidney failure (renal acidosis), when too much sulphuric and phosphoric acids are retained within the body or an excess of bicarbonate is excreted.

ACNE a disorder of the skin, the commonest of which is *acne vulgaris* in adolescents, characterized by the presence of pustules and blackheads. SEBACEOUS GLANDS in the skin become over-active (due to hormonal influence) and there is a greater production of SEBUM and proliferation of bacteria which cause infection. The hair follicles become blocked and pustules form which eventually turn black. The condition usually resolves with time but can be eased with creams and sometimes antibiotics. Other forms of acne also occur, *see* ROSACEA.

ACQUIRED a condition or malady that is not CONGENITAL but arises after birth.

ACTION POTENTIAL *see* NERVE IMPULSE.

ACUTE a disease or condition which is short-lived, and which starts rapidly with severe symptoms.

ADACTYLY describes the absence of fingers or toes (digits).

ADAM'S APPLE a projection of the thyroid cartilage of the LARYNX which is visible beneath the skin of the throat.

ADDICTION a broadly-used term which describes a state of physical and psychological dependence upon a substance or drug.

ADDISON'S DISEASE a disease caused by the failure of the ADRENAL GLANDS to secrete certain substances (the adrenocortical hormones), because the adrenal cortex has been damaged. This damage commonly used to be caused by tuberculosis but now, it may more often result from disturbances in the immune system. The symptoms of the disease are wasting, weakness, low blood pressure and dark pigmentation of the skin. A complete cure can be effected by replacing the deficient hormones with hormone replacement therapy.

ADENITIS refers to inflammation of one or more glands.

ADENOIDECTOMY the removal, by surgery, of the ADENOIDS.

ADENOIDS a clump of lymphoid tissue situated at the back of the nose (in the nasopharynx). The adenoids may become swollen as a result of persistent throat infections, and obstruct breathing through the nose.

ADIPOSE TISSUE a type of loose, fibrous, connective tissue containing a mass of fat cells. Excess food is laid down and stored within the fat cells and adipose tissue is found beneath the skin and around the kidneys. It provides a reserve energy store and also has an insulating function.

ADJUVANT THERAPY a type of drug therapy used in the management of certain cancers following on from radiotherapy, or surgical removal of a primary tumour. The aim is to destroy secondary tumours where there is a risk of these occurring and it is sometimes used in the treatment of breast cancer.

ADRENAL GLANDS each of the two kidneys within the body bears an adrenal gland upon its upper surface. The adrenal glands, also known as suprarenal glands, are important ENDOCRINE organs, producing

HORMONES that regulate various body functions. Each adrenal gland has two parts, an outer cortex and an inner medulla which secrete a variety of hormones. Two of the most important ones are ADRENALINE and CORTISONE.

ADRENALINE a very important hormone produced by the medulla of the adrenal glands which, when released, prepares the body for "fright, flight or fight" by increasing the depth and rate of respiration, raising the heartbeat rate and improving muscle performance. It also has an inhibitive effect on the processes of digestion and excretion. It can be used medically in a variety of ways, for instance in the treatment of bronchial asthma where it relaxes the airways. It may be applied to wounds to check bleeding, as it constricts blood vessels in the skin, and also to stimulate the heart when there is cardiac arrest. Adrenaline is also known as epinephrine. *See* ADDISON'S DISEASE.

ADRENOCORTICOTROPHIC HORMONE (ACTH) is an important substance produced and stored by the anterior PITUITARY GLAND. It regulates the release of corticosteroid hormones from the adrenal glands and is used medically, by injection, to test their function. It is also used in the treatment of asthma and rheumatic disorders.

ADULT RESPIRATORY DISTRESS SYNDROME describes the condition of severe respiratory failure brought about by a number of different disorders. There is a lack of oxygen in the blood, which exhibits itself by imparting a blue tinge to the skin, and rapid breathing and pulse rate. The syndrome may be caused by physical damage to the lungs, by infection or by an adverse reaction following surgery or transfusion. It is often fatal.

AGORAPHOBIA an abnormal fear of public places or open spaces.

AIDS this refers to *A*cquired *I*mmune *D*eficiency *S*yndrome which was first recognized in Los Angeles in the U.S.A. in 1981. The causal agent was identified in 1983 as being the human immunodeficiency virus known as HIV, a ribonucleic acid (RNA) RETROVIRUS. The virus has been found in blood, other body fluids, semen and cervical secretions and is mainly transmitted by sexual activity. The HIV virus affects the T-LYMPHOCYTES of the immune system, and leaves the patient increasingly unable to resist certain infections and tumours which are particularly associated with AIDS. Although they may take a long time to develop, these infections eventually prove to be fatal and at the present time there is no known cure for AIDS.

AIR EMBOLISM a bubble of air in a blood vessel which interferes with the outward flow of blood from the right ventricle of the heart. The air may enter the circulation after an injury, surgery or infusion into a vein. The symptoms are chest pain and breathlessness leading to acute heart failure.

AIR PASSAGES these are all the openings and passages through which air enters and is taken into the lungs. These are the nose, pharynx (throat), larynx, trachea (windpipe) and bronchial tubes. Air entering via this route has dust particles removed, and is warmed and moistened before entering the lungs.

ALIMENTARY CANAL the whole of the passage along which food is passed starting at the mouth and ending at the anus.

ALKALOSIS an abnormal rise in the alkalinity (a decrease in pH) of the blood and body fluids due to a failure or swamping of the mechanisms which regulate the acid-base balance in the body. It may arise through acid loss following prolonged vomiting, or occur in a patient who has been treated for a gastric ulcer with a large amount of alkalis. Respiratory alkalosis may arise if breathing is too deep for the amount of physical exertion being undertaken. The symptoms of alkalosis include muscular cramps and fatigue.

ALLANTOIS a structure which develops

early in the life of an embryo and grows out from the hindgut, becoming attached to the wall of the womb. It later develops into the placenta and umbilical cord.

ALLELE one of several forms of a GENE at a given place on the CHROMOSOME. They are usually present on different chromosomes and are responsible for certain characteristics of the PHENOTYPE. It is the dominance of one allele over another that determines the phenotype of the individual.

ALLERGEN any substance, usually a protein, which causes a hypersensitive (allergic) reaction in a person who is exposed to the allergen. There are a great variety of allergens which cause reactions in different tissues and body functions. The respiratory system and skin are often affected.

ALLERGY a state of hypersensitivity in an affected individual to a particular allergen, which produces a characteristic response whenever the person is exposed to the substance. In an unaffected person, antibodies present in the bloodstream destroy their particular antigens (ALLERGENS). However, in an affected individual this reaction causes some cell damage and there is a release of substances such as histamine and bradykin which cause the allergic reaction. Examples of allergies are dermatitis, hay fever, asthma and the severe response known as ANAPHYLAXIS.

ALOPECIA *see* BALDNESS.

ALPHA FETOPROTEIN a type of protein formed in the liver and gut of the foetus and which is detectable in the amniotic fluid and maternal blood. It is normally present in small amounts in the AMNIOTIC FLUID but when the foetus has a neural tube defect (SPINA BIFIDA and ANENCEPHALY), this level rises higher during the first six months of pregnancy. It can be detected by a maternal blood test at about the 16th week of pregnancy, and confirmed by AMNIOCENTESIS. If a foetus has DOWN'S SYNDROME, the level of alpha fetoprotein may be abnormally

low. Alpha fetoprotein is also produced by some adult tissues if there is an abnormality present such as a type of liver cancer known as HEPATOMA.

ALVEOLUS (*plural* **ALVEOLI**) a small sac or cavity which in numbers forms the alveolar sacs at the end of the BRONCHIOLES in the lungs. Each alveolus is fed by a rich blood supply via capillaries (*see* CAPILLARY) and is lined with a moist membrane where oxygen and carbon dioxide, the respiratory gases, are exchanged. The alveolar sacs provide an enormous surface area for efficient respiration.

ALZHEIMER'S DISEASE the commonest cause of dementia afflicting those in middle or old age, and a degenerative disease of the cerebral cortex for which there is no cure. Symptoms include progressive loss of memory and speech and paralysis. The cause is not understood but is the subject of ongoing research.

AMENORRHOEA an absence of MENSTRUATION which is normal before puberty, during PREGNANCY and while breast-feeding is being carried out and following the MENOPAUSE. Primary amenorrhoea describes the situation where the menstrual periods do not begin at puberty. This occurs if there is a chromosome abnormality (such as TURNER'S SYNDROME) or if some reproductive organs are absent. It can also occur where there is a hormone or imbalance in the secretion of hormones. In secondary amenorrhoea, the menstrual periods stop when they would normally be expected to be present. There are a variety of causes including hormone deficiency, disorders of the HYPOTHALAMUS, psychological and environmental stresses, during starvation, anorexia nervosa or depression.

AMINES naturally-occurring compounds found in the body which have an important role in a variety of functions. They are derived from AMINO ACIDS and ammonia and include such substances as ADRENALINE and HISTAMINE.

AMINO ACIDS the end products of the digestion of PROTEIN foods and are the building blocks from which all the protein components of the body are built up. They all contain an acidic carboxyl group (-COOH) and an amino group (-NH$_2$) which are both bonded to the same central carbon atom. Some can be manufactured within the body whereas others, the ESSENTIAL AMINO ACIDS, must be derived from protein sources in the diet.

AMNESIA loss of memory which may be partial or total. *Anterograde* amnesia is the loss of memory of recent events following a trauma of some kind. *Retrograde* amnesia is the inability to remember events that preceded a trauma. Other types of amnesia are *post-traumatic* and *hysterical* and more than one kind may be experienced by an individual.

AMNIOCENTESIS a procedure carried out to sample the amniotic fluid surrounding a foetus in order to test it in the laboratory. A fine needle is inserted through the abdominal wall of the mother and the amniotic sac is pierced so that a small quantity of fluid can be drawn off. The amniotic fluid contains ALPHA FETOPROTEIN and cells from the embryo, and various disorders such as Down's syndrome and spina bifida can be detected. If performed, it is usually between the 16th and 20th week of pregnancy.

AMNION a fibrous, tough membranous sac which lines the womb and encloses the foetus floating within it surrounded by amniotic fluid. A "caul" is a piece of the amnion.

AMNIOSCOPY the procedure by which an instrument (an endoscope) is inserted either by means of an incision through the mother's abdominal wall or through her cervix, in order to view the foetus. An amnioscope is used if the procedure is carried out abdominally and a fetoscope if through the cervix.

AMNIOTIC CAVITY the cavity, filled with fluid, which is enclosed by the amnion and surrounds the foetus.

AMNIOTIC LIQUID the liquid within the amniotic cavity which is clear and composed mainly of water containing foetal cells, lipids and urine from the foetus. At first it is produced by the amnion but its volume is supplemented by urine from the kidneys of the foetus. It is circulated by being swallowed by the foetus and excreted by the kidneys back into the cavity, and has an important protective function. The amniotic fluid ("waters") is released when the membranes rupture during labour.

AMNIOTOMY this refers to the artificial rupture of membranes or ARM which is carried out surgically by means of an instrument called an amnihook. The amnion is ruptured in order to induce the onset of labour.

AMPHETAMINES a group of drugs that are chemically similar to adrenaline and have a stimulatin effect on the central nervous system. They act on the SYMPATHETIC NERVOUS SYSTEM and produce feelings of mental alertness and well-being, eliminating tiredness. However, they are highly addictive and their medical use (mainly in the treatment of hyperkinetic syndrome, a mental disorder in children) is strictly controlled.

AMPICILLIN a type of semi-synthetic penicillin used to treat various infections and usually given by mouth or injection.

AMPOULE a small plastic or glass bubble which is sterile and sealed, usually containing one dose of a drug to be administered by injection.

ANABOLIC (STEROIDS) refers to the effect of enhancing tissue growth by promoting the build-up of protein e.g. to enhance muscle bulk. Anabolic steroids are synthetic male sex hormones (which mimic ANDROGEN), and are used medically to aid weight gain after wasting illnesses and to promote growth in children with certain types of dwarfism. They may also be used in the treatment of osteo-porosis. Anabolic steroids should not be taken by healthy people as they have serious side effects especially after prolonged use, and have been misused by athletes.

ANAEMIA a decrease in the ability of the blood to carry oxygen due to a reduction in the number of red blood cells or in the amount of haemoglobin which they contain. Haemoglobin is the pigment within the red blood cells which binds to oxygen. There are a number of different types of anaemia and a variety of reasons for it, and treatment depends upon the underlying cause.

ANAESTHESIA a loss of sensation or feeling in the whole or part of the body, usually relating to the administration of ANAESTHETIC drugs so that surgery can be performed.

ANAESTHETIC a substance which, when administered, produces a loss of sensation in the whole (general) or part (local) of the body. General anaesthetics result in a loss of consciousness and usually a combination of drugs are used to achieve an optimum effect. These act to depress the activity of the CENTRAL NERVOUS SYSTEM, have an ANALGESIC effect and relax muscles, enabling surgical procedures to be carried out with no awareness on the part of the patient. Local anaesthetics block the transmission of nerve impulses in the area where they are applied so that no pain is felt. Commonly used ones are cocaine and lignocaine and they are used for minor surgical procedures and in dentistry.

ANAESTHETIST a doctor who is medically specialized in the administration of anaesthetics.

ANALGESIA a state of reduced reaction to pain, but without loss of consciousness. It may be due to drugs (*see* ANALGESICS) or it may happen accidentally should nerves become diseased or damaged.

ANALGESICS drugs or substances which relieve pain varying in potency from mild, such as paracetamol and aspirin, to very strong e.g. pethidine and morphine.

ANAPHYLAXIS a response exhibited by a hypersensitive individual when confronted with a particular ANTIGEN. It results from the release of histamine in body tissues following the antigen-antibody reaction within cells. An allergic reaction is an example of mild anaphylaxis. Anaphylactic shock is a much rarer and more serious condition which can follow the injection of drugs or vaccines, or a bee sting, to which the individual is hypersensitive. Its onset is immediate and results from a widespread release of histamine in the body. The symptoms include severe breathing difficulties, swelling (OEDEMA), a fall in blood pressure, acute URTICARIA and heart failure. Death may follow if the individual is not soon treated with adrenaline by injection.

ANAPLASIA the condition in which cells and tissues become less differentiated and distinctive and revert to a more primitive form. This state is typical in tumours which are malignant and growing very rapidly.

ANASTOMOSIS in surgery this refers to the artificial joining together of two or more tubes which are normally separate e.g. between parts of the intestine or blood vessels. In anatomy, this is the area of communication between the end branches of adjacent blood vessels.

ANATOMY the scientific study of the body structure of man and animals.

ANDROGEN one of a group of hormones which is responsible for the development of the sex organs and also the secondary sexual characteristics in the male. Androgens are steroid HORMONES and the best known example is TESTOSTERONE. They are mainly secreted by the TESTES in the male but are also produced by the adrenal cortex and by the ovaries of females, in small amounts.

ANENCEPHALY a failure in the development of a foetus resulting in the absence of the cerebral hemispheres of the brain and some skull bones. If the pregnancy goes to term the infant dies soon after birth, but spontaneous abortion occurs in about 50% of affected pregnancies. Anencephaly is often associated with SPINA BIFIDA and is the most common developmental defect of the central nervous system. Anencephaly can be detected during the pregnancy by measuring the amount of ALPHA FETO-PROTEIN present, *see also* AMNIOCENTESIS.

ANEUPLOIDY this describes the condition in which an abnormal number of chromosomes are present in the cells of an affected individual. The number of chromosomes is either more or less than the normal exact multiple of the HAPLOID number (half the full complement) and is characteristic of DOWN'S SYNDROME and TURNER'S SYNDROME, *see* EUPLOID.

ANEURYSM a balloon-like swelling of the wall of an artery which occurs when i tbecomes weakened or damaged in some way. There may be a congenital weakness in the muscular wall of the artery involved, as is often the case within the brain. Damage may also be the result of infection, particularly SYPHILIS, or degenerative conditions e.g. ATHEROMA. There is a danger within the brain that an aneurysm may rupture causing a SUB-ARACHNOID HAEMORRHAGE or cerebral haemorrhage. The surgical treatment of aneurysms has greatly advanced and is very successful in many cases.

ANGINA a suffocating, choking pain, usually used in reference to angina pectoris, which is felt in the chest. The pain is felt or brought on by exercise and relieved by rest, and occurs when the blood supply to the heart muscle is inadequate. During exercise the demand for blood (supplied by the coronary arteries) is increased and if the supply is insufficient, because the arteries are damaged, chest pain results. The coronary arteries may be damaged by ATHEROMA, the most common cause. Angina pectoris is usually first treated with drugs but if the condition worsens, coronary-artery by-pass surgery (ANGIOPLASTY) may need to be performed.

ANGIOCARDIOGRAPHY an X-ray examination technique of the activity of the heart involving the injecting of a radio-opaque substance. The X-ray film

obtained is called an angiocardiogram.

ANGIOGRAPHY an examination technique of blood vessels using X-rays, made possible by first injecting a radio-opaque substance. If the blood vessels being examined are arteries it is called arteriography and if veins, venography or phlebography.

ANGIOMA a clump of distended blood vessels pushing onto the surface of the brain. It may cause epilepsy and occasionally a vessel may burst to cause a SUBARACHNOID HAEMORRHAGE.

ANGIONEUROTIC OEDEMA a short-lived painless swelling which may result from infection, allergic reaction to drugs or food, stress or it can be hereditary.

ANGIOPLASTY a surgical method used to widen or re-open a narrowed or blocked blood vessel or heart valve. A balloon is inserted and then inflated to clear the obstruction.

ANGITIS otherwise known as vasculitis, this describes the condition where there is inflammation of the walls of small blood vessels, usually in patches.

ANOXIA the condition when the body tissues do not receive sufficient oxygen. It may be due to high altitudes (and thus lower atmospheric pressure), a lack of red blood cells, or a disease such as PNEUMONIA which limits the amount of oxygen reaching the lung surfaces and therefore reduces that available for transfer to the blood.

ANTACIDS substances which neutralize acidity, usually hydrochloric acid in the digestive juices of the stomach. An example is sodium bicarbonate.

ANTAGONISTIC ACTION an action in which systems or processes act against each other so that the activity of one reduces that of the other. Two muscles may operate in this way, the contraction of one necessitating the relaxation of the other, as in the movement of a limb. In addition, hormones and drugs act antagonistically, the release of one limiting the effect of the other.

ANTENATAL before birth. Pregnant women attend antenatal clinics which monitor the health of both mothers and their unborn babies.

ANTIBIOTIC a substance, derived from a micro-organism which kills or inhibits the multiplication of other micro-organisms, usually bacteria or fungi. Well-known examples are penicillin and streptomycin.

ANTIBODIES protein substances of the GLOBULIN type which are produced by the lymphoid tissue and circulate in the blood. They react with their correspond-ing ANTIGENS and neutralize them, rendering them harmless. Antibodies are produced against a wide variety of antigens and these reactions are responsible for IMMUNITY and ALLERGY.

ANTICHOLINERGIC SIDE EFFECTS the effects that may be experienced when taking anticholinergic drugs. The drugs compete with the NEUROTRANSMITTER ACETYLCHOLINE at the synapses of nerves resulting in typical side effects such as dry mouth, nausea, vomiting, retention of urine, constipation and impaired vision.

ANTICOAGULANTS drugs or substances which delay or tend to prevent blood clotting, examples of which are warfarin and heparin. These are used in the treatment of EMBOLISM and THROMBOSIS to disperse blood clots in vessels.

ANTICONVULSANTS drugs which are used to reduce the severity of epileptic fits (convulsions) or to prevent them from occurring.

ANTIDEPRESSANTS drugs which are administered in order to alleviate depression and its accompanying symptoms.

ANTIDOTE a substance which counter-acts the effect of a particular poison.

ANTIEMETIC a drug taken in order to prevent vomiting, such as are used for travel sickness, and VERTIGO.

ANTIGENS any substances which cause the formation by the body of ANTIBODIES to neutralize their effect.

Antigens are often protein substances, regarded as "foreign" and "invading" by the body, and elicit the production of antibodies against them. *See* ALLERGEN, ALLERGY and ANAPHYLAXIS.

ANTIHISTAMINES drugs which counteract the effects of histamine release in the body. They are widely used to treat allergic reactions of various sorts, particularly to relieve skin conditions. Those taken by mouth have a sedative effect and so care must be taken while they are being used.

ANTI-INFLAMMATORY anything which reduces inflammation. Typical anti-inflammatory drugs are the antihistamines, non-steroidal anti-inflammatory drugs (NSAID types used especially in the treatment of rheumatic disease) and glucocorticoids.

ANTIMETABOLITES a group of drugs used particularly in the treatment of certain cancers which mimic substances (metabolites) present in the cells. The antimetabolites combine with enzymes which would otherwise use the metabolites for cell growth. Hence they reduce the growth of cancer cells but also have attendant side effects which can be severe.

ANTIPERISTALSIS see PERISTALSIS.

ANTISEPTICS substances which prevent the growth of disease-causing micro-organisms such as bacteria, and are applied to the skin to prevent infection and to cleanse wounds. Examples are iodine and crystal violet.

ANTISERUM a serum that is usually prepared from horses, which contains a high concentration of antibody against a particular antigen. It is injected to give immunity against a particular disease or toxin.

ANURIA a failure of the kidneys to produce urine which may result from a number of disorders which cause a prolonged drop in blood pressure. Anuria is typical of increasing URAEMIA and HAEMODIALYSIS may be necessary.

ANUS the opening of the alimentary

canal at the opposite end from the mouth, through which faeces are voided. The anus is at the lower end of the bowel and its opening is controlled by two muscles, the internal and external sphincters.

ANXIETY see NEUROSIS.

AORTA the major large artery of the body which arises from the left ventricle of the heart and which carries blood to all areas. The other arteries of the body are all derived from the aorta.

AORTIC STENOSIS a narrowing of the opening of the aortic valve resulting in the obstruction of bloodflow from the left ventricle to the aorta. A common cause of this is calcium deposits formed on the valve associated with ATHEROMA, or damage may have been caused by previous RHEUMATIC FEVER. Also, the condition may arise CONGENITALLY. The effect is that the left ventricle muscle has to work harder in order to try and maintain the blood flow and becomes thicker as a result. The symptoms of aortic stenosis include ANGINA PECTORIS, breathlessness, and the condition is treated surgically by valve replacement.

APHASIA speechlessness caused by disease or injury to those parts of the brain which govern the activities involved in speech-making. It is caused by THROMBOSIS, EMBOLISM or HAEMORRHAGE of a blood vessel within the brain as in a STROKE, or by a TUMOUR. It may be temporary if the blood supply is not permanently damaged, but often the power of speech continues to be impaired and is associated with other intellectual disorders.

APHONIA loss of the voice which may be caused by disease or damage to the LARYNX or mouth or to nerves controlling throat muscles, or may result from hysteria.

APLASIA a complete or partial failure in the correct development of an organ or tissue.

APNOEA a temporary halt in breathing which may result from a number of different causes. Apnoea is quite common in newborn infants and can be registered by an apnoea monitor which sounds an alarm if the baby ceases to breathe.

APOCRINE the term for sweat glands that occur in hairy parts of the body. The odours associated with sweating are due to bacterial action on the sweat produced (see also PERSPIRATION)

APPENDICECTOMY also APPENDECTOMY, this is the surgical operation to remove the vermiform APPENDIX.

APPENDICITIS inflammation of the vermiform APPENDIX which, in its acute form, is the most common abdominal emergency in the western world, usually requiring treatment by APPENDICECTOMY. It is most common in young people during their first 20 years, and the symptoms include abdominal pain which may move about, appetite loss, sickness and diarrhoea. If not treated the appendix can become the site of an ABSCESS, or gangrenous, which eventually may result in PERITONITIS. This arises because infected material spreads from the burst appendix into the peritoneal cavity. Appendicectomy at an early stage is highly successful and normally results in a complete cure.

APPENDIX a blind-ended tube which is an appendage of various organs within the body. It normally refers to the vermiform appendix which is about 9 to 10 cm long and projects from the CAECUM (a pouch) of the large intestine. It has no known function and can become the site of infection probably as the result of obstruction. See APPENDICECTOMY and APPENDICITIS.

AREOLA means a small space and usually refers to the brown-coloured, pigmented ring around the nipple of the breast.

ARRYTHMIA any disturbance in the normal rhythm of heartbeat. The built-in pacemaker of the heart is the sinoatrial node situated in the wall of the right atrium, which itself is regulated by the AUTONOMIC NERVOUS SYSTEM. The electrical impulses produced by the pacemaker control the rate and rhythm of heartbeat. Arrythmias occur when these electrical impulses are disturbed and there are various different types including EXTRASYSTOLES (ectopic beats), ectopic tachycardias, heart block and FIBRILLATION. Most heart diseases cause arryhmias but they may also arise for no obvious cause.

ARTERIECTOMY the surgical removal of a part or the whole of an artery.

ARTERIOGRAM the recording of an arterial pulse which appears as a trace in wave form. It may be recorded on an oscilloscope screen or on a paper strip by various methods.

ARTERIOGRAPHY the X-ray examination of an artery following the injection of a radio opaque substance.

ARTERIOLE a small branch of an artery leading to a capillary.

ARTERIOPLASTY surgery to reconstruct an artery which is carried out especially in the treatment of ANEURYSMS.

ARTERIOSCLEROSIS a vague term used to describe several degenerative conditions affecting the arteries. *See* ATHEROMA, ATHEROSCLEROSIS.

ARTERITIS inflammation of an artery.

ARTERY a blood vessel which carries blood away from the heart. Oxygenated (bright red) blood is carried by the arteries to all parts of the body. However, the pulmonary arteries carry dark, unoxygenated blood from the heart to the lungs. An artery has thick, elastic walls which are able to expand and contract, and contain smooth muscle fibres. This smooth muscle is uder the control of the SYMPATHETIC NERVOUS SYSTEM.

ARTHRITIS inflammation of the joints or spine, the symptoms of which are pain and swelling, restriction of movement, redness and warmth of the skin. There are many different causes of arthritis including OSTEOARTHRITIS, RHEUMATOID ARTHRITIS, TUBERCULOSIS and RHEUMATIC FEVER.

ARTHROPATHY any joint order or disease.

ARTHROPLASTY the operation to repair a diseased joint by constructing a new one, often involving the insertion of artificial materials.

ARTIFICIAL INSEMINATION SEMEN collected from a donor is inserted by means of an instrument into the vagina of a woman in the hope that she will conceive. The semen may be from her husband or partner (AIH) or from an anonymous donor (AID) and is introduced near the time of ovulation. Usually AIH is used where the partner is impotent and AID when he is sterile.

ARTIFICIAL RESPIRATION an emergency procedure carried out when normal respiration has ceased in order to artificially ventilate the lungs, usually referred to as "mouth-to-mouth resuscitation." In hospital where a seriously ill person is unable to breathe unaided, artificial respiration is achieved by means of a machine known as a ventilator.

ASEPSIS a state of complete absence of harmful pathogenic micro-organisms achieved by various sterilization techniques. This is the optimum state in which operations are carried out.

ASPIRATION the process of removing fluid or gases from cavities in the body by means of suction. The instrument used is called an aspirator and various types exist depending upon site of use.

ASPIRIN a type of drug in widespread use which is correctly called acetylsalicylic acid. It is used to relieve mild pain e.g. headache, neuralgia and that associated with rheumatoid arthritis. It is also used to combat fever, and is also helpful in the prevention of CORONARY THROMBOSIS. In susceptible individuals it may cause irritation and bleeding of the stomach lining and is not normally given to children under the age of 12 years. High doses will cause dizziness and possibly mental confusion.

ASTHMA a condition characterized by breathing difficulties caused by narrowing of the airways (bronchi, *see* BRONCHUS) of the lung.

It is a distressing condition with breathlessness and a paroxysmal wheezing cough and the extent to which the bronchi narrow varies considerably. Asthma may occur at any age but usually begins in early childhood, and is a hypersensitive response which can be brought on by exposure to a variety of ALLERGENS, exercise, stress or infections. An asthma sufferer may have other hypersensitive conditions such as eczema and hay fever, and it may be prevalent within a family. It may or may not be possible for a person to avoid the allergen(s) responsible for an asthma attack. Treatment involves the use of drugs to dilate the airways (bronchodilators) and also inhaled corticosteroids.

ASTRINGENT a substance that causes cells to contract by losing proteins from their surface. They cause localized contraction of blood vessels and are applied to minor wounds of the skin, and are used in mouth washes and eye drops.

ATAXIA a loss of co-ordination in the limbs due to a disorder of the CENTRAL NERVOUS SYSTEM. There may be a disease of the sensory nerves (sensory ataxia) or of the CEREBELLUM (cerebellar ataxia). An ataxic person produces clumsy movements and lacks fine control. See FRIEDREICH'S ATAXIA and LOCOMOTOR ATAXIA.

ATHEROMA a degenerative condition of the arteries. The inner and middle coats of the arterial walls become scarred and fatty deposits (CHOLESTEROL) are built up at these sites. The blood circulation is impaired and it may lead to such problems as ANGINA pectoris, stroke and heart attack. The condition is associated with the western lifestyle. i.e. lack of exercise, smoking, obesity and too high an intake of animal fats.

ATHEROSCLEROSIS similar to ATHEROMA being a degenerative disease of the arteries associated with fatty deposits on the inner walls leading to reduced blood flow.

ATHLETE'S FOOT a fungal infection of the skin particularly occurring between the toes and often due to ringworm.

ATRIUM (pl. ATRIA) one of the two thin-walled, upper chambers of the heart, which receive blood from major veins. The right atrium receives (deoxygenated) blood from the venae cavae and the left atrium is supplied with (oxygenated) blood from the pulmonary vein. (Atria also refers to various other chambers in the body.)

ATROPHY wasting of a body part due to lack of use, malnutrition or as a result of ageing. The ovaries of women atrophy after the menopause and muscular atrophy accompanies certain diseases. See POLIOMYELITIS.

AURAL anything relating to the ear.

AURICLE the external part of the ear of flap known as the pinna. Also, an ear-shaped appendage of the ATRIUM of the heart.

AUTOANTIBODY an antibody produced by the body against one of its own tissues which is a feature of AUTOIMMUNE DISEASE.

AUTOIMMUNE DISEASE one of a number of conditions resulting from the production of antibodies by the body which attack its own tissues. For reasons which are not understood the immune system loses the ability to distinguish between "self" and "non-self". Autoimmune disease is currently thought to be the cause of a number of disorders including acquired haemolytic anaemia (see HAEMOLYSIS), PERNICIOUS ANAEMIA, RHEUMATOID ARTHRITIS, RHEUMATIC FEVER and DIABETES MELLITUS.

AUTOCLAVE equipment used to sterilize surgical equipment and dressings, etc. by means of steam at high pressure. It is one of the most important methods of sterilization.

AUTOGRAFT a graft of skin or tissue taken from one part of a person's body and transferred to another region. Since the graft is "self" it is not rejected by the body's immune system.

AUTOIMMUNITY a failure of the immune system in which the body develops antibodies that attack components or substances belonging to itself. *See* AUTOANTIBODY, AUTOIMMUNE DISEASE.

AUTONOMIC NERVOUS SYSTEM the part of the nervous system which controls body functions that are not under conscious control, e.g. the heartbeat and other smooth muscles and glands. It is divided into the SYMPATHETIC and PARASYMPATHETIC NERVOUS SYSTEMS.

AUTOPSY or *post mortem*, the examination and dissection of a body after death.

AXON *see* NEURON.

BACILLUS (*plural* bacilli) a term for any bacterium that is rod-shaped. Also a genus of gram-positive (*see* GRAM'S STAIN) bacteria that includes *B. anthracis*, the cause of anthrax.

BACKBONE *see* SPINAL COLUMN.

BACTERIA (*singular* bacterium) single-celled organisms that underpin all life sustaining processes. GRAM'S STAIN is a test used to distinguish between the two types (Gram positive and Gram negative). They are also identified by shape: spiral, (spirilli), rod-like (bacilli), spherical (cocci), comma-shaped (vibrid) and the spirochaetal that are corkscrew-like. Bacteria are the key agents in the chemical cycles of carbon, oxygen, nitrogen and sulphur. Some are responsible for disease in plants and animals, e.g. tuberculosis, typhoid, syphilis and cholera.

BACTERICIDE something that kills bacteria, but used especially when referring to drugs and antiseptics.

BACTERIOLOGY the study of bacteria.

BACTERIOPHAGE a virus that attacks a BACTERIUM. The phage replicates in the host which is ultimately destroyed as new phages are released.

Each phage is specific to a certain bacterium and uses are found in genetic engineering in cloning and certain manufacturing processes.

BALDNESS the gradual depletion of hair on the head which is to a great extent hereditary. Baldness is a symptom of some diseases, e.g. SYPHILIS, MYXOEDEMA, and anaemia and *alopecia* is a patchy baldness of the scalp that can affect other areas of the body. Baldness is often preceded (for several years) by SEBORRHOEIC ECZEMA which causes hair follicles to lose their capacity to produce hair in the natural cycle of replacement.

BALSAM one of several resinous substances, in the main derived from evergreens, that contain BENZOIC ACID, e.g. Friar's balsam and balsam of tolu. They are used to alleviate colds and may be applied to abrasions.

BARBITURATE drugs that are derived from barbituric acid and which have anaesthetic, hypnotic or sedative effects. Barbiturates reduce blood pressure and temperature and depress the central nervous system and respiration. TRANQUILLIZERS are replacing barbiturates to lessen drug abuse.

BARIUM SULPHATE a heavy chemical powder used in X-ray examinations. Due to its opaque (to X-rays) nature, it forms a shadow in whatever cavity it lies. It is used for the examination of the stomach and intestines and can be used to trace a meal through the bowels.

BARRIER CREAM a cream, lotion or ointment put on to the skin to provide protection against irritants, allergens, sunlight, etc. Water-repellent silicones are frequently used.

BASAL GANGLION GREY MATTER at the base of the CEREBRUM that is involved in the subconscious control of voluntary movement.

BASE PAIRING linking of the two strands of a DNA molecule between the bases of the constituent NUCLEOTIDES. The bases differ in structure: adenine and guanine being purines; thymine, cytosine and uracil being pyrimidines; and a purine bonds to a pyrimidine, e.g. A - T, C - G. The particular nature of the base pairing produces a highly structured DNA that can be replicated precisely (ensuring accurate transmission of genetic information from parent to daughter cell).

BCG VACCINE Bacillus Calmette-Guérin vaccine, named after the two French bacteriologists and first introduced in France in 1908. It is used as a vaccine against TUBERCULOSIS, usually administered intradermally, and complications are rare. A pre-vaccination test is applied to all save the new-born and vaccination is given to those showing a negative result. Vaccination is usually given to: school children aged 10 to 14; children of Asian origin because tuberculosis has a high incidence in this ethnic group; health workers and others.

BELL'S PALSY a paralysis of the facial muscles on either or both sides of the face caused by infection/inflammation, when it may be temporary. Permanent paralysis may result from a basal skull fracture, stroke, etc. The paralysis results in an inability to open and close the eye, smile, close the mouth on the side affected.

B ENDORPHIN a painkiller released by the PITUITARY in response to pain and stress.

BENEDICT'S TEST a test for glucose and reducing sugars. It consists of a solution of copper sulphate, sodium carbonate and sodium citrate to which the sample is added. The resulting solution is boiled and sugar is indicated by a rust-coloured precipitate. The test is used to detect sugar in urine if DIABETES is suspected.

BENIGN used most frequently with reference to tumours, meaning not harmful.

BENZENE HEXACHLORIDE a rapidly acting insecticide.

BENZHEXOL (or benzhexol hydrochloride, also trihexyphenidyl hydrochloride) a drug prescribed in the treatment of Parkinson's disease (see PARKINSONISM).

BENZOCAINE used in various forms, a local anaesthetic for relief of painful skin conditions including those within the mouth.

BENZODIAZEPINES a group of drugs that act as tranquillizers (e.g. diazepam), hypnotics (flurazepam) and anticonvulsants, depending upon the duration of action.

BENZOIC ACID an antiseptic used to preserve certain pharmaceutical preparations and foodstuffs. It is also used in treating fungal infections of the skin, and urinary tract infections.

BENZOIN a resin used in the preparation of compounds which are inhaled in the treatment of colds, bronchitis (e.g. Friar's BALSAM) etc.

BENZOTHIADIAZINES DIURETIC compounds taken orally, which reduce the reabsorption of chloride and sodium ions in the renal tubules of the KIDNEY. A secondary effect is a lowering of the blood pressure and a primary use is to relieve OEDEMA in heart failure.

BENZOYL PEROXIDE a bactericidal agent used as a bleach in the food industry and also as a treatment for ACNE.

BERI BERI a disease causing inflammation of the nerves and due to a dietary lack of vitamin B_1 (thiamine) which results in fever, paralysis, palpitations and can occasionally precipitate heart failure. Beri beri is most prevalent in south-east Asia, China and Japan and is due to the removal of rice husks in processing.

BETA BLOCKER drugs used to treat ANGINA, reduce high blood pressure and manage abnormal heart rhythms. Certain receptors of nerves in the SYMPATHETIC NERVOUS SYSTEM are blocked, reducing heart activity. A notable side effect is constriction of bronchial passages which ma adversely affect some patients.

BIFURCATION the branching of, for example, a blood vessel into two. Also the TRACHEA where it forms two bronchi (see BRONCHUS).

BIGUANIDES substances, taken orally, that reduce blood sugar level and are used in the treatment of *diabetes mellitus*. The result is that glucose production in the liver is reduced.

BILE a viscous, bitter fluid produced by the LIVER and stored in the GALL BLADDER, a small organ near the liver. It is an alkaline solution of bile salts, pigments (*see* BILIRUBIN), some mineral salts and CHOLESTEROL which aids in fat digestion and absorption of nutrients. Discharge of bile into the intestine is increased after food and of the amount secreted each day (up to one litre), most is reabsorbed with the food, passing back into the blood to circulate back to the liver. If the flow of bile into the intestine is restricted, it stays in the blood, resulting in jaundice.

BILE DUCT a duct that carries BILE from the liver. The main duct is the hepatic which joins the cystic duct from the GALL BLADDER to form the common bile duct which drains into the small INTESTINE.

BILIRUBIN one of the two important BILE pigments, formed primarily from the breakdown of HAEMOGLOBIN from red blood cells. Bilirubin is orange-yellow in colour while its oxidized form biliverdin is green. The majority of bile produced daily is eventually excreted and confers colour to the stools.

BIOAVAILABILITY the term used to describe the amount of a drug that becomes available at its target, after administration and having followed a particular route. The amount may be low for drugs administered by mouth since food affects bioavailability through the alteration of the rate of absorption. Components of food, e.g. calcium, may act as a chelating agent (restricting the amount of the drug that is free), also reducing the absorption of a drug.

BIOPSY an adjunct to diagnosis which involves removing a small sample of living tissue from the body for examination under the microscope. The technique is particularly important in differentiating between benign and malignant tumours. A biopsy can be undertaken with a hollow needle inserted into the relevant organ.

BIOTIN one of a number of vitamins in the B-complex that is synthesized by bacteria in the intestine. It also occurs in liver, meat, eggs, vegetables, milk and cereals. A biotin deficiency can occur only if large amounts of egg white are ingested because a constituent, avidin, binds to the biotin. Serious deficiency results in dermatitis, muscle pains, anorexia and changes in heart activity.

BIRTHMARK (*or* NAEVUS) an agglomeration of dilated blood vessels creating a malformation of the skin and which is present at birth. These may occur as a large port-wine stain which can now be treated by laser, or a strawberry mark which commonly fades in early life (*see also* MOLE).

BISMUTH a metal of which various salts are used in medicine. It occurs in treatments for diarrhoea, haemorrhoids and externally in the management of skin conditions.

BLADDER a sac of fibrous and muscular tissue that contains secretions and which can increase and decrease in capacity. Discharge of the contents is through a narrow opening (*see for example* GALL BLADDER *and* URINARY ORGANS).

BLASTOCYST a spherical mass of cells that forms an early stage in human development and occurs at the time of implantation in the uterus wall.

BLINDNESS being unable to see, a condition which may vary from a total lack of light perception (total blindness) through degrees of visual impairment. The commonest causes of blindness are GLAUCOMA, senile CATARACT, vitamin A deficiency (night blindness) and DIABETES MELLITUS.

BLOOD a suspension of red blood cells (or corpuscles) called erythrocytes, white blood cells (leucocytes) and platelets (small disc-shaped cells involved in BLOOD CLOTTING) in a liquid medium, blood PLASMA. The circulation of blood through the body provides a mechanism for transporting substances. Its functions include:

) carrying oxygenated blood from the heart to all tissues via the arteries while the veins return deoxygenated blood to the heart.

2) carrying essential nutrients, e.g. glucose, fats and amino acids to all parts of the body.

3) removing the waste products of metabolism - ammonia and carbon dioxide, to the liver where urea is formed and then transported by the blood to the kidneys for excretion.

4) carrying important molecules, e.g. hormones, to their target cells.

The red blood cells, produced in the bone marrow, are haemoglobin-containing discs while the white varieties vary in shape and are produced in the marrow and lymphoid tissue. The plasma comprises water, proteins and electrolytes and forms approximately half the blood volume.

BLOOD BANK a unit in which blood is collected, processed and stored prior to its use in transfusions.

BLOOD CLOT a hard mass of blood platelets, trapped red blood cells and fibrin. After tissue damage, blood vessels in the area are constricted and a plug forms to seal the damaged are. The plug formation is initiated by an ENZYME released by the damaged blood vessels and platelets.

BLOOD COUNT (*or* **COMPLETE BLOOD COUNT**, CBC) a count of the numbers of red and white blood cells per unit volume of blood. The count may be performed manually using a microscope, or electronically.

BLOOD GROUPS the division and classification of people into one of four main groups based upon the presence of ANTIGENS on the surface of the red blood cells (corpuscles). The classifying reaction depends upon the SERUM of one person's blood agglutinating (clumping together) the red blood cells of someone else. The antigens, known as agglutinogens react with antibodies (agglutinins) in the serum. There are two agglutinogens

termed A and B and two agglutinins called anti-A and anti-B. This gives rise to four groups: corpuscles with no agglutinogens, group O; with A; with B and with both A and B (hence blood group AB). The agglutinin groups match those of the agglutinogens, thus a person of blood group B has anti-A serum in their blood. It is vital that blood groups are matched for transfusion because incompatibility will produce blood clotting.

The Rhesus factor is another antigen (named after the Rhesus monkey which has a similar antigen), those with it being Rh-positive and those without Rh-negative. About 85% of people are Rh-positive. If a Rh-negative person receives Rh-positive blood, or if a Rh-positive foetus is exposed to antibodies to the factor in the blood of the Rh-negative mother, then HAEMOLYSIS occurs in the foetus and newborn child. This may cause the stillbirth of the child, or jaundice after birth. Testing of pregnant women is thus essential.

BLOOD POISONING *see* SEPTICAEMIA.

BLOOD PRESSURE the pressure of the blood on the heart and blood vessels in the system of circulation. Also the pressure that has to be applied to an artery to stop the pulse beyond the pressure point. Blood pressure peaks at a heart beat (SYSTOLE) and falls in between (DIASTOLE). The systolic pressure in young adults is equivalent to approximately 120mm mercury (and 70mm in diastole). The pressure also depends upon the hardness and thickness of vessel walls and blood pressure tends to increase with age as arteries thicken and harden.

A temporary rise in blood pressure may be precipitated by exposure to cold; a permanent rise by kidney disease and other disorders. A lower blood pressure can be induced by a hot bath or caused by exhaustion. The instrument used to measure blood pressure is the SPHYGMOMANOMETER.

BLOOD SUGAR glucose concentration in the blood for which the typical value is 3.5 to 5.5 mmol/l (millimoles per litre). *See also* HYPOGLYCAEMIA and HYPERGLYCAEMIA.

BLOOD TRANSFUSION the replacement of blood lost due to injury, surgery, etc. A patient may receive whole blood or a component e.g. packed red cells (red blood cells separated from the PLASMA, used to counteract anaemia and restore HAEMOGLOBIN levels). Blood from donors is matched to the recipient for BLOOD GROUP and haemoglobin. Donor blood can be stored for three weeks before use if kept just a few degrees above freezing after which the platelets, leucocytes and some red blood cells become non-viable. Plasma and serum are also transfused and in the dried form, plasma can be stored for up to five years.

BLOOD VESSEL the veins and arteries and their smaller branchings, venules and arterioles, through which blood carried to and from the heart.

BLUE BABY the condition whereby an infant is born with CYANOSIS due to a congenital malformation of the heart. The result is that blue blood (i.e. deoxygenated) does not go through the lungs to be oxygenated but is pumped around the body. Surgery can usually be performed to correct the condition.

BOIL (or furuncle) a skin infection in a hair follicle or gland that produces inflammation and pus. The infection is often due to the bacterium *Staphylococcus*, but healing is generally quick upon release of the pus or administration of antibiotics. Frequent occurrence of boils is usually investigated to ensure the patient is not suffering from DIABETES MELLITUS.

BOLUS a chewed lump of food ready for swallowing.

BONDING the creation of a link between an infant and its parents, particularly the mother. Factors such as eye to eye contact, soothing noises etc. are part of the process.

BONE the hard connective tissue that with CARTILAGE forms the skeleton. Bone has a matrix of COLLAGEN fibres with bone salts (crystalline calcium phosphate

or hydroxyapatite, in which are the bone cells, OSTEOBLASTS and OSTEOCYTES). The bone cells form the matrix.

There are two types of bone: compact or dense, forming the shafts of long bones and spongy or cancellous which occurs on the inside and at the ends of long bones and also forms the short bones. Compact bone is a hard tube covered by the periosteum (a membrane) and enclosing the marrow and contains very fine canals (*see* HAVERSIAN CANALS) around which the bone is structured in circular plates (*see also* BONE DISEASES, BONE MARROW).

BONE DISEASES *see* OSTEOMYELITIS, OSTEOCHONDRITIS, OSTEOSARCOMA and ACHONDROPLASIA.

BONE MARROW a soft tissue found in the spaces of bones. In young animals all bone marrow, the red marrow, produces blood cells. In older animals the marrow in long bones is replaced by yellow marrow which contains a large amount of fat and does not produce blood cells. In mature animals the red marrow occurs in the ribs, sternum, vertebrae and the ends of the long bones (e.g. the femur). The red marrow contains MYELOID tissue with ERYTHROBLASTS from which red blood cells develop. LEUCOCYTES also form from the myeloid tissue and themselves give rise to other cell types.

BOTULISM the most dangerous type of food poisoning, caused by the anaerobic bacterium *Clostridium botulinum*. The bacterium is found in oxygen-free environments, e.g. in contaminated food in bottles or tins. During growth it releases a toxin of which one component attacks the nervous system. It has a very small lethal dose and symptoms commence with a dry mouth, constipation and blurred vision and worsen to muscle weakness. Death is caused by paralysis of the muscles involved in respiration.

BOVINE SPONGIFORM ENCEPHALOPATHY (*or* BSE) a disease of cattle which is similar to scrapies in sheep and CREUTZFELDT-JAKOB DISEASE in humans.

BOW LEGS (or *genu varum*) a deformity

in which the legs curve outwards producing a gap between the knees when standing. Small children may exhibit this to some degree but continuance into adult life or its later formation is due to abnormal growth of the EPIPHYSIS. It can be corrected by surgery.

BRACHIAL adjective meaning 'of the upper arm', hence brachial artery etc.

BRADYCARDIA slowness of the heartbeat and pulse to below 60 per minute.

BRADYKINESIA the condition in which there is abnormally slow movement of the body and limbs and slowness of speech, as may be caused by PARKINSONISM.

BRADYKININ a POLYPEPTIDE derived from plasma proteins that causes smooth muscle to contract. It is also a powerful dilator of veins and arteries.

BRAIN the part of the CENTRAL NERVOUS SYSTEM contained within the cranium. Vertebrates have a highly complex brain which is connected via the spinal cord to the remainder of the nervous system. The brain interprets information received from sense organs and emits signals to control muscles. The brain comprises distinct areas: the CEREBRUM, CEREBELLUM, PONS, MEDULLA OBLONGATA and mid-brain or MESENCEPHALON. GREY MATTER and WHITE MATTER make up the brain, in different arrangements, and a dense network of blood vessels supplies the grey matter and both blood vessels and nerve cells are supported by a fibrous network, the NEUROGLIA. The average female brain weighs 1.25kg, and the male 1.4kg and the maximum size occurs around the age of 20, whereupon it decreases gradually. Three membranes (the MENINGES) separate the brain from the skull and between each pair is a fluid-filled space to cushion the brain. There are twelve nerves connected to the brain mainly in the region of the brain stem and four arteries carrying blood to the brain. Two veins drain the central portion and many small veins open into venous SINUSES which connect with the internal jugular vein.

BRAIN DISEASES many brain diseases are indicated by some impairment of a facility, e.g. a loss of sensation or an alteration in behaviour. *See, amongst others,* APHASIA, CONCUSSION, EPILEPSY, HYDROCEPHALUS *and* MENINGITIS.

BRAINSTEM DEATH (*or* BRAIN DEATH) a complete and continuous absence of the vital reflexes controlled by centres in the brainstem (breathing, pupillary responses, etc.). Tests are performed by independent doctors, repeated after an interval, before death is formally confirmed. At this point, organs may be removed for transplant providing suitable permission has been obtained.

BREAST the MAMMARY GLAND that produces milk. Each breast has a number of compartments with lobules surrounded by fatty tissue and muscle fibres. Milk formed in the lobules gathers in branching tubes or ducts that together form lactiferous ducts. Near the nipple the ducts form ampullae (small 'reservoirs') from which the ducts discharge through the nipple.

BREAST CANCER a CARCINOMA or SARCOMA which is the commonest cancer in women. Incidence is low in countries where breast feeding persists and animal fat intake in the diet is low. The first sign may be a lump in the breast or armpit (the latter being due to spread to the lymph nodes). A localized tumour may be removed surgically and in addition, radio, chemo- and hormone therapy can form part of the treatment.

BREAST SCREENING procedures adopted to detect breast cancer as early as possible. In addition to self-examination, there are many formal programmes of screening.

BREATHLESSNESS is caused fundamentally by any condition that depletes blood oxygen resulting in excessive and/or laboured breathing to gain more air. The causes are numerous, ranging from lung diseases or conditions

(PNEUMONIA, EMPHYSEMA, BRONCHITIS) to heart conditions and obesity. In children, narrowing of the air passages is a cause, as is ASTHMA.

BREECH PRESENTATION the position of a baby in the uterus whereby it would be delivered buttocks first instead of the usual head first delivery. The baby, and possibly the mother, may be at risk in such cases.

BRITTLE BONE DISEASE see OSTEOGENESIS IMPERFECTA.

BRONCHIOLE very fine tubes occurring as branches of the bronchi (see BRONCHUS). The bronchioles end in alveoli (see ALVEOLUS) where carbon dioxide and oxygen are exchanged.

BRONCHITIS occurring in two forms, acute and chronic, bronchitis is the inflammation of the bronchi. Bacteria or viruses cause the acute form which is typified by the symptoms of the common cold initially, but develops with painful coughing, wheezing, throat and chest pains and the production of purulent (pus-containing) mucus. If the infection spreads to the BRONCHIOLES (bronchiolitis) the consequences are more serious as the body is deprived of oxygen. Antibiotics and EXPECTORANTS can relieve the symptoms. Chronic bronchitis is identified by an excessive production of mucus and may be due to recurrence of the acute form. It is a common cause of death among the elderly and there are several parameters of direct consequence to its cause: excessive smoking of cigarettes; cold, damp climate; obesity; respiratory infections. Damage to the bronchi and other complications may occur giving rise to constant breathlessness. Bronchodilator drugs are ineffective in treatment of the chronic form.

BRONCHODILATOR drugs used to relax the SMOOTH MUSCLE of the bronchioles, thus increasing their diameter and the air supply to the lungs. They are used in the treatment of ASTHMA.

BRONCHUS air passages supported by rings of cartilage. Two bronchi branch

off from the TRACHEA and these split into further bronchi. The two main bronchi branch to form five lobar bronchi, then twenty segmental bronchi and so on.

BROWN FAT see ADIPOSE TISSUE.

BRUCELLOSIS a disease of farm animals (pigs, cattle, goats) caused by a species of a gram-negative bacillus, *Brucella* (see GRAM'S STAIN). It may be passed to man through contact with an infected animal or by drinking contaminated, untreated, milk. In cattle the disease causes contagious abortion but in man it is characterized by fever, sweats, joint pains, back and headache. The use of antibiotics and sulphonamides over a period of time is usually effective and although brucellosis itself is rarely fatal, it may have serious complications, e.g. MENINGITIS or PNEUMONIA.

BUCCAL generally pertaining to the mouth, specifically the inside of the cheek or the gum next to the cheek.

BULIMIA an insatiable craving for food.

BULIMIA NERVOSA an overwhelming desire to eat a lot of food followed by misuse of laxatives or induced vomiting to avoid weight gain. Although there is no attempt to hide the condition, it is psychological in origin, and the sufferers have a fear of obesity. There are many similarities with anorexia NERVOSA but little success in treatment.

BURNS burns and scalds show similar symptoms and require similar treatment, the former being caused by dry heat, the latter moist heat. Burns may also be due to electric currents and chemicals. Formerly burns were categorized by degrees (a system developed by Dupuytres, a French surgeon) but are now either superficial, where sufficient tissue remains to ensure skin regrows, or deep where GRAFTING will be necessary. Severe injuries can prove dangerous because of shock due to fluid loss at the burn. For minor burns and scalds, treatment involves holding the affected area under cold water. In more severe cases antiseptic dressings are normally applied and in very severe cases hospitalization is required. Morphine is usually administered to combat the pain. If the burns exceed 9% then a TRANSFUSION is required.

CAECUM an expanded, blind-ended sac at the start of the large intestine between the small intestine and colon. the small intestine and vermiform appendix open into the caecum.

CAESARIAN SECTION a surgical operation to deliver a baby by menas of an incision through the abdomen and uterus. It is performed when there is a risk to the health of the baby or mother through normal delivery, both as a planned and as an emergency procedure.

CAESIUM 137 a radioactive substance produced artificially from caesium which is used in RADIOTHERAPY.

CAFFEINE a substance obtained from coffee and tea which has a stimulating effect on the central nervous system. It is used as a component of medicines given to relieve headache and also has DIURETIC properties. In addition it acts as a cardiac stimulant and has a beneficial effect in the treatment of certain forms of asthma.

CALAMINE zinc carbonate which is a mild astringent and is a component of lotions used to relieve itchy, painful skin conditions such as eczema, urticaria and sunburn.

CALCIFEROL a form of VITAMIN D which is manufactured in the skin in the presence of sunlight or derived from certain foods (e.g. liver and fish oils). Its main role is in calcium metabolism enabling calcium to be absorbed from the gut and laid down in bone. A deficiency of vitamin D leads to the bone disease OSTEOLAMACIA and also RICKETS.

CALCIFICATION the deposition of calcium salts which is normal in the formation of bone but may occur at other sites in the body, *see* OSSIFICATION.

CALCIUM a metallic element which is essential for normal growth and functioning of body processes. It is an important component of bones and teeth and has a role in vital metabolic processes, e.g. muscle contraction, passage of nerve impulses and blood clotting. Its concentration in the blood is regulated by various THYROID HORMONES. Calcium is an essential element in a normal healthy diet and it is found in dairy products such as milk and cheese.

CALCIUM-CHANNEL BLOCKERS also known as calcium antagonists, these are drugs which inhibit the movement of calcium ions into smooth muscle and cardiac muscle cells. Their effect is to relax the muscle and reduce the strength of contraction and to cause vasodilation. They are used in the treatment of high blood pressure and angina.

CALLUS material which forms around the end of a broken bone containing bone-forming cells, cartilage and connective tissue. Eventually this tissue becomes calcified.

CALORIE a term applied to a unit of energy which is the heat required to raise the temperature of one gram of water by one degree centigrade.

CANCER a widely-used term describing any form of malignant tumour. Characteristically, there is an uncontrolled and abnormal growth of cancer cells which invade surrounding tissues and destroy them. Cancer cells may spread throughout the body via the blood stream or lymphatic system, a process known as METASTASIS, and set up secondary growths elsewhere. There are known to be a number of different causes of cancer including cigarette smoking, radiation, ultraviolet light, some viruses and possibly the presence of cancer GENES (oncogenes). Treatment depends upon the site of the cancer but involves radiotherapy, chemotherapy and surgery, and survival rates in affected people are showing encouraging improvements.

CANDIDIASIS those infections caused by *Candida* (a yeast-like fungus), such as THRUSH and VAGINITIS.

CANNULA a hollow tube which is used to draw off fluid from a body cavity. It fits tightly round a solid core, with a sharp pointed end (known as a trocar) which aids insertion. Once the cannula is correctly situated, the trocar is withdrawn so that fluid can run through the tube.

CAPILLARY a fine blood vessel which communicates with an ARTERIOLE or VENULE. Capillaries form networks in most tissues and have walls which are only one cell thick. There is a constant exchange of substances (oxygen, carbon dioxide, nutrients, etc.) between the capillaries, arterioles and venules supplying the needs of the surrounding tissues.

CAPSULE a sheath of connective tissue or membrane surrounding an organ. The adrenal gland, kidney and spleen are all housed within a capsule. A JOINT capsule is a fibrous tissue sheath surrounding various joints. A capsule is also used to describe a small, gelatinous pouch containing a drug, which can be swallowed.

CARBARYL an insecticide substance which is especially used in preparations for the elimination of head lice.

CARBOHYDRATES organic compounds which include sugars and starch and contain carbon, hydrogen and oxygen. They are the most important source of energy available to the body and are an essential part of the diet. They are eventually broken down in the body to the simple sugar, glucose, which can be used by cells in numerous metabolic processes.

CARBOLIC ACID phenol derived from coal tar and the fore-runner of modern antiseptics. A strong disinfectant, it is used in lotions and ointments such as CALAMINE lotion, but is highly poisonous if ingested.

CARBON DIOXIDE also known as carbonic acid, this is a gas formed in the tissues as a result of metabolic processes within the body. Medically, carbon dioxide is used combined with oxygen during anaesthesia. At very low temperatures (-75°C) carbon dioxide forms a snow-like solid known as "dry ice." This is used on the skin to freeze a localized area and also in the treatment of warts.

CARBON MONOXIDE (CO) an odourless and colourless gas which is highly dangerous when inhaled, leading to carbon monoxide poisoning. In the blood it has a very great affinity for oxygen and converts haemoglobin into carboxyhaemoglobin. The tissues of the body are quickly deprived of oxygen because there is no free haemoglobin left to pick it up in the lungs. Carbon monoxide is present in coal gas fumes and vehicle exhaust emissions. The symptons of poisoning include giddiness, flushing of the skin (due to carboxyhaemoglobin in the blood which is bright red), nausea, headache, raised respiratory and pulse rate and eventual coma, respiratory failure and death. An affected person must be taken into the fresh air and given oxygen and artificial respiration if required.

CARCINOGEN any substance which causes damage to tissue cells likely to result in cancer. Various substances are known to be *carcinogenic* including tobacco smoke, asbestos and ionizing radiation.

CARCINOMA a cancer of the EPITHELIUM, i.e. the tissue that lines the body's internal organs and skin.

CARDIAC ARREST the failure and stopping of the pumping action of the heart. There is a loss of consciousness and breathing and the pulse ceases. Death follows very rapidly unless the heart beat can be restored, and methods of achieving this include external CARDIAC MASSAGE, artificial respiration, DEFIBRILLATION and direct cardiac massage.

CARDIAC CYCLE the whole sequence

f events which produces a heart beat which normally takes place in less than one second. The atria (*see* ATRIUM) contract together and force the blood into the ventricles (DIASTOLE). These then also contract (SYSTOLE) and blood exits the heart and is pumped around the body. As the ventricles are contracting the atria relax and fill up with blood once again.

CARDIAC MASSAGE a means of restoring the heart beat if this activity has suddenly ceased. Direct cardiac massage, which is only feasible if the person is in hospital, involves massaging the heart by hand through an incision in the chest wall. Another method, used in conjunction with artificial respiration, is by rhythmic compression of the chest wall while the person is laid on his or her back. The heel of the hand is placed on the chest in the lower region of the breast bone, and firmly compressed between 60 and 80 times a minute, alternating with mouth-to-mouth resuscitation.

CARDIAC MUSCLE specialized muscle unique to the heart, consisting of branching, elongated fibres possessing the ability to contract and relax continuously.

CARDIAC PACEMAKER *see* PACEMAKER and SINOATRIAL NODE.

CARDIOMYOPATHY any disease or disorder of the heart muscle which may arise from a number of different causes including viral infections, congenital abnormalities and chronic alcoholism.

CARDIOPULMONARY BYPASS an artificial mechanism for maintaining the body's circulation while the heart is intentionally stopped in order to carry out cardiac surgery. A "heart-lung" machine carries out the functions of heart and lungs until surgery is completed.

CARDIOVASCULAR SYSTEM the heart and the whole of the circulatory system, which is divided into the *systemic* (arteries and veins of the body), and *pulmonary* (arteries and veins of the lungs). The cardiovascular system is

responsible for the transport of oxygen and nutrients to the tissues, and removing waste products and carbon dioxide from them, taking these to the organs from which they are eventually eliminated.

CAROTID ARTERY one of two large arteries in the neck which branch and provide the blood supply to the head and neck. The paired common carotid arteries arise from the AORTA on the left side of the heart and from the inominate artery on the right. These continue up on either side of the neck and branch into the internal and external carotids.

CAROTID BODY a small area of specialized reddish-coloured tissue situated one on either side of the neck where the common carotid artery branches to form the internal and external carotids. It is sensitive to chemical changes in the blood, containing chemoreceptors which respond to oxygen, carbon dioxide and hydrogen levels. If the oxygen level falls, impulses are transmitted to the respiratory centres in the brain resulting in an increase in the rate of respiration and heart beat.

CARPUS latin for wrist, consisting of eight small bones which articulate with the ULNA and RADIUS of the forearm on one side and with the *metacarpals* (bones of the hand) on the other.

CARTILAGE a type of firm connective tissue which is pliable and forms part of the skeleton. There are three different kinds, hyaline cartilage, fibro-cartilage and elastic cartilage. *Hyaline* cartilage is found at the joints of movable bones and in the trachea, nose, bronchi and as costal cartilage joining the ribs to the breast bone. *Fibro-cartilage*, which consists of cartilage and connective tissue, is found in the intervertebral discs of the spinal column and in tendons. *Elastic* cartilage is found in the external part of the ear (pinna).

CATALEPSY a mental disorder in which the person enters a trance-like state. The body becomes rigid like a statue and the limbs, if moved, stay in the position in which they are placed. There is no sense of recognition or sensation and a loss of voluntary control. The vital body functions are shut down to a minimum level necessary for life and, in fact, may be so low as to resemble death. The condition is brought on by severe mental trauma, either as a result of a sudden shock or by a more prolonged depression. It may last for minutes or hours or, rarely, for several days.

CATARACT a condition in which the lens of the eye becomes opaque, resulting in a blurring of vision. It may arise from a number of different causes including injury to the eye, as a congenital condition (e.g. DOWN'S SYNDROME) or as a result of certain diseases such as DIABETES. However, the commonest cause is advancing age during which changes naturally take place in the lens involving the protein components. This is known as senile cataract. Cataract is treated by surgical removal of the whole or part of the affected lens.

CATATONIA when a patient becomes statue-like, remaining rigid. It is a symptom of mental disease and often a feature of catatonic SCHIZOPHRENIA. Treatment involves tranquillizers and possibly intravenous barbiturates.

CATHETER a fine flexible tube which is passed into various organs of the body either for diagnostic purposes or to administer some kind of treatment. One of the commonest kinds are urethral catheters inserted into the bladder to clear an obstruction, draw off urine or wash out this organ.

CAUTERIZE the application of a heated instrument known as a cautery to destroy living tissue or to stop a haemorrhage. It is used in the treatment of warts and other small growths on the skin.

CELL the basic building block of all life and the smallest structural unit in the body. Human body cells vary in size and function and number several billion. Each cell consists of a cell body surrounded by a membrane. The cell body consists of a substance known as cytoplasm containing various organelles, and also a nucleus. The nucleus contains the CHROMOSOMES composed of the genetic material, the DNA. Most human body cells contain 46 chromosomes (23 pairs), half being derived from the individual's father and half from the mother. Cells are able to make exact copies of themselves by a process known as MITOSIS and a full complement of chromosomes is received by each daughter cell. However, the human sex cells (sperm and ova) differ in always containing half the number of chromosomes. At fertilization, a sperm and ovum combine and a complete set of chromosomes is received by the new embryo. *See* MITOSIS and MEIOSIS.

CENTRAL NERVOUS SYSTEM the brain and the spinal cord which receives and integrates all the nervous information from the peripheral nervous system.

CEPHALOSPORINS a group of semi-synthetic antiobiotics derived from a mould called *Cephalosporium*. They are effective against a broad spectrum of micro-organisms and are used to treat a variety of infections. They are sometimes able to destroy organisms which have become resistant to penicillin.

CEREBELLUM the largest part of the hind brain consisting of a pair of joined hemispheres. It has an outer grey cortex which is a much folded layer of grey matter and an inner core of white matter. The cerebellum co-ordinates the activity of various groups of voluntary muscles and maintains posture and balance.

CEREBRAL CORTEX the outer layer of grey matter of the cerebral hemi-spheres of the CEREBRUM. It is highly folded and contains many millions of nerve cells, and makes up about 40% of the brain by weight. The cerebral cortex controls intellectual processes such as thought, perception, memory and intellect, and is also involved in the senses of sight, touch and hearing. It also controls the voluntary movement of muscles and is connected with all the different parts of the body.

CEREBRAL PALSY an abnormality of the brain which usually occurs before or during birth. It may arise as a development defect in the foetus due to genetic factors, or by a (viral) infection during pregnancy. A lack of oxygen during a difficult labour or other trauma to the infant can result in cerebral palsy. After birth, the condition can result from haemolytic disease of the newborn, or infection of the brain e.g. MENINGITIS. It can also be caused by cerebral thrombosis or trauma. The condition is characterized by spastic paralysis of the limbs, the severity of which is variable. Also, there may be involuntary writhing movements called athetosis, and balance and posture are also affected. There is often mental subnormality and speech impairment and sometimes EPILEPSY. Treatment may involve surgery but also physiotherapy, speech and occupational therapy and special education.

CEREBROSPINAL FLUID a clear, colourless fluid with a similar composition to LYMPH. It fills the ventricles and cavities in the CENTRAL NERVOUS SYSTEM and bathes all the surfaces of the brain and spinal cord. The brain floats in it and it has a protective function acting as a shock absorber helping to prevent mechanical injury to the central nervous system. The cerebrospinal fluid is secreted by the choroid plexuses in the ventricles of the brain and it contains some white blood cells (but no red), salts, glucose and enzymes. It is re-absorbed by veins back into the blood stream.

CEREBRUM the largest and most highly developed part of the brain consisting of a pair of cerebral hemispheres divided from each other by a longitudinal fissure. The cerebral hemispheres are covered by the CEREBRAL CORTEX below which lies white matter in which the BASAL GANGLIA are situated. The cerebrum controls complex intellectual activities and also all the voluntary responses of the body.

CERVICAL relating to the neck but often used in connection with the neck of the womb (uterus).

CERVICAL CANCER cancer of the neck or cervix of the womb which is one of the most common cancers affecting women. In the pre-cancerous stage, readily detectable changes occur in the cells lining the surface of the cervix. These can be identified by means of a CERVICAL SMEAR test and, if treated at this stage, the prevention and cure rates of the cancer are very high. Early cancer is treated by CRYOSURGERY, diathermy, laser treatment and electrocoagulation. The sexual behaviour of a woman influences her risk of contracting cervical cancer. Early sexual intercourse and numerous different partners are now recognized to increase the risk.

CERVICAL SMEAR a simple test, involving scraping off some cells from the cervix and examining them microscopically. The test is carried out every three years to detect early indications of cancer and is a form of preventative medicine.

CERVIX a neck-like structure especially the cervix uteri or neck of the womb. It is partly above and partly within the vagina projecting into it and linking it with the cavity of the uterus via the cervical canal.

CHEMORECEPTOR a cell or number of cells that detect the presence of specific chemical compounds. In the presence of the chemical an electrical impulse is sent along a specialized sensory nerve to the brain where the information is received and de-coded. Chemoreceptors are present in the nose and taste buds. *See also* CAROTID BODY.

CHEMOTHERAPY the treatment of disease by the administration of chemical substances or drugs. It includes the treatment of infectious diseases with antibiotics and other types of drug. Also, the treatment and control of various tropical diseases and, especially in recent years, many different forms of cancer with ANTIMETABOLITE drugs.

CHICKEN POX a highly infectious disease which mainly affects children and is caused by the *Varicella zoster* virus. There is an incubation period of two to three weeks and then usually a child becomes slightly feverish and unwell. Within twenty-four hours an itchy rash appears on the skin which consists of fluid-filled blisters. Eventually these form scabs which fall off after about one week. The treatment consists of the application of calamine lotion to reduce the itching, and isolation from other children.

The disease is uncommon in adults as a childhood attack gives lifelong immunity and most children are exposed to chicken pox at some stage. However, the virus may remain within the system and become active later as shingles (HERPES ZOSTER).

CHILBLAIN a round, itchy inflammation of the skin which usually occurs on the toes or fingers during cold weather, and is caused by a localized deficiency in the circulation. Chilblains may sometimes be an indication of poor health or inadequate clothing and nutrition. Keeping the feet and hands warm, paying attention to the diet and exercise to improve the circulation help to prevent chilblains.

CHLORAL HYDRATE a type of sedative drug which is given mainly to elderly people and children. Within half an hour of being taken by mouth (usually as a syrup), it induces sleep and its effects last for about eight hours. It is useful when used sparingly, but harmful in large doses causing toxic effects and addiction.

CHLORHEXIDINE also known as hibitane, chlorhexidine is an antiseptic substance which is used in preparations to cleanse the skin. It is also used in LOZENGES for mild infections of the mouth and throat. Dilute solutions are effective as mouthwash.

CHOLERA an infection of the small intestine caused by the BACTERIUM *Vibrio cholerae*. It varies in degree from very mild cases to extremely severe illness and death. The disease originated in Asia but spread widely last century when there were great cholera epidemics in Britain and elsewhere. During epidemics of cholera, the death rate is over 50% and these occur in conditions of poor sanitation and overcrowding. The disease is spread through contamination of drinking water by faeces of those affected by the disease, and also by flies landing on infected material and then crawling on food.

Epidemics are rare in conditions of good sanitation but when cholera is detected, extreme attention has to be paid to hygiene including treatment and scrupulous disposal of the body waste of the infected person. The incubation period for cholera is one to five days and then a person suffers from severe vomiting and diarrhoea (known as "cholera diarrhoea" or "rice water stools"). This results in severe dehydration and death may follow within 24 hours. Treatment involves bed rest and the taking by mouth of salt solutions, or these may need to be given intravenously. Tetracycline or other sulphonamide drugs are given to kill the bacteria. The death rate is low (5%) in those given proper and prompt treatment but the risk is greater in children and the elderly. Vaccination against cholera can be given but it is only effective for about 6 months.

CHOLESTEROL a fatty insoluble molecule (sterol), which is widely found in the body and is synthesized from saturated fatty acids in the liver. Cholesterol is an important substance in the body being a component of cell membranes and a precursor in the production of steroid hormones (sex hormones) and bile salts. An elevated level of blood cholesterol is associated with ATHEROMA which may result in high blood pressure and coronary thrombosis, and this is seen in the disease, DIABETES MELLITUS. There appears to be a relationship between the high consumption of saturated animal fats (which contain cholesterol) in the western diet and the greater incidence of coronary heart disease among, for example, Western Europeans and North Americans. It is generally recommended that people in these countries should reduce their consumption of saturated fat and look for alternatives in the form of unsaturated fats which are found in vegetable oils.

CHOLINE an organic compound which is a constituent of some important substances in the body such as phospholipids, lecithin and ACETYL-CHOLINE. It is sometimes classed as part of the vitamin B complex but this essential compound can also be synthesized by the body.

CHOLURIA bile in the urine which occurs when there is an elevated level of bile in the blood. This may result from the condition known as obstructive JAUNDICE when the bile ducts become obstructed so that bile manufactured in the liver fails to reach the intestine. The urine is dark coloured and contains bile salts and pigments.

CHOREA a disorder of the nervous system characterized by the involuntary, jerky movements of the muscles mainly of the face, shoulders and hips. *Sydenham's chorea* or *St. Vitus' Dance* is a disease that mainly affects children and is associated with acute rheumatism. About one third of affected children develop rheumatism elsewhere in the body, often involving the heart, and the disease is more common in girls than in boys. If the heart is affected there may be problems in later life but treatment consists of rest and the giving of mild sedatives. The condition usually recovers over a period of a few months. *Huntington's chorea* is an inherited condition which does not appear until after the age of 40 and is accompanied

by dementia. *Senile chorea* afflicts some elderly people but there is no dementia. *See also* RHEUMATIC FEVER.

CHORION one of two foetal membranes completely surrounding the embryo and forming the placenta.

CHORIONIC GONADOTROPHIC HORMONE a hormone produced during pregnancy by the placenta, large amounts of which are present in the urine of a pregnant woman. The presence of this hormone is the basis of most pregnancy tests. Also known as human chorionic gonadotrophin (HCG), it is given by injection to treat cases of delayed puberty and, with another hormone called follicle stimulating hormone, women who are sterile due to a failure in ovulation. It is also used to treat premenstrual tension.

CHOROID PLEXUS an extensive network of blood vessels present in the ventricles of the brain and responsible for the production of the CEREBROSPINAL FLUID.

CHROMOSOMES the rod-like structures present in the nucleus of every body cell which carry the genetic information or genes. Each human body cell contains twenty-three pairs of chromosomes (apart from the sperm and ova), half derived from the mother and half from the father. Each chromosome consists of a coiled double filament (double helix) of DNA with genes carrying the genetic information arranged linearly along its length. The genes determine all the characteristics of each individual. Twenty-two of the pairs of chromosomes are the same in males and females. The twenty-third pair are the sex chromosomes and males have one X and one Y whereas females have two X chromosomes. *See* CELL and SEX-LINKED INHERITANCE.

CIRCULATION OF THE BLOOD the basic circulation is as follows: all the blood from the body returns to the heart via the veins, eventually entering the right atrium through the inferior and superior venae cavae. This contracts and forces the blood into the right ventricle and from there is driven to the lungs via the pulmonary artery. In the lungs, oxygen is taken up and carbon dioxide is released and the blood then passes into the pulmonary veins and is returned to the left atrium of the heart. Blood is forced from the left atrium into the left ventricle and from there into the aorta. The aorta branches giving off the various arteries which carry the blood to all the different parts of the body. The blood eventually enters the fine network of arterioles and capillaries and supplies all the tissues and organs with oxygen and nutrients. It passes into the venules and veins, eventually returning to the right atrium through the vena cavae to complete the cycle.

CIRCUMCISION a surgical removal of the foreskin (or prepuce) of the penis in males and part or all of the external genitalia (CLITORIS, labia minora, labia majora) in females. In females and usually in males, the procedure is carried out for religious reasons. Male circumcision may be required in the medical conditions known as PHIMOSIS and paraphimosis. Female circumcision is damaging and not beneficial to a woman's health.

CIRRHOSIS a disease of the liver in which fibrous tissue resembling scar tissue is produced as a result of damage and death to the cells. The liver becomes yellow-coloured and nodular in appearance, and there are various types of the disease including alcoholic cirrhosis and postnecrotic cirrhosis caused by viral hepatitis. The cause of the cirrhosis is not always found (cryptogenic cirrhosis) but the progress of the condition can be halted if this can be identified and removed. This particularly is applicable in alcoholic cirrhosis where the consumption of alcohol has to cease.

CLAVICLE the collar bone forming a part of the shoulder girdle of the skeleton. It is the most commonly fractured bone in the body.

CLEFT PALATE a developmental defect in which a fissure is left in the midline of the palate as the two sides fail to fuse. It may also involve the lip (HARELIP) and the condition is corrected by surgery.

CLITORIS a small organ present in females, situated where the labial folds meet below the pubic bone. It contains erectile tissue which enlarges and hardens during sexual stimulation.

CLONE a group of cells that are derived from one cell (by asexual division) and are genetically identical.

CLOSTRIDIUM a group of bacteria which are present in the intestine of man and animals. Some species are responsible for serious diseases such as botulism, tetanus and gas GANGRENE.

CLOT the term applied to a semi-solid lump of blood or other fluid in the body. A blood clot consists of a fine network of FIBRIN in which blood corpuscles are caught, see COAGULATION.

COAGULATION (of the blood) the natural process in which blood is converted from a liquid to a semi-solid state to arrest bleeding (haemorrhage). A substance known as prothrombin and calcium are normally present in the blood, and the enzyme thromboplastin is present in the platelets (see BLOOD). When bleeding occurs, thromboplastin is released and prothrombin and calcium are converted by the enzyme into THROMBIN. A soluble protein called fibrinogen is always present in the blood and is converted by thrombin into FIBRIN which is the final stage in the coagulation process. A fibrous meshwork or clot is produced consisting of fibrin and blood cells which seals off the damaged blood vessel. In normal healthy conditions, thromboplastin is not released and so a clot cannot form. The coagulation or clotting time is the time taken for blood to clot and is normally between three to eight minutes.

COAGULATION FACTORS these are substances present in plasma which are involved in the process of blood coagulation. They are designated by a set of Roman numerals, e.g. Factor VIII, and lack of any of them means that the blood is unable to clot. *See* HAEMOPHILIA.

COBALT-60 an artificial radioisotope which emits gamma radiation and is used in RADIOTHERAPY.

COCAINE an alkaloid substance derived from the leaves of the coca plant which is used as a local anaesthetic in nose, throat, ear and eye surgery. It has a stimulating effect on the central nervous system when absorbed, in which fatigue and breathlessness (caused by exertion) disappear. However, it is highly addictive and damaging to the body if it is used often and hence it is very strictly controlled. It is also one of the drugs given for pain relief in cases of terminal cancer.

COCCYX the end of the backbone, which consists of four fused and reduced vertebrae which correspond to the tail of other mammals. The coccyx is surrounded by muscle and joins with the SACRUM, a further group of fused vertebrae which is part of the pelvis.

COCHLEA a spiral-shaped organ resembling a snail shell forming a part of the inner ear and concerned with hearing. It consists of three fluid-filled canals with receptors which detect pressure changes caused by sound waves. Nerve impulses are sent to the brain where the information is received and decoded.

CODEINE a substance derived from morphine which is used for pain relief and to suppress a cough.

COD LIVER OIL oil derived from the pressed fresh liver of cod which is a rich source of vitamins D and A, and is used as a dietary supplement.

COELIAC DISEASE also known as gluten enteropathy, this is a wasting disease of childhood in which the intestines are unable to absorb fat. The intestinal lining is damaged due to a sensitivity to the protein gluten which is found in wheat and rye flour. An excess of fat is excreted and the child fails to grow and thrive. Successful treatment is by adhering strictly to a gluten-free diet throughout life.

COFACTOR some ENZYMES can only work if their particular cofactor is present. Cofactors may be inorganic (e.g. metal ions) or non-protein organic substances (e.g. coenzymes), and they may activate their enzyme or actually take part in the reaction itself.

COLD (common cold) widespread and mild infection of the upper respiratory tract caused by a virus. There is inflammation of the mucous membranes and symptoms include feverishness, coughing, sneezing, runny nose, sore throat, headache and sometimes face ache due to catarrh in the SINUSES. The disease is spread by coughing and sneezing and treatment is by means of bed rest and the taking of mild ANALGESICS.

COLD SORE *see* HERPES SIMPLEX.

COLECTOMY surgical removal of the colon.

COLIC spasmodic, severe abdominal pain which occurs in waves with brief interludes in between. Intestinal colic is usually the result of the presence of some indigestible food which causes the contraction of the intestinal muscles. Infantile colic, common in young babies, is due to wind associated with feeding. An attack of colic is generally not serious but can result in a twisting of the bowel which must receive immediate medical attention. Colic-type pain may also be caused by an obstruction in the bowel such as a tumour which again requires early medical treatment.

COLITIS inflammation of the colon, the symptoms of which include abdominal pain and diarrhoea, sometimes blood-stained. *Ulcerative colitis* tends to affect young adults and tends to occur periodically over a number of years. There is abdominal discomfort, fever, frequent watery diarrhoea containing mucus and blood, and anaemia. The condition can be fatal but usually there is a gradual recovery.

Treatment is by means of bed rest, drug treatment with corticosteroids and iron supplements, and a bland, low roughage diet. Colitis may be due to infections caused by the organism *Entamoeba histolytica* (amoebic colitis) and by bacteria (infective colitis). It may also occur in CROHN'S DISEASE.

COLLAGEN a protein substance that is widely found in large amounts in the body in connective tissue, tendons, skin, cartilage, bone and ligaments. It plays a major part in conferring tensile strength to various body structures.

COLLAR BONE *see* CLAVICLE.

COLON the main part of the large intestine which removes water and salts from the undigested food passed into it from the small intestine. When water has been extracted the remains of the food (faeces) are passed on to the rectum.

COLOSTOMY a surgical operation to produce an artificial opening of the colon through the abdominal wall. The colostomy may only be temporary, as part of the management of a patient's condition, e.g. to treat an obstruction in the colon or rectum. However, if the rectum or part of the colon have been removed because of cancer the colostomy is permanent and functions as the anus.

COMA a state of deep unconsciousness from which a person cannot be roused. There may be an absence of pupillary and corneal reflexes and no movements of withdrawal when painful stimuli are applied. It may be accompanied by deep, noisy breathing and strong heart action and is caused by a number of different conditions. These include apoplexy, high fever, brain injury, diabetes mellitus, carbon monoxide poisoning and drug overdose. A comatose person may eventually die but can recover depending upon the nature of the coma and its cause.

COMMINUTED FRACTURE a serious injury to a bone in which more than one break occurs accompanied by splintering and damage to the surrounding tissues. It usually results from a crushing force, with damage to nerves, muscles and blood vessels, and the bone is difficult to set.

COMPRESS a pad soaked in hot or cold water, wrung out and applied to an inflamed or painful part of the body. A hot compress is called a fomentation.

COMPUTERIZED TOMOGRAPHY a diagnostic technique in radiology whereby "slices" of the body are recorded using a special X-ray scanner known as a CT scanner. The information is integrated by computer to give an image in cross-section of the tissue under investigation. The technique is used for investigations of the brain, for example if a tumour, haematoma or abscess is present. Whole body scans may be required for a number of conditions, but are particularly useful when malignancy is present, supplying information about the position and outline of a tumour and the extent of spread of cancer.

CONCRETIONS hard, stony masses of various sizes formed within the body. Examples are gall stones and kidney stones and they are usually composed of mineral salts. Also known as calculi (single, *calculus*).

CONCUSSION a loss of consciousness caused by a blow to the head. The sudden knock to the head causes a compression wave which momentarily interrupts the blood supply to the brain. The unconsciousness may last for seconds or hours and when the person comes round there may be some headache and irritability which can last for some time. A mild case of concussion may not involve complete loss of consciousness but be marked by giddiness, confusion and headache. In all cases, the person needs to rest and remain under observation.

CONDYLE a rounded knob that is found at the ends of some bones e.g. on the femur and humerus and articulates with an adjacent bone.

CONE a type of photoreceptor (light-sensitive cell) found in the RETINA of the eye which detects colour. Cones contain the pigment retinene and the protein opsin and there are three different types which react to light of differing wavelengths, (blue, green and red).

CONGENITAL diseases or conditions that are present at birth.

CONJUNCTIVITIS inflammation of the mucous membrane (conjunctiva) that lines the inside of the eyelid and covers the front of the eye. The eyes become pink and watery and the condition is usually caused by an infection which may be bacterial, viral or the micro-organism *Chlamydia* may be responsible. Treatment depends upon cause but a number of drugs are used often in the form of eyedrops.

CONNECTIVE TISSUE supporting or packing tissue within the body which holds or separates other tissues and organs. It consists of a ground material composed of substances called muco-polysaccharides. In this, certain fibres such as yellow elastic, white collagenous and reticular fibres are embedded along with a variety of other cells, e.g MAST CELLS, MACROPHAGES, fibroblasts and fat cells. The constituents vary in proportions in different kinds of connective tissue to produce a number of distinct types. Examples are adipose (fatty) tissue, cartilage, bone, tends and ligaments.

CONSTIPATION the condition in which the bowels are opened too infrequently and the faeces become dry, hard and difficult and painful to pass. The frequency of normal bowel opening varies between people but when constipation becomes a problem, it is usually a result of inattention to this habit or to the diet. To correct the condition a change of lifestyle may be needed including taking more exercise, fluid and roughage in the diet. Laxatives and enemas are also used to alleviate the condition. Constipation is also a symptom of the more serious condition of blockage of the bowel (by a tumour), but this is less common.

CONTRACEPTION prevention of conception. Pregnancy can be prevented by *barrier methods* in which there is a physical barrier to prevent the sperm from entering the cervix. These comprise the condom (sheath) and diaphragm (cap). As well as being a contraceptive the sheath reduces the risk of either partner contracting a sexually transmitted disease including HIV infection. Non-barrier methods do not interpose this physical barrier and include the INTRA-UTERINE CONTRACEPTIVE DEVICE (coil) and oral contraceptives (the Pill) which are hormonal preparations. Depot preparations are also hormonal drugs that are given by injection, planted under the skin (subcutaneous implants) and released from intravaginal rings, and have a long-lasting effect.

Sterilization of either a man or woman provides a means of permanent contraception. It is also possible to give a high dose of oral contraceptives within 72 hours of unprotected intercourse, but this is usually regarded as an emergency method. The rhythm method of contraception involves restricting sexual intercourse to certain days of a woman's monthly cycle when conception is least likely to occur.

CONTROLLED DRUGS those drugs which, in the United Kingdom, are subject to the restrictions of the Misuse of Drugs Act 1971. They are classified into three categories: Class A includes LSD, morphine, cocaine and pethidine. Class B includes cannabis, ampheta-mines and barbiturates and Class C comprises amphetamine-related drugs and some others.

CONVULSIONS also known as fits, these are involuntary, alternate, rapid, muscular contractions and relaxations throwing the body and limbs into contortions. They are caused by a disturbance of brain function and in adults usually result from epilepsy. In babies and young children they occur quite commonly but, although alarming, are generally not serious. Causes include a high fever due to infection, brain diseases such as meningitis and breath-holding, which is quite common in infants and very young children. Convulsions are thought to be more common in the very young because the nervous system is immature. Unless they are caused by the presence of disease or infection which requires to be treated, they are rarely life-threatening.

CORNEA the outermost, exposed layer of the EYE which is transparent and lies over the iris and lens. It refracts light entering the eye, directing the rays to the lens and thus acting as a coarse focus. It is a layer of connective tissue which has no blood supply of its own but is supplied with nutrients from fluid within the eye (the aqueous humour). It is highly sensitive to pain and presence or absence of response if the cornea is touched is used as an indicator of a person's condition, for example in a comatose patient.

CORNEAL GRAFT also known as keratoplasty, this is a surgical procedure to replace a damaged or diseased cornea with one from a donor. Sometimes only the outer layers of the cornea are replaced (lamellar keratoplasty) or the whole structure may be involved (penetrating keratoplasty).

CORONARY ANGIOPLASTY see ANGIOPLASTY.

CORONARY ARTERIES the arteries that supply blood to the heart and which arise from the AORTA.

CORONARY ARTERY DISEASE any abnormal condition that affects the arteries of the heart. The commonest disease is coronary ATHEROSCLEROSIS which is more prevalent in those populations with high fat, saturated fat, refined carbohydrates etc. in their diet. ANGINA is a common symptom of such diseases.

CORONARY BYPASS GRAFT a surgical operation which is carried out when one or more of the coronary arteries have become narrowed by

disease (ATHEROMA). A section of vein from a leg is grafted to bypass the obstruction and this major operation is usually successful and greatly improves a person's quality of life.

CORONARY THROMBOSIS a sudden blockage of one of the coronary arteries by a blood clot or thrombus which interrupts the blood supply to the heart. The victim collapses with severe and agonizing chest pain often accompanied by vomiting and nausea. The skin becomes pale and clammy, the temperature rises and there is difficulty in breathing. Coronary thrombosis generally results from ATHEROMA, and the part of the heart muscle which has its blood supply disrupted dies, a condition known as MYOCARDIAL INFARCTION. Treatment consists of giving strong pain-relieving drugs such as morphine. Also specialist care in a coronary care unit is usually required to deal with ARRHYTHMIA, heart failure and CARDIAC ARREST which are the potentially fatal results of coronary thrombosis.

CORPUS LUTEUM the tissue that forms within the ovary after a Graafian follicle (the structure which contains the egg) ruptures and releases an ovum at the time of OVULATION. It consists of a mass of cells containing yellow, fatty substances, and secretes the hormone PROGESTERONE which prepares the womb to receive a fertilized egg. If the egg is not fertilized and no implantation of an embryo takes place, the corpus luteum degenerates. However, if a pregnancy ensues, the corpus luteum expands and secretes progesterone until this function is taken over by the placenta at the fourth month.

CORTEX the outer part of an organ situated beneath its enclosing capsules or outer membrane. Examples are the adrenal cortex of the adrenal glands, renal cortex of the kidneys and cerebral cortex of the brain.

CORTICOSTEROIDS any steroid hormone manufactured by the adrenal cortex of which there are two main types. Glucocorticosteroids such as cortisol and cortisone are required by the body mainly for glucose metabolism and for responding to stress. Mineralocorticosteroids, e.g. aldosterone regulate the salt and water balance. Both groups are manufactured synthetically and used in the treatment of various disorders. Glucocorticosteroids are potent anti-inflammatory agents and are used in the treatment of conditions where inflammation is involved.

CORTICOSTEROID SIDE EFFECTS those effects that may be experienced when taking corticosteroid drugs. A mineralocorticoid may produce water retention, HYPERTENSION, muscle weakness, loss of potassium and cushingoid changes (*see* CUSHING'S SYNDROME). A glucocorticoid may produce depression, OSTEOPOROSIS, euphoria, peptic ulcer, cushingoid changes.

CORTISONE a glucocorticosteroid hormone produced by the adrenal cortex. It is used medically to treat deficiency of corticosteroid hormones. Deficiency occurs in ADDISON'S DISEASE and if the adrenal glands have had to be surgically removed for some reason. Its use is restricted because it causes severe side effects including damage to the muscle, bone, eye changes, stomach ulcers and bleeding as well as nervous and hormonal disturbances.

COSTAL CARTILAGE a type of cartilage connecting a rib to the sternum (breastbone).

COT DEATH *see* SUDDEN INFANT DEATH SYNDROME.

CRADLECAP a form of seborrhoea or dermatitis of the scalp which affects young babies and responds to an ointment containing white soft paraffin, salicylic acid and sulphur.

CRAMP prolonged and painful spasmodic muscular contraction which often occurs in the limbs but can affect certain internal organs (*see* COLIC and GASTRALGIA). Cramp may result from a salt imbalance as in heat cramp. Working in high temperatures causes excessive sweating and consequent loss of salt. It can be corrected and prevented by an increase of the salt intake. Occupational cramp results from continual repetitive use of particular muscles, e.g. writer's cramp. Night cramp occurs during sleep and is especially common among elderly people, diabetics and pregnant women. The cause is not known.

CRANIAL NERVES twelve pairs of nerves which arise directly from the brain each with dorsal and ventral branches known as *roots*. Each root remains separate and is assigned a roman numeral as well as a name. Some cranial nerves are mainly sensory while others are largely motor and they leave the skull through separate apertures. The cranial and spinal nerves are an important part of the *peripheral nervous system* which comprises all parts lying outside the brain and spinal cord.

CRANIUM the part of the skull that encloses the brain, formed from eight fused and flattened bones that are joined by immovable suture JOINTS.

CREPITUS the grating sound heard when the ends of fractured bones rub together and also from the joints of those suffering from arthritis. It also occurs in *chondromalacia patellae* which is a roughening of the inner surface of the kneecap which produces the grating sound and pain. Crepitus also denotes the sound heard by means of a STETHOSCOPE from an inflamed lung when there is fluid in the alveoli.

CRETINISM a syndrome caused by lack of thyroid hormone which is present before birth and is also called *congenital hyperthyroidism*. It is characterized by dwarfism, mental retardation and coarseness of skin and hair. Early diagnosis and treatment with thyroid extract (thyroxine) is vital as this greatly inproves a child's intellectual and other abilities. In the UK, blood serum from newborn babies is tested for thyroxine level in order to detect this condition.

CREUTZFELDT-JAKOB DISEASE also known as spongiform encephalopathy, this is a fatal disease of the brain thought to be caused by a SLOW VIRUS. There is a spongy degeneration of the brain and rapid progressive dementia. The disease usually strikes in middle and early old age and is usually fatal within a year. Similar diseases in animals are bovine spongiform encephalopathy (BSE) in cattle and scrapie in sheep which, it is alleged by some scientists, may be transmittable to man. Recently there has been alarm that some adults treated in childhood for dwarfism with extracts of pituitary glands obtained from corpses, may be at risk of contracting Creutzfeldt-Jakob disease. It is alleged that some of the pituitary glands obtained may have been infected with the virus and that the disease has been passed on and has already caused some deaths.

CROUP a group of diseases characterized by a swelling, partial obstruction and inflammation of the entrance to the larynx, occurring in young children. The breathing is harsh and strained producing a typical crowing sound, accompanied by coughing and feverishness. Diphtheria used to be the most common cause of croup but it now usually results from a viral infection of the respiratory tract (LARYNGO-TRACHEO BRONCHITIS). The condition is relieved by inhaling steam (a soothing preparation such as tincture of benzoin is sometimes added to the hot water) and also by mild sedatives and/or pain killers. Rarely, the obstruction becomes dangerous and completely blocks the larynx in which case emergency TRACHEOSTOMY or nasotracheal INTUBATION may be required. Usually, the symptoms of croup subside and the child recovers, but then he or she may have a tendency towards attacks on future occasions.

CRYOSURGERY the use of extreme cold to perform surgical procedures, usually on localized areas to remove unwanted tissue. The advantages are that there is little or no bleeding or sensation of pain, and scarring is very much reduced. An instrument called a cryoprobe is used, the fine tip of which is cooled by means of a coolant substance contained within the probe. The coolants used are carbon dioxide ad nitrous oxide gas and liquid nitrogen. Cryosurgery is used for the removal of cataracts, warts and to destroy some bone tumours.

CULTURE a population of bacteria viruses other microorganisms, or cells grown in the laboratory on a nutrient base known as a *culture medium*.

CURARE an extract from the bark of certain South American trees which relaxes and paralyses voluntary muscle. The pure alkaloid substance obtained from the bark is known as d-tubocurarine chloride and it is used as a muscle relaxant in anaesthesia.

CUSHING'S SYNDROME a metabolic disorder which results from excessive amounts of CORTICOSTEROIDS in the body due to an inability to regulate cortisol or adrenocorticotropic hormone (ACTH). The commonest cause is a tumour of the PITUITARY GLAND (producing secretion of ACTH) or a malignancy elsewhere, e.g. in the lung, or adrenal gland requiring extensive therapy with corticosteroid drugs. Symptoms include obesity, reddening of face and neck, growth of body and facial hair, OSTEOPOROSIS, high blood pressure and possible mental disturbances.

CUTICLE another name for the outer layer or EPIDERMIS of the skin and also refers to the outer layer of flattened cells covering a hair.

CYANIDE POISONING poisoning with any of the salts of hydrocyanic acid which paralyses every part of the nervous system and is usually fatal within minutes. The person rapidly becomes unconscious and this is followed by convulsions and death. The antidotes are amyl nitrite sodium thiosulphate and cobalt edetate which may save life if quickly administered.

CYANOCOBALAMIN *see* VITAMIN B12.

CYANOSIS a blue appearance of the skin due to insufficient oxygen within the blood. It is first noticeable on the lips, tips of the ears, cheeks and nails and occurs in heart failure, lung diseases, asphyxia and in "blue babies" who have congenital heart defects.

CYSTIC FIBROSIS a genetic disease, the defective gene responsible for it being located on human chromosome no. 7. The disease affects all the mucus-secreting glands of the lungs, pancreas, mouth and gastro-intestinal tract and also the sweat glands of the skin. A thick mucus is produced which affects the production of pancreatic enzymes and cause the bronchi to widen (bronchiectasis) and become clogged. Respiratory infections are common and the sweat contains abnormally high levels of sodium and chloride. The stools also contain a lot of mucus and have a foul smell. The disease is incurable and cannot be diagnosed by antenatal tests. However, the outlook for affected children has greatly improved and treatment consists of physiotherapy to relieve bronchial congestion, taking pancreatic enzyme tablets, vitamins and prompt treatment of respiratory infections when these occur.

CYSTITIS inflammation of the bladder normally caused by bacterial infection, the causal organism usually being *E. coli*. It is marked by the need to pass urine frequently accompanied by a burning sensation. There may be cramp-like pains in the lower abdomen with dark strong urine which contains blood. The condition is common in females and is usually not serious, but there is a danger that the infection may spread to the kidneys. Treatment is by means of antibiotics and also by drinking a lot of fluid possibly with the addition of bicarbonate of soda. The prevalence of the condition in females is due to the fact that the urethra is much shorter in women than in men, and the bacteria (which are present and harmless in the bowel) are more likely to gain access both to the urinary tract and vagina.

CYSTS small, usually benign, tumours containing fluid (or soft secretions) within a membranous sac. Examples are wens (caused by blockage of sebaceous glands in the skin), cysts in the breasts caused by blocked milk ducts and ovarian cysts which may be large and contain a clear, thick liquid. *Dermoid cysts* are congenital and occur at sites in the body where embryonic clefts have closed up before birth. These may contain fatty substances, hair, skin fragments of bone and even teeth. *Hydatid cysts* are a stage in the life cycle of certain parasites (tapeworm) and may be found in man, especially in the liver.

CYTOMEGALOVIRUSES a number of viruses belonging to the *Herpes* group which give infected cells a swollen appearance. They cause severe effects in those whose immune system is disrupted and are responsible for a serious disease of newborn babies called cytomegalic disease. The virus is transmitted to the baby before or during birth and can cause jaundice, enlargement of the liver and spleen and mental retardation.

CYTOPLASM the jelly-like substance within the cell wall which surrounds the nucleus and contains a number of organelles.

CYTOTOXIC a substance wchich damages or destroys cells. Cytotoxic drugs are used in the treatment of various forms of cancer and act by inhibiting cell division. However, they also damage normal cells and hence their use has to be carefully regulated in each individual patient. Cytotoxic drugs may be used in combination with RADIOTHERAPY or on their own.

DECIDUA the soft epithelial tissue that forms a lining to the uterus during pregnancy and which is shed at birth.

DEFIBRILLATION the application of a large electrick shock to the chest wall of a patient whose heart is fibrillating (*see* FIBRILLATION). The delivery of a direct electric countershock hopefully allows the pacemaker to set up the correct rhythm again.

DEGENERATION the deterioration over time of body tissues or an organ resulting in a lessening of its function. The changes may be structural or chemical and there are a number of types: fatty, FIBROID, calcareous (as with CONCRETIONS), mucoid and so on. Degeneration may be due to ageing, heredity or poor nutrition. Poisons such as alcohol also contribute to degeneration, as with CIRRHOSIS.

DEHYDRATION the removal of water. More specifically, the loss of water from the body through diuresis, sweating etc. or a reduction in water content due to a low intake. Essential body electrolytes (such as sodium chloride and potassium) are disrupted and after the first symptom, thirst, irritability and confusion follow.

DELIRIUM a mental disorder typified by confusion, agitation, fear, anxiety, illusions and sometimes hallucinations. The causal cerebral disfunction may be due to deficient nutrition, stress, toxic poisoning or mental shock.

DELIRIUM TREMENS a form of DELIRIUM due often to partial or total withdrawal of alcohol after a period of excessive intake. Symptoms are varied and include insomnia, agitation, confusion and fever, often with vivid hallucinations. The treatment involves lessening and removing the dependence on alcohol

which is accompanied by sedation with drugs such as BENZODIAZEPINEL.

DEMENTIA a mental disorder typified by confusion, disorientation, memory loss, personality changes and a lessening of intellectual capacity. Dementia occurs in several forms: SENILE DEMENTIA, ALZHEIMER'S DISEASE and MULTI-INFARCT DEMENTIA. The causes are various and include vascular disease, brain tumour, SUBDURAL HAEMATOMA, HYDROCEPHALUS and hyperthyroidism.

DEMYELINATION the process whereby the myelin sheath surrounding a nerve fibre is destroyed, resulting in impaired nerve function. This is associated with MULTIPLE SCLEROSIS but can also happen after a nerve has been injured.

DENATURATION the disruption, usually by heat, of the weak bonds that hold a protein together. Extremes of temperature are fatal to most animals because the ENZYMES (which are proteins) that perform essential catalytic functions in life-sustaining biochemical processes, are irreversibly denatured.

DENDRITE one of numerous thin branching extensions of a nerve cell. The dendrites are at the "receiving end" of the nerve cell (neuron) and they form a network which increases the area for receiving impulses from the terminals of axons of other neurons at the SYNAPSE.

DEPOT with reference to a drug, being injected or implanted for slow absorption into the circulation.

DEPRESSANT a drug which is used to reduce the functioning of a system of the body e.g. a respiratory depressant. Drugs such as opiates, general anaesthetics, etc. are depressants.

DEPRESSION a mental state of extreme sadness dominated by pessimism and in which normal behaviour patterns (sleep, appetite, etc.) are disturbed. Causes are varied: upsetting events, loss, etc. and treatment involves the use of therapy and drugs (*see also* MANIC DEPRESSIVE PSYCHOSIS).

DERMATITIS an inflammation of the

skin which is similar in many respects to, and often interchanged with, ECZEMA. It is characterized by erythema (redness due to dilatation of capillaries near the surface), pain and PRURITIS. Several forms of dermatitis can be identified: Contact dermatitis caused by the skin coming into contact with a substance to which the skin is sensitive. A large range of compounds and materials may cause such a reaction. Treatment usually involves the use of a corticosteroid. Light dermatitis manifests itself as a reddening and blistering of skin exposed to sunlight and this occurs on hands, face and neck and occurs during the summer months. Some individuals become sensitized by drugs or perfumes in cosmetics while others have an innate sensitivity. Erythroderma or exfoliative dermatitis involves patches of reddened skin which thicken and peel off. It is often associated with other skin conditions, e.g. PSORIASIS. Corticosteroids form a central part of the treatment in this case.

DESENSITIZATION the technique whereby an individual builds up resistance to an allergen by taking gradually increasing doses of the allergen over a period of time. Also in the treatment of phobias, where a patient is gradually faced with the thing that is feared and concurrently learns to relax and reduce anxiety.

DIABETES INSIPIDUS a rare condition which is completely different from DIABETES MELLITUS and is characterized by excessive thirst (see POLYDIPSIA) and POLYURIA. It is due to a lack of the antidiuretic hormone or the inability of the kidney to respond to the hormone.

DIABETES MELLITUS a complex metabolic disorder involving carbohydrate, fat and protein. It results in an accumulation of sugar in the blood and urine and is due to a lack of INSULIN produced by the pancreas, so that sugars are not broken down to release energy. Fats are thus used as an alternative energy source. Symptoms include thirst,

POLYURIA, loss of weight and the use of fats can produce KETOSIS and KETONURIA. In its severest form, convulsions are followed by a diabetic coma. Treatment relies upon dietary control with doses of insulin or drugs, long-term effects include thickening of the arteries, and in some cases the eyes, kidneys, nervous system, skin and circulation may be affected (see also HYPOGLYCAEMIA and HYPERGLYCAEMIA).

DIALYSIS the use of a semipermeable membrane to separate large and small molecules by selective diffusion. Starch and proteins are large molecules while salts, glucose and amino acids are small molecules. If a mixture of large and small molecules is separated from distilled water by a semi-permeable membrane, the smaller molecules diffuse into the water which is itself replenished. This principle is the basis of the artificial kidney which, because a patient's blood is processed, is known as HAEMODIALYSIS.

DIAPHRAGM a membrane of muscle and tendon that separates the thoracic and abdominal cavities. It is covered by a SEROUS MEMBRANE and attached at the lower ribs, breastbone and backbone. The diaphragm is important in breathing, when it bulges up to its resting position during exhalation. It flattens during inhalation and in so doing it reduces pressure in the thoracic cavity and helps to draw air into the lungs. Also a rubber bowl-shaped cap used as a contraceptive with spermicidal cream. It fits inside the VAGINA over the neck of the UTERUS.

DIAPHYSIS the central part of shaft of a long bone.

DIARRHOEA increased frequency and looseness of bowel movement, involving the passage of unusually soft faeces. Diarrhoea can be caused by food poisoning, COLITIS, IRRITABLE BOWEL SYNDROME, DYSENTERY, etc. A severe case will result in the loss of water and salts which must be replaced and anti-diarrhoeal drugs are used in certain circumstances.

DIASTASE (amylases) ENZYMES that break down starch into sugar. Specifically, diastase is the part of malt containing â amylase. Diastase is used to help in the digestion of starch in some digestive disorders.

DIASTOLE the point at which the heart relaxes between contractions, when the ventricles fill with blood. This usually lasts about half a second at the end of which the ventricles are about three-quarters full.

DIGESTION the process of breaking down food into substances that can be absorbed and used by the body. Digestion begins with the chewing and grinding of food at which point it is mixed with saliva to commence the process of breakdown. Most digestion occurs in the stomach and small intestine. In the stomach the food is subject to gastric juice which contains pepsins to break down proteins and hydrochloric acid. The food is mixed and becomes totally soluble before passing into the small intestine as chyme, where it is acted upon by pancreatic juice, bile, bacteria and succus entericus (intestinal juices). Water is absorbed in the intestine in a very short time, while the bulk of the food may take several hours. The chyme forms chyle due to the action of bile and pancreatic juice. Fats are removed from this in emulsion form into the lymph vessels (see LACTEAL) and then into the blood. Sugars, salts and amino acids move directly into the small blood vessels in the intestine and the whole process is promoted by microfolding of the intestine wall producing finger-like projections (villi). The food passes down the intestine due to muscle contractions of the intestine wall and ultimately the residue and waste are excreted.

DIGITALIS a powder derived from the leaf of the wild foxglove (*Digitalis purpurea*) which finds use in cases of heart disease. It acts in two ways; strengthening each heartbeat and increasing each pause (DIASTOLE) so that the damaged heart

muscle has longer to rest. It also has a diuretic effect. Digitalis poisoning may occur with prolonged use or an overdose. Symptoms include vomiting, nausea, blurred vision, irregular heartbeat and possible breathing difficulties and unconsciousness.

DILATATION AND CURETTAGE (D & C) the technique whereby the cervix is opened using DILATORS and then the lining is scraped using a curette. Such sampling is performed for the removal of incomplete abortions and tumours, to diagnose disease of the uterus or to correct bleeding, etc.

DIPEPTIDE a compound comprising two amino acids joined by a peptide bond (a characteristic chemical linkage where the amino group - NH_2 - of one amino acid is joined to the carboxyl group - COOH - of another).

DIPHTHERIA a serious, infectious disease caused by the bacterium *Corynebacterium diphtheriae*, and commonest in children. The infection causes a membranous lining on the throat which can interfere with breathing and eating. The toxin produced by the bacterium damages heart tissue and the central nervous system and can be fatal if not treated. The infection is countered by injection of the antitoxin with penicillin or erythromycin taken to kill the bacterium. Diphtheria can be immunized against.

DIPLEGIA paralysis on both sides of the body.

DIPLOPIA double vision. Caused by disfunction in the muscles that move the eyeballs such that rays of light fall in different places on the two retinae. The condition can be due to a nervous disease, intoxication or certain diseases such as diphtheria.

DISC a flattened circular structure, such as the cartilage between vertebrae.

DISINFECTION the process of killing PATHOGENIC organisms (not spores) to prevent the spread of infection. Different compounds are used, appropriate to the surface being disinfected.

DIURESIS an increase in urine production due to disease, drugs, hormone imbalance or increased fluid intake.

DIURETICA a substance that increases urine formation and excretion and which may work specifically within the kidney e.g. by prevention of sodium, and therefore water, reabsorption or outside the kidney.

DIVERTICULITIS the inflammation of diverticula (*see* DIVERTICULUM) in the large intestine. During the condition, there are cramp-like pains in the left side of the abdomen, possibly with constipation and fever. Treatment normally involves complete rest with no solid food, and antibiotics.

DIVERTICULOSIS the condition in which there are DIVERTICULA in the large intestine, occurring primarily in the lower colon. They are caused by the muscles of the bowel forcing the bowel out through weak points in the wall. It is thought that it may be related to diet, but symptoms are not always produced.

DIVERTICULUM in general, a pouch extending from a main cavity. Specifically applied to the intestine, a sac-like protrusion through the wall, many of which usually develop later in life. The formation of diverticula is DIVERTICULOSIS and their inflammation, DIVERTICULITIS.

DNA (deoxyribonucleic acid) a nucleic acid and the primary constituent of CHROMOSOMES. It transmits genetic information from parents to offspring in the form of GENES. It is a very large molecule comprising two twisted nucleotide chains which can store enormous amounts of information in a stable but not rigid way i.e. parental traits and characteristics are passed on but evolutionary changes are allowed to occur.

DONOR INSEMINATION *see* ARTIFICIAL INSEMINATION.

DOPA an amino acid compound formed from tyrosine (an amino acid synthesized in the body) and which is a precursor of DOPAMINE and NORADRENALINE (norepinephrine in America). A drug form, levodopa or l-dopa, is used to treat PARKINSONISM,

as it can increase the concentration of dopamine in the basal ganglia.

DOPAMINE a catecholamine derived from DOPA and an intermediate in the synthesis of NORADRENALINE. (Catecholamines comprise benzene, hydroxyl groups and an amine group and are physiologically important in the functioning of the nervous system, mainly as NEUROTRANSMITTERS). It is found mainly in the basal ganglia of the brain and a deficiency is typical in PARKINSONISM.

DOSAGE the overall amount of a drug administered, determined by size, frequency and number of doses and taking into account the patient's age, weight and possible allergic reactions. Modern techniques enable controlled dosage using transdermals (drugs absorbed from a plaster on the skin) and implantable devices. The latter are polymeric substances containing the drug and placed just beneath the skin which deliver the correct dose at any predetermined rate.

DOWN'S SYNDROME (formerly called mongolism) a syndrome created by a CONGENITAL CHROMOSOME disorder which occurs as an extra chromosome 21, producing 47 in each body cell. Characteristic facial features are produced - a shorter, broader face with slanted eyes (similar to the Mongolian races, hence the term mongolism). It also results in a shorter stature, weak muscles and the possibility of heart defects and respiratory problems. The syndrome also confers mental retardation.

Down's syndrome occurs once in approximately 600 to 700 live births and although individuals may live beyond middle age, life expectancy is reduced and many die in infancy. The incidence increases with the age of the mother from 0.04% of children to women under 30 to 3% to women at 45. It is therefore likely that above 35 an AMNIOCENTESIS test would be made.

DRUG BINDING when a drug is attached to a protein, fat or component of tissues.

DRUG CLEARANCE is defined as the volume of blood which in one minute is completely cleared of a drug.

DRUG INTERACTIONS when a patient is prescribed several drugs, there is the possibility for interactions between some or all of the medications. There are several ways in which the interaction may occur e.g. one drug displacing another at the site of action thus affecting its effectiveness; as alteration in the rate of destruction of one drug by another (by altering the activity of liver enzymes); prevention of absorption.

DRUG METABOLISM the process by which a drug is altered by the body into a metabolite (i.e. necessary for metabolic action), which may be the active agent and the process which ultimately results in the removal of the drug and thus determines the length of time over which it is active.

DUBLIN-JOHNSON SYNDROME a rare, chronic and hereditary condition in which there is an excess of BILIRUBIN in the blood leading to gall bladder disorders, jaundice and abnormal pigmentation of the liver.

DUCT a narrow tube-like structure joining a gland with an organ or the body surface, through which a secretion passes e.g. sweat ducts opening onto the skin.

DUCTLESS GLAND a gland which releases the secretion directly into the blood for transport around the body, e.g. the pituitary and thyroid. Some glands, such as the PANCREAS, operate as a ductless gland (for INSULIN), but secrete a digestive juice via ducts into the small intestine.

DUCTUS ARTERIOSUS when a foetus is in the uterus, the lungs do not function and the foetal blood bypasses the lungs by means of the ductus arteriosus which takes blood from the pulmonary artery to the aorta. The vessel stops functioning soon after birth.

DUODENAL ULCER the commonest type of PEPTIC ULCER. Duodenal ulcers may occur after the age of 20 and are more common in men. The cause is open

to debate but probably results from an abrasion or break in the duodenum lining which is then exacerbated by gastric juice. Smoking seems to be a contributory but not causal factor.

The ulcer manifests itself as an upper abdominal pain roughly two hours after a meal that also occurs during the night. Food (e.g. milk) relieves the symptom and a regime of frequent meals and milky snacks, with little or no fried food and spices and a minimum of strong tea and coffee is usually adopted. Recent drug treatments enable the acid secretion to be reduced, thus allowing the ulcer to heal. Surgery is required only if there is no response to treatment, if the PYLORUS is obstructed or if the ulcer becomes perforated. The latter is treated as an emergency.

DUODENUM the first part of the small intestine where food (chyme) from the stomach is subject to action by BILE and pancreatic enzymes. The duodenum also secretes a hormone secretion that contributes to the breakdown of fats, proteins and carbohydrates. In the duodenum, the acid conditions pertaining from the stomach are neutralized and rendered alkaline for the intestinal enzymes to operate.

DURA MATER *see* MENINGES and BRAIN.

DWARFISM an abnormal under-development of the body manifested by small stature. There are several causes including incorrect functioning of the PITUITARY or THYROID glands. Pituitary dwarfism produces a small but correctly proportioned body and if diagnosed sufficiently early, treatment with growth hormone can help. A defect in the thyroid gland may results in CRETINISM or in the activity of digestive organs and their secretions. RICKETS may also be responsible for dwarfism.

DYSENTERY an infection and ulceration of the lower part of the bowels that causes severe diarrhoea with the passage of mucus and blood. There are two forms of dysentery caused by different organisms. Amoebic dysentery is due to *Entamoeba histolytica* which is spread via infected food or water and occurs mainly in the tropics and sub-tropics. The appearance of symptoms may be delayed but in addition to diarrhoea there is indigestion, anaemia and weight loss. Drugs are used in treatment.

Bacillary dysentery is caused by the bacterium *Shigella* and spreads by contact with a carrier or contaminated food. Symptoms appear from one to six days after infection and include diarrhoea, cramp, nausea, fever and the severity of the attack varies. Antibiotics may be given to kill the bacteria but recovery usually occurs within one to two weeks.

DYSLEXIA a disorder that renders reading or learning to read difficult. There is usually an associated problem in writing and spelling correctly. A very small number of children are affected severely and boys are more prone than girls by a factor of three.

DYSPEPSIA (or indigestion) after eating there may be discomfort in the upper abdomen/lower chest with heartburn, nausea and flatulence accompanying a feeling of fullness. The causes are numerous and include GALLSTONES, PEPTIC ULCER, HIATUS HERNIA and diseases of the liver or pancreas.

DYSPHASIA a general term for an impairment of speech whether it is manifested as a difficulty in understand-ing language or in self-expression. There is a range of conditions with varying degrees of severity. *Global aphasia* is a total inability to communicate, however some individuals partially understand what is said to them. *Dysphasia* is when thoughts can be expresed up to a point. *Non-fluent dysphasia* represents poor self-expression but good understanding while the reverse is called *fluent dysphasia*. The condition may be due to a stroke or other brain damage and can be temporary or permanent.

EAR the sense organ used for detection of sound and maintenance of balance. It comprises three parts, the external or outer, middle and inner ear, the first two acting to collect sound waves and transmit them to the inner ear, where the hearing and balance mechanisms are situated.

The outer ear (*auricle* or *pinna*) is a cartilage and skin structure which is not actually essential to hearing in man. The middle ear is an air-filled cavity that is linked to the PHARYNX via the EUSTACHIAN TUBE. Within the middle ear are the ear (or auditory) ossicles, three bones called the *incus, malleus* and *stapes* (anvil, hammer and stirrup respectively). Two small muscles control the bones and the associated nerve (the chorda tympani). The ossicles bridge the middle ear, connecting the eardrum with the inner ear and in so doing convert sound (air waves) into mechanical movements which then impinge upon the fluid of the inner ear.

The inner ear lies within the temporal bone of the skull and contains the apparatus for hearing and balance. The COCHLEA is responsible for hearing and balance is maintained by the semi-circular canals. The latter are made up of three loops positioned mutually at right angles and in each is the fluid endolymph. When the head is moved the fluid moves accordingly and sensory cells produce impulses that are transmitted to the brain.

EARACHE pain in the ear may be due directly to inflammation of the middle ear but is often referred pain from other conditions, e.g. infections of the nose, larynx or tooth decay.

EATING DISORDERS *see* BULIMIA

ECG *see* ELECTROCARDIOGRAM

ECHOCARDIOGRAPHY the use of

ULTRASOUND to study the heart and its movements.

ECHOGRAPHY (or ultrasonography) the use of sound waves (ULTRASOUND) to create an image of the deeper structures of the body, based upon the differences in reflection of the sound by various parts of the body.

ECLAMPSIA convulsions that occur during pregnancy, usually at the later stages or during delivery. Although the cause is not known the start of convulsions may be associated with cerebral OEDEMA or a sudden rise in blood pressure. Kidney function is usually badly affected. The condition is often preceded for days or weeks by symptoms such as headache, dizziness and vomiting and seizures follow. The fits differ in severity and duration and in the one in twelve fatalities, there may be a cerebral haemorrhage, pneumonia or the breathing may gradually fade. The condition requires immediate treatment as it threatens both mother and baby. Treatment is by drugs and reduction of outside stimuli, and a CAESARIAN section is undertaken.

ECZEMA an inflammation of the skin that causes itching, a red rash and often small blisters that weep and become encrusted. This may be followed by the skin thickening and then peeling off in scales. There are several types of eczema, *atopic* being one of the most common. (Atopic is the hereditary tendency to form allergic reactions due to an antibody in the skin). A form of atopic eczema is infantile eczema that starts at 3 or 4 months and it is often the case that eczema, hay fever and asthma is found in the family history. However, many children improve markedly as they approach the age of 10 or 11. The treatment for such conditions usually involves the use of HYDROCORTISONE and other steroid creams and ointments.

EEG *see* ELECTROENCEPHALOGRAM

ELECTROCARDIOGRAM a record of the changes in the heart's electrical potential, on an instrument called an electrocardiograph. The subject is connected to the equipment by leads on the chest and legs or arms. A normal trace has one wave for the activity of the atria and others relating to the ventricular beat. Abnormal heart activity is often indicated in the trace and it therefore forms a useful diagnostic aid.

ELECTROCONVULSIVE THERAPY a somewhat drastic treatment for severe DEPRESSION and sometimes SCHIZOPHRENIA. An electric current is passed through the brain, producing a convulsion. The convulsion is controlled by administering an anaesthetic and a muscle relaxant. There is no memory of the shock and there may be temporary amnesia, with headache and confusion - symptoms that usually dissipate within a few hours. It is a treatment that is used much less than was the case and even then it is considered suitable for only very carefully chosen patients.

ELECTROENCEPHALOGRAM (EEG) a record of the brain's electrical activity measured on an electroencephalograph. Electrodes on the scalp record the charge of electric potential - or brain waves. There are four main types of waves: alpha, beta, theta and delta. Alpha waves, with a frequency of ten per second, occur when awake and delta waves (seven or less per second) occur in sleeping adults. The occurrence of delta waves in wakeful adults indicates brain damage or cerebral tumours.

ELECTROLYTES *sensu stricto* - a compound that dissolves in water to produce a solution containing ions that is able to conduct an electrical charge. In the body, electrolytes occur in the blood plasma, all fluid and interstitial fluid and normal concentrations are imperative for normal metabolic activity. Some diseases alter the electrolyte balance either through vomiting or diarrhoea or because the kidney is malfunctioning. The correct balance can be restored through oral or intravenous dosage or by DIALYSIS.

EMBOLECTOMY the surgical, and

often emergency, removal of an EMBOLUS or clot to clear an arterial obstruction.

EMBOLISM the state in which a small blood vessel is blocked by an EMBOLUS, or fragment of material which the circulatory system has carried through larger vessels. This plug may be fragments of a clot, a mass of bacteria, air bubbles that have entered the system during an operation, or a fragment of tumour. The blockage leads usually to the destruction of that part of the organ supplied by the vessel. The most common case is a pulmonary embolism. Treatment utilises an anticoagulant drug such as warfarin or heparin, EMBOLECTOMY or streptokinase. The latter is an enzyme capable of dissolving blood clots.

EMBOLUS material carried by the blood which then lodges elsewhere in the body (*see* EMBOLISM). The material may be a blood clot, fat, air, a piece of tumour etc.

EMBRYO the stage of development from 2 weeks, when the fertilized ovum is implanted in the uterus, to 2 months.

EMBRYOLOGY the study of the embryo, its growth and development from fertilization to birth.

EMBRYO TRANSFER (*see also* IN VITRO FERTILIZATION) the fertilization of an ovum by sperm and its development into an early embryo, outside the mother, and its subsequent implantation in the mother's uterus. Such procedures result in what is popularly termed a "test-tube baby."

EMESIS is the medical term for vomit.

EMETICS a substance that causes vomiting. Direct emetics such as mustard in water, copper sulphate, alum or a lot of salty water irritate the stomach, while indirect emetics such as apomorphine and ipecacuanha act on the centre of the brain that controls the act of vomiting. Tickling the throat is also classed as an emetic (indirect). Emetics tend to be used little nowadays, but great care must be exercised if their use is advocated.

EMOLLIENTS substances that soften or soothe the skin whether in the form of a powder, oil or preparation, often used in the treatment of eczema. Examples are olive oil, glycerin and French chalk.

EMPHYSEMA refers, in the main, to an abnormal condition of the lungs where the walls of the are over-inflated and distended and changes in their structure occur. This destruction of parts of the walls produces large air-filled spaces which do not contribute to the respiratory process. Acute cases of emphysema may be caused by whooping cough, bronchopneumonia and chronic cases often accompany chronic bronchitis which itself is due in great part to smoking. Emphysema is also developed after tuberculosis when the lungs are stretched until the fibres of the alveolar walls are destroyed. Similarly in old age, the alveolar membrane may collapse producing large air sacs, with decreased surface area.

ENCEPHALINS PEPTIDES that act as NEUROTRANSMITTERS. Two have been identified, both acting as analgesics when their release controls pain. They are found in the brain and in nerve cells of the spinal cord.

ENCEPHALITIS Inflammation of the brain. It is usually a viral infection and sometimes occurs as a complication of some common infectious diseases, e.g. measles or chickenpox. There are several forms of the disease including *Encephalitis lethargica* (sleepy sickness or epidemic encephalitis) which attacks and causes swelling in the basal ganglia, cerebrum and brain stem that may result in tissue destruction; Japanese encephalitis, which is caused by a virus carried by mosquitoes and tick-borne encephalitis which occurs in Europe and Siberia. In most cases there is no readily available treatment under the causative virus is *Herpes*.

ENCEPHALOGRAPHY any technique used to record brain structure or activity e.g. electroencephalography (*see* EEG).

ENCEPHALOID the term given to a form of cancer that superficially resembles brain tissue.

ENCEPHALOMYELITIS inflammation of the brain and spinal cord typified by headaches, fever, stiff neck and back pain, with vomiting. Depending upon the extent of the inflammation and the patient's condition, encephalomyelitis may cause paralysis, personality changes, coma or death.

ENCEPHALOPATHY any disease affecting the brain or an abnormal condition of the brain's structure and function. It refers in particular to degenerative and chronic conditions such as Wernicke's encephalopathy which is caused by a THIAMINE deficiency and associated with alcoholism.

ENDEMIC the term used to describe, for example, a disease that is indigenous to a certain area.

ENDOCARDITIS inflammation of the ENDOCARDIUM, heart valves and muscle, caused by a bacterium, virus or rheumatic fever. Those at greatest risk are patients with some damage to the endocardium from a CONGENITAL deformity or alteration of the immune system by drugs. Patients suffer fever, heart failure and/or EMBOLISM. Large doses of an antibiotic are used in treatment and surgery may prove necessary to repair heart valves that become damaged. If not treated the condition is fatal.

ENDOCARDIUM a fine membrane lining the heart which forms a continuous membrane with the lining of veins and arteries. At the cavities of the heart it forms cusps on the valves and its surface is very smooth to facilitate blood flow.

ENDOCRINE GLANDS DUCTLESS GLANDS that produce HORMONES for secretion directly into the bloodstream (or lymph). Some organs e.g. the PANCREAS also release secretions via a DUCT. In addition to the pancreas the major endocrine glands are the THYROID, PITUITARY, PARATHYROID, OVARY and TESTIS. Imbalances in the secretions of endocrine glands produce a variety of diseases (see individual entries).

ENDOCRINOLOGY the study of the ENDOCRINE GLANDS, the hormones secreted by the glands and the treatment of any problems.

ENDOGENOUS referring to within the body, whether growing within, or originating from within or due to internal causes.

ENDOMETRIOSIS the occurrence of ENDOMETRIUM in other parts of the body e.g. within the muscle of the uterus, in the ovary, FALLOPIAN TUBES, PERITONEUM and possibly the bowel. Because of the nature of tissue, it acts in a way similar to that of the uterus lining and causes pelvic pain, bleeding, painful menstruation. The condition occurs between puberty and the menopause and ceases during pregnancy. The treatment required may include total hysterectomy, but occasionally the administration of a steroid hormone will alleviate the symptoms.

ENDOMETRITIS inflammation of the ENDOMETRIUM caused commonly by bacteria but can also be due to a virus, parasite or foreign body. It is associated with fever and abdominal pain and occurs most after abortion or childbirth or women with an INTRAUTERINE CONTRACEPTIVE DEVICE.

ENDOMETRIUM the womb's mucous membrane lining that changes in structure during the menstrual cycle, becoming thicker with an increased blood supply later in the cycle. This is in readiness for receiving an embryo but if this does not happen, the endometrium breaks down and most is lost in menstruation.

ENDORPHINS a group of compounds, PEPTIDES that occur in the brain and have pain-relieving qualities similar to morphine. They are derived from a substance in the PITUITARY and are involved in endocrine control. In addition to their opiate effects, they are involved in urine output, depression of respiration, sexual activity and learning (see also ENCEPHALINS).

ENDOSCOPE the general term for an instrument used to inspect the interior of a body cavity or organ, e.g. the gastroscope is for viewing the stomach. The instrument is fitted with lenses and a light source and is usually inserted through a natural opening although an incision can be used.

ENEMA the procedure of putting fluid into the rectum for purposes of cleansing or therapy. An evacuant enema removes faeces and consists of soap in water or olive oil while a barium enema is given to permit an X-ray of the colon to be taken. The compound barium sulphate is opaque to X-rays. The insertion of drugs into the rectum is a therapeutic enema.

ENTERAL the term meaning relating to the intestine.

ENTERAL FEEDING the procedure of feeding a patient who is very ill through a tube via the nose, to the stomach. Through the tube is given a liquid, low waste food and there are a number of proprietary brands, some containing whole protein, some amino acids. This is a particularly useful technique when a patient suffers tissue damage with an ensuing reduction of muscle and plasma proteins after a major operation, burns, renal failure etc.

ENTERIC FEVERS *see* TYPHOID FEVER and PARATYPHOID FEVER.

ENTERITIS inflammation of the intestine, due usually to a viral or bacterial infection, causing diarrhoea.

ENTEROVIRUS a virus that enters the body via the gut where it multiplies and from where they attack the central nervous system. Examples are POLIOMYELITIS and the Coxsackie viruses (the cause of severe throat infections, MENINGITIS, and inflammation of heart tissue, some muscles and the brain).

ENZYME any protein molecule that acts as a catalyst in the biochemical processes of the body. They are essential to life ad are highly specific, acting on certain substrates at a set temperature and pH. Examples are the digestive enzymes amylase, lipase and trypsin. Enzymes act by providing active sites

(one or more for each enzyme) to which substrate molecules bind, forming a short-lived intermediate. The rate of reaction is increased, and after the product is formed, the active site is freed. Enzymes are easily rendered inactive by heat and some chemicals. The names of most enzymes end in *-ase*, and this is added onto the name of the substrate thus a peptidase breaks down peptides. Enzymes are vital for the normal functioning of the body and their lack or inactivity can produce metabolic disorders.

EPIDEMIC a disease that affects a large proportion of the population at the same time. Usually an infectious disease that occurs suddenly and spreads rapidly, e.g. today there are influenza epidemics.

EPIDERMIS the outer layer of the skin which comprises four layers and overlies the dermis. The top three layers are continually renewed as cells from the innermost germinative layer (called *the Malpighian layer or stratum germinativum*) are pushed outwards. The topmost layer (*stratum corneum*) is made up of dead cells where the CYTOPLASM has been replaced by KERATIN. This layer is thickest on the palms and soles of the feet.

EPIDURAL ANAESTHESIA anaesthesia in the region of the pelvis, abdomen or genitals produced by local anaesthetic injected into the epidural space of the spinal column (the epidural space is that space between the vertebral canal and the dura mater of the spinal cord).

EPIGLOTTIS situated at the base of the tongue, a thin piece of cartilage enclosed in MUCOUS MEMBRANE that covers the LARYNX. It prevents food from passing into the larynx and TRACHEA when swallowing. The epiglottis resembles a leaf in shape.

EPIGLOTTITIS inflammation of the mucous membrane of the EPIGLOTTIS. Swelling of the tissues may obstruct the airway and swift action may be necessary i.e. a TRACHEOSTOMY to avoid a fatality. The other symptoms of epiglottitis are sore throat, fever, a croup-like cough and it occurs mainly in children, usually during the winter.

EPILEPSY a neurological disorder involving convulsions, seizures and loss of consciousness. There are many possible causes or associations of epilepsy, including cerebral trauma, brain tumour, cerebral haemorrhage and metabolic imbalances as in HYPOGLYCAEMIA. Usually an epileptic attack occurs without warning, with complete unconsciousness and some muscle contraction and spasms. Some drugs are used in treatment although little can be done during the fit itself.

EPIPHYSIS the softer end of a long bone that is separated from the shaft by a plate (the epiphyseal plate) of cartilage. It develops separately from the shaft but when the bone stops growing it disappears as the head and shaft fuse. Separation of the epiphysis is a serious fracture because the growing bone may be affected.

EPISIOTOMY the process of making an incision in the PERINEUM to enlarge a woman's vaginal opening to facilitate delivery of a child. The technique is used to prevent tearing of the perineum.

EPITHELIOMA an epithelial (*see* EPITHELIUM) tumour used formerly to describe any carcinoma.

EPITHELIUM (*plural* **EPITHELIA**) tissue made up of cells packed closely

FACE the front-facing part of the head which extends from the chin to the forehead. There are fourteen bones in the skull, supporting the face, and numerous fine muscles are responsible for movements around the eyes, nose and mouth producing expression. These are under the control of the 7th cranial nerve which is a mixed sensory and motor nerve known as the FACIAL NERVE.

FACIAL NERVE the cranial nerve which has a number of branches and supplies the muscles which control facial expression. It also has branches to the middle ear, taste buds, salivary glands and lacrimal glands. Some branches are motor and others sensory in function.

FACIAL PARALYSIS paralysis of the facial nerve, which leads to a loss of function in the muscles of the face producing a lack of expression in the affected side. It occurs in the condition known as *Bell's palsy* in which there may also be a loss of taste and inability to close the eye. The condition is often temporary, if caused by inflammation which recovers in time. However, if the nerve itself is damaged by injury or if the person has suffered a stroke, the condition is likely to be permanent.

FACTOR VIII this is one of the COAGULATION FACTORS normally present in the blood and is known as antihaemophilic factor. If the factor is deficient in males it results in HAEMOPHILIA.

FAECES the end waste product of digestion which is formed in the colon and discharged from the bowels via the ANUS. Also known as stools, it consists of undigested food (chiefly cellulose), bacteria, mucus and other secretions, water and bile pigments which are responsible for the colour. The condition and colour of the faeces are indicators of general health e.g. pale stools are produced in JAUNDICE and COELIAC DISEASE and black stools often indicate the presence of digested blood.

FALLOPIAN TUBES a pair of tubes, one of which leads from each ovary to the womb. At the ovary, the tube is expanded to form a funnel with fingerlike projections, known as fimbriae, surrounding the opening. This funnel does not communicate directly with the ovary but is open to the abdominal cavity. However, when an egg is released from the ovary the fimbriae move and waft it into the fallopian tube. The tube is about 10 to 12cm long and leads directly in to the womb at the lower end through a narrow opening.

FALSE RIB see RIB.

FARMER'S LUNG an allergic condition caused by sensitivity to inhaled dust and fungal spores that are found in mouldy hay or straw. It is a form of allergic alveolitis (inflammation of the ALVEOLI of the lungs) characterized by increasing breathlessness. The condition may be treated by CORTICOSTEROID drugs but can only be cured by avoidance of the allergen.

FAT see ADIPOSE TISSUE.

FATTY ACIDS a group of organic compounds each consisting of a long, straight hydrocarbon chain and a terminal carboxylic acid (COOH) group. The length of the chain varies from one to nearly thirty carbon atoms and the chains may be *saturated* or *unsaturated*. Some fatty acids can be synthesized within the body but others, the ESSENTIAL FATTY ACIDS, must be obtained from food. Fatty acids have three major roles within the body.

(1) They are components of glycolipids (lipids containing carbohydrate) and phospholipids (lipids containing phosphate). These are of major importance in the structure of tissues and organs.

(2) Fatty acids are important constituents of triglycerides (lipids which have three fatty acid molecules joined to a glycerol molecule). They are stored in the cytoplasm of many cells and are broken down when required to yield energy. They are the form in which the body stores fat.

(3) Derivatives of fatty acids function as hormones and intracellular messengers.

FAVISM an inherited disorder which takes the form of severe haemolytic ANAEMIA (destruction of red blood cells) brought on by eating broad beans. A person having this disorder is sensitive to a chemical present in the beans and also to certain drugs, particularly some antimalarial drugs. It is caused by the lack of a certain enzyme, glucose 6-phosphate dehydrogenase, which plays an important role in glucose metabolism. The

defective gene responsible is passed on as a SEX-LINKED dominant characteristic and appears to persist in populations where it occurs, because it also confers increased resistance to malaria. Favism is found in American negroes, Yemenite Jews in Israel and in some people living in the Mediterranean region and in Iran.

FEBRILE having a fever.

FEMORAL describing the femur or area of the thigh e.g. femoral artery, vein, nerve and canal.

FEMUR the thigh bone which is the long bone extending from the hip to the knee and is the strongest bone in the body. It is the weight-bearing bone of the body and fractures are common in old people who have lost bone mass. It articulates with the pelvic girdle at the upper end, forming the hip joint and at the lower end with the patella (knee cap) and tibia to form the knee joint.

FERTILIZATION the fusion of SPERM (-ATOZOON) and OVUM to form a zygote which then undergoes cell division to become an embryo. Fertilization in humans takes place high up in the FALLOPIAN TUBE near the ovary and the fertilized egg travels down and becomes implanted in the womb.

FEVER an elevation of body temperature above the normal which accompanies many diseases and infections. The cause of fever is the production by the body of endogenous pyrogen which acts on the thermo-regulatory centre in the hypothalamus of the brain. This responds by promoting mechanisms which increase heat generation and lessen heat loss, leading to a rise in temperature. Fever is the main factor in many infections caused by bacteria or viruses and results from toxins produced by the growth of these organisms. Examples of these *primary* or *specific* fevers are diphtheria, scarlet fever and typhoid fever. An *intermittent fever* describes a fluctuating body temperature, which commonly accompanies MALARIA, in which the temperature sometimes returns to normal. In a *remittent fever* there is also a fluctuating body temperature but this does not return to normal. In a *relapsing fever*, caused by bacteria of the genus *Borella*, transmitted by ticks or lice, there is a recurrent fever every 3 to 10 days following the first attack which lasts for about one week.

Treatment of fever depends upon the underlying cause. However, it may be necessary to reduce the temperature by direct methods such as sponging the body with tepid water, or by giving drugs such as ASPIRIN. As well as a rise in body temperature, symptoms of fever include headache, shivering, nausea, diarrhoea or constipation. Above 105°F, there may be delirium or convulsions, especially in young children.

FIBREOPTIC ENDOSCOPY a method of viewing internal structures such as the digestive tract and tracheo-bronchial tree using fibreoptics. Fibreoptics uses illumination from a cold light source which is passed down a bundle of quartz fibres. The instruments used are highly flexible compared to the older form of endoscope and can be employed to illuminate structures which were formerly inaccessible. Using fibreoptic endoscopy, direct procedures can be carried out, such as BIOPSY and polypectomy (surgical removal of a POLYP).

FIBRILLATION The rapid non-synchronized contraction or tremor of muscles in which individual bundles of fibres contract independently. It applies especially to heart muscle and disrupts the normal beating so that the affected part is unable to pump blood. Two types of fibrillation may occur depending upon which muscle is affected. Atrial fibrillation, often resulting from ATHEROSCLEROSIS or rheumatic heart disease, affects the muscles of the atria and is a common type of arrhythmia. The heart beat and pulse are very irregular and cardiac output is maintained by the contraction of the ventricles alone. With ventricular fibrillation the heart stops

pumping blood so that this, in effect, is cardiac arrest. The patient requires immediate emergency resuscitation or death ensues within minutes.

FIBRIN the end product of the process of blood COAGULATION, comprising threads of insoluble protein formed from a soluble precursor, FIBRINOGEN, by the activity of the enzyme thrombin. Fibrin forms a network which is the basis of a blood clot, *see* COAGULATION.

FIBRINOGEN a COAGULATION FACTOR present in the blood which is a soluble protein and the precursor of FIBRIN, *see* COAGULATION.

FIBROCYSTIC DISEASE OF THE PANCREAS *see* CYSTIC FIBROSIS.

FIBROID a type of benign tumour found in the womb (uterus) composed of fibrous and muscular tissue and varying in size from one or two mm to a mass weighing several pounds. They more commonly occur in childless women and those over the age of thirty five. Fibroids may present no problems but alternatively can be the cause of pain, heavy and irregular menstrual bleeding, urine retention or frequency of MICTURITION and sterility. Fibroids can be removed surgically but often the complete removal of the womb (HYSTERECTOMY) is carried out.

FIBROMA a benign tumour composed of fibrous tissue.

FIBROSIS the formation of thickened connective or scar tissue usually as a result of injury or inflammation. This may affect the lining of the ALVEOLI of the lungs (pulmonary interstitial fibrosis) and causes breathlessness, *see also* CYSTIC FIBROSIS.

FIBROSARCOMA a malignant tumour of connective tissue particularly found in the limbs and especially the legs.

FIBROSITIS inflammation of fibrous connective tissue, muscles and muscle sheaths, particularly in the back, legs and arms causing pain and stiffness.

FIBROUS TISSUE a tissue type which occurs abundantly throughout the body. *White fibrous tissue* consists of collagen fibres, a protein with a high tensile strength and unyielding structure, that forms ligaments, sinews and scar tissue, and occurs in the skin. *Yellow fibrous tissue* is composed of the fibres of another protein, elastin. It is very elastic and occurs in ligaments which are subjected to frequent stretching, such as those in the back of the neck. It also occurs in arterial walls and in the walls of the alveoli (*see* ALVEOLUS), and in the dermis layer of the skin.

FIBULA the outer, thin, long bone which articulates with the larger tibia in the lower leg.

FISSURE a natural cleft or groove or abnormal break in the skin or mucous membrane e.g. an anal fissure.

FISTULA an abnormal opening between two hollow organs or between such an organ or gland and the exterior. These may arise during development so that a baby may be born with a fistula. Alternatively, they can be produced by injury, infection or as a complication following surgery. A common example is an anal fistula, which may develop if an abscess present in the rectum bursts and produces a communication through the surface of the skin. An operation is normally required to correct a fistula, but healing is further complicated in the case of an anal fistula because of the passage of waste material through the bowels.

FIT any sudden convulsive attack; a general term which is applied to an epileptic seizure, convulsion or bout of coughing.

FLATULENCE a build-up of gas in the stomach or bowels which is released through the mouth or anus.

FLEXOR any muscle that causes a limb or other body part to bend.

FLUTTER an abnormal disturbance of heart beat rhythm which may affect the atria or ventricles but is less severe than FIBRILLATION. The causes are the same as those of fibrillation and the treatment is also similar.

FLUX an excessive and abnormal flow from any of the natural openings of the body e.g. alvine flux which is diarrhoea.

FOETUS an unborn child after the eighth week of development.

FOLLICLE any small sac, cavity or secretory gland. Examples are hair follicles and the Graafian follicles of the ovaries in and from which eggs mature and are released

FONTANELLE openings in the skull of newborn and young infants in whom the bone is not wholly formed and the sutures are incompletely fused. The largest of these is the *anterior fontanelle* on the top of the head which is about 2.5cm square at birth.

The fontanelles gradually close as bone is formed and are completely covered by the age of 18 months. If a baby is unwell, for example with a fever, the fontanelle becomes tense. If an infant is suffering from diarrhoea and possibly dehydrated, the fontanelle is abnormally depressed.

FOOD POISONING an illness of the digestive system caused by eating food contaminated by certain bacteria, viruses or by chemical poisons (insecticides) and metallic elements such as mercury or lead. Symptoms include vomiting, diarrhoea, nausea and abdominal pain and these may arise very quickly and usually within 24 hours. Bacteria are the usual cause of food poisoning and proliferate rapidly producing toxins which cause the symptoms of the illness. Those involved include members of the genera *Salmonella, Staphylococcus, Campylobacter* and also *Clostridium botulinum,* the causal organism of botulism. Food poisoning may be fatal, the old and the young being especially at risk.

FORAMEN a hole or opening which usually refers to those which occur in some bones. For example the *foramen magnum* is a large hole at the base of the skull (in the *occipital bone*) through which the spinal cord passes out from the brain.

FORCEPS surgical instruments, of which there are many different types, which are used as pincers.

FORESKIN the PREPUCE which is a fold of skin growing over the end (glans) of the penis.

FOSSA a natural hollow or depression on the surface or within the body. Examples include the fossae within the skull which house different parts of the brain, and the cubital fossa, a hollow at the front of the elbow joint.

FOVEA any small depression, often referring to the one which occurs in the RETINA of the EYE in which a large number of the light-sensitive cells called CONES are situated. It is the site of greatest visual acuity being the region in which the image is focused when the eyes are fixed on an object.

FRACTURE any break in a bone which may be complete or incomplete. In a *simple fracture* (or *closed fracture*) the skin remains more or less intact but in a *compound fracture* (or *open fracture*) there is an open wound connecting the bone with the surface. This type of fracture is more serious as it provides a greater risk of infection and more blood loss. If a bone which is already diseased suffers a fracture, (such as often occurs in older women who have OSTEOPOROSIS), this is known as a *pathological fracture*. A *fatigue fracture* occurs in a bone which suffers recurrent, persistent stress, e.g. the *March fracture* sometimes seen in the second toe of soldiers after long marches. A GREENSTICK FRACTURE only occurs in young children whose bones are still soft and tend to bend. The fracture occurs on the opposite side from the causal force. A *complicated fracture* involves damage to surrounding soft tissue including nerves and blood vessels. A *depressed fracture* refers only to the skull when a piece of bone is forced inwards and may damage the brain. *See also* COMMINUTED FRACTURE.

FRECKLES small, brown spots occurring on the skin, especially in people with red hair or with a fair complexion. They often occur after exposure to the sun as a result of an increased production of the skin pigment, melanin.

FRIEDREICH'S ATAXIA an inherited disorder caused by degeneration of nerve cells in the brain and spinal cord. It appears in children, usually in adolescence. The symptoms include unsteadiness during walking and a loss of the knee-jerk reflex, leading progressively to tremors, speech impairment and curvature of the spine. The symptoms are increasingly disabling and may be accompanied by heart disease. *See also* ATAXIA.

FRONTAL LOBE the anterior part of the *cerebral hemisphere* of the CEREBRUM of the brain, extending back to a region called the central sulcus which is a deep cleft on the upper, outer surface.

FROZEN SHOULDER painful stiffness of the shoulder joint which limits movement and is more common in older people between the ages of 50 and 70. It may result from injury but often there is no apparent cause. Treatment involves exercises and sometimes injections of corticosteroid drugs, and usually there is a gradual recovery.

FUNDUS the enlarged base of an organ farthest away from its opening or a point in the RETINA of the EYE opposite the pupil.

FUNGAL DISEASES diseases or infections caused by fungi.

GALACTORRHOEA flow of milk from the breast, not associated with childbirth or nursing. It may be a symptom of a tumour in the pituitary gland.

GALL another term for BILE.

GALL BLADDER a sac-like organ situated on the underside of the liver which stores and concentrates BILE. It is approximately 8cm long and 2.5cm at its widest and its volume is a little over 30cm³. When fats are digested, the gall bladder contracts, sending bile into the

DUODENUM through the common bile duct. GALLSTONES, the most common gall bladder disease, may form in certain circumstances.

GALLSTONES stones of varying composition, that form in the GALL BLADDER. Their formation seems to be due to a change in bile composition rendering cholesterol less soluble. Stones may also form around a foreign body. There are three types of stone: cholesterol, pigment and mixed, the latter being the most common. Calcium salts are usually found in varying proportions. Although gallstones may be present for years without symptoms, they can cause severe pain and may pass into the common bile duct to cause, by the resulting obstruction, jaundice.

GAMETE a mature germ or sexual cell, male or female, that can participate in fertilization e.g. OVUM and SPERMATOZOON.

GAMMA GLOBULIN (or immune gamma GLOBULIN) a concentrated form of the antibody part of human blood. It is used for immunization against certain infectious diseases, e.g. measles, poliomyelitis, hepatitis A, etc. It is of no use when the disease is diagnosed but can prevent or modify it if given before.

GANGLION (*plural* **GANGLIA**) 1. a mass of nervous tissue containing nerve cells and SYNAPSES. Chains of ganglia are situated on each side of the spinal cord while other ganglia are sited near to or in the appropriate organs. Within the central nervous system some well-defined masses of nerve cells are called ganglia e.g. basal ganglia (*see* BASAL GANGLION). 2. a benign swelling that often forms in the sheath of a tendon and is fluid-filled. It occurs particularly at the wrist, and may disappear quite suddenly.

GANGRENE death of tissue due to loss of blood supply or bacterial infection. There are two types of gangrene, *dry* and *moist*. Dry gangrene is caused purely by loss of blood supply and is a late stage complication of DIABETES MELLITUS in which ATHEROSCLEROSIS is present. The affected part becomes cold and turns brown and black and there is an obvious line between living and dead tissue. In time the gangrenous part drops off. Moist gangrene is the more common type and is due to bacterial infection which leads to putrefaction and issuing of fluids from the tissue, accompanied by an obnoxious smell. The patient may suffer from fever and ultimately die of blood poisoning. (*See also* GAS GANGRENE.)

GAS GANGRENE a form of GANGRENE that occurs when wounds are infected with soil bacteria of the genus *Clostridium*. The bacterium produces toxins that cause decay and putrefaction with the generation of gas. The gas spreads into muscles and connective tissue causing swelling, pain, fever and possibly toxic delirium, and if untreated the condition quickly leads to death. Some of these bacteria are anaerobic (exist without air or oxygen) hence surgery, oxidizing agents and penicillin can all be used in treatment.

GASTRALGIA term meaning pain in the stomach.

GASTRECTOMY the surgical removal of, usually, part of the stomach. This may be performed for stomach cancer, severe peptic ulcers or to stop haemorrhaging.

GASTRIC anything relating to the stomach.

GASTRIC GLANDS glands that are situated in the MUCOUS MEMBRANE of the stomach and secrete GASTRIC JUICE. The glands are the *cardiac*, *pyloric* and *fundic*.

GASTRIC JUICE the secretion from the GASTRIC GLANDS in the stomach. The main constituents are hydrochloric acid, rennin, mucin and pepsinogen, the latter forming pepsin in the acid conditions. The acidity (which is around pH 1 to 1.5) also destroys unwanted bacteria.

GASTRIC ULCER an erosion of the stomach MUCOSA caused by such agents as acid and bile. It may penetrate the muscle and perforate the stomach wall (*see* PERFORATION). Typical symptoms include burning pain, belching and possibly nausea when the stomach is empty or soon after eating. Relief may be found with antacid compounds, but surgery may be necessary.

GASTRITIS inflammation of the stomach lining (MUCOSA). It may be due to bacteria or excessive alcohol intake.

GASTROENTERITIS inflammation of both the stomach and intestines leading to vomiting, diarrhoea. It is most commonly due to viral or bacterial infection and fluid loss can be serious in children.

GASTROENTEROLOGY the study of diseases that affect the gastrointestinal tract including the pancreas, gall bladder and bile duct in addition to the stomach and intestines.

GASTROENTEROSTOMY an operation undertaken to reroute food from the stomach to enable an obstruction to be relieved. It consists of making an opening in the stomach and the nearby small intestine and joining the two together. It is often performed with a gastrectomy.

GASTROSCOPE a flexible instrument comprising fibre optics or a miniature video camera that permits internal visual examination of the stomach. It is possible to see all areas of the stomach and take specimens using special tools. The tube is introduced via the mouth and oesophagus.

GASTROSTOMY the creation, usually by surgery, of an opening into the stomach from the outside. This permits food to be given to a patient who cannot swallow due to oesophageal cancer, post-oesophageal surgery or who may be unconscious for a long time.

GENE the fundamental unit of genetic material found at a specific location on a CHROMOSOME. It is chemically complex and responsible for the transmission of information between older and younger generations. Each gene contributes to a particular trait or characteristic. There are more than 100,000 genes in man and gene size varies with the characteristic e.g. the gene that codes for the hormone INSULIN is 1700 BASE PAIRS long.

There are several types of gene, depending upon their function and in addition genes are said to be dominant or recessive. A dominant characteristic is one that occurs whenever the gene is present while the effect of a recessive gene (say a disease) requires that the gene be on both members of the chromosome pair that is, it must be HOMOZYGOUS (*see also* SEX-LINKED DISORDERS).

GENETIC CODE specific information carried by DNA molecules that controls the particular AMINO ACIDS and their positions in every protein and thus all the proteins synthesized within a cell. Because there are just four nucleotides a unit of three bases becomes the smallest unit that can produce codes for all 20 amino acids. The transfer of information from gene to protein is based upon three consecutive nucleotides called *codons*. A change in the genetic code results in an amino acid being inserted incorrectly in a protein, resulting in a mutation.

GENETIC COUNSELLING the provision of advice to families about the nature and likelihood of inherited disorders and the options available in terms of prevention and management. With modern techniques of antenatal diagnosis it is possible to determine at an early stage of a pregnancy whether a child will be abnormal.

GENETIC ENGINEERING (or recombinant DNA technology) the artificial modification of an organism's genetic make-up. More specifically for example, the insertion of GENES from a human cell which are inserted into a bacterium where they perform their usual function. Thus it is possible to produce, on a commercial scale, hormones such as INSULIN and GROWTH HORMONE by utilizing a bacterium with a human gene. The organism often used is *Escherichia coli*. The process has other applications, including production of monoclonal antibodies.

GENETIC FINGERPRINTING the technique that utilises an individual's DNA to identify that person. DNA can be extracted from body tissues and used in settling issues of a child's maternity or paternity. In forensic medicine samples of blood etc. at the scene of a crime are taken to match a suspect to the criminal.

GENETICS the study of heredity and variation in individuals and the means whereby characteristics are passed from parent to offspring. The classical aspects of the subject were expounded by Mendel, an Austrian monk, in the early 19th century. Now there are several subdisciplines, including population genetics and molecular genetics.

GENETIC SCREENING the procedure whereby individuals are tested to determine whether their gene make-up suggests they carry a particular disease or condition. If it is shown that someone carries a genetically-linked disease then decisions can be taken regarding future children (*see also* SEX-LINKED DISORDERS).

GENITAL the term describing anything relating to reproduction or the reproductive organs.

GENITALIA the male or female reproductive organs, often referring to the external parts only.

GENITO-URINARY MEDICINE the subdiscipline concerned with all aspects of sexually transmitted diseases.

GENITO-URINARY TRACT (urogenital in U.S.) the genital and urinary organs and associated structures: kidneys, ureter, bladder, urethra and genitalia.

GERIATRICS the subdiscipline of medicine that deals with all aspects of diseases and conditions that affected the aged.

GERMAN MEASLES (*or* RUBELLA) a highly infectious viral disease occurring mainly in childhood, but which is mild in effect. Spread occurs through close contact with infected individuals and there is an incubation period of two to three weeks. The symptoms are headache, shivering and sore throat with a slight fever. There is some swelling of the neck and soon after the onset a rash of pink spots

appears, initially on the face and/or neck, and subsequently spreading over the body. The rash disappears in roughly one week but the condition remains infectious for 3 or 4 more days. Immunity is usually conferred by the infection and although it is a mild disease it is important because an attack during the early stages of pregnancy may cause foetal abnormalities. Girls are therefore immunized around the age of 12 or 13.

GERMS microorganisms. The term is used particularly for microorganisms that are PATHOGENIC.

GESTATION the length of time from fertilization of the ovum to birth (*see also* PREGNANCY).

GIARDIASIS the disease caused by the parasite *Giardia lamblia* which inhabits the small intestine. Although usually harmless, it may cause diarrhoea. It is contracted from untreated drinking water but is readily treated with medication.

GIDDINESS *see* VERTIGO.

GINGIVITIS inflammation of the gums.

GLAND an organ or group of cells that secretes a specific substance or substances. ENDOCRINE GLANDS secrete directly into the blood while *exocrine* glands secrete onto an epithelial surface via a duct. Some glands produce fluids, e.g. milk from the mammary glands, saliva from the sublingual bland and others. The THYROID gland is an endocrine gland releasing hormones into the bloodstream. A further system of glands, the lymphatic glands, occur throughout the body in association with the lymphatic vessels (*see* LYMPH).

GLANDULAR FEVER (*also known as* INFECTIOUS MONONUCLEOSIS) an infectious viral disease caused by the Epstein-Barr virus. It produces a sore throat and swelling in neck lymph nodes (also those in the armpits and groin). Other symptoms include headache, fever and a loss of appetite. The liver may be affected and the SPLEEN may become enlarged or even ruptured which then requires surgery. The disease is diagnosed by the large number of MONOCYTES in the blood and although complications tend to be rare, total recovery may take many weeks.

GLAUCOMA a condition which results in loss of vision due to high pressure in the EYE, although there is usually no associated disease of the eye. There are several types of glaucoma which occur at differing rates but all are characterized by high intra-ocular pressure (due to the outflow of AQUEOUS HUMOUR being restricted) which damages nerve fibres in the RETINA and optic nerve. Treatment involves reduction of the pressure with drops and tablets (to reduce production of aqueous humour) and if necessary surgery is undertaken to create another outlet for the aqueous humour.

GLEET discharge due to chronic GONORRHOEA.

GLIA (NEUROGLIA or **GLIAL CELLS)** CENTRAL NERVOUS SYSTEM connective tissue composed of a variety of cells. The *macroglia* are divided into astrocytes that surround brain capillaries and oligodendrocytes that form MYELIN sheaths. The *microglia* perform a mainly scavenging function. Glial cells are present in ten to fifty times the number of neurons in the nervous system.

GLOBULIN a group of globular proteins that occur widely in milk, blood, eggs and plants. There are four types in blood SERUM: a_1, a_2, b, and g. The alpha and beta types are carrier proteins like haemoglobin and gamma globulins include the IMMUNOGLOBULINS involved in the immune response.

GLOTTIS the opening between the VOCAL CHORDS. Also used for the part of the LARYNX involved with sound production.

GLUCAGON a hormone important in maintaining the level of the body's blood sugar. It works antagonistically with INSULIN, increasing the supply of blood sugar through the breakdown of GLYCOGEN to glucose in the liver. Glucagon is produced by the ISLETS OF LANGERHANS when blood sugar level is low.

GLUE EAR (or **SECRETORY OTITIS MEDIA)** a form of OTITIS, common in children, which occurs as an inflammation of the middle ear with the production of a persistent sticky fluid. It can cause deafness and may be associated with enlarged adenoids. In treatment of the condition the adenoids may be removed and GROMMETS inserted.

GLUTEAL the term given to the buttocks or the muscles forming them.

GLUTEUS one of the three muscles of each buttock. The *gluteus maximus* shapes the buttock and extends the thigh, the *gluteus medius* and *minimus* abduct (move the limb away from the body) the thigh while the former also rotates it.

GLYCOGEN sometimes called animal starch, is a carbohydrate (poly-saccharide) stored mainly in the liver. It acts as an energy store which is liberated upon hydrolysis (*see* GLUCAGON).

GLYCOSURIA the presence of sugar (glucose) in the urine which is usually due to DIABETES MELLITUS.

GOITRE swelling of the neck due to THYROID GLAND enlargement. The thyroid tries to counter the dietary lack of iodine necessary to produce thyroid hormone, by increasing the output, thereby becoming larger. The endemic or simple goitre is due to this cause. Other types are caused by HYPERPLASIA and auto-immune diseases, for example when antibodies are produced against antigens in the thyroid gland.

GOLD SALTS (or **gold compound)** chemicals containing gold that are used in minute quantities to treat RHEUMATOID ARTHRITIS. It is given by injection into muscles and because side effects may include skin reactions, blood disorders, mouth ulcers and inflammation of the kidneys, very careful control is kept on the dosage.

GONAD the reproductive organs that produce the GAMETES and some hormones. In the male and female the gonads are the testes and ovaries respectively.

GONADOTROPHIN (or **GONADO-TROPHIC HORMONE)** hormones

secreted by the anterior PITUITARY GLAND. Follicle-stimulating hormone (FSH) is produced by males and females as is luteinizing hormone, LH, (interstitial cell-stimulating hormone, ICSH, in males). FSH controls, directly or indirectly, growth of the ova and sperm, while LH/ICSH stimulates reproductive activity in the GONADS.

GONORRHOEA the most common VENEREAL DISEASE which is spread primarily by sexual intercourse but may be contracted through contact with infected discharge on clothing, towels etc. The causative agent is the bacterium *Neisseria gonorrhoeae* and it affects the mucous membrane of the vagina, or in the male, the urethra. Symptoms develop approximately one week after infection and include pain on urinating with a discharge of pus. Inflammation of nearby organs may occur (testicle, prostate in men; uterus, Fallopian tubes and ovaries in women) and prolonged inflammation of the urethra may lead to formation of fibrous tissue causing STRICTURE. Joints may also be affected and later complications include ENDOCARDITIS, arthritis and CONJUNCTIVITIS.

If a baby is born to a woman with the disease, the baby's eyes may become infected, until recently a major cause of blindness (called *ophthalmia neonatorum*). Treatment is usually very effective through the administration of penicillin, sulphonamides or tetracycline.

GOUT a disorder caused by an imbalance of URIC ACID in the body. Uric acid is normally excreted by the kidneys but sufferers of gout have an excess in their bloodstream which is deposited in joints as salts (urates) of the acid. This causes inflammation of the affected joints and painful gouty arthritis with destruction of the joints. The kidneys may also be damaged, with formation of stones. Deposits of the salts (called *tophi*) may reach the stage where they prohibit further use of the joints, causing hands and feet to be set in a particular

position. Treatment of gout is through drugs that increase the excretion of the urate salts or slow their formation.

GRAAFIAN FOLLICLE see FOLLICLE.

GRAFT the removal of some tissue or an organ from one person for application to or implantation into the same person or another individual. For example, a skin graft involves taking healthy skin from one area of the body to heal damaged skin, and a kidney (or renal) graft (or transplant) is the removal of the organ from one person (usually a recently dead individual) to another. Numerous types of graft are now feasible, including skin, bone, cornea, cartilage, nerves and blood vessels, and whole organs such as kidney, heart and lung.

GRAM'S STAIN a technique described by H.C.J. Gram, the Danish bacteriologist in 1884, which involves using a stain to differentiate between certain bacteria. Bacteria on a microscope slide are first stained with a violet dye and iodine, then rinsed in ethanol to decolorize and a second red stain added. *Gram-positive* bacteria keep the first stain and appear violet when examined under the microscope, while *Gram-negative* forms lose the first but take up the second stain, thus appearing red. The difference in staining is due to the structure of the bacteria cell walls.

GRAND MAL a convulsive epileptic fit involving involuntary muscular contractions and lack of respiration. The latter produces bluish skin and lips (CYANOSIS) during the *tonic* phase. Convulsive movements follow and often the tongue is bitten and bladder control is lost (the *clonic* phase). Upon awakening the patient has no recall of the event.

GRANULOCYTE see LEUCOCYTE. GRANULOCYTOSIS is when the blood has an abnormally high number of granulocytes (see LEUCOCYTE).

GRAVE'S DISEASE a disorder typified by thyroid gland overactivity (see HYPERTHYROIDISM), an enlargement of the gland, and protruding eyes. It is due to antibody production and is probably an auto-immune response (*see* AUTO-IMMUNE DISEASE). Patients commonly exhibit excess metabolism (because thyroid hormones control the body's metabolism); nervousness, tremor, hyperactivity, rapid heart rate, an intolerance of heat, breathlessness and so on. Treatment may follow one of three courses; drugs to control the thyroid's production of hormones; surgery to remove part of the thyroid; or radioactive iodine therapy.

GRAVID another term for pregnant.

GREENSTICK FRACTURE a fracture occurring in bones with some flexibility (and therefore in children) where the bone is not broken right across but just on the outer arc of the bend.

GREY MATTER a part of the CENTRAL NERVOUS SYSTEM comprising the central part of the spinal cord and the cerebral cortex and outer layer of the cerebellum in the brain. It is brown-grey in colour and is the co-ordination point between the nerves of the central nervous system. It is composed of nerve cell bodies, DENDRITES, SYNAPSES, glial cells (supporting cells, *see* GLIA) and blood vessels.

GROIN the areas where the abdomen joins the thighs.

GROMMET a small tube with a lip at either end that is inserted into the eardrum to permit fluid to drain from the middle ear. It is used in the treatment of secretory otitis media (GLUE EAR).

GROWING PAINS pains similar to rheumatism that occur in the joints and muscles of children. They are usually insignificant and may be due to fatigue or bad posture but must be dealt with in case the cause is more serious e.g. bone disease, or rheumatic fever.

GROWTH HORMONE (soma-totrophin or FH) a HORMONE produced and stored by the anterior PITUITARY GLAND that controls protein synthesis in muscles and the growth of long bones in legs and arms. Low levels result in DWARFISM in children and over-production produces gigantism.

GULLET another term for the OESOPHAGUS.

GYNAECOLOGY the subdiscipline of medicine that deals with diseases of women, particularly concerning sexual and reproduction function and diseases of reproductive organs.

GYNAECOMASTIA the abnormal enlargement of breasts in men which may be due to drugs, hormone imbalance, testicular or pituitary cancer.

HAEM a compound containing iron, composed of a pigment which is known as a *porphyrin* which confers colour. It combines with a protein called globin in the blood to form HAEMOGLOBIN. The prefix *haem* also indicates anything relating to blood.

HAEMANGIOMA a benign tumour of the blood vessels. It may be visible on the skin as a type of NAEVUS (birthmark) e.g. a *strawberry haemangioma*.

HAEMARTHROSIS bleeding into a joint which causes swelling and pain and may be the result of injury or disease. It can be a symptom of HAEMOPHILIA.

HAEMATEMESIS vomiting of blood which may occur for a number of different reasons. Common causes are ulcers, either gastric or duodenal, or gastritis, especially when this is caused by irritants or poisons such as alcohol. Also blood may be swallowed and subsequently vomited as a result of a nosebleed.

HAEMATINIC a substance which increases the amount of haemoglobin in the blood e.g. ferrous sulphate. Haematinic drugs are often prescribed during pregnancy.

HAEMATOCOELE leakage of blood into a cavity causing a swelling. A haematocoele usually forms as a result of an injury due to the rupture of blood vessels and the leaking of blood into a natural body cavity.

HAEMATOLOGY the scientific study of blood and its diseases.

HAEMATOMA a collection of blood forming a firm swelling-a bruise. It may occur as a result of injury, a clotting disorder of the blood or if blood vessels are diseased.

HAEMATURIA the presence of blood in the urine which may have come from the kidneys, ureters, bladder or urethra. It indicates the presence of inflammation or disease such as a stone in the bladder or kidney.

HAEMODIALYSIS the use of an *artificial kidney* to remove waste products from a person's blood using the principle of DIALYSIS. It is carried out when a person's kidneys have ceased to function and involves passing blood from an artery into the dialyser on one side of a semi-permeable membrane. On the other side of the membrane, a solution of electrolytes of similar composition to the blood is circulated. Water and waste products pass through the membrane into this solution while cells and proteins are retained within the blood. The purified blood is then returned to the patient's body through a vein.

HAEMOGLOBIN the respiratory substance contained within the red blood cells which contains a pigment responsible for the red colour of blood. It consists of the pigment HAEM and the protein globin and is responsible for the transport of oxygen around the body. Oxygen is picked up in the lungs by arterial blood and transported to the tissues where it is released. This (venous) blood is then returned to the lungs to repeat the process, see OXYHAEMOGLOBIN.

HAEMOGLOBINOPATHY any of a number of inherited diseases in which there is an abnormality in the formation of haemoglobin. Examples are THALASSAEMIA and sickle-cell ANAEMIA.

HAEMOGLOBINURIA the presence

of haemoglobin in the urine caused by disintegration of red blood cells, conferring a dark red or brown colour. It can sometimes result from strenuous exercise or after exposure to cold in some people. It is also caused by the ingestion of poisons such as arsenic, and is a symptom of some infections, particularly *blackwater fever*, a severe and sometimes fatal form of MALARIA.

HAEMOLYSIS the destruction (lysis) of red blood cells which may result from infection, poisoning or as an antibody response.

HAEMOLYTIC DISEASE OF THE NEWBORN a serious disease affecting foetuses and newborn babies which is characterized by HAEMOLYSIS leading to anaemia and severe jaundice. In severe cases the foetus may die due to heart failure and OEDEMA (termed *hydrops foetalis*). The usual cause is incompatibility between the blood of the mother and that of the foetus. Generally the foetus has Rh positive red blood cells (i.e. they contain the rhesus factor) while that of the mother is Rh negative. The mother produces antibodies to the Rh factor present in the foetal blood and these are passed to the foetus in the placental circulation. This then produces the haemolysis of the foetal red blood cells. The incidence of the disease has been greatly reduced by giving a Rh negative mother an injection of anti-D immunoglobulin, following the birth of a Rh positive baby. This prevents the formation of the antibodies which would harm a subsequent baby and is also given to Rh negative women following miscarriages or abortions.

HAEMOPHILIA an hereditary disorder of blood coagulation in which the blood clots very slowly. It is a sex-linked recessive condition carried on the X chromosome and hence it affects males with females being the carriers. There are two types of haemophilia due to a deficiency of either one of two COAGULATION FACTORS in the blood.

Haemophilia A is caused by deficiency of factor VIII and haemophilia B by deficiency of factor IX, called *Christmas factor*. The severity of the disease depends upon how much less of the coagulation factor than normal is present in the blood. The symptoms of haemophilia are prolonged bleeding from wounds and bleeding into joints, muscles and other tissues. In the past, the outlook for haemophiliacs was poor with few surviving into adult life. However, now the condition can be treated by injections or transfusions of plasma containing the missing coagulation factor and, with care, a sufferer can hope to lead a much more normal life. *See* SEX-LINKED DISORDERS.

HAEMOPOIESIS formation of blood cells (particularly *erythrocytes*, the red blood cells) and platelets, which takes place in the bone marrow in adults but in a foetus it occurs in the liver and spleen.

HAEMORRHAGE bleeding - a flow of blood from a ruptured blood vessel which may occur externally or internally. A haemorrhage is classified according to the type of vessels involved: *Arterial H* - bright red blood spurts in pulses from an artery. *Venous H* - a darker coloured steady flow from a vein. *Capillary L* - blood oozes from torn capillaries at the surface of a wound. In addition, a haemorrhage may be *primary* i.e. it occurs at the moment of injury. It is classed as *reactionary* when it occurs within 24 hours of an injury and results from a rise in blood pressure. Thirdly, a *secondary haemorrhage* occurs after a week or ten days as a result of infection (sepsis). Haemorrhage from a major artery is the most serious kind as large quantities of blood are quickly lost and death can occur within minutes. Haemorrhages at specific sites within the body are designated by special names e.g. *haematuria* (from the kidney or urinary tract), *haemoptysis* (from the lungs) and *haematemesis* (from the stomach).

HAEMORRHOIDS (piles) varicose and inflamed veins around the lower end of the bowel situated in the wall of the anus. They are classified as internal, external and mixed depending upon whether they appear beyond the anus. They are commonly caused by constipation or diarrhoea, especially in middle and older age, and may be exacerbated by a sedentary life style. They may also occur as a result of child-bearing. Symptoms of haemorrhoids are bleeding and pain, and treatment is by means of creams, injections and suppositories. Attention to diet (to treat constipation) and regular exercise are important, but in severe cases, surgery to remove the haemorrhoids may be necessary.

HAEMOSTASIS the natural process to arrest bleeding involving blood coagulation and contraction of a ruptured blood vessel. The term is also applied to a number of surgical procedures designed to arrest bleeding such as the use of ligatures and diathermy. A haemostatic substance stops or prevents haemorrhage e.g. phytomenadone.

HAEMOTHORAX a leakage of blood into the pleural cavity of the chest, usually as a result of injury.

HALLUCINOGEN a substance or drug which causes HALLUCINATIONS e.g. mescaline and lysergic acid diethylamide.

HAMSTRING any of four tendons at the back of the knee which are attached to the *hamstring muscles* and anchor these to the TIBIA and FIBULA. The hamstring muscles are responsible for the bending of the knee joint.

HAND the extremity of the upper limb below the wrist which has a highly complex structure and an "opposable" thumb which is unique to man. The human hand is highly developed in terms of structure, nervous supply and function and communicates with a large area on the surface of the brain. It is capable of performing numerous functions with a high degree of precision. When there is brain damage and paralysis, the uses of the hand tend to be lost early and more permanently compared to movements in the leg and face. The skeletal structure of the hand consists of eight small *carpal* bones in the wrist, five *metacarpal* bones in the region of the palm and three *phalanges* in each finger.

HAPLOID the description for a cell nucleus or organism with half the normal number of chromosomes. This is the case with GAMETES and is important at fertilization to ensure the *diploid* chromosome number is restored.

HARE LIP a congenital developmental deformity which results in the presence of a cleft in the upper lip. It is brought about by a failure in the fusion of three blocks of embryonic tissue and is often associated with a CLEFT palate.

HARTMANN'S SOLUTION a solution of salts which is given to replace lost fluid in cases of dehydration, acidosis and after HAEMORRHAGE while awaiting cross-matched blood for transfusion.

HAY FEVER an allergic reaction to pollen e.g. that of grasses, trees and many other plants which affects numerous individuals. The symptoms are a blocked and runny nose, sneezing and watering eyes due to the release of histamine. Treatment is by means of antihistamine drugs and, if the allergen can be identified, *desensitization* may be successful. This involves injecting or exposing the individual to controlled and gradually increasing doses of the allergen until antibodies are built up.

HEADACHE pain felt within the head which is thought to be caused by dilation of intracranial arteries or pressure upon them. Common causes are stress, tiredness, feverishness accompanying an infection such as a cold, an excess of close work involving the eyes, dyspepsia, rheumatic diseases, high blood pressure and uraemia. Headache may indicate the presence of disease or disorder in the brain e.g. an infection such as MENINGITIS, TUMOUR or ANEURYSM and also as a result of injury and concussion.

HEART the hollow, muscular organ which acts as a pump and is responsible for the circulation of the blood. The heart is cone-shaped with the point downwards and is situated between the lungs and slightly to the left of the midline. The heart projects forwards and lies beneath the fifth rib. The wall consists mainly of CARDIAC MUSCLE lined on the inside by a membrane known as the ENDOCARDIUM. An external membrane known as the PERICARDIUM surrounds the heart. A SEPTUM divides the heart into right and left halves, each of which is further divided into an upper chamber known as an ATRIUM and a lower one called a VENTRICLE. Four valves control the direction of blood flow at each outlet, comprising the aortic, pulmonary, tricuspid and mitral (bicuspid). These valves prevent backflow once the blood has been forced from one chamber into the next. *See* CIRCULATION OF THE BLOOD.

HEART ATTACK *see* CARDIAC ARREST.

HEART BLOCK a condition describing a failure in the conduction of electrical impulses from the natural pacemaker (the sinoatrial node) through the heart, which can lead to slowing of the pumping action.

There are three types: in first degree (partial or incomplete) heart block there is a delay in conduction between atria (*see* ATRIUM) and VENTRICLES but this does not cause slowing. In second degree heart block, there is intermittent slowing because not all the impulses are conducted between atria and ventricles. In third degree (or complete) heart block there is no electrical conduction, the heartbeats are slow and the ventricles beat at their own intrinsic slow rhythm. This causes blackouts (*see* STOKES ADAMS SYNDROME) and can lead to heart failure. Heart block is more common in elderly people where degenerative changes have occurred. However, it may also be CONGENITAL or result from other forms of heart disease such as MYOCARDITIS, CORONARY THROMBOSIS, CARDIOMYOPATHY and VALVE DISEASE. For second and third degree heart block, treatment involves the use of an artificial pacemaker.

HEARTBURN a burning pain or discomfort felt in the region of the heart and often rising upwards to the throat. It is caused by regurgitation of the stomach contents, the burning being caused by the acid in gastric juice or by OESOPHAGI-TIS. It is relieved by taking antacid tablets or alkaline substances such as sodium bicarbonate.

HEAT EXHAUSTION exhaustion and collapse due to overheating of the body and loss of fluid following unaccustomed or prolonged exposure to excessive heat. It is more common in hot climates and results from excessive sweating leading to loss of fluids and salts and distur-bance of the electrolyte balance in body fluids. In the mildest form which is *heat collapse*, blood pressure and pulse rate fall accompanied by fatigue, light-headedness and there may be muscular cramps. Treatment involves taking drinks of salt solution, or these may be given intravenously and avoidance by gradual acclimatization to the heat, especially if hard physical work is to be carried out.

HEAT STROKE or **HEAT HYPER-PYREXIA** a severe condition following exposure of the body to excessive heat characterized by a rise in temperature and failure of sweating and temperature regulation. There is a loss of conscious-ness, followed by coma and death which can occur rapidly. The body must be cooled by sponging and salt solutions given either by mouth or intravenously.

HEEL the part of the foot behind the ankle joint formed by the *calcaneus* or heel bone.

HEIMLICH'S MANOEUVRE a procedure to dislodge a foreign body which is blocking the larynx causing choking. The person carrying out the procedure encircles the patient from behind with his arms. A fist is made with one hand slightly above the patient's navel and below the ribs. With the free hand, the fist is thrust firmly into the abdomen with a rapid upward push which may need to be repeated several times. As a result of this, the foreign particle is expelled through or into the patient's mouth.

HENLE'S LOOP *see* KIDNEY.

HEPARIN an anticoagulant substance naturally present in the body, and produced by liver and some white blood cells and in some other sites. It acts by inhibiting and neutralizing the action of the enzyme thrombin (*see* BLOOD COAGULATION) and is a polysaccharide (carbohydrate) containing sulphur and amino groups. It is used medically to prevent blood coagulation in patients with thrombosis and also in blood collected for sampling.

HEPATECTOMY surgical removal of the whole or part of the liver.

HEPATIC VEIN one of the veins which drains blood from the liver leading to the inferior vena cava.

HEPATITIS inflammation of the liver due to the presence of toxic substances or infection caused by viruses. *Acute hepatitis* produces abdominal pain, jaundice, itching, nausea and fever. *Chronic hepatitis* has a similar range of symptoms which may persist for years and lead eventually to CIRRHOSIS. Alcohol abuse is a common cause of hepatitis which may also result as a side effect from a number of drug treatments or from overdose. Many virus infections can cause hepatitis such as HIV and GLANDULAR FEVER.

However, the so-called hepatic viruses are designated A, B, C, D, and E. Hepatitis A causes *infectious hepatitis* (epidemic hepatitis) and is transmitted by eating food contaminated by a person who has the virus, and is common in conditions of poor hygiene and sanitation. Hepatitis E acts in a similar way and both produce symptoms of fever, sickness and jaundice. Recovery is usually complete unless the symptoms are acute and immunity from a future attack is conferred. *Serum hepatitis* is caused by viruses B, C and D, the route of infection being blood or blood products. Serum hepatitis is most common where infected needles have been used among drug addicts. The infection may also be passed on by tattooing needles and also through sexual intercourse with an infected individual. The mortality rate is 5 - 20%, but many patients make a gradual recovery from the illness which is characterized by fever, chills, fatigue, headaches and jaundice. All these viruses may persist in the blood for a long time and if B is involved, the condition is known as *chronic type - B hepatitis*. Cancer (hepatocellular carcinoma) is common in populations where the B virus is prevalent. Various drugs are used to combat viral hepatitis including interferon.

HEPATOMA a malignant tumour of the liver which is rare in Western countries except among those with CIRRHOSIS. It is common in parts of the Far East and Africa and a suspected cause is the *aflatoxin* or poison produced by a fungus which contaminates stored peanuts and cereals. The cancer often produces alpha fetoprotein which is detectable in the blood and is an indicator of the presence of the malignancy.

HEREDITY the principle applied to the passing on of all bodily characteristic from parents to offspring. See GENETICS.

HERMAPHRODITE an individual possessing both male and female sex organs or in whom ovarian and testicular cells are present in the gonads (*ovotestis*). This condition is extremely rare and the individual is usually sterile with reduced SECONDARY SEXUAL CHARACTERISTICS.

HERNIA the protrusion of a part or whole of an organ from out of its normal position within the body cavity. Most commonly, a hernia involves part of the bowel. A *congenital hernia* is present at birth, a common one being an *umbilical hernia* in which abdominal organs protrude into the umbilical cord. This is due to a failure during foetal development and can be corrected by surgery. An *acquired hernia* occurs after birth, a common example being an *inguinal hernia* in which part of the bowel bulges through a weak part of the abdominal wall, (known as the inguinal canal). Another common type is a *hiatus hernia* in which the stomach passes through the hiatus (a hole allowing passage of the oesophagus), from the abdomen into the chest cavity. A *reducible hernia* is freely movable and can be returned by manipulation into its rightful place. An *irreducible hernia* describes the opposite situation and an *incarcerated hernia* is one which has become swollen and fixed in its position. An *obstructed hernia* is one involving the bowel. The contents of the hernia are unable to pass further down and are held up and obstructed. The most dangerous situation is a *strangulated hernia* in which the blood supply has been cut off due to the protrusion itself. This becomes painful and eventually gangrenous and requires immediate surgery as it is life-threatening. Strenuous physical activity can lead to the production of a hernia which usually develops gradually. Although short-term measures are employed to control a hernia or reduce its size, the usual treatment is by means of surgery to return and retain the protrusion in its proper pace. See HERNIOPLASTY.

HERNIOPLASTY the surgical operation to repair a hernia.

HEROIN a white crystalline powder, also known as dimorphine hydrochloride, which is derived from morphine. It is a very potent analgesic (painkiller), but is highly addictive and dangerous.

HERPES infectious inflammation of the skin and mucous membranes, characterized by the development of small blisters, and caused by a number of different *Herpes viruses*. The *Herpes simplex* virus, types I and II, are the cause of cold sores which usually affect the lips, mouth and face. The virus is usually acquired in childhood and once present persists for life. It can be contracted without causing any symptoms but tends to flare up from time to time producing the cold sores.

Herpes simplex is also the cause of genital herpes in which the blisters affect the genital region. *Herpes zoster* or shingles is produced by a virus which causes chicken pox in children. The virus affects the course of a nerve producing severe pain and small yellowish blisters on the skin. Often the affected areas are the abdomen, back, face and chest and although the disease subsides after about three weeks, the blisters form scabs which eventually drop off and the pain can persist for months. This is known as *post-herpetic neuralgia* and pain-relieving drugs are needed to help relieve the condition. Other Herpes viruses are the CYTOMEGA-LOVIRUS and EPSTEIN BARR virus.

HETEROSEXUAL describes sexual behaviour between individuals of opposite sexes.

HETEROZYGOUS the situation in which each member (ALLELE) of a pair of genes determining a certain characteristic is dissimilar. Usually one is dominant and this is the form exhibited in the individual's body, but either type can be passed on in the gametes (sex cells). *Compare* HOMOZYGOUS.

HEXACHLOROPHANE an antiseptic, disinfectant substance similar to phenol, the use of which is now limited in soaps and creams as it may produce toxic effects when absorbed through the skin.

HIATUS HERNIA *see* HERNIA.

HINDBRAIN the part of the brain which consists of the MEDULLA OBLONGATA, PONS and CEREBELLUM.

HIP the region on either side of the body where the FEMUR (thigh bone) articulates with the pelvis.

HIRSUTISM the growth of dark, coarse hair on the body of a female on the face, chest, abdomen and upper back. This is either due to a greater sensitivity of hair follicles to a normal level of male hormones (androgens) producing hair of a more masculine type. Or, there may be

an excessive production of androgens responsible for the growth of the hair. The condition may be the result of an underlying disorder such as an ADRENAL tumour but there is a wide normal variation in the amount of body hair present in individuals and between females of different races.

HISTAMINE a substance derived from histidine which is an amino acid. It is widely found throughout all the body tissues and is responsible for the dilation of blood vessels (arterioles and capillaries) and the contraction of smooth muscle, including that of the bronchi of the lungs. Histamine is released in great quantities in allergic conditions and ANAPHYLAXIS (*see also* ALLERGY).

HISTOLOGY the scientific study of tissues, involving such techniques as light and electron microscopy and the use of dyes and stains.

HIV the human immunodeficiency virus responsible for the condition known as AIDS. The virus affects and destroys a group of lymphocytes (T-lymphocytes) which are part of the body's natural defences (the IMMUNE SYSTEM).

HIVES a common name for urticaria or nettle rash.

HLA ANTIGENS these are the human leucocyte antigens. There are four genes responsible for their production (A, B, C, D) which are located on chromosome 6 which make up the HLA system. One GENE or set of genes is inherited from each parent and produce the HLA antigens on the surfaces of cells throughout the body. These antigens are the means by which the IMMUNE SYSTEM recognizes "self" and rejects "non-self," and this is very important in organ transplantation. The closer the match of HLAs between donor and recipient, the greater the chances of success. If two individual shave identical HLA types, they are described as being *histocompatible*.

HODGKIN'S DISEASE a malignant disease of unknown cause affecting the lymphatic system in which there is a gradual and increasing enlargement of lymph glands and nodes throughout the body. The accompanying symptoms include loss of weight, sweating, anaemia and a characteristic type of fever (known as Pel-Ebstein fever). The person becomes gradually weaker and the glands may attain a very large size. The outlook is good, especially if the disease is detected early, and treatment is by means of surgery, radiotherapy and chemotherapy (with a combination of drugs) one or more of these being employed.

HOMEOPATHY a system of medicine devised by Samuel Hahnemann (1755 - 1843) which is part of "alternative" medicine in the U.K. It is based on the premise that "like cures like" and so a patient is given minute quantities of drugs that can, in themselves, produce symptoms of the disease or malady being treated.

HOMOSEXUAL describes sexual behaviour between individuals of the same sex. The adjective is usually now applied to males, lesbian being the corresponding term for females.

HOMOZYGOUS the situation in which each member (ALLELE) of a pair of genes determining a certain characteristic is the same. Hence only one form of the GENE can be passed on in the gametes (sex cells) to the offspring. Genes which are normally recessive can be expressed in the body of a person who is homozygous for that particular characteristic e.g. albinism. Compare HETEROZYGOUS.

HRT see MENOPAUSE.

HORMONE a naturally-produced chemical substance produced by the body which acts as a messenger. A hormone is produced by cells or glands in one part of the body and passes into the bloodstream. When it reaches another specific site, its "target organ," it causes a reaction there, modifying the structure or function of cells, perhaps by causing the release of another hormone. Hormones are secreted by the ENDOCRINE GLANDS and examples are the sex hormones, e.g. TESTOSTERONE secreted by the testes and oestradiol and PROGESTERONE secreted by the ovaries.

HUMAN CHORIONIC GONADO-TROPHIN a hormone secreted by the PLACENTA during early pregnancy under the influence of which the CORPUS LUTEUM of the OVARY produces OESTROGEN, PROGESTERONE and relaxin. These are essential for the maintenance of pregnancy. Pregnancy can be detected early on by a laboratory procedure which tests for the presence of human chorionic gonadotrophin in the urine.

HUMAN LEUCOCYTE ANTIGEN see HLA.

HUMAN T-CELL LYMPHO-CYTOTROPHIC VIRUS (HTLV) a group of viruses including the AIDS (HIV) virus which is HTLV III. These viruses are responsible for LYMPHOMAS.

HUMERUS the bone of the upper arm which articulates with the shoulder blade (SCAPULA) of the PECTORAL GIRDLE and the ULNA and RADIUS at the elbow.

HUMOUR a natural fluid in the body, the best known examples being the aqueous and vitreous humours of the EYE.

HUNTINGTON'S CHOREA see CHOREA.

HYDROCEPHALUS an abnormal collection of cerebrospinal fluid within the skull which causes, in babies and children, a great increase in the size of the head. Hydrocephalus results either from an excessive production of fluid or from a defect in the mechanism for its reabsorption, or from a blockage in its circulation. The cause may be CONGENITAL, and it often accompanies SPINA BIFIDA in babies, or infection (meningitis) or the presence of a TUMOUR. Hydrocephalus causes pressure on the brain with drowsiness, irritability and mental subnormality in children. Treatment involves surgery to redirect the fluid but is not always successful. About 50% of children survive if the progress of the condition is halted and one third of these go on to enjoy a normal life with little or no physical or mental impairment.

HYDROCORTISONE a STEROID glucocorticoid hormone, produced and released by the cortex of the ADRENAL GLANDS (a CORTICOSTEROID). It is closely related to cortisone being released in response to stress and playing a significant part in carbohydrate metabolism. Medically it has a number of uses especially in the treatment of ADDISON'S DISEASE, inflammatory, allergic and rheumatic conditions e.g. eczema and rheumatoid arthritis. Hydrocortisone is contained in ointments in creams or given by mouth or injection depending upon the condition under treatment. Prolonged use may cause side effects including peptic ulcers, stunting of growth in children, CUSHING'S SYNDROME and damage to bone and muscle tissue.

HYDROXOCOBALAMIN this is a cobalt-containing (cobalamin) substance used in the treatment of vitamin B_{12} deficiencies, such as pernicious ANAEMIA.

HYMEN a thin membrane that covers the lower end of the VAGINA at birth which usually tears to some extent before a girl reaches puberty.

HYPERADRENALISM a condition in which the adrenal glands are overactive producing the symptoms of CUSHING'S SYNDROME.

HYPERALGESIA an extreme sensitivity to pain.

HYPERCALCAEMIA a high blood calcium level often associated with bone tumours, hyperparathyroidism (*see* PARATHYROID) and OSTEOPOROSIS. Symptoms include anorexia, muscle pain and weakness.

HYPERGLYCAEMIA the presence of excess sugar (glucose) in the blood, as in DIABETES MELLITUS caused by insufficient INSULIN to cope with carbohydrate intake. The condition can lead to a diabetic coma.

HYPERKALAEMIA a high blood potassium level often seen with kidney failure of which the signs are diarrhoea, nausea and muscle weakness.

HYPERLIPIDAEMIA (hyperlipaemia) the presence of an excess concentration of fat in the blood. An excess of CHOLESTEROL in the blood may lead to CORONARY ARTERY DISEASE and ATHEROMA. An excess of triglycerides may lead to pancreatitis.

HYPERPLASIA increased growth in size and number of the normal cells of a tissue so that the affected part enlarges e.g. the breasts during pregnancy. *Compare* HYPERTROPHY and NEOPLASM.

HYPERSENSITIVITY abnormal allergic response to an ANTIGEN to which the person has previously been exposed. Hypersensitive responses vary from quite mild such as hay fever to very severe and life-threatening e.g. ANAPHYLACTIC SHOCK (*see also* ALLERGY).

HYPERTENSION high blood pressure (in the arteries). *Essential* hypertension may be due to an unknown cause, or kidney disease or endocrine diseases. *Malignant* hypertension will prove fatal if not treated. It may be a condition itself or an end stage of essential hypertension. It tends to occur in a younger age group and there is high diastolic blood pressure (*see* DIASTOLE) and kidney failure. Previously a rapidly fatal condition, antihypertensive drugs have revolutionized treatment and given sufferers a near-normal life.

HYPERTHERMIA extremely high and abnormal body temperature i.e. a fever. Also, a method of treatment of certain diseases by artificially inducing a state of fever achieved by a variety of techniques.

HYPERTHYROIDISM excessive activity of the thyroid gland - an over-active thyroid. It may be caused by increased growth of the gland, by the presence of a tumour or due to GRAVES DISEASE.

HYPERTROPHY increase in size of an organ due to enlargement of its cells (rather than in their number) often in response to a greater demand for work. An example is the increase in size of the remaining kidney if the other is removed for some reason. *Compare* HYPERPLASIA.

HYPERVENTILATION breathing at

an abnormally rapid rate when at rest, which may be a response to stress and, if not checked, results in unconsciousness because the concentration of carbon dioxide in the blood falls. If the carbon dioxide level in the blood is abnormally high, due to impaired gas exchange in the lungs, e.g. in pulmonary OEDEMA and pneumonia, hyperventilation may occur. (See also HYPOVENTILATION.)

HYPNOTICS substances or drugs that induce sleep e.g. BARBITURATES and chloral hydrate.

HYPNOSIS a state of altered attention resembling sleep in which the mind is more receptive to recall of memories of past events and to suggestion. The person who induces this state in another is known as a *hypnotist*. One of the ways of inducing hypnosis is to ask the patient to fix his eyes on a given point or source of light and then rhythmically repeat soothing words in a low voice. Some people appear to be more easily *hypnotized* than others and there are three merging levels of hypnosis, *light, medium* and *deep*. It is a useful form of treatment in psychiatry and also in pain relief e.g. during labour and dental repair. It is also used in the treatment of asthma and alcoholism.

HYPOCALCAEMIA a low blood calcium level possibly resulting from kidney failure, pancreatitis, vitamin D deficiency, hypoparathyroidism and producing heart ARRHYTHMIAS, TETANY, reduction of the sense of touch (lips, tongue, feet and hands).

HYPOCHONDRIA an abnormal pre-occupation by an individual with the state of his or her health. In its severest form the person wrongly believes that he or she is suffering from a number of illnesses and is extremely anxious and depressed. Treatment is by means of psychotherapy and anti-depressant drugs but the condition tends to be difficult to cure.

HYPODERMIC beneath the skin. The term is usually used in reference to injections given by means of a *hypodermic syringe*.

HYPOGLYCAEMIA a lack of sugar in the blood which occurs in starvation and also with DIABETES MELLITUS when too much insulin has been given and insufficient carbohydrates have been eaten. The symptoms include weakness, sweating, light-headedness and tremors and can lead to coma. The symptoms are alleviated by taking in glucose either by mouth, or injection in the case of hypoglycaemic coma.

HYPOKALAEMIA a low blood potassium level producing weakness, abnormal ECG and may be caused by ADRENAL tumour, starvation, treatment of diabetic acidosis or diabetic therapy.

HYPOPLASIA underdevelopment of a tissue or organ such as can occur in the teeth due to illness or starvation (dental hypoplasia). It is marked by lines across the teeth of brown enamel.

HYPOTHALAMUS an area of the forebrain in the floor of the third ventricle, having the thalamus above and pituitary gland below. It contains centres controlling vital processes, e.g. fat and carbohydrate metabolism, thirst and water regulation, hunger and eating, thermal regulation and sexual function. It also plays a part in the emotions and in the regulation of sleep. It controls the sympathetic and parasympathetic nervous systems and secretions from the pituitary gland.

HYPOTHERMIA describes the bodily state when the core temperature falls below 35°C due to prolonged exposure to cold. At first, shivering occurs and the heart works harder to increase the flow of blood around the body. However, eventually shivering ceases and, with increasing chilling, the function of the body organs becomes disturbed and cardiac output falls. The tissues require less oxygen as their functions start to fail, but eventually the heart is unable to supply even this reduced demand. The symptoms of hypothermia are fatigue and confusion followed by unconsciousness and death. The elderly are particularly at risk through inadequate domestic heating.

Occasionally, a state of artificial hypo-thermia is induced during surgery to reduce the oxygen requirements of the tissues and enable the circulation to be briefly halted.

HYPOTHYROIDISM reduced activity of the THYROID gland which may be caused by surgical removal, lower activity of the thyroid releasing hormone from the HYPOTHALAMUS or lower secretion from the PITUITARY of thyroid stimulating hormone. Typical symptoms include dry skin, weight gain, constipation, arthritis, general sluggishness. Ultimately, if untreated, it leads to coma and death.

HYPOVENTILATION an abnormally slow rate of shallow breathing which may result from injury or the effects of drugs on the respiratory centre in the brain. The effect is to increase the amount of carbon dioxide in the blood and lessen that of oxygen. Eventually this leads to death due to a lack of oxygen supply to cells and tissues.

HYSTERECTOMY the surgical removal of the womb either by means of an abdominal incision or through the VAGINA. It is commonly carried out if fibroids are present or if the womb is cancerous, and also if there is excessive bleeding.

ICHTHYOSIS a generally hereditary skin condition in which the skin is very dry and looks cracked producing a resemblance to fish scales. There is particular medication to take but vitamin A may help. The treatment is thus external and involves special baths and the application of ointments.

IDIOPATHIC the term given to a disease indicating that its cause is not known.

ILEITIS inflammation of the ILEUM with pain, bowel irregularity and loss of weight.

The intestine may become thickened and if the tract becomes blocked, surgery is required immediately. The specific cause is not known but it may occur in association with tuberculosis, bacterial infection (by *Yersinia enterocolitica*), Crohn's disease (chronic inflammation of the bowel) and typhoid.

ILEECTOMY removal by surgery of all or part of the ILEUM.

ILEOSTOMY a surgical procedure in which an opening is made in the abdominal wall, to which the ileum is joined. This creates an artificial anus through which the waste contents of the intestines are collected in a special bag. This procedure is undertaken to allow the COLON to heal after surgery or colitis, or in association with other surgery in treating cancer of the rectum.

ILEUM the lower part of the small intestine between the JEJUNUM and the CAECUM.

ILEUS an obstruction of the intestine (often the ILEUM) which may be mechanical due to worms or a gallstone from the gall bladder, or it can be due to loss of the natural movement of the intestines (peristalsis). This latter condition may be caused by surgery, injury to the spine or PERITONITIS.

ILIAC ARTERIES those arteries supplying blood to the lower limbs and pelvic region.

ILIUM the largest of the bones that form each half of the pelvic girdle. It ha a flattened wing-like part fastening to the SACRUM by means of ligaments.

IMMUNE the state of being protected against an infection by the presence of antibodies specific to the organism concerned.

IMMUNITY the way in which the body resists infection due to the presence of ANTIBODIES and white blood cells. Antibodies are generated in response to the presence of ANTIGENS of a disease. There are several types of immunity: *active immunity* is when the body produces antibodies and continues to be able to do so, during the course of a disease whether occurring naturally (also called *acquired immunity*) or by deliberate stimulation. *Passive immunity* is short-lived and due to the injection of ready-made antibodies from someone who is already immune.

IMMUNIZATION producing immunity to disease by artificial means. Injection of an antiserum will produce temporary passive immunity. Active immunity is produced by making the body generate its own antibodies and this is done by the use of treated antigens (vaccination or inoculation). vaccine is used for immunization and it may be treated live bacteria or viruses or dead organisms or their products.

IMMUNOGLOBULINS a group of high molecular weight proteins that act as antibodies and are present in the serum body. Designated Ig, there are five groups each with different functions identified by a particular letter. Immunoglobulin A (Ig A) is most common and occurs in all secretions of the body. It is the main antibody in the mucous membrane of the intestines, bronchi, saliva and tears. It defends the body against microorganisms by combining with a protein in the mucosa. Ig D is found in the serum in small amounts but increases during allergic reactions.

Ig E is found primarily in the lungs, skin and mucous membrane cells and is an anaphylactic antibody (*see* anaphylaxis). Ig G is synthesized to combat bacteria and viruses in the body.

Ig M (or macroglobulin) has a very high molecular weight (about five or six times that of the others) and is the first produced by the body when antigens occur. It is also the main antibody in blood group incompatibilities.

IMMUNOLOGY the study of immunity, the immune system of the body and all aspects of the body's defence mechanisms.

IMMUNOSUPPRESSION the use of

drugs (immunosuppressives) that affect the body's immune system and lower its resistance to disease. These drugs are used in transplant surgery to maintain the survival of the transplanted organ, and to treat autoimmune diseases. The condition may also be produced as a side effect, e.g. after chemotherapy treatment for cancer. In all instances, there is an increased risk of infection.

IMMUNOTHERAPY the largely experimental technique of developing the body's immunity to a disease by administering drugs or gradually increasing doses of the appropriate allergens thereby modifying the immune response. The most widely studied disease is cancer where this forms an auxiliary treatment to drug therapy.

IMPACTION a descriptive term for things being locked or wedged together; or stuck in position. For example a wisdom tooth is impacted when it cannot erupt normally because of other tissues blocking it. Also impacted faeces form a block in the colon or rectum and an impacted fracture is where the adjacent ends are locked together.

IMPETIGO a staphylococcal and infectious skin disease found primarily in children. It spreads quickly over the body, starting as a red patch which forms pustules that join to create crusted yellowish sores. It is easily spread by contact or through towels etc. and must be treated quickly otherwise it may continue on an individual for months. Treatment with antibiotics is usually effective.

IMPLANT a drug, tissue or artificial object inserted or grafted into the skin or an organ. Drugs are often inserted into the skin for controlled release and in radiotherapy, treatment of prostate tumours, or head/neck cancers can include embedding a capsule of radio-active material in the tissue. A surgical implant covers a tissue graft (e.g. a blood vessel), insertion of a pacemaker or a hip prosthesis.

IMPLANTATION 1. the placing of an

IMPLANT. 2. the attachment of the BLASTOCYST to the uterus wall during the very early stages of embryo development.

IMPOTENCE when a man is unable to have sexual intercourse through lack of penile ERECTION, or less commonly to ejaculate having gained an erection. The cause may be *organic* and due to a condition or disease (DIABETES, endocrine gland disorder) or more commonly *psychogenic*, i.e. due to psychological or emotional problems such as anxiety, fear, guilt.

INCISION a surgical cut into tissue or organ, and the act of making the cut.

INCISOR the tooth with a chisel edge to it, used for biting. They form the four front teeth in each jaw.

INCONTINENCE an inability to control bowel movements or passage of urine. Urinary incontinence may be due to a LESION in the brain or spinal cord, injury to the sphincter, or damage to the nerves of the bladder. Stress incontinence occurs during coughing or straining and is common in women due to weakening of muscles through childbirth. There are other categories of incontinence depending on the cause or the frequency of urine passage and the stimulus causing urination.

INCUBATION 1. the time between a person being exposed to an infection and the appearance of symptoms. Incubation periods for diseases tend to be quite constant, some commoner ones being; measles, 10 to 15 days; German measles, 14 to 21; chicken pox, 14 to 21; mumps, 18 to 21 and whooping cough, 7 to 10 days. 2. the time taken to start and grow microorganisms in culture media. 3. the process of caring for a premature baby in an incubator.

INCUBATOR 1. the transparent box-like container in which premature babies are kept in controlled, infection-free conditions. 2. a heated container for growth of bacterial cultures in laboratories.

INDIGESTION *see* DYSPEPSIA.

INDUCTION the commencement of labour by artificial means, either by administering drugs to produce uterine contractions, or by AMNIOTOMY.

In anaesthesia, it is the process prior to the required state of anaesthesia and includes premedication with a sedative.

INFANT a child from birth to 12 months.

INFANT MORTALITY (*or* **INFANT MORTALITY RATE**) a statistical measure of infant deaths, calculated as the number of deaths of infants under one year, per 1000 live births (in any given year). The figure is regarded as a measure of social conditions in a country rather than a guide to the medical services.

INFARCTION the formation of an *infarct* or dead area of tissue in an organ or vessel due to the obstruction of the artery supplying blood. The obstruction may be caused by a blood clot or an EMBOLUS.

INFECTION when PATHOGENS invade the body causing disease. Bacteria, viruses, fungi etc. are all included and they enter the body, multiply and after the INCUBATION period symptoms appear. The organisms reach the body in many ways: airborne droplets, direct contact, sexual intercourse, by VECTORS, from contaminated food or drink etc.

INFERTILITY when a couple are unable to produce offspring naturally. Female infertility may be because of irregular or no ovulation, blocked FALLOPIAN TUBES, ENDOMETRIOSIS; while a low sperm count or other deficiency in the spermatozoa can lead to male infertility. Treatment can include drug therapy, surgery, or more recently the technique of *in vitro* fertilization.

INFESTATION when animal parasites occur on the skin, in the hair or within the body (e.g. parasitic worms).

INFLAMMATION the response of the body's tissues to injury which involves pain, redness, heat and swelling (*acute* inflammation). The first sign when the tissues are infected or injured physically or chemically is a dilation of blood vessels in the affected area increasing blood flow resulting in heat and redness.

The circulation then slows a little and white blood cells migrate into the tissues producing the swelling. The white blood cells engulf invading bacteria, dead tissue, foreign particles. After this either the white blood cells migrate back to the circulation, or there is the production and discharge of pus, as healing commences. *Chronic* inflammation is when repair is not complete and there is formation of scar tissue.

INFLUENZA a highly infectious disease caused by virus that affects the respiratory tract. Symptoms include headache, weakness and fever, appetite loss and general aches and pains. Sometimes there is the complication of a lung infection which requires immediate treatment. There are three main strains of influenza virus, designated A, B and C. The viruses quickly produce new strains which is why an attack of one is unlikely to provide protection against a later bout of the disease. Epidemics occur periodically and in Britain virus A is responsible for the majority of outbreaks.

INGESTION the process of chewing and swallowing food and fluid which then goes into the stomach. Also the means whereby a *phagocyte* (a cell that can surround and break down cell debris, foreign particles and microorganisms) takes in particles.

INHALANTS substances taken into the body by INHALATION. The substances can be in several forms: inhaling the steam of a hot solution; as a pressurized aerosol of droplets of particles; or as a non-pressurized passive inhaler where powdered medication is drawn into the body by inhaling deeply. Sufferers of asthma use inhalers to deliver drugs to the bronchi (bronchodilator drugs) for relief from attacks.

INHALATION 1. (*or* **INSPIRATION**) the act of drawing air into the lungs. 2. the medication breathed in, whether in gas, vapour of particulate form, to ensure contact with and/or treatment of conditions of the throat, bronchi or lungs.

INJECTION the means whereby a liquid (often a drug) is introduced into the body using a syringe when it would otherwise be destroyed by digestive processes. The location of the injection depends upon the speed with which the drug is to be absorbed and the target site. Thus injections may go into the skin (*intradermal*), beneath the skin (*subcutaneous*, as with INSULIN). For slow absorption an *intramuscular* injection would be used, and *intravenous* for fast delivery.

INNER EAR *see* EAR.

INNERVATION the nerves serving a particular organ, tissue or area of the body which carries MOTOR impulses to the target and sensory impulses away from it and towards the brain.

INOCULATION the process whereby a small quantity of material is introduced into the body to produce or increase immunity to the disease related to the injected material (*see* IMMUNIZATION *and* VACCINATION).

INSEMINATION injection of semen into the vagina whether by sexual intercourse or artificial means (*see* ARTIFICIAL INSEMINATION).

INSOMNIA being unable to remain asleep or to fall asleep in the first instance, resulting in debilitating tiredness. It may be caused by a painful condition but is more likely to be due to anxiety.

INSULIN a pancreatic hormone produced in the ISLETS OF LANGERHANS that initiates uptake of glucose by body cells and thereby controls the level of glucose in the blood. It works by stimulating proteins on cell surfaces within muscles and other tissues to take up the glucose for their activity. A lack of hormone results in the sugar derived from food being excreted in the urine - the condition DIABETES MELLITUS. For such cases, insulin can be administered by injection.

INTERCOSTAL the term given to nerves, muscles etc. that are situated between the ribs.

INTERFERON glycoproteins released

from cells infected with a virus which restrict, or *interfere* with, the growth of viruses, and they limit the growth of cells, hence their use in cancer treatment (which is as yet of indeterminate value). There are three human interferons: a from white blood cells, b from connective tissue and g from lymphocyte (*see* INTERLEUKINS). Sufficient quantities of interferon can now be produced by GENETIC ENGINEERING.

INTERLEUKINS one of several cytokines (molecules secreted by a cell to regulate other cells nearby e.g. see INTERFERON) that act between LEUCOCYTES. There are eight interleukins currently recognized and some are involved in functions such as the recognition of ANTIGENS, enhancing the action of MACROPHAGES and the production of other cytokines e.g. interleukin 2 promotes the production of g-interferon and is used in the treatment of MELANOMA.

INTERVERTEBRAL DISC fibrous cartilaginous discs that connect adjacent vertebrae and permit rotational and bending movements. The discs make up approximately 25% of the backbone length and they act as shock absorbers providing cushioning for the brain and spinal cord. With age the discs lose their effectiveness and may be displaced.

INTESTINAL FLORA the bacteria usually found in the intestine, some of which synthesize vitamin K. An acidic surrounding is produced by the bacteria and this helps lessen infection by pathogens unable to withstand the acidic conditions.

INTESTINE the part of the ALIMENTARY CANAL or tract between stomach and anus where final digestion and absorption of food matter occur in addition to the absorption of water and production of faeces. The intestine is divided into the small intestine comprising DUODENUM, ILEUM and JEJUNUM, and the large intestine made up of the CAECUM, vermiform APPENDIX, COLON and RECTUM. The length of the intestine in man is about 30 feet.

INTOLERANCE when a patient is unable to metabolize a drug. There is usually an associated drug reaction.

INTOXICATION being poisoned by drugs, alcohol or other toxic substances.

INTRACRANIAL term meaning within the skull and applied to diseases, structures etc.

INTRACRANIAL PRESSURE the pressure within the cranium, more specifically the pressure as maintained by all tissues: brain, blood, cerebrospinal fluid etc. An increase in the pressure can occur through injury, haemorrhage, tumour and treatment will be necessary.

INTRAMUSCULAR term meaning within a muscle, as with an intramuscular injection.

INTRAUTERINE CONTRACEPTIVE DEVICE (IUD) a plastic or metal device, often in the shape of a coil about 25mm long, that is placed in the uterus. The device probably prevents conception by interfering with potential implantation of the embryo. There are sometimes side effects e.g. back pain and heavy menstrual bleeding, but it is a reasonably effective method.

INTRAVENOUS term meaning relating to the inside of a vein hence intravenous injections are made into a vein, and blood transfusions are intravenous.

INTUBATION the insertion of a tube into the body through a natural opening. It is commonly, though not exclusively, used to keep an airway open by insertion into the mouth or nose into the larynx. The same technique may be adopted to enable an anaesthetic gas, or oxygen to be delivered.

INTUMESCENCE swelling, of an organ.

INTUSSUSCEPTION an eventual obstruction of the bowel caused by one part of the bowel slipping inside another part beneath it, much as a telescope closes up. The commonest sufferers are young children and the symptoms include pain, vomiting and the passage of a jelly-like blood-stained mucus. If the condition does not right itself corrective treatment is essential either by a barium enema or surgery.

INVASION when bacteria enter the body; but more commonly used to describe the process whereby malignant cancer cells move into nearby normal and deeper tissues and gain access to the blood vessels.

IN VITRO referring to a biological or biochemical reaction or process that occurs literally 'in glassware' i.e. in test-tube or a similar piece of laboratory apparatus.

IN VITRO FERTILIZATION (IVF) the process of fertilizing an OVUM outside the body. The technique is used when a woman has blocked FALLOPIAN TUBES or when there is some other reason for sperm and ovum not uniting. The woman produces several ova (due to hormone therapy treatment) which are removed by laparoscopy (see LAPAROSCOPE) and these are mixed with sperm and incubated in culture medium until the ova are fertilized and at the BLASTOCYST stage these are implanted in the mother's uterus. The first successful live birth utilizing this technique was in 1978 and the phrase 'test-tube baby' was coined.

IN VIVO referring to biological processes that occur in a living organism.

INVOLUNTARY MUSCLE one of two types of muscle not under voluntary or conscious control such as the blood vessels, stomach and intestines. The heart muscle is slightly different (see CARDIAC MUSCLE).

INVOLUTION the process whereby an organ decreases in size e.g. the return of the uterus to its normal size after childbirth. Also applied to degeneration of organs in old age i.e. atrophy.

IRIDECTOMY the surgical removal of part of the IRIS, often undertaken to correct the blockage of aqueous humour (see EYE) associated with GLAUCOMA. It may also be necessary for removal of a foreign body or as part of CATARACT surgery.

IRIDOTOMY an incision into the IRIS.

IRIS the part of the EYE that controls the amount of light to enter. It is in effect a muscular disc and to reduce the amount of light entering circular muscles contract, and to increase the aperture in dim light, radiating muscles contract. The varying sized hole is the PUPIL. The iris can be seen through the CORNEA which is transparent and is the coloured part of the eye, this latter feature is due to pigment cells containing melanin (blue is little; brown is more).

IRRADIATION the use in treatment of any form of radiating energy i.e. electromagnetic radiation in the form of X-rays, a, b or g radiation, also heat and light. Some radiations are used in diagnosis or cancer treatments, others for relief of pain (heat treatment) etc.

IRRIGATION the washing out of a wound or body cavity with a flow of water or other fluid.

IRRITABLE BOWEL SYNDROME a condition caused by abnormal muscular contractions (or increased motility) in the COLON producing effects in the large and small intestines. Symptoms include pain in the abdomen which changes location, disturbed bowel movements with diarrhoea then normal movements or constipation, heartburn and a bloated feeling due to wind. The specific cause is unknown and as no disease is present treatment is limited to relief of anxiety or stress (which may be a contributory factor), some drug therapy to reduce muscle activity and careful choice of diet, to include a high fibre content.

IRRITANT a general term encompassing any agent that causes irritation of a tissue e.g. nettle stings, chemicals and gases etc.

ISCHAEMIC relating to a decrease in blood supply to a part of the body or an organ, caused by a blockage or narrowing of the blood vessels. It is often associated with pain.

ISCHIUM one of the three bones that comprise each half of the pelvis. It is the most posterior and it supports the weight of the body when sitting.

ISLETS OF LANGERHANS clusters of cells within the PANCREAS which are the ENDOCRINE part of the gland. There are three types of cells termed alpha, beta and delta, the first two producing GLUCAGON and INSULIN respectively, both vital hormones in the regulation of blood sugar levels. The third hormone produced is somatostatin (also released by the HYPOTHALAMUS) which works antagonistically against growth hormone by blocking its release by the pituitary gland. The islets are named after Paul Langerhans, a German pathologist.

ISOTOPES atoms that differ from other atoms of the same element due to a different number of neutrons in the nucleus. Isotopes have the same number of protons and therefore the same atomic number, but a different mass number (total number of protons and neutrons). Radioactive isotopes decay into other elements or isotopes through the emission of alpha, beta or gamma radiation, and some radioactive isotopes can be produced in the laboratory. RADIOTHERAPY uses such isotopes in the treatment of cancer.

ITCHING a skin condition or sensation prompting scratching to obtain relief. The causes are numerous and include mechanical irritation e.g. by clothing or lice, skin diseases or conditions such as ECZEMA, allergies etc.

JAUNDICE a condition characterized by the unusual presence of bile pigment (BILIRUBIN) in the blood. The BILE produced in the liver passes into the blood instead of the intestines and because of this there is a yellowing of the skin and the whites of the eyes. There are several types of jaundice: *obstructive* due to bile not reaching the intestine due to an obstruction e.g. a GALLSTONE; *haemolytic* where red blood cells are destroyed by HAEMOLYSIS; *hepatocellular* due to a liver disease such as HEPATITIS which results in the liver being unable to use the bilirubin. *Neonatal jaundice* is quite common in newborn infants when the liver is physiologically immature but it usually lasts only a few days. The infant can be exposed to blue light which converts bilirubin to biliverdin, another (harmless) bile pigment.

JAW a term for the bones that carry the teeth and associated soft tissues. More specifically, they are the upper jaw (*maxilla*) and the lower jaw (*mandible*). The maxillae are fixed, while the mandible (which is one bone after the age of about 12 months) hinges on part of the temporal bone, in front of the ear.

JEJUNUM the part of the small intestine lying before the ILEUM and after the DUODENUM. Its main function is the absorption of digested food and its lining has numerous finger-like projections (villi) that increase the surface area for absorption. The villi are longer in the jejunum than elsewhere in the small intestine.

JOINTS connections between bones (and cartilages). Joints can be divided upon their structure and the degree to which they permit movement. *Fibrous* joints are fixed by fibrous tissue binding bones together e.g the bones of the skull. *Cartilaginous* joints are slightly movable. These have discs of cartilage between bones so that only limited movement is permitted over one joint but over several adjacent joints, considerable flexure is achieved, as with the spine. The final category is *synovial* joints which can move freely. Each synovial joint comprises the bones, cartilage over the ends, then a *capsule* (sheath of fibrous tissue) from which the ligaments form, and a SYNOVIAL MEMBRANE with synovial fluid to lubricate the joint.
This type of joint then occurs in two forms: hinge joints allowing planar

movement (e.g. the knee) and ball and socket joints permitting all-round movement (e.g. the hip). Joints are subject to various conditions and diseases including SYNOVITIS, epiphysitis (inflammation of the EPIPHYSIS), GOUT, RHEUMATISM and dislocations.

JUGULAR a general term for structures in the neck.

JUGULAR VEIN any of the veins in the neck, particularly the anterior, internal and external. The anterior jugular vein is an offshoot of the external jugular and runs down the front of the neck. The external jugular itself drains the scalp, face and neck while the larger internal jugular drains the face, neck and brain and is sited vertically down the side of the neck.

KAOLIN (or china clay) a white powder form of aluminium silicate used in cases of skin irritation. It is also an adsorbent taken internally to treat DIARRHOEA.

KAPOSI'S SARCOMA a condition involving malignant skin tumours which form from the blood vessels. Purple lumps, due to the tumours, form on the feet and ankles, spreading to arms and hands. The disease is common in Africa but less so in western countries, although it is associated with AIDS. Radiotherapy is the primary treatment but chemotherapy may also be required.

KELOID (*also* **CHELOID**) scar tissue which forms due to the growth of fibrous tissue over a burn or injury creating a hard, often raised patch with ragged edges.

KERATIN a fibrous, sulphur-rich protein made up of coiled POLYPEPTIDE chains. It occurs in hair, fingernails and the surface layer of the skin.

KERATOSIS a condition of the skin whereby there is a thickening and over-growth of the horny layer (or *stratum corneum*) of the SKIN. The condition is usually induced by excessive sunlight and can occur as scales and patchy skin pigmentation (*actinic keratosin*) or as yellow/brown warts (*seborrhoeic keratosis*). It is essential to avoid over-exposing skin to sunlight if the condition is to be prevented or treated.

KERNIG'S SIGN the inability of someone with MENINGITIS to straighten his legs at the knee when the thighs are at right angles to be body. It is symptomatic of the disease.

KETOACIDOSIS acidosis resulting from a disorder in the metabolism of carbohydrates which produces a build-up of KETONES in the body. It is mainly a complication of DIABETES mellitus and produces a fruity smell on the breath, also symptoms such as nausea, vomiting, dehydration, shortness of breath, weight loss and coma if untreated.

KETOGENESIS the normal production of KETONES in the body due to metabolism of fats. Excess production leads to KETOSIS.

KETONE an organic compound that contains a carbonyl group (C=O) within the compound. Ketones can be detected in the body when fat is metabolized for energy when food intake is insufficient.

KETONE BODY one of several compounds (e.g. acetoacetic acid) produced by the liver due to metabolism of fat deposits. These compounds normally provide energy, via KETOGENE-SIS, for the body's peripheral tissues. In abnormal conditions, when carbohydrate supply is reduced, ketogensis produces excess ketone bodies in the blood (KETOSIS) which may then appear in the urine (KETONURIA).

KETONURIA (acetonuria, or ketoaciduria) the presence of ketone bodies (*see* KETONE and KETONE BODY) in the urine due to starvation or DIABETES MELLITUS causing excessive KETOGENESIS and KETOSIS.

KETOSIS the build-up of ketones in the body and bloodstream due to a lack of carbohydrates for metabolism, or failure to use fully available carbohydrates resulting in fat breakdown (*see* KETOGENESIS and KETONURIA). It is induced by starvation, DIABETES MELLITUS or any condition in which fats are metabolized quickly and excessively.

KIDNEY one of two glands/organs that remove nitrogenous wastes, mainly UREA, from the blood and also adjust the concentrations of various salts. The kidney measures approximately 10cm long, 6cm wide and 4cm thick, and is positioned at the back of the abdomen, below the diaphragm. Blood is supplied to the kidney by the renal artery and leaves via the renal vein. Each kidney is held in place by fat and connective tissue and comprises an inner medulla and outer cortex. The kidneys produce and eliminate URINE by a complex process of filtration and reabsorption. The 'active' parts are the nephrons which filter blood under pressure, reabsorbing water and other substances. A nephron comprises a renal tubule and blood vessels. The tubule expands into a cup shape (*Bowman's capsule*) that contains a knot of capillaries (the *glomerulus*) and the latter bring the water, urea, salts, etc. Filtrate passes from the glomerulus through three areas of the tubule (proximal convoluted tubule; the loop of Henle, distal convoluted tube, which together form a shape resembling a hairpin) leaving as urine.

The kidneys contain roughly two million nephrons and receive between one and two thousand litres of blood each day, processing 150 - 200 litres of filtrate, resulting in roughly 1° litres of urine.

KININ one of a group of POLYPEPTIDES that lower blood pressure through dilation of the blood vessels and cause SMOOTH MUSCLE to contract. They are associated with inflammation, causing local increases in the permeability of tissue capillaries. In addition they play some part in the allergic response and ANAPHYLAXIS. Kinins do not normally occur in the blood but form under these conditions or when the tissue is damaged (*see also* BRADYKININS).

KLINEFELTER'S SYNDROME a genetic imbalance in males in which there are 47 rather than 46 CHROMOSOMES, the extra one being an X chromosome producing a genetic make-up of XXY instead of the usual XY. The physical manifestations are small testes which atrophy resulting in a lack of sperm production, enlargement of the breasts, long thin legs and little or no facial or body hair. There may be associated mental retardation and pulmonary disease.

KNEE the joint connecting the thigh to the lower leg and formed by the femur, tibia and kneecap (PATELLA). It is a hinge type of synovial JOINT with very strong ligaments binding the bones together. Although the knee is a strong joint, it is complex and injuries can be serious.

KNEE JERK *see* REFLEX ACTION.

KNOCK-KNEE (*or* GENU VALGUM) an abnormal curvature of the legs such that when the knees are touching, the ankles are spaced apart. When walking, the knees knock and severe cases can lead to stress on the joints in the legs, with arthritis. Surgery may be performed to correct the condition which in the past was commonly due to RICKETS but is now due mainly to poor muscles.

KORSAKOFF'S SYNDROME a neurological disorder described by the Russian neuropsychiatrist Sergei Korsakoff (1854-1900) characterized by short-term memory loss, disorientation and confabulation (the invention and detailed description of events, situations and experiences to cover gaps in the memory). The condition is caused primarily by alcoholism and a deficiency of thiamine (vital in converting carbohydrate to glucose).

KWASHIORKOR a type of malnutrition seen especially among children in Africa. It is due to a deficiency in dietary protein and foods normally eaten for energy. It occurs when a child is weaned from the breast onto an adult diet that is inadequate such that the child cannot eat enough to get sufficient protein. The result is appetite loss, diarrhoea, OEDEMA, anaemia, and other conditions due to, for example, VITAMIN deficiencies. Initially the condition responds well to first-class protein, but it is less straightforward with more prolonged cases.

KYPHOSIS an abnormal outward curvature of the spine causing the back to be hunched. There is an increased curvature of the spine which may be caused by weak musculature or bad posture (mobile kyphosis) or it may be due to collapsed vertebrae (fixed kyphosis) as in OSTEOPOROSIS of the aged.

LABIA (*singular* **LABIUM**) meaning lips as in the folds of skin enclosing the VULVA (the *labia majora* and *minora*).
LABIAL pertaining to the lips. Also the tooth surface next to the lips.
LABOUR the process of giving birth from dilatation of the CERVIX to expulsion of the afterbirth. It usually commences naturally although some labours are induced (*see* INDUCTION). The cervix expands and at the same time the muscles of the uterus will contract pushing part of the AMNION down into the opening. The amnion ruptures releasing the "waters" but these two events do not necessarily occur at the same time. The second stage is the actual delivery of the child which passes through the bony girdle of the pelvis, via the VAGINA to the outside. Initially the head appears at the cervix and the uterine contractions strengthen. These contractions are augmented by abdominal muscular contractions when the baby is in the vagina. When the baby's head is clear, the whole body is helped out and the umbilical cord

severed. The final stage, accomplished by some contractions is expulsion of the PLACENTA and membranes.
On average, labour lasts 12 hours (less for subsequent pregnancies) and in the second stage an EPISIOTOMY may be necessary to facilitate the emergence of the head. In most cases, the baby lies head down at delivery although some are delivered feet or buttocks first (BREECH PRESENTATION). Other complications tend to be rare and maternal mortality is very low in the west.
LABYRINTH part of the inner ear (*see* EAR) consisting of canals, ducts and cavities forming the organs of hearing and balance. There are two parts; the *membranous labyrinth* comprising the semi circular canals and associated structures and the central cavity of the cochlea, and the *bony labyrinth*, a system of canals filled with perilymph and surrounding the other parts.
LACERATION a wound with jagged edges.
LACRIMAL relating to, or about tears.
LACRIMAL GLAND one of a pair of glands situated above and to the side of each eye that secrete saline and slightly alkaline tears that moisten the conjunctiva (the mucous membrane lining the inside of the eyelid). The glands comprise part of the *lacrimal apparatus*, the remainder being the lacrimal ducts (or canaliculi) through which the tears drain, to the lacrimal sacs and the nasal cavity.
LACTATION the process of milk secretion by the MAMMARY GLANDS in the breast which begins at the end of pregnancy. colostrum is produced and secreted before the milk. Lactation is controlled by hormones and stops when the baby ceases to be breast fed.
LACTASE the enzyme that acts on milk sugar (LACTOSE) to produce glucose and galactose.
LACTEAL vessels forming part of the lymphatic system. They occur as projections with a closed end extending

into villi (*see* VILLUS) in the small intestine and take up digested fats as a milky fluid called chyle.

LACTOSE milk sugar found only in mammalian milk and produced by the MAMMARY GLANDS. It is made up of one molecule of glucose and one molecule of galactose. People with a low level of activity of the enzyme LACTASE, or none at all, cannot absorb lactose, a condition called lactose intolerance.

LACUNA (*plural* **LACUNAE**) an anatomical term meaning a small depression, cavity or pit, especially in compact bone.

LAMINECTOMY the surgical procedure in which access is gained to the spinal cord by the removal of the arch of one or more vertebrae. It is adopted when a tumour is to be removed, or a slipped disc is to be treated.

LARGE INTESTINE *see* INTESTINE.

LARYNGECTOMY surgical excision of all or part of the LARYNX. This procedure is adopted for cancer of the larynx.

LARYNGITIS inflammation of the mucous membrane that lines the LARYNX and vocal cords. It is due to viral infection in the main, but also bacteria, chemical irritants, heavy smoking or excessive use of the voice. *Acute* laryngitis accompanies infections of the upper respiratory tract and the symptoms include pain, a cough, difficulty in swallowing. *Chronic* laryngitis may be due to recurrence of the acute form, but is often attributable to excessive smoking worsened by alcohol. Changes occurring in the vocal cords are more permanent and the symptoms are as for the acute form, but longer lasting.

LARYNGOSCOPE a type of endoscope used to examine the larynx.

LARYNGOTRACHEOBRONCHITIS an acute inflammation of the major parts of the respiratory tract, causing shortness of breath, a croup-like cough and hoarseness. It occurs usually through viral infection and particularly in young children where there may be some obstruction of the LARYNX (*see also* CROUP). The main airways, bronchi, become coated with fluid generated by the inflamed tissues resulting in the shortness of breath. Treatment is through inhalations, antibiotics if appropriate and if the obstruction is serious, hospitalization may be necessary for INTUBATION, TRACHEOSTOMY etc.

LARYNX part of the air passage connecting the PHARYNX with the TRACHEA and also the organ producing vocal sounds. It is situated high up in the front of the neck and is constructed of cartilages with ligaments and muscles. The ligaments bind together the cartilages and one pair of these form the VOCAL CORDS. The larynx is lined with mucous membrane and in all is about 5cm long.

LASER (*Light Amplification by Stimulated Emission of Radiation*) a device that produces a powerful and narrow beam of light where the light is of one wavelength in phase. This produces a beam of high energy light which can be used in surgery. Different lasers can be used for different procedures for example the argon laser heats and coagulates tissues because haemoglobin absorbs the energy - this is therefore used to seal bleeding vessels. The carbon-dioxide laser is used to make incisions because water in cells absorbs the energy, thus destroying the cells. Lasers are also used in retina surgery, and in the removal of birthmarks.

LAUDANUM a NARCOTIC ANALGESIC prepared from opium, used widely in the past.

LAUGHING GAS the common name for NITROUS OXIDE.

LAXATIVE a substance that is taken to evacuate the bowel or to soften stools. Typical laxatives include castor oil, senna, and its derivatives (*see also* PURGATIVE).

LEGIONNAIRE'S DISEASE a bacterial infection and a form of pneumonia caused by *Legionella pneumophila*. It produces an illness similar to influenza with symptoms appearing after a two to ten day incubation period. Fever, chills, head and muscular aches may progress to PLEURISY and chest pains. Antibiotic treatment is usually effective (e.g. erythromycin).

The disease was named after an outbreak in America in 1976 at the American Legion convention. The bacterium is found in nature, particularly in water, and static water provides ideal conditions for multiplication. Inhalation of an aerosol of water is the likeliest way of becoming infected and air conditioning cooling towers are a particular source of infected water. It is vital that infected systems be cleaned and chlorinated.

LENS the part of the eye that focuses incoming light onto the RETINA. It is composed of a fibrous protein, crystallin, and is enclosed in a thin capsule.

LEPROSY a serious disease caused by the bacterium *Mycobacterium leprae* that attacks the skin, nerves and mucous membranes and has an incubation period of several years. There are two forms of the disease, *tuberculoid* and *lepromatous*, depending upon the resistance of the host (the former occurs in those with a higher degree of immunity). The tuberculoid form produces discoloured patches of skin with some numbness but is generally benign and often heals untreated.

Lepromatous leprosy is a much more serious and progressively destructive form of the disease, creating lumps in the skin, thickening of skin and nerves, inflammation of the iris, numbness of the skin with muscle weakness and paralysis. The more serious cases show deformity and considerable disfigurement and sometimes blindness. There is also an intermediate form with symptoms of both types (indeterminate leprosy). Although many millions of people are affected, drugs therapy is quite effective, providing a combination of antibiotics is used (because the bacterium develops resistance to one of the sulphone drugs commonly used).

LEPTOMENINGITIS inflammation of

two of the three MENINGES surrounding the brain and spinal cord. Specifically, the inner two (pia mater and arachnoid) are affected.

LEPTOSPIROSIS an acute infectious disease caused by bacteria in the genus *Leptospira*. The disease varies from the mild form of an influenza type of illness to the more serious cases involving fever, liver disease and therefore jaundice, and possibly kidney disease or meningitis. In such cases there may be fatalities. The organism occurs in the urine of rats and dogs and this renders workers on farms, sewage works etc. more susceptible, but it can be contracted by bathing or immersion in contaminated water (e.g. canals). Antibiotics can be given but must be administered at an early stage to be effective.

One particular species *L. icterohaemorrhagiae*, which is transmitted by rats, is responsible for the type called Weil's disease.

LESBIAN see HOMOSEXUAL.

LESION a wound or injury to body tissues. Also an area of tissue which because of damage due to disease or wounding does not function fully. Thus primary lesions include tumours and ulcers, and from primary lesions secondaries may form.

LETHARGY the state of being inactive mentally and physically and one that approaches the unconscious. The cause may be psychological or physical. The lethargy associated with the aftermath of glandular fever is well-known but it may also be due to ANAEMIA, DIABETES MELLITUS or malnutrition, amongst others.

LEUCOPENIA a fall in the number of LEUCOCYTES (white blood cells) in the blood.

LEUCOCYTE (or leukocyte) a white blood cell, so called because it contains no HAEMOGLOBIN. It also differs from red blood cells in having a nucleus.

Leucocytes are formed in the bone marrow, spleen, thymus and lymph nodes and there are three types: granulocytes, comprising 70% of all white blood cells, lymphocytes (25%) and monocytes (5%). Granulocytes help combat bacterial and viral infection and may be involved in allergies. LYMPHOCYTES destroy foreign bodies either directly or through production of antibodies and MONOCYTES ingest bacteria and foreign bodies by the process called *phagocytosis* (engulfing micro-organisms and cell debris to remove them from the body). In disease, immature forms of leucocytes may appear in the blood (ultimately forming both red and white blood cells).

LEUCOCYTOSIS except for pregnancy, menstruation and during exercise an abnormal and temporary increase in the number of white blood cells in the blood. It usually accompanies bacterial but not viral infections, because the body's defence mechanism is fighting the bacteria by producing leucocytes. A blood sample may thus form a useful diagnostic tool for a condition which has not yet manifested any physical symptoms.

LEUCORRHEA a discharge of white or yellow-coloured mucus from the vagina. It may be a normal condition, increasing before and after menstruation but a large discharge probably indicates an infection somewhere in the genital tract. A common cause is the infection called THRUSH but it may also be due to GONORRHOEA in which case the treatment will differ.

LEUKAEMIA a cancerous disease in which there is an uncontrolled proliferation of LEUCOCYTES in the bone marrow. The cells fail to mature to adult cells and thus cannot function as part of the defence mechanism against infections. This leads to anaemia, bleeding, easy bruising, with enlargement of the spleen, liver and lymph nodes. Acute leukaemia has a sudden onset and development while the chronic form may take years to develop the same symptoms.
The cause of leukaemia is unknown although it has been attributed to viruses, exposure to toxic chemicals or ionizing radiations. In addition to the acute and chronic forms, it is further classified by the predominant white blood cells thus acute lymphoblastic leukaemia, acute myeloblastic leukaemia (myeloblast is an early form of granulocytes, *see* LEUCOCYTE), chronic lymphatic leukaemia. The treatment involves radiotherapy, chemotherapy and bone marrow transplants and although there is no cure, the outlook has improved over recent years. The survival or remission rate varies with the type of leukaemia.

LIBIDO the sexual drive, often associated with psychiatric illnesses. Lack of libido may be due to illness or a lack of sex hormones due to an endocrine disorder.

LICE (*singular* **LOUSE**) insects parasitic on man. Lice are wingless and attach themselves to hair or clothing by means of their legs and claws. They suck blood and are particularly resistant to crushing and have to be removed using special shampoos and combs (*see also* PEDICULOSIS).

LIGAMENT bands of fibrous connective tissue composed chiefly of COLLAGEN, that join bones together, restricting movement and preventing dislocation. Ligaments strengthen joints and most joints are surrounded by a capsular ligament. Also, a layer of SEROUS MEMBRANE e.g. the PERITONEUM that supports or links organs.

LIGATION the procedure of tying off a duct or blood vessel to prevent flow during surgery etc. The application of a LIGATURE.

LIGATURE material for tying firmly around a blood vessel or duct to stop bleeding or prevent flow. The material may be wire, silk, catgut etc.

LIGHTENING a sensation experienced by many pregnant women, normally towards the last month of the pregnancy, whereby the foetus settles lower in the pelvis. This lessens the pressure on the diaphragm and breathing becomes easier.

LIGHT REFLEX the mechanism whereby the PUPIL of the EYE opens in response to direct light or consensual pupillary stimulation (i.e. stimulation of one pupil with light results in a response from the other pupil).

LIGNOCAINE a commonly used local anaesthetic. It is given by injection for minor surgery and dental treatment and it can be applied directly to the eyes, throat etc. because it is absorbed directly through mucous membranes. It is also used in the treatment of some disorders in heart rhythm.

LINCTUS a medicine, particularly to treat coughs, that is thick and syrup-like.

LINGUAL term meaning relating to the tongue, or something close to the tongue e.g. lingual nerve, or the lingual surface of a tooth.

LINIMENT a creamy/oily substance for rubbing onto the skin to alleviate irritation or pain. Many of the compounds are poisonous and contain such substances as camphor, turpentine and even belladonna.

LINKAGE two or more GENES are said to be linked together if they occur close to each other on the same CHROMOSOME. The genes are thus likely to be inherited together as will be characteristics that they represent. This is because the linked genes are more likely to be together in nuclei formed as a result of meiosis (the chromosomal division that produces the GAMETES).

LINT a cotton fabric (formerly linen) used for surgical dressings which has one fluffy side and one smooth, the latter being placed against the skin.

LIPOLYSIS the breakdown of lipids into FATTY ACIDS via the action of the enzyme lipase.

LIPOMA a benign tumour made up of fat cells which can occur in the fibrous tissues of the body, often beneath the skin. The only problem associated with such structures may be their size and position.

LIPOSARCOMA a malignant tumour of fat cells which is very rare, particularly under the age of 30. It occurs in the buttocks or thighs.

LIPOSOME a spherical droplet of microscopic size comprising fatty membranes around an aqueous vesicle. Liposomes are created in the laboratory by adding an aqueous solution to a phospholipid gel (phospholipids are compounds containing FATTY ACIDS and a phosphate group). Liposomes bear some resemblance to living cell components and are studied on this basis. Additionally, they can be introduced into living cells and are used to transport toxic drugs to a specific treatment site. The liposomes retain the drug while in the blood and on passing through the chosen organ the membrane is melted by selectively heating the organ and the drug is released. This technique is used for certain forms of cancer.

LISTERIOSIS an infectious disease caused when the Gram-positive (*see* GRAM'S STAIN) bacterium *Listeria monocytogenes* which attacks animals is contracted by man through eating infected products. It produces symptoms similar to influenza or it may cause MENINGITIS or ENCEPHALITIS. The old and frail are more susceptible as are the newborn. It may terminate a pregnancy or damage the foetus if contracted during a pregnancy. Antibiotics such as penicillin provide an effective treatment.

LITTLE'S DISEASE CEREBRAL PALSY on both sides of the body but where the legs are affected more than the arms.

LIVER a very important organ of the body, with many functions critical in regulating metabolic processes. It is also the largest gland in the body weighing around 1 kg. It occupies the top right hand part of the abdominal cavity and is made up of four lobes. It is fastened to the abdominal wall by ligaments and sits beneath the DIAPHRAGM, and upon the right kidney, large intestine, DUODENUM and stomach.

There are two blood vessels supplying the liver: the hepatic artery delivers oxygenated blood, while the hepatic portal vein conveys digested food from the stomach. Among its functions, the liver converts excess glucose to GLYCOGEN for storage as a food reserve; excess amounts of AMINO ACIDS are converted to urea for excretion by the kidneys; BILE is produced for storage in the GALL BLADDER and LIPOLYSIS occurs; some poisons are broken down (detoxified) hence the beneficial effect of the hepatic portal vein carrying blood to the liver rather than it going around the body first. The liver also synthesizes blood-clotting substances such as FIBRINOGEN and prothrombin and the anti-coagulant HEPARIN; it breaks down red blood cells at the end of their life and processes the haemoglobin for iron, which is stored; vitamin A is synthesized and stored and it also stores vitamins B_{12}, D, E and K. In the embryo it forms red blood cells. Such is the chemical and biochemical activity of the liver that significant heat energy is generated and this organ is a major contributor of heat to the body.

LOBE certain organs are divided by fissures into large divisions which are called lobes, e.g. the brain, liver and lungs.

LOBECTOMY the removal of a lobe of an organ e.g. lung or brain. A lobe of a lung may be removed for cancer or other disease.

LOBULE a small lobe. Also a division of an organ that is smaller than a lobe, e.g. the lobules of the liver.

LOCKJAW see TETANUS.

LOCOMOTOR ATAXIA an unsteady gait which is one symptom of TABES DORSALIS, a form of SYPHILIS. The organism destroys sensory nerves producing further symptoms such as pains in the legs and body, loss of bladder control and blurred vision due to optic nerve damage.

LOIN that area of the back between the lower ribs and pelvis.

LUMBAGO pain of any sort in the lower back. It can be muscular, skeletal or neurological in origin. A severe and sudden case may be due to a strained muscle or slipped disc and the latter is usually the cause of lumbago with SCIATICA.

LUMBAR a general term for anything relating to the LOINS, e.g. lumbar vertebrae.

LUMBAR PUNCTURE the procedure whereby a hollow needle is inserted into the spinal canal in the lumbar region (usually between the 3rd and 4th lumbar vertebrae) to obtain a sample of cerebro-spinal fluid. The fluid is used in diagnosis of diseases of the nervous system, or to introduce drugs, anaesthetics, etc.

LUMBAR VERTEBRAE numbering five, the lumbar vertebrae are between the SACRUM and the thoracic vertebrae at the lowest part of the back. These vertebrae are not fused and have strong attachments points (processes) for the muscles of the lower back.

LUMPECTOMY the surgical removal of a tumour with the tissue immediately around it but leaving intact the bulk of the tissue and the lymph nodes. This applies particularly to breast cancer when the procedure is often followed by radio-therapy and is undertaken for patients with a small tumour (less than 2cm) and no metastases (see METASTASIS) to nearby lymph nodes or organs elsewhere in the body.

LUNGS the sac-like, paired organs of respiration situated with their base on the DIAPHRAGM and the top projecting into the neck. Each lung consists of fibrous, elastic sacs that are convoluted to provide a large surface area for gaseous exchange. Air enters the body through the windpipe or TRACHEA which branches into two bronchi (see BRONCHUS), one to each lung. Further branching then occurs, into numerous BRONCHIOLES. The bronchioles divide further and then end in alveoli (see ALVEOLUS) which are tiny sac-like structures where the gaseous exchange occurs. The exchange of oxygen and carbon dioxide occurs between the many blood capillaries on one side of the membrane and the air on the other. The lungs are served by the pulmonary arteries and pulmonary veins.
The *total lung capacity* of an adult male is five to six litres although only about half a litre (500ml) is exchanged in normal breathing (called the *tidal volume*).

LYME DISEASE an arthritic disease with rashes, fever and possibly carditis inflammation of the heart) and ENCEPHALITIS. It is caused by a spirochaete a type of BACTERIUM) that is transmitted by tick bite. Symptoms may not appear until some time after the bite but antibiotics can be used in treatment.

LYMPH a colourless, watery fluid that surrounds the body tissues and circulates in the lymphatic system. It is derived from blood and is similar to plasma comprising 95% water, with protein, sugar, salts and LYMPHOCYTES. The lymph is circulated by muscular action and it passes through LYMPH NODES which act as filters, and is eventually returned to the blood via the thoracic duct (one of the two main vessels of the lymphatic system).

LYMPHADENECTOMY removal of LYMPH NODES when, for example, a node has become cancerous due to it draining the area around an organ with a malignancy.

LYMPHADENITIS inflammation of the LYMPH NODES which become enlarged, hard and tender. The neck lymph nodes are commonly affected in association with another inflammatory condition.

LYMPHADENOMA see HODGKIN'S DISEASE.

LYMPHANGIOGRAPHY the technique of injecting a radio-opaque substance into the lymphatic system to render it visible on an X-ray, used primarily in investigating the spread of cancer.

LYMPHATIC GLAND see GLAND.

LYMPHATICS (or LYMPHATIC SYSTEM) the network of vessels, valves, nodes etc. that carry lymph from the tissues to the bloodstream and help maintain the internal fluid environment of the body. Lymph drains into capillaries and larger vessels, passing through nodes and going eventually into two large vessels the thoracic duct and right lymphatic duct) which return it to the bloodstream by means of the innominate veins.

LYMPH NODE small oval structures that occur at various points in the LYMPHATICS. They are found grouped in several parts of the body, including the neck, groin and armpit and their main functions are to remove foreign particles and produce LYMPHOCYTES, important in the IMMUNE response.

LYMPHOCYTE a type of white blood cell (LEUCOCYTE) produced in the bone marrow and also present in the SPLEEN, THYMUS GLAND and lymph nodes, which forms a vital component of the immune system. There are two types: B cells and T cells. B cells produce antibodies and search out and bind with particular antigens. T cells circulate through the thymus gland where they differentiate. When they contact an antigen, large numbers of T cells are generated which secrete chemical compounds to assist the B cells in destroying, e.g. bacteria.

LYMPHOCYTOSIS when the blood contains an increased number of lymphocytes as during many diseases or lymphocytic LEUKAEMIA.

LYMPHOEDEMA the build-up of LYMPH in soft tissues causing swelling. It may be due to obstruction of the vessels by parasites, tumour or inflammation. A secondary form of lymphoedema may occur after removal of lymph vessels in surgery, or by blocking. The condition occurs most in the legs and treatment comprises use of elastic bandages and DIURETIC drugs.

LYMPHOGRAPHY see LYMPHANGIOGRAPHY.

LYMPHOID TISSUE tissues that are involved in the formation of lymph, lymphocytes and antibodies such as the spleen, thymus and lymph nodes.

LYMPHOMA a tumour, usually malignant, of the lymph nodes. Often several lymph nodes become enlarged and subsequent symptoms include fever, anaemia, weakness and weight loss. If much of the lymphoid tissue is involved, there may be enlargement of the liver and spleen. Life expectancy is often very low although treatment with drugs often produces a marked response. Radiotherapy may be used for localized varieties (*see also* HODGKIN'S DISEASE).

LYMPHOSARCOMA a tumour of the lymphatics resulting in enlargement of the glands, spleen and liver. In general an older term applied to lymphomas other than HODGKIN'S DISEASE.

LYSIS the destruction of cells by antibodies called *lysins*, thus haemolysis is the break-up of red blood cells by haemolysin. Also, more generally, the destruction of cells or tissues due to breakdown of the cell membranes.

LYSOZYME an enzyme present in tears, nasal secretions and on the skin that has an antibacterial action (by breaking the cell wall of the bacterium). Lysozyme also occurs in egg white.

MACROCEPHALY an abnormal enlargement of the head when compared with the rest of the body, *see* MICROCEPHALY, HYDROCEPHALUS.

MACROCYTE a red blood cell (erythrocyte) which is abnormally large. Macrocytes are characteristic of PERNICIOUS ANAEMIA.

MACROCYTOSIS the condition in which abnormally large red blood cells (erythrocytes) are present in the blood. It is characteristic of macrocytic anaemias such as those caused by the deficiency of vitamin B_{12} (*see* CYANOCOBALAMIN and PERNICIOUS ANAEMIA) and folic acid. Macrocytes are also produced in those anaemias in which there is an increased rate of production of erythrocytes.

MACROPHAGE a large scavenger cell (PHAGOCYTE), numbers of which are found in various tissues and organs including the LIVER, SPLEEN, BONE MARROW, LYMPH NODES, CONNECTIVE TISSUE and the *microglia* of the CENTRAL

NERVOUS SYSTEM. They remove foreign bodies such as bacteria from blood and tissues. *Fixed macrophages* remain in one place in the connective tissue, *free microphages* are able to migrate between cells and gather at sites of infection to remove bacteria and other foreign material.

MACULA a small area or spot of tissue that is distinct from the surrounding region e.g. the *yellow spot* in the retina of the eye.

MACULES spots of small pigmented areas in the skin which may be thickened. They appear as a result of pregnancy, sunburn, eczema, psoriasis and may be symptomatic of other diseases such as syphilis and those affecting internal organs.

MALABSORPTION SYNDROME a group of diseases in which there is a reduction in the normal absorption of digested food materials in the small intestine. The food materials involved are commonly fats, vitamins, minerals, amino acids and iron. The diseases include COELIAC DISEASE, PANCREATITIS, CYSTIC FIBROSIS, sprue and STAGNANT LOOP SYNDROME and also surgical removal of a part of the small intestine.

MALARIA an infectious disease caused by the presence of minute parasitic organisms of the genus *Plasmodium* in the blood. The disease is characterized by recurrent bouts of fever and anaemia, the interval between the attacks depending upon the species . The parasite is transmitted to man by the *Anopheles* mosquito, (common in sub-tropical and tropical regions) being present in the salivary glands and passed into the bloodstream of a person when the insect bites. Similarly, the parasite is ingested by the mosquito when it takes a blood meal from an infected person. Efforts to control malaria have centred on destruction of the mosquito and its breeding sites. Once injected into the blood, the organisms concentrate in the liver where they multiply and then re-enter the bloodstream destroying red blood cells. This releases the parasites causing shivering, fever, sweating and anaemia. The process is then repeated, with hours or days between attacks. Drugs are used both to prevent infection, although these may not be totally effective, and to cure the disease once present.

MALIGNANT a term used in several ways but commonly referring to a tumour that proliferates rapidly and destroys surrounding healthy tissue, and which can spread via the lymphatic and blood system to other parts of the body. The term is also applied to a more serious form of a disease than the usual one which is life-threatening such as *malignant smallpox* and malignant HYPERTENSION.

MALPOSITION (*and* **MALPRESEN-TATION)** the situation in which the head of an unborn baby before and near delivery is not in the usual (occipitoanterior) position. In *malposition* the baby is head down but a wider part of the skull is presented to the pelvic opening due to the angle of the head. In *malpresentation* the baby is not head down. Both these conditions prolong and complicate labour and, in the latter case especially, are likely to require delivery by CAESARIAN SECTION.

MAMMARY GLAND a gland present in the female breast which produces milk after childbirth.

MAMMOGRAPHY a special X-ray technique used to determine the structure of the breast and useful in the early detection of tumours and in distinguishing between benign and malignant tumours.

MAMMOPLASTY plastic surgery of the breasts to decrease or increase size and other shape.

MANIA a form of mental illness characterized by great excitement and euphoria which then gives way to irritability as in MANIC DEPRESSIVE PSYCHOSIS.

MANIC DEPRESSIVE PSYCHOSIS a form of severe mental illness in which there are alternating bouts of MANIA and great depression. During the manic phase, the person may be incoherent in thought and speech and outrageous and sometimes violent in behaviour. Drug treatment is required for both phases of the illness and there seems to be an inherited tendency towards acquiring it. Drugs are also helpful in reducing the frequency of attacks between which the person is normally quite well.

MANTOUX TEST a test for the presence of a measure of immunity to tuberculosis. A protein called *tuberculin*, extracted from the tubercle bacilli (bacteria) is injected in a small quantity beneath the skin of the forearm. If an inflamed patch appears within 18 to 24 hours it indicates that a measure of immunity is present and that the person has been exposed to tuberculosis. The size of the reaction indicates the severity of the original tuberculosis infection although it does not mean that the person is actively suffering from the disease at that time.

MASTALGIA pain in the breast.

MAST CELL a large cell, many of which are found in loose connective tissue. The cytoplasm contains numerous granules with chemicals important in the body including histamine, serotonin, heparin and the antibody immunoglobulin E. All are important in allergic and inflammatory responses.

MASTECTOMY surgical removal of the breast usually performed because of the presence of a tumour. Mastectomy may be *simple* leaving the skin (and possibly the nipple) so that an artificial breast (prosthesis) can be inserted. Or it may be *radical* in which case the whole breast, pectoral muscles and lymph nodes beneath the armpit are all removed, generally performed because a cancer has spread.

MASTICATION chewing of food in the mouth, the first stage in the digestive process.

MASTITIS inflammation of the breast

usually caused by bacterial infection during breast feeding, the organisms responsible gaining access through cracked nipples. *Cystic mastitis* does not involve inflammation, but the presence of cysts (thought to be caused by hormonal factors), causes the breast(s) to be lumpy.

MASTOIDECTOMY surgical removal of the inflamed cells in the MASTOID PROCESS of the temporal bone of the skull, which is situated behind the ear, when these have become infected. *See* MASTOIDITIS.

MASTOIDITIS inflammation of the mastoid cells and mastoid antrum usually caused by bacterial infection which spreads from the middle ear. Treatment is by means of antibiotic drugs and sometimes surgery. *See* MASTOID PROCESS and MASTOIDECTOMY.

MASTOID PROCESS a *breast-like* projection of the temporal bone of the skull which contains numerous air spaces (mastoid cells) and is situated behind the ear. It provides a point of attachment for some of the neck muscles and communicates with the middle ear through an air-filled channel called the *mastoid antrum*. *See* MASTOIDITIS.

MEASLES an extremely infectious disease of children caused by a virus and characterized by the presence of a rash. It occurs in epidemics every two or three years. After an incubation period of 10 to 15 days the initial symptoms are those of a cold with coughing, sneezing and high fever. It is at this stage that the disease is most infectious and spreads from one child to another in airborne droplets before measles has been diagnosed. This is the main factor responsible for the epidemic nature of the disease. Small red spots with a white centre (known as *Koplik spots*) may appear in the mouth on the inside of the cheeks. Then a characteristic rash develops on the skin, spreading from behind the ears and across the face and also affecting other areas. The small red spots may be grouped together in patches and the child's fever is usually at its height while these are developing. The spots and fever gradually decline and no marks are left upon the skin, most children making a good recovery. However, complications can occur, particularly pneumonia and middle ear infections, which can result in deafness. A vaccine now available has reduced the incidence and severity of measles in the United Kingdom.

MEATUS a passage or opening, e.g. the *external auditory meatus* linking the *pinna* of the outer ear to the eardrum.

MEDIA the middle layer of a tissue or organ. Usually it is applied to the middle layer of the wall of a vein or artery comprising alternating sheaths of smooth muscle and elastic fibres.

MEDIASTINUM the space in the chest cavity between the two lungs which contains the heart, aorta, oesophagus, trachea, thymus gland and phrenic nerves.

MEDICATION any substance introduced into or on the body for the purposes of medical treatment, e.g. drugs and medicated dressings.

MEDULLA refers to the inner portion of a tissue or organ when there are two distinct parts. Examples include the adrenal medulla and the medulla of the kidneys. *Compare* CORTEX.

MEDULLA OBLONGATA the lowest part of the brain stem which extends through the FORAMEN *magnum* to become the upper part of the spinal cord. It contains important centres which govern respiration, circulation, swallowing and salivation.

MEGALOBLAST an abnormally large form of any of the cells that go on to produce erythrocytes (red blood cells). In certain forms of anaemia (megaloblastic anaemias) they are found in the bone marrow and their presence is due to a deficiency of vitamin B_{12} or of folic acid. They indicate a failure in the maturation process of erythrocytes which results in anaemia.

MEGALOBLASTIC ANAEMIA a blood disorder in which there are a large number of large but immature red blood cells. It is usually found when there is a vitamin B_{12} deficiency or PERNICIOUS ANAEMIA.

MEGALOMANIA a form of insanity in which a person suffers from delusions of grandeur about his or her greatness and power. It can accompany certain mental illnesses such as schizophrenia.

MEIOSIS a type of cell division which occurs in the maturation process of the gametes (sperm and ova) so that the sex cells eventually contain only half the number of chromosomes of the parent cells from which they are derived. The daughter cells also have genetic variation from the parent cell, brought about by a process known as "crossing over" which occurs during meiosis. When sperm and ovum fuse at fertilization, the full chromosome number is restored in a unique combination in the embryo. There are two phases of division in meiosis each of which is divided into four stages namely *prophase, metaphase, anaphase* and *telophase.*

MELANIN a dark brown pigment found in the skin and hair and also in the choroid layer of the eye. Melanin is contained and produced within cells known as *melanocytes* in the dermis layer of the skin. When the skin is exposed to hot sunshine, more melanin is produced giving a "suntan." In dark-skinned races more melanin is produced by greater activity of the melanocytes and it helps to protect the skin from harmful ultra violet radiation.

MELANOMA an extremely malignant tumour of the melanocytes, the cells in the skin which produce melanin. Melanomas are also found, although less commonly, in the mucous membranes and in the eye. There is a link between the occurrence of melanoma of the skin and exposure to harmful ultra violet light during sunbathing. A highly malignant form can also arise from the pigmented cells of moles. Melanoma can be successfully treated by surgery if it is superficial and caught at an early stage. However, it commonly spreads, especially to the liver and lymph nodes, in which case the outlook is poor. The incidence of malignant melanoma is increasing and has attracted much attention in connection with the formation of holes in the ozone layer, which screens the earth from harmful UV radiation. Most experts recommend that people should cover exposed skin, use sunscreen creams and avoid the sun at the hottest part of the day .

MEMBRANE a thin composite layer of lipoprotein surrounding an individual cell or a thin layer of tissue surrounding an organ, lining a cavity or tube or separating tissues and organs within the body.

MENIÈRE'S DISEASE a disease first described by the Frenchman, Prosper Menière in 1861, which affects the inner ear causing deafness and TINNITUS (ringing in the ears), vertigo, vomiting and sweating. The disease is most common in middle-aged men, with severe attacks of vertigo followed by vomiting. The time interval between attacks varies from one week to several months, but the deafness gradually becomes more pronounced. The symptoms are caused by an over-accumulation of fluid in the labyrinths of the inner ears, but the reason for this is not known. Treatment is by a variety of drugs and surgery, neither of which are completely successful.

MENINGES the three connective tissue membranes which surround the spinal cord and brain. The outermost layer (meninx) is called the *dura mater* which is fibrous, tough and inelastic, and also called the *pachymeninx,* closely lining the inside of the skull and helping to protect the brain. It is thicker than the middle layer, the *arachnoid mater,* which surrounds the brain. The innermost layer, the *pia mater*, is thin and delicate and lines the brain. Cerebrospinal fluid circulates between it and the arachnoid mater and both these inner layers are richly supplied with blood vessels which supply the surface of the brain and skull. These two inner membranes are sometimes collectively called the *pia-arachnoid* or *leptomeninges*.

MENINGIOMA a slow-growing tumour affecting the MENINGES of the brain or spinal cord which exerts pressure on the underlying nervous tissue. It may cause paraplegia if present in the spinal cord or other losses of sensation. In the brain it causes increasing neurological disability. A meningioma can be present for many years without being detected. The usual treatment is surgical removal if the tumour is accessible. Malignant meningiomas, known as *meningeal sarcomas*, can invade surrounding tissues. These are treated by means of surgery and also radiotherapy.

MENINGITIS inflammation of the meninges (membranes) of the brain (*cerebral meningitis*) or spinal cord (*spinal meningitis*) or the disease may affect both regions. Meningitis may affect the *dura mater* membrane in which case it is known as *pachymeningitis*, although this is relatively uncommon. It often results as a secondary infection due to the presence of disease elsewhere, as in the case of *tuberculous meningitis* and *syphilitic meningitis*. Meningitis which affects the other two membranes, (the *pia-arachnoid* membranes) is known as *leptomeningitis* and this is more common and may be either a primary or secondary infection. Meningitis is also classified according to its causal organism and may be either viral or bacterial. *Viral meningitis* is fairly mild and as it does not respond to drugs, treatment is by means of bed rest until recovery takes place. *Bacterial meningitis* is much more common and is caused by the organisms responsible for

tuberculosis, pneumonia and syphilis. Also, the *meningococcus* type of bacteria causes one of the commonest forms of the disease, *meningococcal meningitis*. The symptoms are a severe headache, sensitivity to light and sound, muscle rigidity especially affecting the neck, KERNIG'S SIGN, vomiting, paralysis, coma and death. These are caused by inflammation of the meninges and by a rise in INTRACRANIAL PRESSURE. One of the features of meningitis is that there is a change in the constituents and appearance of the cerebrospinal fluid, and the infective organism can usually be isolated from it and identified. The onset of the symptoms can be very rapid and death can also follow swiftly. Treatment is by means of antibiotic drugs and sulphonamides.

MENOPAUSE also known as the climacteric this is the time in a woman's life when the ovaries no longer release an egg cell every month and ceases. The woman is normally no longer able to bear a child and the age at which the menopause occurs is usually between 45 to 55. The menopause may be marked by a gradual decline in menstruation or in its frequency, or it may cease abruptly. There is a disturbance in the balance of sex hormones and this causes a number of physical symptoms including palpitations, hot flushes, sweats, vaginal dryness, loss of libido and depression. In the long term, there is a gradual loss of bone (OSTEOPOROSIS) in post-menopausal women which leads to greater risk of fractures, especially of the femur in the elderly. All these symptoms are relieved by HORMONE REPLACEMENT THERAPY involving oestrogen and progesterone which is now generally recognized to be of great benefit.

MENORRHAGIA when menstruation is unusally long or heavy which may result in anaemia.

MENSTRUAL CYCLE AND MENSTRUATION the cyclical nature of the reproductive life of a sexually mature female. One OVUM develops and matures within a GRAAFIAN FOLLICLE in one of the ovaries. When mature, the follicle ruptures to release the egg which passes down the FALLOPIAN TUBE to the uterus. The ruptured follicle becomes a temporary ENDOCRINE GLAND called the CORPUS LUTEUM which secretes the HORMONE, PROGESTERONE. Under the influence of progesterone the uterus wall (ENDOMETRIUM), thickens and its blood supply increases in readiness for the implantation of a fertilized egg. If the egg is not fertilized and there is no pregnancy, the thickened endometrium is shed along with a flow of blood through the vagina (menstruation). The usual age at which menstruation starts is 12 to 15 but it can be as early as 10, or as late as 20. The duration varies and can be anything from 2 to 8 days, the whole cycle usually occupying about 29 to 30 days.

MERCAPTOPURINE a type of ANTIMETABOLITE, CYTOTOXIC drug which prevents the proliferation of malignant cancer cells and is used in the treatment of certain kinds of LEUKAEMIA, and Crohn's disease (a disease of the digestive tract).

MESENCEPHALON otherwise known as the mid-brain which connects the PONS and CEREBELLUM with the *cerebral hemispheres.*

MESENTERY a double layer of the peritoneal membrane (PERITONEUM) which is attached to the back wall of the abdomen. It supports a number of abdominal organs including the stomach, small intestine, spleen and pancreas and contains associated nerves, lymph and blood vessels.

MESOTHELIOMA a malignant tumour of the PLEURA of the chest cavity and also of the PERICARDIUM or PERITONEUM. It is usually associated with exposure to asbestos dust but may arise independently with no known cause. Most mesotheliomas are in sites which render them inoperable, and chemotherapy and radiotherapy are used but often with limited success.

METABOLISM the sum of all the physical and chemical changes within cells and tissues that maintain life and growth. The breakdown processes which occur are known as *catabolic* (*catabolism*), and those which build materials up are called *anabolic* (*anabolism*). The term may also be applied to describe one particular set of changes e.g. *protein metabolism*. *Basal metabolism* is the minimum amount of energy required to maintain the body's vital processes e.g. heartbeat and respiration and is usually assessed by means of various measurements taken while a person is at rest.

METACARPAL BONE one of the five bones of the middle of the hand between the phalanges of the fingers and the CARPAL bones of the wrist forming the *metacarpus*. The heads of the metacarpal bones form the knuckles, *see* HAND.

METAPLASIA an abnormal change which has taken place within a tissue e.g. *myeloid metaplasia* where elements of bone marrow develop within the spleen and liver. Also *squamous metaplasia* which involves a change in the EPITHELIUM lining the BRONCHI of the lungs.

METASTASIS the process by which a malignant tumour spreads to a distant part of the body, and also refers to the secondary growth that results from this. The spread is accomplished by means of three routes, the blood circulation, lymphatic system and across body cavities.

METATARSAL BONE one of the five bones in the foot lying between the toes and the TARSAL bones of the ankle, together forming the *metatarsus*. The metatarsal bones are equivalent to the METACARPAL BONES in the hand.

METHYLDOPA a drug that is used to reduce high blood pressure especially in pregnancy.

METRITIS inflammation of the womb.

MHC major histocompatibility complex - a group of genes located on chromosome 6 which code for the HLA ANTIGENS.

MICROCEPHALY the condition in which there is abnormal smallness of the head compared to the rest of the body, *see* MACROCEPHALY.

MICROSURGERY surgery performed with the aid of an operating microscope using high precision miniaturized instruments. It is routine for some operations on the eye, larynx and ear and increasingly in areas inaccessible to normal surgery e.g. parts of the brain and spinal cord. Microsurgery is also performed in the re-joining of severed limbs, fingers, toes etc. where very fine suturing of minute blood vessels and nerves is required.

MICROWAVE THERAPY the use of very short wavelength electromagnetic waves in the procedure known as diathermy.

MICTURITION the act of urination.

MIDDLE EAR *see* EAR.

MIDWIFERY the profession devoted to the care of mothers during pregnancy and childbirth and of mothers and babies during the period after delivery. A member of the profession is known as a *midwife*.

MIGRAINE a very severe throbbing headache, usually on one side of the head, which is often accompanied by disturbances in vision, nausea and vomiting. Migraine is a common condition and seems to be triggered by any one or several of a number of factors. These include anxiety, fatigue, watching television or video screens, loud noises, flickering lights (e.g. strobe lights) and certain foods such as cheese and chocolate or alcoholic drinks. The cause is unknown but thought to involve constriction followed by dilation of blood vessels in the brain and an outpouring of fluid into surrounding tissues. The attack can last up to 24 hours and treatment is by means of bed rest in a darkened, quiet room and pain-relieving drugs.

MISCARRIAGE *see* ABORTION.

MITOBRONITOL a type of drug used in the treatment of leukaemia which prevents the growth of cancer cells.

MITOCHONDRION a tiny rod-like structure, numbers of which are present in the CYTOPLASM of every CELL. *Mitochondria* contain enzymes and ATP involved in cell METABOLISM.

MITOSIS the type of cell division undergone by most body cells by means of which growth and repair of tissues can take place. Mitosis involves the division of a single cell to produce two genetically identical daughter cells each with the full number of chromosomes, *compare* MEIOSIS.

MITRAL INCOMPETENCE also known as *mitral regurgitation*, this is the condition in which the MITRAL VALVE of the heart is defective and allows blood to leak back from the left ventricle into the left atrium. It is often caused by rheumatic fever, as a congenital defect or as a result of a heart attack. The left ventricle is forced to work harder and enlarges, but eventually may be unable to cope and this can result in left-sided heart failure. Other symptoms include atrial FIBRILLATION, breathlessness and embolism. Drug treatment and/or surgery to replace the defective valve may be required (*mitral prosthesis, see* MITRAL STENOSIS *and* HEART.

MITRAL STENOSIS the condition in which the opening between the left atrium and left ventricle is narrowed due to scarring and adhesion of the MITRAL VALVE. This scarring is often caused by rheumatic fever and the symptoms are similar to those of MITRAL INCOMPETENCE, accompanied also by a *diastolic murmur*. It is treated surgically by widening the stenosis (mitral VALVOTOMY) or by valve replacement - *mitral prosthesis*.

MITRAL VALVE formerly known as the *bicuspid valve*, this is located between the atrium and ventricle of the left side of the heart attached to the walls at the opening between the two. It has two cusps or flaps and normally allows blood to pass into the ventricle from the atrium, but prevents any back flow.

MMR VACCINE a recently-introduced vaccine (1988) which protects against MEASLES, MUMPS and RUBELLA (German measles) and is normally given to children during their second year.

MOLE a dark-coloured pigmented spot in the skin which is usually brown. It may be flat or raised and may have hair protruding from it. Some types can become malignant, see MELANOMA.

MONOCYTE the largest type of white blood cell (leucocyte) with a kidney-shaped nucleus found in the blood and lymph. It ingests foreign bodies such as bacteria and tissue particles.

MONONUCLEOSIS see GLANDU-LAR FEVER.

MONOZYGOTIC TWINS also known as *identical twins*, these are children who are derived from a single fertilized egg.

MORBIDITY the state of being diseased, the *morbidity rate* being expressed as the number of cases of a disease occurring within a particular number of the population.

MORIBUND dying.

MORNING SICKNESS vomiting and nausea, most common during the first three months of pregnancy.

MORPHINE a narcotic and very strong analgesic drug which is an alkaloid derived from opium. It is used for the relief of severe pain but tolerance and dependence may occur, see ADDICTION.

MOTOR NERVE a nerve containing motor neurone fibres which carries electrical impulses outwards from the central nervous system to a muscle or gland to bring about a response there.

MOTOR NEURONE one of the units or fibres of a MOTOR NERVE. An *upper motor neurone* is contained entirely within the central nervous system having its cell body in the brain and its *axon* (a long process) extending into the spinal cord where it SYNAPSES with other neurones. A *lower motor neurone* has its cell body in the spinal cord or brain stem and an axon that runs outwards via a spinal or cranial MOTOR NERVE to an effector muscle or gland, see NERVE.

MOTORNEURONE DISEASE a disease of unknown cause which most commonly occurs in middle age and is a degenerative condition affecting elements of the central nervous system (i.e. the corticospinal fibres, motor nuclei in the brain stem and the cells of the anterior horn of the spinal cord). It causes increasing paralysis involving nerves and muscles and is ultimately fatal.

MOUTH the opening which forms the beginning of the alimentary canal and in which food enters the digestive process. The entrance is guarded by the lips behind which lie the upper and lower sets of teeth embedded in the jaw. The roof of the mouth is called the palate, the front part being hard and immobile while behind lies the mobile soft palate. The tongue is situated behind the lower teeth and SALIVARY GLANDS which are present secrete saliva into the mouth through small ducts. Saliva contains the enzyme ptyalin which begins the breakdown of starch while the chewing action of the teeth and manipulation with the tongue reduces the food to a more manageable size so that it can be swallowed.

MUCOSA another term for MUCOUS MEMBRANE.

MUCOUS MEMBRANE a moist membrane which lines many tubes and cavities within the body and is lubricated with MUCUS. The structure of a mucous membrane varies according to its site and they are found, for example, lining the mouth, respiratory, urinary and digestive tracts. Each has a surface EPITHELIUM, a layer containing various cells and glands which secrete mucus. Beneath this lie connective tissue and muscle layers, the *laminae propria* and *muscularis mucosa* respectively, the whole forming a pliable layer.

MUCUS a slimy substance secreted by MUCOUS MEMBRANES as a lubricant, and composed mainly of glycoproteins of which the chief one is *mucin*. It is a clear viscous fluid which may contain enzymes and has a protective function. It is normally present in small amounts but the quantity increases if inflammation and/or infection is present.

MULTIPLE BIRTHS twins, triplets, quadruplets, quintuplets and sextuplets born to one mother. While naturally-occurring twins are relatively common, other multiple births are normally rare. Their incidence has increased with the advent of *fertility drugs* although often some of the infants do not survive.

MULTIPLE SCLEROSIS a disease of the brain and spinal cord which affects the MYELIN sheaths of nerves and disrupts their function. It usually affects people below the age of 40 and its cause is unknown, but is the subject of much research. The disease is characterized by the presence of patches of hardened (sclerotic) connective tissue irregularly scattered through the brain and spinal cord. At first the fatty part of the nerve sheaths breaks down and is absorbed, leaving bare nerve fibres, and then connective tissue is laid down. Symptoms depend upon the site of the patches in the central nervous system and the disease is characterized by periods of progression and remission. However, they include unsteady gait and apparent clumsiness, tremor of the limbs, involuntary eye movements, speech disorders, bladder disfunction and paralysis. The disease can progress very slowly but generally there is a tendency for the paralysis to become more marked.

MUMPS an infectious disease of childhood usually occurring in those between the ages of 5 to 15, and caused by a virus which produces inflammation of the *parotid salivary glands*. The incubation period is two to three weeks followed by symptoms including feverishness, headache, sore throat and vomiting, before or along with a swelling of the parotid gland on one side of the face. The swelling may be confined to one side or spread to the other side of the face and also may go on to include the *submaxillary* and *sublingual salivary glands* beneath the jaw. Generally after a few days the swelling subsides and the child recovers but remains infectious until the glands have returned to normal. The infection may spread to the pancreas and, in 15 to 30% of males, to the testicles. In adult men this infection can cause sterility. More rarely, inflammation in females can affect the ovaries and breasts, and MENINGITIS is another occasional complication, especially in adults. A protective vaccine is now available, see MMR.

MUNCHAUSEN'S SYNDROME a rare mental disorder in which a person tries to obtain hospital treatment for a non-existent illness. The person is adept at simulating symptoms and may self-induce these or cause self-inflicted injury to add authenticity. The person may end up having unnecessary treatment and operations and is resistant to psychotherapy.

MURMUR a characteristic sound which can be heard using a STETHOSCOPE, caused by uneven blood flow through the heart or blood vessels when these are diseased or damaged. Heart murmurs can also be present in normal individuals, especially children, without indicating disease. Murmurs are classified as *diastolic* (when the ventricles are relaxed and filling with blood) or *systolic*, when they are contracting.

MUSCLE the contractile tissue of the body which produces movements of various structures both internally and externally. There are three types of muscle: 1. *striated* or *voluntary muscle* which has a striped appearance when viewed under a microscope and is attached to the skeleton. It is called "voluntary" because it is under the control of the will and produces movements, for example, in the limbs. 2. *smooth* or *involuntary muscle* which has a plain appearance when viewed microscopically and is not under conscious control but is supplied by the autonomic nervous system. Examples are the muscles which supply the digestive and respiratory tracts. 3. *cardiac muscle*, the specialized muscle of the walls of the heart which is composed of a network of branching, elongated fibres which rejoin and interlock, each having a nucleus. It has a somewhat striated appearance and where there are junctions between fibres, irregular transverse bands occur known as *intercalated discs*. This muscle is involuntary and contracts and expands rhythmically throughout a person's life. However, rate of heart beat is affected by activity within the vagus nerve.

MUSCLE CRAMP *see* CRAMP.

MUSCLE RELAXANTS substances or drugs which cause muscles to relax. They are mainly used in anaesthesia to produce relaxation or paralysis of muscles while surgery is being carried out, e.g. tubocurarine and gallamine. Others are administered to counteract muscular spasms, which are a feature of spastic conditions such as PARKINSONISM, e.g. diazepam.

MUSCULAR DYSTROPHY also known as *myopathy*, this is any of a group of diseases which involve wasting of muscles and in which an hereditary factor is involved. The disease is classified according to the groups of muscles which it affects and the age of the person involved. The disease usually appears in childhood and causes muscle fibres to degenerate and to be replaced by fatty and fibrous tissue. The affected muscles eventually lose all power of contraction causing great disability and affected children are prone to chest and other infections which may prove fatal in their weakened state. The cause of the disease is not entirely understood but the commonest form, *Duchenne muscular dystrophy*, is sex-linked and recessive. Hence it nearly always affects boys, with the mother as a carrier, and appears in

very early childhood, *see also* SEX-LINKED DISORDERS.

MUTAGEN any substance or agent which increases the rate of mutation in body cells, examples being various chemicals, viruses and radiation. Mutagens increase the number rather than the range of mutations beyond that which might be expected.

MUTATION a change which takes place in the DNA, (the genetic material) of the CHROMOSOMES of a cell which is normally a rare event. The change may involve the structure or number of whole chromosomes or take place at one GENE site. Mutations are caused by faulty replication of the cell's genetic material at cell division. If normal body (*somatic*) cells are involved there may be a growth of altered cells or a tumour, or these may be attacked and destroyed by the immune system. In any event, this type of mutation cannot be passed on - if the sex cells (ova or sperm) are involved in the mutation, the alteration may be passed on to the offspring producing a changed characteristic.

MUTISM the refusal or inability to speak which may result from brain damage or psychological factors. Speechlessness is most common in those who have been born deaf (deaf-mutism).

MYALGIA pain in a muscle.

MYALGIC ENCEPHALOMYELITIS (ME) a disorder characterized by muscular pain, fatigue, general depression and loss of memory and concentration. The cause is not understood, but seems to follow on from viral infections such as influenza, hence it is also called post-viral fatigue syndrome. Recovery may be prolonged and there is no specific treatment.

MYASTHENIA GRAVIS a serious and chronic condition of uncertain cause which may be an auto-immune disease. It is more common among young people, especially women (men tend to be affected over 40). Rest and avoidance of unnecessary exertion is essential to conserve muscle strength as there is a reduction in the ability of the neurotransmitter, ACETYLCHOLINE, to effect muscle contraction. There is a weakening which affects skeletal muscles and those for breathing and swallowing etc. However, there is little wasting of the muscles themselves. It seems the body produces antibodies which interfere with the acetylcholine receptors in the muscle, and that the THYMUS GLAND may be the original source of these receptors. Surgical removal of the thymus gland is one treatment. Other treatment is by means of drugs, e.g. Pyridodstigmine, which inhibit the activity of the enzyme *cholinesterase* which destroys excess acetylcholine. Other *immunosuppressive* drugs are used to suppress production of the antibodies which interfere with the receptors.

MYCOSIS any disease which is caused by fungi, e.g. thrush and ringworm.

MYELIN a sheath of phospholipid and protein that surrounds the axons of some NEURONS. It is formed by specialized cells known as *Schwann cells*, each of which encloses the axon in concentric folds of its cell membrane. Thesse folds then condense to form myelin, the neuron then being described as *myelinated*. Schwann cells produce myelin at regular intervals along the length of the axon and electrical impulses pass more rapidly along myelinated nerve fibres than along non-myelinated ones.

MYELITIS 1. any inflammatory condition of the spinal cord such as often occurs in MULTIPLE SCLEROSIS. 2. bone marrow inflammation, *see* OSTEOMYELITIS.

MYELOFIBROSIS a disease, the cause of which is unknown, in which FIBROSIS takes place within the bone marrow, and many immature red and white blood cells appear in the circulation because of the resultant anaemia. There is an enlargement of the SPLEEN, and blood-producing (myeloid) tissue is abnormally found both here and in the liver.

MYELOGRAPHY a specialized X-ray technique involving the injection of a radio-opaque dye into the central canal of the spinal cord in order to distinguish the presence of disease. The X-rays are called *myelograms*.

MYELOID means like or relating to bone marrow or, like a *myelocyte*. This is a cell which is an immature type of granulocyte responsible for the production of white blood cells.

MYELOMA a malignant disease of the bone marrow in which tumours are present in more than one bone at the same time. The bones may show "holes" when X-rayed due to typical deposits, and certain abnormal proteins may be present in the blood and urine. Treatment is by chemotherapy and radiotherapy. *Myelomatosis* is the production of myeloma which is usually fatal.

MYOCARDIAL INFARCTION *see* CORONARY THROMBOSIS.

MYOCARDITIS inflammation of the muscle in the wall of the heart.

MYOCARDIUM the middle of the three layers of the HEART wall which is the thick, muscular area. The outer layer is the *epicardium* (forming part of the *pericardium*) and the inner the *endocardium*.

MYOGLOBIN an iron-containing pigment which is similar to HAEMOGLOBIN, and occurs in muscle cells. It binds oxygen from haemoglobin and releases it in the muscle cells.

MYOMA a benign tumour in muscle, often in the WOMB.

MYOMECTOMY surgical removal of FIBROIDS from the muscular wall of the WOMB (UTERUS).

MYOMETRIUM the muscular tissue of the WOMB, composed of smooth muscle and surrounding the ENDOMETRIUM. Its contractions are influenced by the presence of certain hormones and are especially strong during LABOUR.

MYOPATHY *see* MUSCULAR DYSTROPHY.

MYOPIA short-sightedness corrected by wearing spectacles with concave lenses.

MYXOEDEMA a disease caused by under-activity of the thyroid gland (HYPOTHYROIDISM). There is a characteristic development of a dry, coarse skin and swelling of subcutaneous tissue. There is intellectual impairment with slow speech and mental dullness, lethargy, muscle pain, weight gain and constipation. The hair thins and there may be increased sensitivity to cold. As the symptoms are caused by the deficiency of thyroid hormones, treatment consists of giving THYROXINE in suitable amounts.

NAEVUS see BIRTHMARK.

NARCOSIS a state induced by narcotic drugs in which a person is completely unconscious or nearly so but can respond a little to stimuli. It is due to the depressant action of the drugs on the body.

NARCOTIC a drug that leads to a stupor and complete loss of awareness. In particular opiates derived from morphine or produced synthetically produce various conditions: deep sleep, euphoria, mood changes and mental confusion. In addition, respiration and the cough reflex are depressed and muscle spasms may be produced. Because of the dependence resulting from the use of morphine-like compounds, they have largely been replaced for sleeping drugs.

NASAL CAVITY one of two cavities in the nose, divided by a SEPTUM, which lie between the roof of the mouth and the floor of the cranium.

NASOGASTRIC TUBE a small diameter tube passed through the nose into the stomach for purposes of introducing food or drugs or removing fluid (ASPIRATION).

NAUSEA a feeling of being about to vomit. It may be due to motion sickness, early pregnancy, pain, food poisoning or a virus.

NEBULA a slight opacity or scar of the cornea that does not obstruct vision but may create a haziness. Also an oily substance that is applied in a fine spray.

NEBULIZER a device for producing a fine spray. Many inhaled drugs are administered in this way, and it is an effective method of delivering a concentrated form of medication e.g. bronchodilators.

NECROPSY an autopsy (post-mortem) which results in little disfigurement.

NECROSIS death of tissue in a localized area or organ, caused by disease, injury or loss of blood supply.

NEOMYCIN an antibiotic, usually applied as a cream and which is effective against a wide spectrum of bacteria. Its main use is as a skin treatment.

NEONATAL term meaning relating to the first 28 days of life.

NEOPLASM a new and abnormal growth of cells i.e. a tumour, which may be benign or malignant.

NEPHRECTOMY surgical removal of all (*radical*) or part of the kidney (*partial*). It may be necessary to remove a tumour (in which case the surrounding fat and adrenal gland will probably also be removed) or to drain an ABSCESS.

NEPHRITIS inflammation of the KIDNEY, which may be due to one of several causes. Types of nephritis include glomerulonephritis (when the glomerulus is affected), acute nephritis, hereditary nephritis, etc.

NEPHRON see KIDNEY.

NERVE a bundle of nerve fibres comprising NEURONS and glial (supporting) cells (see GLIA), all contained in a fibrous sheath, the perineurium. Motor nerves carry (efferent) impulses in motor neurons from the brain (or spinal cord) to muscles or glands and a sensory nerve carries (afferent) impulses in sensory neurons from sensory organs to the brain or spinal cord. Most large nerves are mixed nerves containing both motor and sensory nerves.

NERVE BLOCK (*or* **CONDUCTION ANAESTHESIA**) the technique of blocking sensory nerves sending pain impulses to the brain, thus creating anaesthesia in that part of the body. It is achieved by injecting the tissue around a nerve with local anaesthetic (e.g. LIGNOCAINE) to permit minor operations.

NERVE INJURY nerves may be injured by being severed, pressure may damage a nerve directly or push it against a bone. Damage to a sensory nerve results in a lack of or lessening in sensation, while paralysis of muscles will result from damage to the associated motor nerve.

NERVE IMPULSE the transmission of information along a nerve fibre by electrical activity which has its basis in the formation of chemical substances and the generation of the *action potential*. This is a change in electrical potential across the cell membrane (between inside and outside) of an axon (nerve cell) as an impulse moves along. It is a temporary and localized occurrence caused by a stimulus which travels down the axon and the voltage is caused by sodium ions (Na^+) entering the axon and changing the potential across the cell membrane from -65mV to +45mV (millivolts). When the stimulus has passed the membrane is restored to its resting potential. When a stimulus is continually received, several hundred pulses travel along the nerve per second.

NERVOUS SYSTEM the complete system of tissues and cells including NERVES, NEURONS, SYNAPSES and receptors (a special cell sensitive to a particular stimulus which then sends an impulse through the nervous system). The nervous system operates through the transmission of impulses (*see* NERVE IMPULSE) that are conducted rapidly to and from muscles, organs etc. It consists of the central nervous system (brain and spinal cord) and the peripheral nervous

system that includes the cranial and spinal nerves (*see* AUTONOMIC NERVOUS SYSTEM).

NEURALGIA strictly, pain in some part or the whole of a nerve (without any physical change in the nerve) but used more widely to encompass pain following the course of a nerve or its branches, whatever the cause. Neuralgia often occurs at the same time each day and is frequently an agonizing pain. It occurs in several forms and is named accordingly, e.g. SCIATICA, trigeminal neuralgia (affecting the face, *see* TRIGEMINAL NERVE) and intercostal neuralgia (affecting the ribs). Treatment often involves the application of ointments, and the taking of pain-killing drugs. If such treatments do not bring relief, it is possible to freeze the nerve or destroy part of it by surgery.

NEURITIS inflammation of a nerve or nerves which may be due to inflammation from nearby tissues, or a more general condition in which the nerve fibres degenerate. This latter condition (*polyneuritis*) is due to a systemic poison such as alcohol or long-term exposure to solvents such as naphtha.

NEUROENDOCRINE SYSTEM one of a number of dual control systems regulating bodily functions through the action of nerves and hormones.

NEUROGLIA the fine web of tissues that support nerve fibres (*see* GLIA).

NEUROHORMONE a hormone that is secreted by the nerve endings of specialized nerve cells (i.e. neurosecretory cells) and not by an endocrine gland. They are secreted into the bloodstream or directly into the target tissue. Included are NORADRENALINE and VASOPRESSIN (produced in the HYPOTHALAMUS and secreted by the pituitary gland-active in the control of water reabsorption in the kidneys).

NEUROLEPTIC any drug that induces neurolepsis, that is, reduced activity, some indifference to the surroundings and possibly sleep. They are used to quieten disturbed patients suffering from delirium, brain damage or behavioural disturbances.

NEUROLOGY the subdiscipline of medicine that involves the study of the brain, spinal cord and peripheral nerves, their diseases and conditions and the treatment of those conditions.

NEUROMUSCULAR BLOCKADE the blocking of impulses at the NEUROMUSCULAR JUNCTION to paralyse a part of the body for surgery (*see also* NERVE BLOCK).

NEUROMUSCULAR JUNCTION the area of membrane between a muscle cell and a motor NEURON forming a SYNAPSE between the two. Nerve impulses travel down the neuron and each releases ACETYLCHOLINE which depolarizes the enlarged end of the neuron (the motor end plate) slightly. These small depolarization are totalled until a threshold of -50mV is reached and this results in the production of an ACTION POTENTIAL that crosses the synapse into the muscle fibre producing a muscle contraction.

NEURON a nerve cell, vital in the transmission of impulses. Each cell has an enlarged portion (the cell body) from which extends the long, thin axon for carrying impulses away. Shorter, more numerous dendrites receive impulses. The transmission of impulses is faster in axons that are covered in a sheath of MYELIN.

NEUROPATHY any disease that affects the peripheral nerves, whether singly (mononeuropathy) or more generally (polyneuropathy). The symptoms depend upon the type and the nerves affected.

NEUROSIS (*plural* **NEUROSES**) a mental disorder, but one where the patient retains a grasp on reality (unlike PSYCHOSIS). Neuroses may be due to depression, phobia, hysteria or hypochondria. Anxiety is the commonest version, although this does respond to treatment. In practice, the boundary between neurosis and psychosis is vague.

NEUROSURGERY surgical treatment of the brain, spinal cord or nerves,

including dealing with head injuries, intracranial pressure, haemorrhages, infections and the treatment of tumours.

NEUROTIC someone afflicted with a neurosis. More generally a nervous person who acts on emotions more than reason.

NEUROTRANSMITTER one of several chemical substances released in minute quantities by axon tips into the SYNAPSE to enable a nerve impulse to cross. It diffuses across the space and may depolarize the opposite membrane allowing the production of an action potential (*see* NERVE IMPULSE). Outside the central nervous system ACETYLCHOLINE is a major neurotransmitter, and NORADRENALINE is released in the SYMPATHETIC NERVOUS SYSTEM. Acetylcholine and noradrenaline also operate within the central nervous system as does DOPAMINE, amongst others.

NEUTROPENIA a fall in the number of neutrophils (a type of granulocyte or white blood cell) in the blood resulting from bone marrow tumours, acute leukaemia, and other conditions.

NIFEDIPINE a drug used in the treatment of ANGINA and high blood pressure.

NIGHT BLINDNESS (NYCTALOPIA) poor vision in dim light or at night due to a deficiency within the cells responsible for such vision (*see* ROD). The cause may be a lack of VITAMIN A in the diet or a congenital defect.

NITROUS OXIDE formerly called laughing gas, a colourless gas used for anaesthesia over short periods. Longer effects require its use with oxygen and it may be used as a 'carrier' for stronger anaesthetics.

NON-STEROIDAL ANTI-INFLAM-MATORY DRUGS (*see* NSAID).

NORADRENALINE (norepinephrine in U.S.) a NEUROTRANSMITTER of the SYMPATHETIC NERVOUS SYSTEM secreted by nerve endings and also the adrenal glands. It is similar to ADRENALINE in structure and function. It increases blood pressure by constricting the vessel, slows the heartbeat, increases breathing both in rate and depth.

NOSE the olfactory organ and also a pathway for air entering the body, by which route it is warmed, filtered and moistened before passing into the lungs. The 'external' nose leads to the NASAL CAVITY which has a mucous membrane with olfactory cells.

NOTIFIABLE DISEASES diseases that must be reported to the health authorities to enable rapid control and monitoring to be undertaken. The list varies between countries but in the U.K. includes acute poliomyelitis, AIDS, cholera, dysentery, food poisoning, measles, meningitis, rabies, rubella, scarlet fever, smallpox, tetanus, typhoid fever, viral hepatitis and whooping cough.

NSAID (Non-Steroidal Anti-Inflammatory Drugs) a large group of drugs used to relieve pain, and also inhibit inflammation. They are used for conditions such as rheumatoid arthritis, sprains etc. and include aspirin. The main side-effect is gastric ulcer or haemorrhage but the synthesis of new compounds has led to some with milder side-effects.

NUCLEAR MAGNETIC RESONANCE an analytical technique based upon the absorption of electromagnetic radiation over specific frequencies for those nuclei that spin about their own axes. The result is a change in orientation of the nuclei and certain elements are particularly susceptible (hydrogen, fluorine and phosphorus). The technique has been developed into a medical imaging tool which can create an image of soft tissues in any part of the body.

NUCLEIC ACID a linear molecule that occurs in two forms: DNA (deoxyribonucleic acid) and RNA (ribonucleic acid), composed of four NUCLEOTIDES. DNA is the major part of CHROMOSOMES in the cell nucleus while RNA is found outside the nucleus and is involved in protein synthesis.

NUCLEOTIDE the basic molecular building block of the nucleic acids RNA and DNA. A nucleotide comprises a five-carbon sugar molecule with a phosphate group and an organic base. The organic base can be a *purine*, e.g. adenine and guanine or a *pyrimidine* e.g. cytosine and thymine as in DNA. In RNA uracil replaces thymine.

NUCLEUS the large organelle (a membrane-bounded cell constituent) that contains the DNA. Unless it is dividing a nucleolus with RNA is present. During cell division the DNA, which is normally dispersed with protein (as chromatin), forms visible CHROMOSOMES.

OBESITY the accumulation of excess fat in the body, mainly in the subcutaneous tissues, caused by eating more food than is necessary to produce the required energy for each day's activity. The effects of obesity are serious, being associated with increased mortality or cause of illness from cardio-vascular disease, diabetes, gall bladder complaints, hernia and many others. Treatment involves a low energy diet but more drastic measures (e.g. stapling of the stomach) may be necessary.

OBSTETRICS the subdiscipline of medicine that deals with pregnancy and childbirth and the period immediately after birth; midwifery.

OCCIPITAL BONE a bone of the SKULL which is shaped like a saucer and forms the back of the cranium and part of its base. Arising from the base of thin bone are two occipital condyles that articulate with the first cervical vertebrae (the atlas) of the spinal column.

OCCLUSION the closing or blocking of an organ or duct. In dentistry it is the way the teeth meet when the jaws are closed.

OCCULT a term meaning not easily

seen; not visible to the naked eye.

OCCUPATIONAL DISEASES (or industrial diseases) diseases, specific to a particular occupation, and to which workers in that occupation are prone. There are many lung conditions including: PNEUMOCONIOSIS (from coal mining); SILICOSIS (mining, stone dressing, etc.); ASBESTOSIS; FARMER'S LUNG (from fungal spores), and so on. In addition there are dangers from excessive noise, irritant chemicals, occupations resulting in musculo-skeletal disorders, decompression sickness (*see also* BENDS) radiation and infections from either animals or humans.

OCCUPATIONAL THERAPY the treatment of both psychiatric and physical conditions by encouraging patients to undertake activities to enable them use what skills they have and to achieve some independence and self-confidence. The activities may vary enormously from craft and woodwork to social and community activities.

OCULOMOTOR NERVE either of a pair of cranial nerves which are involved in eye movements including movement of the eyeball, and alterations in the size of the pupil and lens.

OEDEMA an accumulation of fluid in the body, possibly beneath the skin or in cavities or organs. With an injury the swelling may be localized or more general as in cases of kidney or heart failure. Fluid can collect in the chest cavity, abdomen or lung (PULMONARY OEDEMA). The causes are numerous, e.g. CIRRHOSIS of the liver, heart or kidney failure, starvation, acute NEPHRITIS, allergies or drugs. To alleviate the symptom, the root cause has to be removed. Subcutaneous oedema commonly occurs in women before menstruation, as swollen legs or ankles, but does subside if the legs are rested in a raised position.

OESOPHAGOSCOPE an instrument for inspecting the oesophagus. It has a light source and can be used to open the tube if narrowed, remove material for biopsy or remove an obstruction.

OESOPHAGUS the first part of the ALIMENTARY CANAL lying between the PHARYNX and stomach. The mucous membrane lining produces secretions to lubricate food as it passes and the movement of the food to the stomach is achieved by waves of muscular movement called *peristalsis*.

OESTRADIOL the major female sex hormone. It is produced by the ovary and is responsible for development of the breasts, sexual characteristics and premenstrual uterine changes.

OESTROGEN one of a group of STEROID hormones secreted mainly by the ovaries and to a lesser extent by the adrenal cortex and placenta. (The testes also produce small amounts). Oestrogens control the female secondary sexual characteristics, i.e. enlargement of the breasts, change in the profile of the pelvic girdle, pubic hair growth and deposition of body fat. High levels are produced at ovulation and with PROGESTERONE they regulate the female reproductive cycle. Naturally-occurring oestrogens include OESTRADIOL, oestriol and oestrone. Synthetic varieties are used in the contraceptive pill and to treat gynaeco-logical disorders.

OLFACTION the sense of smell, *see* NOSE.

OLFACTORY NERVE one of a pair of sensory nerves for smell. It is the first cranial nerve and comprises many fine threads connecting receptors in the mucous membrane of the olfactory area which pass through holes in the skull, fuse to form one fibre and then pass back to the brain.

ONCOGENE any GENE directly involved in cancer, whether in viruses or in the individual.

ONCOGENIC any factor that causes cancer. This may be an organism, a chemical or some environmental condition. Some viruses are oncogenic and have the result of making a normal cell become a cancer cell.

ONCOLOGY the subdiscipline of medicine concerned with the study and treatment of tumours, including medical, surgical aspects and their treatment with radiation.

OOCYTE a cell in the OVARY that undergoes MEIOSIS to produce an OVUM, the female reproductive cell. A newborn female already has primary oocytes, of which only a small number survive to puberty, and even then only a fraction will be ovulated (*see* OVULATION).

OPERCULUM a lid, plug or flap. A term used in several areas of medicine e.g. it is a plug of mucus blocking the cervix in a pregnant woman; it is also used in neurology and dentistry.

OPHTHALMOLOGY the branch of medicine dealing with the structure of the eye, its function, associated diseases and treatment.

OPHTHALMOPLEGIA paralysis of the muscles serving the EYE, which may be internal (affecting the iris and ciliary muscle) or external (those muscles moving the eye itself).

OPHTHALMOSCOPE an instrument, with a light source, used to examine the interior of the EYE. Some focus a fine beam of light into the eye and the point upon which it falls can be seen, while others form an image of the inside of the eye which can be studied.

OPIATE one of several drugs, derived from opium and including morphine and codeine. They act by depressing the central nervous system, thus relieving pain and suppressing coughing. Morphine and heroin, its synthetic derivative, are narcotics.

OPIUM a milky liquid extracted from the unripe seed capsules of the poppy, *Papaver somniferum* which has almost 10% of anhydrous morphine. Opium is a NARCOTIC and ANALGESIC.

OPPORTUNISTIC an infection that is contracted by someone with a lower resistance than usual. This may be due to

drugs or another disease such as DIABETES MELLITUS, cancer or AIDS. In normal circumstances, in a healthy person, the infecting organism would not cause the disease.

OPTIC ATROPHY a deterioration and wasting of the optic disc due to degeneration of fibres in the optic nerve. It may accompany numerous conditions including DIABETES, ARTERIOSCLEROSIS, GLAUCOMA or may be due to a congenital defect, inflammation or injury, or toxic poisoning from alcohol, lead, etc.

OPTIC CHIASMA (OPTIC COMMISSURE) the cross-shaped structure formed from a crossing over of the optic nerves running back from the eyeballs to meet beneath the brain in the midline.

ORCHIDECTOMY removal of one or both (castration) testes, usually to treat a malignant growth.

ORCHIDOPEXY the operation performed to bring an undescended testis into the scrotum. It is undertaken well before puberty to ensure normal development subsequently.

ORGAN any distinct and recognizable unit within the body that is composed of two or more types of tissue and that is responsible for a particular function or functions. Examples are the liver, kidney, heart and brain.

ORGASM the climax of sexual arousal which in men coincides with ejaculation and comprises a series of involuntary muscle contractions. In women there are irregular contractions of the vagina walls.

ORTHODONTICS a part of dentistry dealing with development of the teeth and the treatment of (or prevention of) any disorders.

ORTHOPAEDICS the subdiscipline of medicine concerned with the study of the skeletal system and the joints, muscles etc. It also covers the treatment of bone damage or disease whether CONGENITAL or acquired.

ORTHOPNOEA a severe difficulty in

breathing that is so bad that a patient cannot lie and has to sleep in a sitting position. It usually only occurs with serious conditions of the heart and lungs.

OSMOSIS the process whereby solvent molecules (usually water) move through a semi-permeable membrane to the more concentrated solution. Cell membranes function as semi-permeable membranes and osmosis is important in regulating water content in living systems.

OSSICLE the term for a small bone, often applied to those of the middle ear, the auditory ossicles (*see* EAR), that transmit sound to the inner ear from the eardrum.

OSSIFICATION (*or* **OSTEOGENE-SIS**) bone formation, which occurs in several stages via special cells called OSTEOBLASTS. COLLAGEN fibres form a network in connective tissue and then a cement of polysaccharide is laid down. Finally, calcium salts are distributed among the cement as tiny crystals. The osteoblasts are enclosed as bone cells (OSTEOCYTES).

OSTEITIS inflammation of bone, caused by damage, infection or bodily disorder. Symptoms include swelling, tenderness, a dull aching sort of pain and redness cover the affected area.

OSTEOARTHRITIS a form of ARTHRITIS involving joint cartilage with accompanying changes in the associated bone. It usually involves the loss of cartilage and the development of OSTEOPHYTES at the bone margins. The function of the joint (most often the thumb, knee and hip) is affected and it becomes painful. The condition may be due to overuse, and affects those past middle age. It also may complicate other joint diseases. Treatment usually involves administering ANALGESICS, possibly anti-inflammatory drugs and the use of corrective or replacement surgery.

OSTEOBLAST a specialized cell responsible for the formation of bone.

OSTEOCHONDRITIS inflammation of bone and cartilage.

OSTEOCHONDROSIS a disease affecting the OSSIFICATION centres of bone in children. It begins with degeneration and NECROSIS but it regenerates and calcifies again.

OSTEOCYTE a bone cell formed from an osteoblast that is no longer active and has become embedded in the matrix of the bone.

OSTEOGENESIS IMPERFECTA (BRITTLE BONE DISEASE) an hereditary disease which results in the bones being unusually fragile and brittle. It may have associated symptoms, namely, transparent teeth, unusually mobile joints, dwarfism, etc. It may be due to a disorder involving COLLAGEN, but there is little that can be done in treatment.

OSTEOMALACIA a softening of the bones, and the adult equivalent of rickets, which is due to a lack of VITAMIN D. This vitamin is obtained from the diet and is produced on exposure to sunlight, and it is necessary for the uptake of calcium from food.

OSTEOMYELITIS bone marrow inflammation caused by infection. This may happen after a compound fracture or during bone surgery. It produces pain, swelling and fever and high doses of antibiotics are necessary.

OSTEOPHYTE bony projections that occur near joints or intervertebral discs where cartilage has degenerated or been destroyed (*see* OSTEOARTHRITIS). Osteophytes may in any case occur with increasing age with or without loss of cartilage.

OSTEOPOROSIS a loss of bone tissue due to it being resorbed, resulting in bones that become brittle and likely to fracture. It is common in menopausal women and results from long-term steroid therapy. It is also a feature of CUSHING'S SYNDROME. Hormone replacement therapy is a treatment available to women.

OSTEOSARCOMA the commonest and most malignant bone tumour that is found most in older children. The femur is usually affected but metastases are common (*see* METASTASIS). It produces pain and swelling and although amputation used to be the standard treatment, surgery is now possible, with replacement of the diseased bone and associated chemotherapy and/or radiotherapy. It remains, nevertheless, a serious cancer with a relatively poor survival rate.

OSTEOSCLEROSIS a condition in which the density of bone tissue increases abnormally. It is due to tumour, infection or poor blood supply and may be due to an abnormality involving osteoclasts, cells that resorb calcified bone.

OTITIS inflammation of the ear. This may take several forms depending upon the exact location which produces diverse symptoms e.g. inflammation of the inner ear (*otitis interna*), affects balance, causing vertigo and vomiting while *otitis media* is usually a bacterial infection of the middle ear resulting in severe pain, and a fever requiring immediate antibiotic treatment. *Secretory otitis media* is otherwise known as GLUE EAR.

OTOLOGY the subdiscipline of medicine concerned with the ear, its disorders, diseases and their treatment.

OTOSCLEROSIS the hereditary condition in which there is overgrowth of bone in the inner ear which restricts and then stops sound being conducted to the inner EAR from the middle ear. The person affected becomes progressively more deaf, often beginning with TINNITUS, but surgery is effective.

OVARIAN CYST a sac filled with fluid that develops in the ovary. Most are benign but their size may cause swelling and pressure on other organs. For those cysts that do become malignant, it is possible that its discovery comes too late to allow successful treatment. ULTRASOUND scanning can be adopted to detect tumours at an early stage.

OVARIOTOMY literally cutting into an ovary, but more generally used for surgical removal of an ovary or an ovarian tumour.

OVARY the reproductive organ of females which produces eggs (ova) and hormones (mainly OESTROGEN and PROGESTERONE). There are two ovaries, each the size of an almond, on either side of the uterus and each contains numerous Graafian FOLLICLES in which the eggs develop. At OVULATION an egg is released from a follicle. The follicles secrete oestrogen and progesterone which regulate the menstrual cycle and the uterus during pregnancy.

OVULATION the release of an egg from an OVARY (i.e. from a mature Graafian follicle) which then moves down the FALLOPIAN TUBE to the uterus. Ovulation is brought about by secretion of *luteinizing hormone* secreted by the anterior PITUITARY GLAND.

OVUM (*plural* **OVA**) the mature, unfertilized female reproductive cell which is roughly spherical with an outer membrane and a single nucleus.

OXYGENATOR a machine for oxygenating blood outside the body. It is used during heart surgery and the patient's blood is pumped through the machine.

OXYTOCIN a hormone from the PITUITARY GLAND that causes the uterus to contract during LABOUR and prompts lactation due to contraction of muscle fibres in the milk ducts of the breasts.

PACEMAKER the part of the heart that regulates the beat - the SINOATRIAL NODE. Also, in patients with a HEART BLOCK, a device inserted into the body to maintain a normal heart rate. There are different types of pacemaker, some being permanent, others temporary; some stimulate the beat while others are activated only when the natural rate of the heart falls below a certain level.

PAEDIATRICS the branch of medicine that deals with children.

PAEDOPHILIA an abnormal sexual attraction to children.

PALLIATIVE a medicine or treatment that is given to effect some relief from symptoms, if only temporarily, but does not cure the ailment. This is often the case in the treatment of cancer.

PALLOR an abnormal paleness of skin because of a reduced blood flow, or a lack of the normal pigments. It may be due directly to ANAEMIA or SHOCK to spending an excessive amount of time indoors.

PALPATION examination of the surface of the body by carefully feeling with hands and fingertips. It is often possible to distinguish between solid lumps or swelling and cystic swellings.

PALPITATION when the heart beats noticeably or irregularly and the person becomes aware of it. The heartbeat is not normally noticed but with fear, emotion or exercise it may be felt, unpleasantly so. Palpitations may also be due to neuroses, ARRHYTHMIA, heart disease and a common cause is too much tea, coffee, alcohol or smoking. Where an excess is the cause (tea, coffee etc.) this can be eliminated. For disease-associated palpitations, drugs can be used for control.

PALSY the term used formerly for paralysis and retained for the names of some conditions.

PANCREAS a gland with both ENDOCRINE and exocrine functions. It is located between the DUODENUM and SPLEEN, behind the stomach, and is about 15cm long. There are two types of cells producing secretions, the *acini* which produce pancreatic juice which goes to the intestine via a system of ducts. This contains an alkaline mixture of salt and enzymes - trypsin and chymotrypsin to digest proteins, amylase to break down

starch and lipase to aid digestion of fats. The second cell types are in the ISLETS OF LANGERHANS and these produce two hormones, INSULIN and GLUCAGON, secreted directly into the blood for control of sugar levels (*see also* DIABETES MELLITUS, HYPO- and HYPERGLYCAEMIA).

PANCREATECTOMY surgical removal of the PANCREAS (or part of it) to deal with tumours or chronic PANCREATITIS. After *total* or *subtotal* pancreatectomy (where all or almost all is removed) the pancreatic secretions to aid digestion and control blood sugar have to be administered.

PANCREATITIS inflammation of the PANCREAS, occurring in several forms, but often associated with gallstones or alcoholism. Any bout of the condition that interferes with the function of the pancreas may lead to DIABETES and MALABSORPTION.

PANDEMIC an epidemic that is so widely spread that it affects large numbers of people in a country or countries.

PAPANICOLAOU TEST (Pap test) another name for a CERVICAL SMEAR.

PAPILLA any small protuberance such as the papillae on the tongue.

PAPILLOMA usually benign growths on the skin surface or mucous membrane e.g. WARTS.

PARACENTESIS the procedure of tapping or taking off (excess) fluid from the body by means of a hollow needle or CANNULA.

PARACETAMOL a drug that has analgesic effects and also reduces fever. It is taken for mild pain (headache, etc.). It may cause digestive problems and large doses are very dangerous. Excessive doses can produce liver failure, causing progressive NECROSIS in a matter of days and very large doses are fatal. In the early stages of poisoning the stomach can be washed out and drugs administered to protect the liver.

PARAINFLUENZA VIRUSES a group of viruses that cause respiratory tract infections with usually mild influenza-like symptoms. Infants and young children seem to be affected most. There are four types of the virus, virulent at different times of the year.

PARALYSIS muscle weakness or total loss of muscle movement which varies depending upon the causal disease and its effect on the brain. Various descriptive terms are used to qualify the parts of the body affected, thus hemiplegia affects one side of the body (*see also* DIPLEGIA, PARAPLEGIA, QUADRIPLEGIA). Paralysis is really a symptom of another condition or disease e.g. brain disease such as a cerebral haemorrhage or THROMBOSIS causing hemiplegia; disease or injury of the spinal cord leading to paraplegia; and POLIOMYELITIS (infantile paralysis). In addition there is the paralysis associated with MOTOR NEURONE DISEASE.

PARAMEDICAL a term for professions working closely with medics e.g. nurses, radiographers and dietitians.

PARANOIA an abnormal mental condition typified by delusions associated with a certain, complicated system which usually involves feelings of persecution or grandeur. The complex web of delusion may develop with time, and with some logic, so that it may appear plausible and the person seems normal in other aspects and behaviour, save for that involving the delusions.

PARAPLEGIA PARALYSIS of the legs. It may be caused by injury or disease of the spinal cord and often bladder and rectum are also affected.

PARASITE any organism that obtains its nutrients by living in or on the body of another organism (the *host*). The extent to which the host is damaged by the parasite ranges from virtually no effect to, in extreme cases, death. Parasites in humans include worms, viruses, fungi, etc.

PARASYMPATHETIC NERVOUS SYSTEM one of the two parts of the AUTONOMIC NERVOUS SYSTEM that acts antagonistically with the SYMPATHETIC NERVOUS SYSTEM. The parasympathetic nerves originate from the brain and lower portion of the spinal cord (sacral region). The AXONS of this system tend to be longer than sympathetic nerves and SYNAPSES with other neurons are close to the target organ. The parasympathetic system contracts the bladder, decreases heart rate, stimulates the sex organs, promotes digestion, etc.

PARATHYROIDECTOMY removal of the PARATHYROID GLANDS, usually in treatment of hyperparathyroidism (hyperactivity of one or all of the glands).

PARATHYROID GLANDS four small glands located behind or within the thyroid gland, that control the metabolism of calcium and phosphorus (as phosphate) in the body. The hormone responsible, parathormone (or simply parathyroid hormone) is produced and released by the glands. A deficiency of the hormone leads to lower levels of calcium in the blood with a relative increase in phosphorus. This produces tetany, a condition involving muscular spasms, which can be treated by injection. This is also known as *hypoparathyroidism* and is often due to removal or injury of the glands during thyroidectomy. If the hormone is at high levels calcium is transferred from bones to the blood, causing weakness and susceptibility to breaks.

PARATYPHOID FEVER a bacterial infection caused by *Salmonella paratyphi A, B* or *C*. Symptoms resemble those of typhoid fever and include diarrhoea, a rash and mild fever. It can be treated with antibiotics and temporary immunity against the *A* and *B* form is gained by vaccination with TAB vaccine.

PARENTERAL NUTRITION provision of food by any means other than by the mouth. For patients with burns, renal failure etc. or after major surgery, this mode of feeding may be necessary and is accomplished intravenously. Protein, fat and carbohydrate can all be delivered as special solutions containing all the essential compounds. The main hazard of such a system is the risk of infection and reactions to the solutions introduced e.g. HYPERGLYCAEMIA can result.

PARKINSONISM a progressive condition occurring in mid to late life which results in a rigidity of muscles affecting the voice and face rather than those in the limbs. A tremor also develops possibly in one hand initially and then spreading to other limbs and it appears most pronounced when sitting. The disease is usually due to a deficiency in the NEUROTRANSMITTER dopamine, due to degeneration of the basal ganglia of the brain (*see* BASAL GANGLION). There is no cure available, but a number of drugs are able, to varying degrees, to control the condition.

PAROTID GLAND one of a pair of salivary glands situated in front of each ear and opening inside on the cheek near the second last molar of the upper jaw.

PAROTITIS inflammation of the PAROTID GLAND, which as epidemic or infectious parotitis is called MUMPS.

PAROXYSM a sudden attack. A term used especially about convulsions.

PARTURITION *see* LABOUR.

PATCH TEST a test undertaken to identify the substances causing a person's allergy. Different allergens are placed in very small amounts on the skin. A red flare with swelling will develop if the person is allergic. This commonly happens within 15 minutes but may take up to 72 hours.

PATELLA the kneecap. An almost flat bone, shaped somewhat like an oyster shell, that lies in front of the knee in the tendon of the thigh muscle.

PATELLAR REFLEX *see* REFLEX ACTION.

PATHOGEN the term applied to an organism that causes disease. Most pathogens affecting humans are bacteria and viruses.

PATHOLOGY the study of the causes, characteristics and effects of disease on the body by examining samples of body fluids and products whether from a living patient or at autopsy.

PECTORAL the descriptive term for anything relating to the chest.

PECTORAL GIRDLE (or shoulder girdle) the skeletal structure to which the bones of the upper limbs are attached. It is composed of two shoulder blades (SCAPULAE) and two collar bones (CLAVICLES) attached to the vertebral column and breastbone (sternum) respectively.

PEDICULOSIS a deficiency disease caused by a lack of nicotinic acid, part of the VITAMIN B complex. It occurs when the diet is based on maize (rather than wheat) with an associated lack of first-class protein (meat and milk). The reason is that although maize contains nicotinic acid it is in an unusable form and also it does not contain the amino acid tryptophan which the body can use to produce nicotinic acid. The symptoms are dermatitis, diarrhoea and depression.

PELVIC GIRDLE (or hip girdle) the skeletal structure to which the bones of the lower limbs are attached. It is made up of the two hip bones, each comprising the ilium, pubis and ischium, fused together.

PELVIC INFLAMMATORY DISEASE an acute or chronic infection of the UTERUS, ovaries or FALLOPIAN TUBES. It is due to infection elsewhere e.g. the appendix, which spreads or as infection carried by the blood. It produces severe abdominal pain which usually responds to antibiotics but surgery may sometimes be necessary to remove diseased tissue.

PENICILLIN the antibiotic derived from the mould *Penicillium notatum* which grows naturally on decaying fruit, bread or cheese. The genus used for production of the drug is *P. chrysogenum*. Penicillin is active against a large range of bacteria and it is non-toxic. It is usually given by injection but can be taken orally. There are many semi-synthetic penicillins acting in different ways including Ampicillin and Propicillin. Some patients are allergic to penicillin but there tend to be very few serious side-effects.

PENIS the male organ through which the URETHRA passes, carrying urine or semen. It is made up of tissue that is filled with blood during sexual arousal, producing an erection which enables penetration of the vagina and ejaculation of semen. The glans is the end part normally covered by the FORESKIN (prepuce).

PEPTIC ULCER an ulcer in the stomach (GASTRIC ULCER), oesophagus, duodenum (DUODENAL ULCER), or JEJUNUM. It is caused by a break in the mucosal lining due to the action of acid and pepsin (an enzyme active in protein breakdown) either because of their high concentrations or due to other factors affecting the mucosal protective mechanisms.

PEPTIDE an organic compound made up of two or more amino acids and collectively named by the number of amino acids. A dipeptide therefore contains two, and a polypeptide many.

PERCUSSION the diagnostic aid which involves tapping parts of the body (particularly on back and chest) with the fingers to produce a vibration and note-like sound. The sound produced gives an indication of abnormal enlargement of organs, and the presence of fluid in the lungs.

PERFORATION when a hole forms in a hollow organ, tissue or tube, e.g. the stomach, eardrum etc. In particular, it is a serious development of an ulcer in the stomach or bowels because on perforation the intestine contents, with bacteria, enter the peritoneal (*see* PERITONEUM) cavity causing PERITONITIS. This is accompanied by severe pain and shock and usually corrective surgery is required.

PERICARDITIS inflammation of the PERICARDIUM. It may be due to URAEMIA, cancer or viral infection and produces fever, chest pain and possible accumulation of fluid.

PERICARDIUM the smooth membrane surrounding the heart. The outer *fibrous* part covers the heart and is connected to the large vessels coming out of the heart. The inner *serous* part is a closed SEROUS MEMBRANE attached both to the fibrous pericardium and the heart wall. Some fluid in the resulting sac enables smooth movement as the heart beats.

PERINATAL MORTALITY foetal deaths after week 28 of pregnancy and newborn deaths during the first week or two of life. The main causes of perinatal mortality are brain injuries during birth, congenital defects and lack of oxygen in the final stages of pregnancy (called *antepartum anoxia*). Perinatal *deaths* are due to complications involving the placenta, congenital defects and birth asphyxia.

PERINEUM the area of the body between anus and urethral opening.

PERIODONTAL descriptive term relating to the tissues surrounding the teeth.

PERIPHERAL NERVOUS SYSTEM those parts of the nervous system excluding the central nervous system (brain and spinal cord). It comprises the afferent (sensory) and efferent (motor) cells which include 12 pairs of cranial nerves and 31 pairs of spinal nerves. The motor nervous system then comprises the somatic nervous system carrying impulses to the skeletal muscles, and the autonomic nervous system which is further divided into the sympathetic and the parasympathetic nervous system (*see individual entries*).

PERIPHERAL NEURITIS inflammation of the nerves of the peripheral system.

PERITONEUM the SEROUS MEMBRANE that lines the abdominal cavity. That lining the abdomen walls is the *parietal* peritoneum while the *visceral* peritoneum covers the organs. The folds of peritoneum from one organ to another are given special names, e.g. MESENTERY. Both are continuous and form a closed sac at the back of the abdomen in the male, while in the female there is an opening from the Fallopian tube on either side.

PERITONITIS inflammation of the peritoneum. It may be caused by a primary infection due to bacteria in the bloodstream (e.g. tuberculous peritonitis) resulting in pain and swelling, fever and weight loss. Secondary infection results from entry into the abdominal cavity of bacteria and irritants (e.g. digestive juices) from a perforated or ruptured organ e.g. duodenum or stomach. This produces severe pain and shock and surgery is often necessary.

PERNICIOUS ANAEMIA a type of ANAEMIA due to VITAMIN B$_{12}$ deficiency which results from dietary lack or the failure to produce the substance that enables B$_{12}$ to be absorbed from the bowel. This in turn results in a lack of red blood cell production and MEGALOB-LASTS in the bone marrow. The condition is easily treated by regular injections of the vitamin.

PERSPIRATION (*or* SWEAT) the excretion from millions of tiny sweat glands in the skin. Sweat that evaporates from the skin immediately is *insensible*, while that forming drops is *sensible perspiration*. Sweat is produced in two types of sweat glands. The *eccrine* glands are found mainly on the soles of the feet and palms of the hands. The *apocrine* glands are in the armpits, around the anus and genitalia and sweat is produced in response to stimuli such as fear and sexual arousal. The major function of sweating, however, is the regulation of body temperature.

PERTHES' DISEASE a hip condition in children between the ages of four and ten, and which is self-healing. Due to OSTEOCHONDROSIS of the EPIPHYSIS of the femur a limp is developed with associated pain. Rest is essential as is traction, until the pain subsides and then a special splint is fitted to permit walking until the condition is fully healed.

PERTUSSIS *see* WHOOPING COUGH.

PESSARY an instrument that fits into the vagina to treat a PROLAPSE. Also a soft solid that is shaped for insertion into the vagina and contains drugs for some gynaecological disorder (also used for inducing labour).

PETHIDINE a drug with ANALGESIC and mild sedative action for relief of moderate pain. It may be given by mouth or injection but side-effects include nausea, dizziness and dry mouth, and also prolonged use may create dependence.

PETIT MAL the lesser type of epileptic seizure which is IDIOPATHIC. It consists of brief periods (seconds) of unconscious-ness when the eyes stare blankly but posture is maintained. Children suffering frequently may have learning difficulties but the condition may disappear in adult life.

PHAEOCHROMOCYTOMA a small vascular tumour (usually benign) of the inner part of the ADRENAL GLAND. It causes uncontrolled secretion of adrenaline and noradrenaline producing increased heart rate, palpitations, high blood pressure, sweating, weight loss and there may be heart failure.

PHAGOCYTOSIS *see* LEUCOCYTE.

PHALLUS penis, or a penis-like object. Also the term used for the embryonic penis before the final development of the urethral duct.

PHANTOM LIMB the feeling that a limb or part of a limb is still attached to the body after it has been amputated. This is probably due to stimulation of the severed nerves and usually wears off with time.

PHARMACEUTICAL relating to pharmacy or drugs.

PHARMACIST a trained, qualified and registered person who is authorized to keep and dispense medicines.

PHARMACOLOGY the branch of medicine concerning the preparation, properties, uses and effects of drugs.

PHARMACY the preparation of drugs (and their dispensing); or the place where this function is undertaken.

PHARYNGECTOMY surgical excision of part of the pharynx.

PHARYNGITIS inflammation of the PHARYNX and therefore throat, commonly due to a virus, and resulting in a sore throat. It is often associated with TONSILLITIS.

PHARYNX the region extending from the beginning of the oesophagus up to the base of the skull at the cavity into which nose and mouth open. It is muscular, with a mucous membrane and acts as the route for both food (to the oesophagus) and air (to the larynx). The EUSTACHIAN TUBES open from the upper part of the pharynx.

PHENOBARBITONE a very widely used BARBITURATE. It can be given orally or by injection and is taken as an anticonvulsant in epilepsy and to treat insomnia or anxiety. It may produce drowsiness and some skin reactions and continued use should be avoided, lest dependence ensue.

PHENOTYPE the detectable, observable characteristics of an individual that are determined by the interaction of his GENES (genotype) and the environment in which he develops. The expression of the dominant gene masks the presence of a recessive one, as only the expressed gene affects the phenotype.

PHENYL KETONURIA a genetic disorder that results in the deficiency of an ENZYME that converts phenylalanine, an ESSENTIAL AMINO ACID, to tyrosine. Children can be severely mentally retarded by an excess of phenylalanine in the blood damaging the nervous system. The responsible gene is recessive therefore the condition occurs only if both parents are carriers. However, there is a test for newborn infants (the Guthrie test) that ensures the condition can be detected and the diet can be modified to avoid phenylalanine and thus any brain damage.

PHIAL a small glass bottle-like receptacle for storing medicines.

PHIMOSIS a condition in which the edge of the FORESKIN is narrowed and cannot be drawn back over the glans of the PENIS. To avoid inflammation and an exacerbation of the problem, circumcision may be necessary.

PHLEBECTOMY removal of a vein, or part of a vein, sometimes undertaken in the treatment of VARICOSE VEINS.

PHLEBITIS inflammation of a vein. This commonly occurs as a complication of VARICOSE VEINS, producing pain and a hot feeling around the vein, with possible THROMBOSIS development. Drugs and elastic support are used in treatment.

PHLEBOTHROMBOSIS the obstruction of a vein by a blood clot, common in the deep veins of the leg (in particular the calf) and resulting from heart failure, pregnancy, injury and surgery, which may change the clotting factors in the blood. The affected leg may swell and there is the danger that the clot may move, creating a PULMONARY EMBOLISM. Large clots may be removed surgically, otherwise the treatment involves anticoagulant drugs and exercise.

PHLEBOTOMY the opening of a vein, or its puncture, to remove blood or to infuse fluids.

PHLEGM a general term (non-medical) for sputum, mucus.

PHOBIA an anxiety disorder and irrational fear of certain objects, animals, situations, events, etc. Avoiding the situation can lead to significant disruption, restriction of normal life or even suffering. There is a variety of phobias including animal, specific and social phobias and treatment involves through behaviour therapy.

PHONATION the production of speech sounds.

PHOTOPHOBIA an atypical sensitivity to light. Exposure produces discomfort and actions to evade the light source. The condition may be associated with medications, or migraine, meningitis, etc.

PHRENIC NERVE the nerve to the

muscles of the DIAPHRAGM, arising from the 3rd, 4th and 5th cervical spinal nerves.

PHYSICAL concerning the body as opposed to the mind.

PHYSICIAN a registered medical practitioner who deals with non-surgical practice.

PHYSIOLOGY the study of the functions of and processes within the body and its various organs.

PHYSIOTHERAPY the use of physical methods to help healing. It may involve exercise, massage and manipulation, heat treatment and the use of light and ultraviolet radiation, etc.

PIA MATER *see* BRAIN and MENINGES.

PIGMENT an organic colouring agent e.g. the blood pigment HAEMOGLOBIN, BILE pigments, rhodopsin (found in the RODS of the RETINA) and MELANIN.

PILES *see* HAEMORRHOIDS.

PILUS a hair or structure like a hair.

PIMPLES (papules) small swellings on the skin that are inflamed and may contain pus. The cause is often infection of a pore that is blocked with fatty secretions from the SEBACEOUS GLANDS. On the face, the condition is called ACNE.

PITUITARY GLAND (*or* HYPOPHYSIS) a small, but very important endocrine gland at the base of the HYPOTHALAMUS. It has two lobes, the anterior *adenohypophysis* and the posterior *neurohypophysis*. The pituitary secretes hormones that control many functions and is itself controlled by hormonal secretions from the hypothalamus. The neurohypophysis stores and releases peptide hormones produced in the hypothalamus namely OXYTOCIN and VASOPRESSIN. The adenohypophysis secretes GROWTH HORMONE, GONADOTROPHIN, prolactin (involved in stimulating lactation), ACTH and THYROID stimulating hormones.

PLACEBO an inactive substance, taken as medication, that nevertheless may help to relieve a condition. The change occurs because the patient expects some treatment (even if nothing need, in reality, be done) and an improvement reflects the expectations of the patient. New drugs are tested in trials against placebos when the effect of the drug is measured against the placebo response which happens, even when there is no active ingredient in the placebo.

PLACENTA the organ attaching the embryo to the UTERUS. It is a temporary feature comprising maternal and embryonic tissues and it allows oxygen and nutrients to pass from the mother's blood to the embryo's blood. There is, however, no direct contact of blood supplies. The embryo also receives salt, glucose, amino acids, some peptides and antibodies, fats and vitamins. Waste molecules from the embryo are removed by diffusion into the maternal circulation. It also stores GLYCOGEN for conversion to glucose if required and secretes hormones to regulate the pregnancy. It is expelled after birth.

PLACENTA PRAEVIA when the placenta is situated in the bottom part of the uterus next to or over the cervix. In the later stages of pregnancy there may be placental separation causing bleeding which will require attention. In the more extreme cases, a Caesarian section will be necessary for delivery.

PLANTAR descriptive term meaning relating to the sole of the foot.

PLAQUE a surface layer on teeth formed from bacteria and food debris and later, calcium salts.

PLASMA a light-coloured fluid component of BLOOD and in which the various cells are suspended. It contains inorganic salts with protein and some trace substances. One protein present is FIBRINOGEN.

PLASTIC SURGERY a branch of surgery that deals with the repair or rebuilding of damaged, deformed or missing parts of the body. *Cosmetic* plastic surgery is merely for the improvement of appearance but most is to repair burns, accident damage or congenital defects.

PLATELET (*or* THROMBOCYTE) a

disc like structure in the blood involved in the halting of bleeding.

PLEURA the SEROUS MEMBRANE that covers the lungs (*visceral*) and the inside of the chest wall (*parietal*). The membranes have a smooth surface which is moistened to allow them to slide over each other.

PLEURAL CAVITY the small space between the PLEURA which slide over each other when breathing in and out. Should gas or fluid enter the cavity due to infection or injury the space increases and may hinder breathing.

PLEURECTOMY removal, by surgery, of part of the PLEURA to overcome PNEUMOTHORAX or to excise diseased areas.

PLEURISY (or PLEURITIS) inflammation of the PLEURA resulting in pain from deep breathing, and resulting shortness of breath. There is a typical frictional rub heard through a stethoscope. Pleurisy is often due to pneumonia in the adjacent lung and is always associated with disease in the lung, diaphragm, chest wall or abdomen e.g. tuberculosis, abscesses, bronchial carcinoma etc.

PLEXUS a network formed from intersecting nerves and/or blood vessels, or lymphatic vessels.

PNEUMOCONIOSIS a general term for a chronic form of lung disease caused by inhaling dust while working. Most of the cases are anthracosis (coal miner's pneumoconiosis), SILICOSIS and asbestosis.

PNEUMONECTOMY the surgical removal of a lung performed mainly for cancer but also for tuberculosis.

PNEUMONIA a bacterial infection of the lungs resulting in inflammation and filling of the ALVEOLI with pus and fluid. As a result the lung becomes solid and air cannot enter. The symptoms vary depending upon how much of the lung is unavailable for respiration, but commonly there will be chest pain, coughing, breathlessness, fever and possibly CYANOSIS. Pneumonia may be caused by several bacteria, viruses or fungi, but bacterial infection is commonest. Bronchopneumonia affects the bronchi and bronchioles; lobar pneumonia the whole lobes of the lung(s). Antibiotic treatment is usually effective although it helps to know which is the infecting organism, to provide the most specific treatment. (*See also* VIRAL PNEUMONIA).

PNEUMONITIS inflammation of the lungs by chemical or physical agents.

PNEUMOTHORAX air in the PLEURAL CAVITY, which enters via a wound in the chest wall or lung. When this happens, the lung collapses but if the air is absorbed from the pleural cavity the lung reinflates.

POCK a small eruption on the skin, which may contain pus, typical of chickenpox and smallpox.

POLIOMYELITIS (or INFANTILE PARALYSIS, POLIO) an infectious disease, caused by a virus, which attacks the central nervous system. The virus is taken in by mouth, passes through the digestive system, is excreted with the faeces and hands may be contaminated, leading to further spread. The incubation period is 7 to 12 days and there are several types of condition, depending upon the severity of the attack. In some cases the symptoms resemble a stomach upset or influenza; in others there is in addition some stiffness of muscles. Paralytic poliomyelitis is less common, resulting in muscle weakness and paralysis while the most serious cases involve breathing when the diaphragm and related muscles are affected (bulbar poliomyelitis). Treatment of the disease involves relief of the symptoms including bed rest, and for the bulbar form, a respirator may be required. Immunization is highly effective and the disease has almost been eradicated in most countries. However, booster doses are advisable when visiting countries with a high incidence of the disease.

POLYDACTYLY the condition in

which there are extra fingers or toes.

POLYDIPSIA an intense thirst, abnormally so. It is a characteristic symptom of DIABETES MELLITUS and certain other diseases.

POLYP a growth from a mucous membrane and attached to it by a stalk. Most are benign but may cause obstructions or infections. They commonly occur in the sinuses, nose, or possibly the bladder or bowels. Their removal is usually straightforward, unless a more extensive operation proves necessary to reach the affected organ.

POLYURIA the passing of a larger than normal quantity of urine which is also usually pale in colour. It may be due merely to a large fluid intake, or to a condition such as DIABETES, or a kidney disorder.

PONS tissue that joins parts of an organ, e.g. the *pons Varolii*, a part of the brainstem links various parts of the brain including the medulla oblongata and thalamus.

PORE a small opening, e.g. sweat pores.

PORPHYRIA a group of disorders that are hereditary in which there is increased production of porphyrins (natural pigments as found in e.g. haemoglobin) leading to abdominal pain, sensitivity to light and neuropathy (disease of the peripheral nerves).

PORTAL VEIN a vein within the hepatic portal system that carries blood to the liver from other abdominal organs (stomach, spleen, intestine, etc.). It is atypical in that it does not take blood directly to the heart but ends in a capillary network.

POSSETTING the term for the normal habit of some quite healthy babies to regurgitate small amounts of a recently-taken meal.

POST MORTEM *see* AUTOPSY and NECROPSY.

POSTPARTUM the term meaning relating to the first few days after birth.

POULTICE (*or* **FOMENTATION**) hot, moist material applied to the body to soften the skin, soothe irritations, ease pain or increase the circulation locally.

POX pus-filled pimples as in chicken-pox or smallpox. Also the small pit-like depressions that are scars of smallpox.

PRECANCEROUS any condition that is not malignant but is known will become so if left untreated.

PRE-ECLAMPSIA the development of high blood pressure in pregnancy, sometimes with OEDEMA which unless treated may result in ECLAMPSIA.

PREGNANCY the period of time, lasting approximately 280 days from the first day of the last menstrual period, during which a woman carries a developing foetus. Signs of a pregnancy include cessation of menstruation, increase in size of the breasts, MORNING SICKNESS, and later in the pregnancy the obvious sign of enlargement of the abdomen. A foetal heart beat and movements also follow later. Many of these changes are hormone-controlled, by progesterone (from the OVARY and PLACENTA).

PREGNANCY TEST various tests are used to check for pregnancy, most based on the presence of CHORIONIC GONADO-TROPHIN HORMONE in the urine.

PREMATURE BIRTH a birth occurring before the end of the normal full term. The definition refers to babies weighing less than 2° kilograms. In many cases the cause is unknown but in some it may be due to PRE-ECLAMPSIA, kidney or heart disease or multiple pregnancy. Premature babies often require incubator care.

PREMEDICATION drugs given to a patient before an operation in which an anaesthetic will be used. It is usually a sedative and a drug to reduce secretions of the lungs which could be inhaled otherwise.

PREMENSTRUAL TENSION (or syndrome) the occurrence for up to ten days before menstruation, of such symptoms as headache, nervousness and irritability, emotional disturbance, depression, fatigue with other physical manifestations such as swelling of legs and breasts, and constipation. The condition usually disappears soon after menstruation begins. The cause is not known although the hormone PROGESTER-ONE is probably involved in some way.

PREMOLAR two teeth between the canines and molars on each side of the jaw.

PRENATAL DIAGNOSIS see AMNIOCENTESIS.

PREPUCE See FORESKIN.

PRESENTATION the point, during LABOUR, at which some part of the foetus lies at the mouth of the womb. In the majority of cases the head presents, but see BREECH PRESENTATION.

PRESSURE SORES see BED SORES.

PRICKLY HEAT (heat rash or miliaria) an itchy rash due to small red spots which are minute vesicles caused by the blocking of sweat or sebaceous glands in the skin. Scratching may produce infection but the condition itself is not serious.

PRIMA GRAVIDA the technical term for a woman in her first pregnancy.

PROGESTERONE a steroid hormone that is vital in pregnancy. It is produced by the CORPUS LUTEUM of the OVARY when the lining of the uterus is prepared for the implanting of an egg cell. Progester-one is secreted under the control of other hormones (prolactin from the anterior PITUITARY, and luteinizing hormone also from the pituitary which stimulates ovulation and formation of the corpus luteum) until the placenta adopts this role later in the pregnancy. The function of progesterone is to maintain the uterus and ensure no further eggs are produced. Small amounts of this hormone are also produced by the testes.

PROGNOSIS a forecast of the likely outcome of a disease, based upon the patient's condition and the course of the disease in other patients at other times.

PROLAPSE a moving down of an organ or tissue from its normal position due to the supporting tissues weakening. This may happen to the lower end of the bowel (in children) or the uterus and vagina in women who have sustained some sort of injury during childbirth. In the latter case prolapse may result in the uterus itself showing on the outside. Surgery can shorten the supporting ligaments and narrow the vaginal opening.

PROLAPSED INTERVERTEBRAL DISC (SLIPPED DISC) the interverte-bral disc provides cushioning for the brain and spinal cord and is composed of an outer fibrous layer over a pulpy centre. A slipped disc is caused by the inner layer being pushed through the fibrous layer to impinge upon nerves, causing pain (commonly lumbago or sciatica). The prolapse usually occurs during sudden twisting or bending of the backbone and is more likely to occur during middle age. Treatment involves bed rest on a flat, firm surface, probably with manipulation and physiotherapy at a later stage. If absolutely necessary, the disc can be removed, but this is now less common.

PRONE lying face downwards.

PROPHYLACTIC some treatment or action that is taken to avoid disease or a condition, e.g. taking a medication to prevent angina.

PROPRIETARY NAME the trade name given to a drug by the company manufacturing it.

PROSTAGLANDIN (PG) a group of compounds derived from essential fatty acids that act in a way that is similar to hormones. They are found in most body tissues (but especially semen) where they are released as local regulators (in the uterus, brain, lungs, etc.). A number have been identified, two of which act antagonistically on blood vessels. PGE causing dilation, PGF constriction. Certain prostaglandins cause uterine contraction in labour, and others are involved in the body's defence mechanisms.

PROSTATECTOMY surgical excision of the PROSTATE GLAND, performed to relieve urine retention caused by enlargement of the prostate. It is also done to counter poor flow of urine or frequent urination. The operation can be undertaken from several approaches: via the urethra, from the bladder, or from the PERINEUM (for a BIOPSY).

PROSTATE GLAND a gland in the male reproductive system which is located below the bladder, opening into the URETHRA. Upon ejaculation, it secretes an alkaline fluid into the semen which aids sperm motility. In older men, the gland may become enlarged, causing problems with urination (*see* PROSTATECTOMY).

PROSTATITIS inflammation of the PROSTATE GLAND due to bacterial infection. The symptoms tend to be similar to a urinary infection although in the chronic form obstructions may form necessitating PROSTATECTOMY.

PROSTHESES (*singular* **PROSTHESIS**) artificial devices fitted to the body, ranging from dentures to hearing aids, pacemakers and artificial limbs.

PROTEIN a large group of organic compounds containing carbon, hydrogen, oxygen, sulphur and nitrogen, with individual molecules built up of AMINO ACIDS in long POLYPEPTIDE chains. Globular protein includes ENZYMES, ANTIBODIES, carrier proteins (e.g. HAEMOGLOBIN) some HORMONES, etc. Fibrous proteins have elasticity and strength and are found in muscle, connective tissue and also chromosomes. Proteins are thus vital to the body and are synthesized from their constituent amino acids, which are obtained from digestion of dietary protein.

PROTEINURIA the condition in which protein (usually albumin) is found in the urine. It is important because it may signify heart or kidney disease. Proteinuria may also occur with fever, severe anaemia and intake of certain drugs or poisons.

PRURITUS another term for itching, of whatever origin.

PSITTACOSIS a bacterial infection of parrots and budgerigars that can be transmitted to man. It causes headache,

shivering, nosebleeds, fever and lung problems. It is treatable with antibiotics.

PSORIASIS a chronic skin disease for which the cause is unknown and the treatment is palliative. The affected skin appears as itchy, scaly red areas, starting usually around the elbows and knees. It often runs in families and may be associated with anxiety, commencing usually in childhood or adolescence. Treatment involves the use of ointments and creams with some drugs and vitamin A.

PSYCHEDELIC DRUGS drugs that affect the mind and consciousness, and which are often hallucinogens.

PSYCHIATRIST a qualified physician who deals with mental disorders including emotional and behavioural problems.

PSYCHIATRY the study of mental disorders, their diagnosis, treatment/management and prevention.

PSYCHOANALYSIS a method of treating mental ill-health by uncovering repressed fears, and dealing with them in the conscious mind. This school of psychology began with Sigmund Freud.

PSYCHOGERIATRICS the branch of psychiatry dealing with mental ill-health in old people.

PSYCHOLOGY the study of the mind, its working and resulting behaviour patterns. There are many schools of psychology including experimental (laboratory experiments to study topics such as learning), PSYCHOANALYSIS, ethology (study of animal behaviour in the natural environment) and behaviourism.

PSYCHOPATHIC when a person has a mental disorder resulting in antisocial behaviour with little or no guilt for any such acts committed. In addition, psychopaths do not show any ability for showing affection, sympathy or love to others and punishment does not deter a repeat of any criminal act.

PSYCHOSIS a very serious state of mental ill-health, essentially insanity. The sufferer loses touch with reality and may suffer delusions and hallucinations. Schizophrenia and manic depressive psychosis are two important psychoses.

PSYCHOSOMATIC the term meaning relating to both mind and body and used most often for illnesses and conditions that result from the effects of excessive emotional stress upon the body. Numerous physical ailments can be triggered in this way, from nausea, abdominal pains, ulcer and asthma to dizziness, insomnia and ARRHYTHMIA. The causes of the stress may be even more numerous but essentially fall into categories such as personal/marital; occupational; social. Although psychological treatment may help, attention to the physical symptoms is more effective.

PSYCHOTHERAPY the treatment of mental disorders, or the mental part of an ailment by psychological means, i.e. by concentrating upon and working through the mind. There are several approaches to this method of treatment including psychoanalysis, group therapy and behavioural therapy.

PSYCHOTROPIC DRUGS drugs that affect the mind and its moods, e.g. anti-depressants, sedatives and stimulants.

PUBERTY the changes that occur in boys and girls around the age of 10 to 14 which signify the beginnings of sexual maturity, and the subsequent functioning of reproductive organs. It is apparent through the appearance of secondary sexual characteristics such as a deepening of the voice in boys and growth of breasts in girls. In addition, girls commence menstruation and in boys the size of testicles increases. In both sexes body shape changes noticeably and body hair grows. The changes are initiated by PITUITARY GLAND hormones acting on the ovaries and testes.

PUBIS one of three bones, and the most anterior, that makes up each half of the pelvic girdle.

PUERPERAL FEVER an infection, now rare in developed countries, which occurs within two or three days of childbirth when a mother is susceptible to disease. Because the body's resources are low and the genital tract after childbirth provides ready access for bacteria, it is essential that clean conditions are maintained to avoid infection. A mild infection of the genital tract may cause fever, high temperature and pulse. Inflammation, and possibly PERITONITIS may result from infection of local lymph and blood vessels while access to the general circulation can cause septicae-mia. Serious cases are, however, rare. Preventive measures are vital, but infections respond to antibiotic treatment.

PULMONARY relating to the lungs.

PULMONARY EMBOLISM a condition involving the blocking of the pulmonary artery or a branch of it by an EMBOLUS (usually a blood clot). The clot usually originates from PHLEBOTHROMBO-SIS of the leg. The seriousness of the attack relates to the size of the clot. Large pulmonary emboli can be immediately fatal. Smaller ones may cause death of parts of the lung, PLEURISY and coughing up of blood. Anticoagulant drugs are used in minor cases; streptokinase may be used to dissolve the clot or immediate surgery may be necessary. Several embolisms may produce PULMONARY HYPERTENSION.

PULMONARY HYPERTENSION an increase in blood pressure in the pulmonary artery due to increased resistance to the flow of blood. The cause is usually disease of the lung (such as BRONCHITIS, EMPHYSEMA, *see also* PULMONARY EMBOLISM) and the result is that the pressure increases in the right ventricle, enlarging it, producing pain with the possibility of heart failure.

PULMONARY OEDEMA gathering of fluid in the lungs caused by, for example, MITRAL STENOSIS.

PULMONARY STENOSIS a narrowing of the outlet from the heart to the pulmonary artery via the right ventricle which may be congenital or due, more rarely, to rheumatic fever. Severe cases can produce ANGINA, fainting and enlargement of the heart with eventual heart failure. Surgery is necessary to clear the obstruction.

PULSE the regular expansion and contraction of an artery as a fluid wave of blood passes along, originating with the contraction of the heart and blood leaving the left ventricle. It is detected on arteries near the surface, e.g. the radial artery on the wrist and decreases with a reduction in the size of artery so that the capillaries are under a steady pressure (hence the reason why venous flow is also steady).

PUPIL the circular opening in the IRIS which permits light into the lens in the EYE.

PURGATIVE DRUGS or other treatments taken to evacuate the bowels. These may be grouped by their mode of action, LAXATIVES providing a gentle effect. Purgatives work by increasing the muscular contractions of the intestine or by increasing the fluid in the intestine.

PUS the liquid found at an infected site (abscess, ulcer, etc.). It is coloured white, yellow or greenish and consists of dead white blood cells, living and dead bacteria and dead tissue.

PUTRID FEVER a former name for TYPHUS FEVER.

PYELITIS inflammation of part of the kidney, the pelvis. (This is the area from which urine drains into the ureter). The cause is usually a bacterial infection (commonly *E. coli*) and sometimes occurs as a complication of pregnancy. The symptoms include pain in the loins, high temperature, loss of weight, but it does respond to antibiotics. It is usually the case that the infection is not limited to the pelvis but all the kidney hence a more accurate term is *pyelonephritis*.

PYLORIC STENOSIS a narrowing of the PYLORUS which limits the movement of food from the stomach to the duodenum, resulting in vomiting. It may be accompanied by distension and peristalsis of the stomach, visible through the abdominal wall. A continuation of the condition causes weight loss, dehydration and ALKALOSIS. It is often due to an ulcer or cancer near the pylorus which requires surgery.

PYLORUS the lower end of the stomach where food passes into the duodenum and at which there is a ring of muscle, the *pyloric sphincter*.

PYREXIA another term for FEVER.

Q FEVER an infectious disease which produces symptoms resembling pneumonia including a severe headache, high fever and breathing problems. It is caused by the organism *Coxiella burnetti* and is a disease of sheep, goats and cattle which can be passed to man mainly through unpasteurized milk. The disease is treated with the drug, tetracycline and also chloramphenicol and is of about two weeks duration.

QUADRICEPS the large thigh muscle, which is divided into four distinct parts, and is responsible for movements of the knee joint.

QUADRIPLEGIA paralysis of all four limbs of the body.

QUARANTINE a period of time in which a person (or animal) who has, or is suspected of having, an infectious disease is isolated from others to prevent the spread of the infection.

QUARTAN FEVER the recurrent fever, which usually occurs every fourth day, associated with *Malaria*.

QUICKENING the first movements of a baby in the womb which are perceived by the mother usually around the fourth month of pregnancy.

QUININE a colourless alkaloid derived from the bark of certain (cinchona) trees which is a strong antiseptic especially effective against the malarial parasite. It was formerly widely used in the treatment of malaria but has now largely been replaced because it is toxic in larger doses. In small amounts it has a stimulating effect and is used in "tonic" water.

QUINSY the medical name for this condition is *pentonsillar abscess* and it is a complication of TONSILLITIS. A pus-filled abscess occurs near the tonsil, causing great difficulty in swallowing, and this may require surgical lancing.

RABIES (also known as *hydrophobia*) a very severe and fatal disease affecting the central nervous system which occurs in dogs, wolves, cats and other canine animals. Human beings are infected through the bite of a *rabid* animal, usually a dog. The onset of symptoms varies from ten days to up to a year from the time of being bitten. Characteristically, the person becomes irritable and depressed, swallowing and breathing difficulties develop, there are periods of great mental excitement, increased salivation and muscular spasms of the throat. Eventually, even the sight of water causes severe muscular spasms, convulsions and paralysis, and death follows within about four days. Treatment consists of thorough cleansing of the bite and injections of rabies vaccine, antiserum and immunoglobulin. As the UK is currently free of rabies, vigilant quarantine and other regulations involving the movement of animals, are in force.

RADIOGRAPH an image produced by x-rays on a film. *Radiography* is the diagnostic technique used to examine the body using X-rays.

RADIOLOGIST a doctor specialized in the interpretation of X-rays and other diagnostic records.

RADIOLOGY the branch of medicine concerned with the use of X-rays.

RADIOTHERAPY the therapeutic use of penetrating radiation including X-rays, beta rays and gamma rays. These may be derived from X-ray machines or radioactive isotopes and are especially employed in the treatment of cancer. The main disadvantages of radiotherapy is that there may be damage to normal, healthy surrounding tissues.

RADIUM a radioactive metallic element which occurs naturally and emits alpha, beta and gamma rays as it decays. The gamma rays derived from radium are used in the treatment of cancer.

RADIUS the shorter outer bone of the forearm the other being the *ulna*

RASH an eruption of the skin which is usually short-lived and consists of reddened, perhaps itchy area or raised red spots.

RADON a radioactive gas produced when RADIUM decays. *Radon seeds* are small, sealed capsules which are used in radiotherapy for cancer.

RECESSIVE GENE a gene whose character will only be expressed if paired with a similar gene (allele).

RECOMBINANT DNA DNA (deoxyribonucleic acid) containing genes which have been artificially combined by the techniques of GENETIC ENGINEERING. Recombinant DNA technology has become synonymous with genetic engineering.

RECTUM the final portion of the large intestine between the colon and anal canal in which faeces are stored prior to elimination.

RED BLOOD CELL *see* ERYTHROCYTE.

REFERRED PAIN (SYNALGIA) pain felt in another part of the body at a distance from the site at which it might be expected. An example is certain heart conditions which cause pain in the left arm and fingers. The condition arises because some sensory nerves share common routes in the central nervous system hence stimulation of one causes an effect in another.

REFLEX ACTION an unconscious movement which is brought about by relatively simple nervous circuits in the central nervous system. In its simplest form it involves a single *reflex arc* of one receptor and sensory nerve which forms a *synapse* in the BRAIN or SPINAL cord with a motor nerve which then transmits the impulse to a muscle or gland to bring about a response. However some reflex actions are more complicated than this, involving several neurones. Examples are the *plantar reflex* of the toes, when the sole of the foot is stroked, the *knee jerk reflex* and the reflex pupil of the eye which contracts suddenly when a light is directed upon its surface. The presence or absence of reflexes give an indication of the condition of the nervous system and are pointers to the presence or absence of disease or damage.

REFRACTORY a condition which does not respond to treatment.

REFRACTORY PERIOD the time taken for a nerve or muscle cell to recover after an electrical impulse has passed along, or following contraction. During this time, the nerve or muscle cell is unable to respond to a further stimulus.

REGIMEN a course of treatment which usually involves several elements including drugs, diet and lifestyle (such as the taking of exercise), aimed at curing a disease or promoting good health.

REGISTRAR a relatively senior hospital doctor responsible for the care of patients and working with consultants.

REGRESSION in psychiatry, this refers to a reversion to a more immature form of behaviour. In medicine the term refers to the stage in the course of a disease when symptoms cease and the patient recovers.

REGURGITATION the bringing up of swallowed undigested food from the stomach to the mouth (*see also* POSSETTING).

The term is also used to describe the backward flow of blood in the heart if one or more valves is diseased and defective.

REHABILITATION the process of restoring (as far as possible), back to normal life a person who has been disabled by injury or physical and/or mental illness. Rehabilitation usually involves various different kinds of therapy and re-training.

REITER'S SYNDROME a disease of unknown cause, affecting men, which produces symptoms of URETHRITIS, CONJUNCTIVITIS and ARTHRITIS. It may also produce other symptoms including fever and diarrhoea and it is suspected that the cause may be a virus.

REJECTION this is a term used in transplant medicine describing the situation in which the immune system of the recipient individual rejects and destroys an organ or tissue grafted from a donor. Various drugs, e.g. *cyclosporin A*, are given to the recipient to dampen down the immune system and reduce the risk of rejection.

RELAPSE the return of the symptoms of a disease from which a person had apparently recovered or was in the process of recovery.

RELAPSING FEVER a disease caused by spirochaete bacteria of the genus *Borrelia* which is transmitted to man by lice and ticks. The disease is characterized by recurrent bouts of fever accompanied by headache, joint and muscle pains and nosebleeds. The first attack lasts for about two to eight days and further milder bouts occur after 3 to ten days. Treatment is by means of bed rest and with erythromycin and tetracycline drugs.

REMISSION a period during the course of a disease when symptoms have lessened or disappeared.

REM SLEEP this stands for *Rapid Eye*

Movement SLEEP and describes a phase when the eyeballs move rapidly behind closed eyelids. This appears to be the phase during which dreaming occurs.

RENAL describing or relating to the kidneys.

REPETITIVE STRAIN INJURY *see* TENDINITIS.

REPRODUCTIVE SYSTEM the name given to all the organs involved in reproduction. In males these comprise the testes, vasa deferentia, prostate gland, seminal vesicles, urethra and penis. In females, the reproductive system consists of the ovaries, Fallopian tubes, womb (uterus), vagina and vulva (*see individual entries*).

RESECTION a surgical operation in which part of an organ, or any body part, is removed.

RESISTANCE the degree of natural immunity which an individual possesses against a certain disease or diseases. The term is also applied to the degree with which a disease or disease-causing organism can withstand treatment with drugs such as a course of antibiotics.

RESONANCE the quality and increase of sound produced by striking the body over an air-filled structure. If resonance is decreased compared to normal this is termed *dullness* and if increased *hyper-resonance*. Tapping the body, often the chest, to determine the degree of resonance, is called *percussion*. An opinion may be formed about the condition of underlying organs, i.e. the amount of air present or fluid (e.g. in the lungs) or if there is any enlargement.

RESPIRATION the whole process by which air is drawn into and out of the lungs during which oxygen is absorbed into the bloodstream and carbon dioxide and water are given off. *External respiration* is the actual process of breathing and the exchange of gases which takes place in the lungs. *Internal respiration* is the process by which oxygen is given up from the blood circulation to the tissues, in all parts of

the body, and carbon dioxide is taken up to be transported back to the lungs and eliminated.

The process of drawing air into the lungs is known as *inhalation* or *inspiration* and expelling it out as *exhalation* or *expiration*. The rate at which this occurs is known as the *respiratory rate* and it is about 18 times a minute in a static healthy adult.

RESPIRATOR one of a number of different devices used to assist or take over RESPIRATION, especially when the muscles which should normally be involved are paralysed, as in some forms of POLIOMYELITIS.

RESPIRATORY DISTRESS SYNDROME this usually refers to a condition arising in newborn babies, especially those which are premature, being particularly common in infants born between 32-37 weeks gestation. It is also known as *hyaline membrane disease* and is characterized by rapid shallow laboured breathing. It arises because the lungs are not properly expanded and lack a substance (known as surfactant) necessary to bring their expansion about.

Adults may suffer from *adult respiratory distress syndrome* in which there is PULMONARY OEDEMA and a high mortality rate.

RESPIRATORY SYNCITIAL VIRUS generally called RS Virus, this is the main cause of BRONCHIOLITIS and pneumonia in babies under the age of 6 months

RESPIRATORY SYSTEM all the organs and tissues involved in RESPIRATION including the nose, pharynx, larynx, trachea, bronchi, bronchioles, lungs and diaphragm, along with the muscles which bring about respiratory movements (*see individual entries*).

RESUSCITATION reviving a person in whom heart beat and breathing has ceased. see ARTIFICIAL RESPIRATION and CARDIAC MASSAGE.

RETARDATION the slowing down of an

activity or a process, often referring to mental subnormality or "backwardness".

RETINA the layer which lines the interior of the eye. The retina itself consists of two layers the inner one next to the cavity of the eyeball containing the light-sensitive cells, the RODS and CONES, and also nerve fibres. This layer receives light directed onto its surface by the lens. The outer layer of the retina next to the *choroid* contains pigmented cells which prevent the passage of light (*See also* EYE).

RETINOL *see* VITAMIN A.

RETRACTOR one of a number of different surgical instruments designed to pull apart the cut edges of an incision to allow greater operating access.

RETROFLEXION the bending backwards of a part of an organ, particularly the upper portion of the uterus (*compare* RETROVERSION).

RETROVERSION an abnormal position of the uterus in which the whole organ is tilted backwards instead of forwards, as is normally the case. A *retroverted uterus* occurs in about 20% of women (*see* RETROFLEXION).

RETROVIRUS a type of virus containing RNA (ribonucleic acid) which is able to introduce its genetic material into the DNA of body cells. These viruses are suspected causal agents in the development of certain cancers.

REYE'S SYNDROME a rare disorder, of unknown cause, which affects children and seems to follow on from a viral infection such as chickenpox, often manifesting itself during the recovery phase. The symptoms include vomiting, high fever, delirium, convulsions leading to coma and death, the mortality rate being about 25%. Among those who survive, about half suffer some brain damage. It has been suggested that aspirin may be implicated in the development of this condition and this drug is not now recommended for children under the age of 12.

RHESUS FACTOR *see* BLOOD GROUP.

RHEUMATIC FEVER a severe disease affecting children and young adults which is a complication of upper respiratory tract infection with bacteria known as *Haemolytic streptococci*. The symptoms include fever, joint pain and ARTHRITIS which progresses from joint to joint, a characteristic red rash known as *Erythema marginatum* and also painless nodules which develop beneath the skin over bony protuberances such as the elbow, knee and back of the wrist. In addition there is CHOREA and inflammation of the heart including the muscle, valves and membranes. The condition may lead to rheumatic heart disease in which there is scarring and inflammation of heart structures. There is sometimes a need for heart valves to be replaced in later life.

The initial treatment consists of destroying the streptococci which cause the disease with antibiotic drugs such as penicillin. Other drugs are also used such as non-steroidal anti-inflammatory drugs (*see* NSAID) and corticosteroids. Surgery may be required later in life to replace damaged heart valves.

RHEUMATISM a general term used to describe aches and pains in joints and muscles.

RHEUMATOID ARTHRITIS the second most common form of joint disease after OSTEOARTHRITIS which usually affects the feet, ankles, fingers and wrists. The condition is diagnosed by means of X-rays which show a typical pattern of changes around the inflamed joints known as *rheumatoid erosions*. At first there is swelling of the joint and inflammation of the SYNOVIAL MEMBRANE (the membraneous sac which surrounds the joint), followed by erosion and loss of cartilage and bone. In addition, a blood test reveals the presence of *serum rheumatoid factor antibody* which is characteristic of this condition. The condition varies greatly in its degree of severity but at its worst can be progressive and seriously

disabling. In other people, after an initial active phase, there may be a long period of remission.
A number of different drugs are used to treat the disease including analgesics and anti-inflammatory agents.

RHEUMATOLOGY the branch of medicine concerned with diseases of the joints and associated tissues and structures. The medical specialist in this field is known as a *rheumatologist*.

RHINITIS inflammation of the mucous membrane of the nose such as occurs with colds and allergic reactions.

RHINOPLASTY any one of a large number of RNA - containing viruses which cause upper respiratory tract infections including the common cold.

RIBS 12 pairs of thin, slightly twisted and curved bones which form the thoracic rib cage which protects the lungs and heart. The *true ribs* are the first seven pairs which are each connected to the STERNUM at the front by a costal CARTILAGE. The *false ribs* are the next three pairs are indirectly connected to the sternum as each is attached by its cartilage to the rib above. The *floating ribs* are the last two pairs which are unattached and end freely in the muscle of the thoracic wall. At the backbone, the head of each rib articulates with one of the 12 thoracic vertebrae.

RICKETS this is a disease affecting children which involves a deficiency of VITAMIN D. Vitamin D can be manufactured in the skin in the presence of sunlight but dietary sources are important especially where sunlight is lacking. The disease is characterized by soft bones which bend out of shape and cause deformities. Bones are hardened by the deposition of calcium salts and this cannot happen in the absence of vitamin D. Treatment consists of giving vitamin D, usually in the form of calciferol, and ensuring that there is an adequate amount in the child's future diet. Vitamin D deficiency in adults causes the condition called OSTEOMALACIA.

RICKETTSIAE a group of microorganisms, which share characteristics in common with both bacteria and viruses and are parasites which occur in lice, fleas and ticks and other arthropods. They can be passed to man by the bites of these animals and are the cause of several serious diseases including TYPHUS, *Rocky Mountain spotted fever* and Q FEVER.

RIGIDITY especially used to describe stiffness in a limb which is being moved passively, which is a symptom of Parkinson's disease (*see* PARKINSONISM).

RIGOR a sudden bout of shivering and feeling of coldness which often accompanies the start of a fever.

RIGOR MORTIS the stiffening of the body that occurs within eight hours of death due to chemical changes in the muscles.

RINGWORM this is an infection caused by various species of fungi and is known medically as Tinea. It is classified according to the area affected e.g. *Tinea capitis* which is ringworm of the scalp. Other areas affected are the beard, groin, (dhobie itch), nails and feet (athletes foot).
The infection is typically slightly raised, itchy and with a ring-like appearance. It is highly contagious and the commonest form is athletes foot which usually begins between the toes. The antibiotic drug griseofulvin, taken by mouth, is the normal treatment for ringworm and also anti-fungal creams applied to the affected areas.

RINNE'S TEST a type of hearing test that uses a vibrating tuning fork which helps to determine whether deafness is perceptive (nervous) or *conductive* (indicating an obstruction within the ear).

RNA ribonucleic acid which is a complex nucleic acid present mainly in the CYTOPLASM of cells but also in the NUCLEUS. It is involved in the production of proteins and exists in three forms, ribosomal (r), transfer (t) and messenger (m) RNA. In some viruses it forms the genetic material (*see also* DNA).

ROD one of the two types of light sensitive cell present in the RETINA of the EYE. The rods enable vision in dim light due to a pigment called *rhodopsin* (*visual purple*). This pigment degenerates or bleaches when light is present and regenerates during darkness. In bright light all the pigment bleaches and the rods cannot function. Bleaching of the pigment gives rise to nerve impulses which are sent to the brain and interpreted.

RODENT ULCER a slow-growing malignant ulcer which occurs on the face in elderly people usually near the lips, nostrils or eyelids. Skin and underlying tissues and bone are destroyed if the ulcer is untreated. Normally, treatment is by means of surgery and possibly radiotherapy.

ROSACEA a disease of the skin of the face characterized by a red, flushed appearance and enlargement of the SEBACEOUS GLANDS in the skin. The nose may also enlarge and look red and lumpy (rhinophyma). The cause is unknown but may be aggravated by certain foods or drinks such as an excess of alcohol. Treatment is by means of *tetracycline drugs*

ROSEOLA any rose-coloured rash such as accompanies various infectious diseases e.g. measles.

ROSE-WAALER REST a diagnostic blood test which is used to detect RHEUMATOID ARTHRITIS.

ROTAVIRUS one of a number of viruses which commonly cause gastroenteritis and diarrhoea in young children under the age of 6 years. They infect the lining cells of the SMALL INTESTINE.

ROTOR SYNDROME a rare inherited liver condition similar to the DUBLIN-JOHNSON SYNDROME.

ROUGHAGE dietary fibre which is necessary to maintain the healthy functioning of the bowels and helps to prevent constipation and DIVERTICULOSIS. The eating of sufficient dietary fibre is thought to be important in the prevention of cancer of the colon.

RUBELLA *see* GERMAN MEASLES.

RUPTURE the bursting open of an organ, tissue or structure, e.g. ruptured APPENDIX. Also, a popular name for a HERNIA.

SABIN VACCINE an oral vaccine for POLIOMYELITIS. The appropriate virus is cultured but rendered non-violent while retaining its ability to stimulate production of antibodies.

SAC a structure resembling a bag, e.g. the lungs.

SACRAL NERVES nerves that serve the legs, anal and genital region and which originate from the sacral area of the spinal column. There are five pairs of sacral nerves.

SACRAL VERTEBRAE the five vertebrae that are fused together form the SACRUM.

SACRUM the lower part of the spinal column comprising five fused vertebrae (SACRAL VERTEBRAE) in a triangular shape. The sacrum forms the back wall of the pelvis and articulates with the coccyx below, lumbar vertebrae above and the hips to the sides.

SAFE PERIOD the days in a woman's menstrual cycle when conception is least likely. OVULATION usually occurs mid-way through the cycle, about 15 days before onset of menstruation, and the fertile period is about 5 days before and 5 after ovulation. Providing periods are regular, it can be calculated when intercourse is unlikely to result in pregnancy.

SALIVA an alkaline liquid present in the mouth to keep the mouth moist, aid swallowing of food and through the presence of amylase enzymes (ptyalin) to digest starch. It is secreted by the SALIVARY GLANDS and in addition to ptyalin, contains water, mucus and buffers (to minimise changes in acidity).

SALIVARY GLANDS three pairs of glands; parotid, submandibular and sublingual, that produce saliva. The stimulus to produce saliva can be the taste, smell, sight or even thought of food.

SALK VACCINE a vaccine against POLIOMYELITIS administered by injection. The virus is treated with formalin which renders it unable to cause the disease but it still prompts the production of antibodies.

SALMONELLA INFECTIONS FOOD POISONING due to *Salmonella*, a genus of Gram-negative (*see* GRAM'S STAIN) rodlike bacteria.

SALPINGECTOMY the surgical excision of a FALLOPIAN TUBE. The removal of both produces sterilization.

SALPINGITIS inflammation of a tube, usually the Fallopian tube by bacterial infection. It may originate in the vagina or uterus, or be carried in the blood. Peritonitis can ensue. Severe cases may cause a blockage of the Fallopian tubes resulting in sterility.

SALPINGOSTOMY the clearing of a blocked FALLOPIAN TUBE, which the blocked part is removed surgically.

SANATORIUM a hospital or similar institution for convalescence or rehabilitation.

SANGUINEOUS containing blood, covered or stained with blood.

SARCOMA *see* CANCER.

SCABIES a skin infection causing severe itching. It is due to the mite *Sarcoptes scabiei* which burrows into the skin, lays eggs, and the resulting larvae cause the itching. The areas of the body affected are the skin between fingers, wrists, buttocks and genitals. An application of special cream is necessary to kill the mites.

SCALDS *see* BURNS.

SCALP the covering of the skull around the top of the head which comprises several layers, from the skin with hair on the outside through fat and fibrous tissue to another fibrous layer (the pericranium) that is attached closely to the skull.

SCALPEL a small surgical knife with renewable blades, used for cutting tissues.

SCAN examination of the body using one of a number of techniques, such as COMPUTERIZED TOMOGRAPHY AND ultrasonography (*see* ULTRASOUND). Also the image produced by a scanning technique

SCAPHOID BONE a bone of the wrist, the outside one on the thumb side of the hand.

SCAPULA the shoulder blade. A triangular bone and one of a pair forming the shoulder girdle.

SCAR the mark left after a wound heals. It is due to the damaged tissues not repairing completely, and being replaced by a fibrous connective tissue.

SCARLET FEVER an infectious disease, mainly of childhood, caused by the bacterium *Streptococcus*. Symptoms show after a few days and include sickness, sore throat, fever and a scarlet rash that may be widespread. Antibiotics are effective and also prevent any complications e.g. inflammation of the kidneys.

SCHIZOPHRENIA any one of a large group of severe mental disorders typified by gross distortion of reality, disturbance in language and breakdown of thought processes, perceptions and emotions. Delusions and hallucinations are usual, as are apathy, confusion, incontinence and strange behaviour. No single cause is known but genetic factors are probably important. Drug therapy has improved the outlook markedly over recent years.

SCIATICA pain in the sciatic nerve, and therefore felt in the back of the thigh, leg and foot. The commonest cause is a PROLAPSED INTERVERTEBRAL DISC pressing on a nerve root, but it may also be due to ankylosing SPONDYLITIS and other conditions.

SCLERA the outer layer of the eyeballs which is white and fibrous same at the front of the eye when it becomes the transparent CORNEA.

SCLERITIS inflammation of the white of the eye (SCLERA).

SCLERODERMA a condition in which connective tissue hardens and contracts. The tissue may be the skin, heart, kidney, lung etc. and the condition may be localized or it may spread throughout the body, eventually being fatal. If the skin is affected, it becomes tough and patchily pigmented and may lead to stiff joints and wasting muscles.

SCLEROSIS hardening of tissue, usually after inflammation leading to parts of organs being hard and of no use. It is applied commonly to such changes in the nervous system (MULTIPLE SCLEROSIS); in other organs it is termed FIBROSIS or CIRRHOSIS.

SCLEROTHERAPY a treatment for VARICOSE VEINS. An irritant solution is injected, causing FIBROSIS of the vein lining and its eventual removal by THROMBOSIS and scarring.

SCREENING TEST a programme of tests carried out on a large number of apparently healthy people to find those who may have a particular disease, e.g. cervical smears to detect the precancerous stage of cervical cancer.

SCROFULA TUBERCULOSIS of the LYMPH NODES in the neck which form sores and scars after healing. It is now an uncommon condition, but drug treatment is effective.

SCROTUM the sac that contains the testicles and holds them outside the body, to permit production and storage of sperm at a temperature lower than that of the abdomen.

SCRUB TYPHUS a disease prevalent in S.E. Asia, caused by a parasitic microorganism *Rickettsia*, transmitted from rodents to man by the bite of mites. It causes chills, headaches, high temperatures, rashes and possibly delirium. An ulcer develops at the initial bite. The condition can be treated with antibiotics.

SCRUM-POX a bacterial (IMPETIGO) or viral (HERPES SIMPLEX) infection of the face, common to rugby players occurring probably through facial contact in the scrum or communal changing facilities.

SCURVY a deficiency disease caused by a lack of VITAMIN C (ascorbic acid) due to a dietary lack of fruit and vegetables. Symptoms begin with swollen, bleeding gums and then subcutaneous bleeding, bleeding into joints, ulcers, anaemia and then fainting, diarrhoea and trouble with major organs. Untreated, it is fatal, but nowadays it is easily prevented, or cured should it arise, through correct diet or administration of the vitamin.

SEBACEOUS CYST a cyst formed in the duct of a SEBACEOUS GLAND of the skin.

SEBACEOUS GLAND any of the minute glands in the skin that secrete an oily substance called SEBUM. The glands open into hair follicles. Activity of the glands varies with age, puberty being the most active period.

SEBORRHOEA excessive production of SEBUM by the SEBACEOUS GLANDS producing either a build up of dry scurf or oily deposits on the skin. The condition often leads to the development of ACNE.

SEBUM the secretion formed by the SEBACEOUS GLANDS, which forms a thin oily film on the skin, preventing excessive dryness. It also has an antibacterial action.

SECONDARY SEXUAL CHARACTERISTICS the physical features that develop at puberty. In girls, the breasts and genitals increase in size and pubic hair grows. Boys grow pubic hair and facial hair, the voice breaks and the genitals become adult size.

SECRETIN a polyPEPTIDE hormone produced by the lining of the DUODENUM and JEJUNUM in response to acid from the stomach. It stimulates production of alkaline pancreatic juice, and BILE secretion by the liver.

SECRETION the material produced by a gland.

SECTION cutting in surgery, e.g. an abdominal section.

Also a thin slice of a specimen as used in microscopy.

SEDATIVE a drug that lessens tension and anxiety. Sedatives are hypnotic drugs, e.g. barbiturates, given in doses lower than would bring on sleep. They may be used to combat pain, sleeplessness, spasms, etc.

SEMEN the fluid that contains the sperm which is ejaculated from the penis during copulation.

SENILE DEMENTIA an organic mental disorder of the elderly involving generalized atrophy of the brain. The result is a gradual deterioration with loss of memory, impaired judgement, confusion, emotional outbursts and irritability. The degree of the condition may vary considerably.

SENSATION a feeling. The result of stimulation of a sensory receptor producing a nerve impulse which travels on an afferent fibre to the brain.

SENSITIVITY with reference to a SCREENING TEST, the proportion of people with the disease who are identified by the test.

SENSITIZATION a change in the body's response to foreign substances. With the development of an allergy, a person becomes sensitized to a certain ALLERGEN and then becomes hypersensitive. Similarly it may be an acquired reaction when ANTIBODIES develop in response to an ANTIGEN.

SEPSIS the destruction of tissues through putrefaction by bacteria-causing disease, or toxins produced by bacteria.

SEPTAL DEFECT a hole in the SEPTUM or partition between the left and right sides of the heart, whether in the atria (*see* ATRIUM) or VENTRICLES. This condition is a CONGENITAL disorder caused by an abnormal development of the foetal heart. Whether the defect is atrial or ventricular, it allows incorrect circulation of the blood from left to right, from higher pressure to lower. This is called a *shunt*, and results in too much blood flowing through the lungs.

PULMONARY HYPERTENSION results and a large shunt may cause heart failure. Surgery can correct the defect, although a small one may not require any treatment.

SEPTIC affected with SEPSIS.

SEPTICAEMIA a term used loosely for any type of blood poisoning. Also a systemic infection with PATHOGENS from an infected part of the body circulating in the bloodstream.

SEPTIC SHOCK a form of shock that occurs due to SEPTICAEMIA. The toxins cause a drastic fall in blood pressure due to tissue damage and blood clotting. Kidneys, heart and lungs are affected and related symptoms include fever, TACHYCARDIA or even coma. The condition occurs most in those who already have a serious disease such as cancer, DIABETES, or CIRRHOSIS. Urgent treatment is vital, with antibiotics, oxygen and fluids given intravenously.

SEPTUM a planar dividing feature within a structure of the body; a partition.

SEROLOGY a laboratory medical subdiscipline involving the study of blood serum and its constituents, including ANTIGEN-ANTIBODY reactions.

SEROSITIS inflammation of a SEROUS MEMBRANE.

SEROUS MEMBRANE a membrane lining a large cavity in the body. The membranes are smooth and transparent and the surfaces are moistened by fluid derived from blood or lymph serum (hence the name). Examples are the PERITONEUM and the PERICARDIUM. Each consists of two layers, the *visceral* which surrounds the organs and the *parietal* which lines the cavity. The two portions are continuous and the surfaces are close together, separated by fluid which permits free movement of the organs.

SERUM a serous fluid. More specifically the clear, sticky fluid that separates from blood and lymph when clotting occurs. In addition to water, serum contains albumin and GLOBULIN with salts, fat, sugar, UREA and other compounds important in disease prevention.

Also, a VACCINE prepared from the serum of a hyperimmune donor for use in protection against a particular infection.

SERUM SICKNESS a hypersensitive reaction that occasionally occurs several days after injection of foreign SERUM, producing rashes, joint pains, fever and swelling of the lymph nodes. It is due to circulating antigen material to which the body responds. It is not a serious condition.

SESSILE in description of a tumour or growth, one having no stalk.

SEX CHROMOSOMES CHROMOSOMES that play a major role in determining the sex of the bearer. Sex chromosomes contain GENES that control the characteristics of the individual, e.g. testes in males, ovaries in females. Women have two X chromosomes while men have one X and one Y chromosomes (*see individual entries*).

SEX HORMONES steroid hormones responsible for the control of sexual development (primary and SECONDARY SEXUAL CHARACTERISTICS) and reproductive function. The ovaries and testes are the organs primarily involved in hormone production, of which there are three main types: ANDROGENS, the male sex hormones; OESTROGENS and PROGESTERONE, the female sex hormones.

SEX-LINKED DISORDERS conditions produced because the genes controlling certain characteristics are carried on the SEX CHROMOSOMES, usually the X chromosome. Some result from an abnormal number of chromosomes, e.g. KLINEFELTER'S SYNDROME affecting only men, and TURNER'S SYNDROME affecting only women. Other disorders such as HAEMOPHILIA are carried on the X chromosome and these manifest themselves in men because although the genes are recessive, there is no other X chromosome to mask the recessive type, as is the case with women.

SEXUALLY-TRANSMITTED DISEASES *see* VENEREAL DISEASES.

SHINGLES the common name for herpes zoster (*see* HERPES).

SHOCK acute circulatory failure, when the arterial blood pressure is too low to provide the normal blood supply to the body. The signs are a cold, clammy skin, pallor, CYANOSIS, weak rapid pulse, irregular breathing and dilated pupils. There may also be a reduced flow of urine and confusion or lethargy. There are numerous causes of shock from a reduction in blood volume as after burns, external bleeding, dehydration etc. to reduced heart activity as in CORONARY THROMBOSIS, PULMONARY EMBOLISM, etc. Certain other circumstances may produce shock, including severe allergic reactions (anaphylactic shock, *see* ANAPHYLAXIS), drugs overdose, emotional shock and so on.

SHORT SIGHT *see* MYOPIA.

SHOULDER BLADE *see* SCAPULA.

SHOULDER GIRDLE *see* PECTORAL GIRDLE.

SICKLE-CELL ANAEMIA a type of inherited, haemolytic ANAEMIA (*see* HAEMOLYSIS) that is genetically-determined and which affects people of African ancestry. It is caused by a recessive gene and is manifested when this gene is inherited from both parents. One AMINO ACID in the HAEMOGLOBIN molecule is substituted causing the disease which results in an abnormal type of haemoglobin being precipitated in the red blood cells during deprivation of oxygen. This produces the distortion of the cells which are removed from the circulation causing anaemia and jaundice. Many people are carriers due to inheritance of just one defective GENE and because this confers increased resistance to malaria, this gene remains at a high level.

SIDE-EFFECT the additional and unwanted effect(s) of a drug above the intended action. Sometimes side-effects are harmful and may be stronger than anticipated results of the drug, or something quite different.

SIGMOID COLON the end part of the COLON which is S-shaped.

SIGMOIDECTOMY surgical excision of the SIGMOID COLON, performed usually for tumours, diverticular disease (*see* DIVERTICULITIS, DIVERTICULOSIS) or a long and twisted sigmoid colon.

SIGMOIDOSCOPY the examination of the SIGMOID COLON and rectum with a special viewing device. The instrument is tubular, with illumination, although modern forms use fibre optics, which are flexible.

SILICOSIS a type of PNEUMOCONIOSIS caused by the inhalation of silica as particles of dust. The silica promotes FIBROSIS of the lung tissue resulting in breathlessness and a greater likelihood to contract tuberculosis. Workers in quarrying, mineral mining, sand blasting, etc. are most susceptible.

SINEW the TENDON of a muscle.

SINOATRIAL NODE the natural heart PACEMAKER which consists of specialized muscle cells in the right atrium. These cells generate electrical impulses, contract and initiate contractions in the muscles of the heart. The AUTONOMIC NERVOUS SYSTEM supplies the node and certain hormones also have an effect.

SINUS in general terms a cavity or channel. Specifically air cavities in bone as in the bones of the face and skull. Also a channel, as in the DURA MATER and which drains venous blood from the brain.

SINUSITIS inflammation of a SINUS. It usually refers to the sinuses in the face which link with the nose and may therefore be due to a spread of infection from the nose. Headaches and a tenderness over the affected sinus are typical symptoms with a pus-conaining discharge from the nose. Persistent infection may necessitate surgery to drain the sinus.

SJÖGREN'S SYNDROME dryness of the mouth and eyes associated with rheumatoid arthritis. The syndrome is due to the destruction of the salivary glands (and lacrimal glands).

SKELETON the rigid, supporting framework of the body that protects organs and tissues, provides muscle attachments, facilitates movement, and produces red blood cells. There are 206 bones divided into the axial skeleton (head and trunk) and the appendicular skeleton (limbs). The types of bone are: long (e.g. humerus), short (e.g. carpals), flat (parts of the cranium) and irregular (e.g. the vertebrae).

SKIN the outer layer of the body comprising an external EPIDERMIS itself made up of a *stratum corneum* (horny layer) formed of flat cells that rub off, being replaced from below. Beneath this are two more layers (*stratum lucidum* and *stratum granulosum*) which act as intermediate stages between the stratum corneum and a still lower layer, the Malpighian layer.

The Malpighian layer is where the epidermis is produced. The dermis lies beneath the epidermis and then follows subcutaneous tissue composed mainly of fat. The subcutaneous tissue contains glands (sweat, SEBACEOUS, etc.), sensory receptors for pain, pressure and temperature, nerves, muscles and blood capillaries.

The skin is a protective layer against injury and parasites and it moderates water loss. It is a medium of temperature control by means of the sweat glands and blood capillaries and also the hairs (which provide insulation).

SKIN GRAFT (*see also* GRAFT) a piece of skin taken from another site on the body to cover an injured area, commonly due to burns. The graft is normally taken from elsewhere on the patient's body (*autograft*) but occasionally from someone else (*homograft*). A variety of thicknesses and graft types are used, depending upon the wound.

SKULL the part of the SKELETON that forms the head and encloses the brain. It is made up of 22 bones, forming the cranium (eight bones) and fourteen in the face and all except the mandible are fused along sutures creating immovable joints. The mandible (lower jaw) articulates close to the ears. A large opening at the base of the skull (FORAMEN magnum) allows the spinal cord to pass from the brain to the trunk of the body.

SLEEP a state of lower awareness accompanied by reduced metabolic activity and physical relaxation. When falling asleep, there is a change in the brain's electrical activity. This activity can be recorded by an ELECTROENCEPHALOGRAM (EEG). There are high amplitude, low frequency waves (slow-wave sleep) interrupted by short periods of low amplitude, high frequency waves. The periods of high frequency waves are typified by restless sleep with dreams and rapid eye movements, hence the name REM SLEEP, and the EEG is similar to that of a waking person. REM sleep comprises about 25% of the time asleep.

SLEEPING SICKNESS (AFRICAN TRYPANOSOMIASIS) a parasitic disease found in tropical Africa which is spread through the bite of tsetse flies. The organism responsible is a minute protozoan, *Trypanosoma*, and initially the symptoms consist of a recurring fever, a slight rash, headache and chills. Then follows ANAEMIA, enlarged LYMPH NODES and pain in joints and limbs. Then after some time (possibly years), sleeping sickness itself develops. This is due to the parasites occupying minute blood vessels in the brain resulting in damage, and symptoms of drowsiness and lethargy. Death may follow from weakness or an associated disease. The early stages are curable with drugs. When the brain is affected, arsenic-containing drugs are used and although they are highly active against the parasites, care is necessary due to the toxicity of the compounds.

SLING a bandage so arranged as to support an injured limb, usually an arm.

SLIPPED DISC *See* PROLAPSED INTERVERTEBRAL DISC.

SLOUGH dead tissue, usually of limited extent, that after infection separates from the healthy tissue of the rest of the body. In cases of GANGRENE it is possible for limbs to be lost.

SLOW VIRUS one of several viruses that show their effects some time after infection, by which time considerable damage of nerve tissue has occurred, resulting ultimately in death. Some years ago such a virus was found to cause scrapie in sheep and recently bovine spongiform encephalopathy in cows. In man a slow virus is thought to be the cause of CREUTZFELDT-JAKOB DISEASE and a type of MENINGITIS.

SMALL INTESTINE *see* INTESTINE.

SMALLPOX a highly infectious viral disease that has nonetheless been eradicated. Infection results, after about two weeks, in a high fever, head and body aches and vomiting. Eventually red spots appear which change to water and then pus-filled vesicles which on drying out leave scars. The person stays infectious until all scabs are shed. Fever often returns, with DELIRIUM, and although recovery is usual, complications often ensue, e.g. PNEUMONIA.

The last naturally-occurring case was in 1977.

SMOOTH MUSCLE *see* INVOLUNTARY MUSCLE.

SNELLEN CHART the chart commonly used for testing distant vision. It comprises rows of capital letters that become progressively smaller.

SOLAR PLEXUS a network of sympathetic nerves and ganglia (*see* GANGLION) behind the stomach, surrounding the coeliac artery. It is a major autonomic PLEXUS of the body where nerves of the sympathetic and parasympathetic nervous system combine (*see* individual terms).

SOMATIC descriptive term meaning relating to the body, as opposed to the mind. More specifically, concerning the *nonreproductive* parts of the body.

SOMNAMBULISM (sleep-walking) walking and performing other functions during sleep with no recollection upon waking.

SOPORIFIC sleep-inducing (*see also* HYPNOTICS).

SORE a common term for an ulcer or open skin wound.

SOUND an instrument resembling a rod, with a curved end, that is used to explore a body cavity, e.g. the bladder, or to dilate STRICTURES.

SOUTHEY'S TUBES very fine tubes for drawing off fluid, e.g. from subcutaneous tissue. They are rarely used today.

SPASM a muscular contraction that is involuntary. Spasms may be part of a more major disorder (e.g. spastic paralysis, convulsions) or they may be specific such as cramp, colic, etc. A heart spasm is known as ANGINA.

SPASMOLYTIC a drug that reduces spasms (in SMOOTH MUSCLE) in a number of ways. It may generally depress the CENTRAL NERVOUS SYSTEM, act directly on the muscles in question, or modify the nerve impulses causing the spasm. Spasmolytics are used in the treatment of ANGINA, colic and as BRONCHODILATORS.

SPASTICITY muscular hypertonicity (i.e. an increase in the state of readiness of muscle fibres to contract; an increase in the normal partial contraction) with an increased resistance to stretch. Moderate cases show movement requiring great effort and a lack of normal coordination while slight cases show exaggerated movements that are coordinated.

SPASTIC COLON see IRRITABLE BOWEL SYNDROME.

SPASTIC PARALYSIS weakness of a limb characterized by involuntary muscular contraction and loss of muscular function. As with SPASTICITY it is due to disease of the nerve fibres that usually control movement and reflexes.

SPATULA a knife-like instrument with a flat, blunt blade used for spreading or mixing ointments and materials. It is also used to hold down the tongue when the throat is being examined.

SPECULUM an instrument for use in examination of an opening in the body. The speculum holds open the cavity and may also provide illumination.

SPERMATIC the term given to any vessel or structure associated with the testicle.

SPERMATOZOON (plural **SPERMATOZOA**) the mature male reproductive cell, or gamete. It has a head with the HAPLOID nucleus containing half the CHROMOSOME number, and an acrosome (a structure that aids penetration of the egg). Behind the head comes a midpiece with energy-producing MITOCHONDRIA, and then a long tail which propels it forward. A few millilitres of SEMEN is ejaculated during intercourse, containing many millions of spermatozoa.

SPERMICIDE a cream, foam, jelly, etc. that kills spermatozoa and which is used in conjunction with a DIAPHRAGM as a contraceptive.

SPHENOID BONE a bone in the skull that lies behind the eyes.

SPHINCTER a circular muscle around an opening. The opening is closed totally or partially by contraction of the muscle, e.g. the anal sphincter around the anus.

SPHYGMOMANOMETER the instrument used to measure arterial blood pressure. An inflatable rubber tube is put around the arm and inflated until the blood flow in a large artery stops. This pressure is taken as the SYSTOLIC PRESSURE (i.e. the pressure at each heart beat). The pressure is then released slowly and the point at which the sound heard in the artery changes suddenly is taken as the diastolic pressure (see DIASTOLE).

SPINA BIFIDA a CONGENITAL malformation in new born babies in which part of the spinal cord is exposed by a gap in the backbone. Many cases are also affected with HYDROCEPHALUS. The symptoms usually include paralysis, incontinence, a high risk of MENINGITIS and mental retardation. There is usually an abnormally high level of ALPHA FETOPROTEIN in the amniotic fluid and since this can be diagnosed and then confirmed by AMNIOCENTESIS, it is possible to terminate these pregnancies.

SPINAL ANAESTHESIA generating

anaesthesia by injecting the cerebrospinal fluid around the spinal cord. Of the two types, the epidural (*see* EPIDURAL ANAESTHESIA) involves injecting into the outer lining of the spinal cord, while *subarachnoid anaesthesia* is produced by injecting between vertebrae in the LUMBAR region of the vertebral column. Spinal anaesthesia is useful for patients who have a condition that precludes a general anaesthetic (e.g. a chest infection or heart disease).

The term is also used for a loss of sensation in a part of the body due to spinal injury.

SPINAL COLUMN (SPINE, BACK-BONE, VERTEBRAL COLUMN) the bony and slightly flexible column that forms a vital part of the SKELETON. It encloses the SPINAL CORD, articulates with other bones, e.g. the skull and ribs, and provides attachments for muscles.

It consists of bones, the vertebrae, between which are discs of fibrocartilage (the intervertebral discs). From the top, the column comprises 7 cervical, 12 thoracic, 5 lumbar, 5 sacral and 4 coccygeal vertebrae. In adults the last two groups are fused to from the sacrum and coccyx, respectively.

SPINAL CORD the part of the CENTRAL NERVOUS SYSTEM that runs from the brain, through the SPINAL CORD. Both GREY and WHITE MATTER are present, the former as an H-shaped core within the latter. A hollow core in the grey matter forms the central canal which contains the cerebrospinal fluid. The cord is covered by MENINGES and it contains both sensory and motor NEURONS. Thirty-one pairs of spinal nerves arise from the cord, passing out between the arches of the vertebrae.

SPIROMETER an instrument used to test how the lungs are working, by recording the volume of air inhaled and exhaled.

SPLEEN a roughly ovoid organ, coloured a deep purple, which is situated on the left of the body, behind and below the stomach. It is surrounded by a peritoneal membrane and contains a mass of lymphoid tissue. MACROPHAGES in the spleen destroy microorganisms by PHAGOCYTOSIS. The spleen produces lymphocytes, leucocytes, plasma cells and blood platelets (*see individual entries*). It also stores red blood cells for use in emergencies. Release of red blood cells is facilitated by SMOOTH MUSCLE under the control of the SYMPATHETIC NERVOUS SYSTEM, and when this occurs, the familiar pain called *stitch* may be experienced. The spleen removes worn out red blood cells, conserving the iron for further production in the bone marrow. Although the spleen performs many functions, it can be removed without detriment and as a result there is an increase in size of the lymphatic glands.

SPLENECTOMY removal of the SPLEEN possibly because of rupture and bleeding.

SPLENOMEGALY an abnormal enlargement of the SPLEEN which occurs commonly with blood disorders and parasitic infections.

SPLINT a support that holds a broken bone in the correct and stable position until healing is complete.

SPONDYLITIS inflammation of the spinal vertebrae - arthritis of the spine. *Ankylosing spondylitis* is a rheumatic disease of the spine and sacroiliac joints (i.e. those of the sacrum and ilium), causing pain and stiffness in the hip and shoulder. It may result in the spine become rigid (*see* KYPHOSIS).

SPONDYLOSIS degeneration of joints and the intervertebral discs of the spine, producing pain in the neck and LUMBAR region where the joints may actually restrict movement. OSTEOPHYTES are commonly formed and the space occupied by the discs reduced. Physiotherapy may help sufferers, and collars or surgical belts can prevent movement and give support. Surgery may be required occasionally to relieve pressure on nerves, or to fuse joints.

SPONGIFORM ENCEPHALOPATHY a neurological disease caused by a SLOW

VIRUS and resulting in a spongy degeneration of the brain with progressive dementia. Examples are CREUTZFELDT-JAKOB DISEASE and kuru (a progressive and fatal viral infection seen in New Guinea highland natives which has decreased with the decline in cannibalism).

SPRAIN an injury to ligaments (or muscles, or tendons) around a joint, caused by a sudden overstretching. Pain and swelling may occur and treatment comprises, in the main, avoiding use of the affected joint.

SPUTUM saliva and mucus from the respiratory tract.

SQUINT (or STRABISMUS) an abnormal condition in which the eyes are crossed. There are two types, paralytic and non-paralytic. The paralytic type is due to a muscular or neurological malfunction, while a non-paralytic squint is caused by a defect in the actual relative position of the eyes. Some squints can be corrected by surgery.

STAMMERING (or STUTTERING) when normal speech falters, with a repetition of the initial consonant of words. Usually it appears first in childhood but often responds to therapy.

STAGNANT LOOP SYNDROME when a segment of the SMALL INTESTINE is discontinuous with the rest or when there is an obstruction, either of which causes slow movement through the intestines. The result is bacterial growth with malabsorption and steatorrhoea (passage of fatty stools).

STENOSIS the abnormal narrowing of a blood vessel, heart valve or similar structure.

STENT a device used in surgery to help the healing of two structures that have been joined, by draining away the contents.

STERILIZATION the process of destroying all microorganisms on instruments and other objects by means of heat, radiation, etc.
Also, a surgical operation to render someone incapable of producing children.

Men usually undergo a VASECTOMY while in women it can be achieved by cutting and tying the FALLOPIAN TUBES, or removing them. The latter operation is performed via an incision in the abdominal wall or through the vagina.

STERNUM the breastbone.

STEROID one of a group of compounds resembling cholesterol, that are made up of four carbon rings fused together. The group includes the sterols (e.g. cholesterol), BILE acids, some HORMONES, and VITAMIN D. Synthetic versions act like steroid hormones and include derivatives of the glucocorticoids used as anti-inflammatory agents for RHEUMATOID ARTHRITIS; oral contraceptives, usually OESTROGEN and PROGESTERONE derivatives; anabolic steroids such as testosterone used to treat OSTEOPOROSIS and wasting.

STERTOR noisy breathing, similar to snoring, often heard in patients who are deeply unconscious.

STETHOSCOPE an instrument used to listen to sounds within the body, particularly the lungs and heart. The simplest type consists of earpieces for the examiner, leading via a tube to a diaphragm placed on the body.

STEVENS-JOHNSON SYNDROME a common hypersensitivity reaction to SULPHONAMIDE antibiotics, and a form of ERYTHEMA. It produces skin lesions and the eyes and mucosa may ulcerate.

STIFFNESS a condition with numerous causes, that results in a reduced movement in joints and muscles. The cause may be quite straightforward, e.g. physical injury, or it may be due to disease such as RHEUMATISM, MENINGITIS or central nervous system diseases.

STIGMA a mark or impression upon the skin, possibly one that is typical of a particular disease.

STILBOESTROL a synthetic OESTROGEN (female sex hormone) with several uses. It relieves menstrual disorders and meno-pause symptoms. It also proves helpful in treating breast and prostate cancers.

STILLBIRTH the birth of any child that provides no evidence of life.

STILL'S DISEASE a chronic ARTHRITIS affecting children and causing arthritis in several joints, with fever and a red rash. Some cases develop into ankylosing SPONDYLITIS and there is often muscle wasting. Illness may affect the whole body, complicated by other conditions, e.g. enlargement of the SPLEEN, and PERICARDITIS.

STIMULANT any drug or other agent that increases the rate of activity of an organ or system within the body. This assumes that the target organ is capable of increased activity which merely requires the necessary stimulus.

STITCH a sharp pain in the side often due to cramp after hard exertion (see also SPLEEN).

STOMA (plural **STOMATA**) an opening made in the abdominal surface to accommodate a tube from the colon or ileum. This operation is undertaken because of malignancy or inflammatory bowel diseases, e.g. Crohn's disease.

STOMACH an expansion of the alimentary canal that lies between the OESOPHAGUS and the DUODENUM. It has thick walls of SMOOTH MUSCLE that contract to manipulate the food, and its exits are controlled by SPHINCTERS, the cardiac anteriorly and the pyloric at the junction with the duodenum (see PYLORUS). Mucosal cells in the lining secrete GASTRIC JUICE. The food is reduced to an acidic semi-liquid which is moved on to the duodenum. The stomach varies in size but its greatest length is roughly 12 inches and the breadth 4 or 5 inches. Its capacity is approximately 1 to 1" litres.

STOOLS see FAECES.

STRANGULATION the constriction or closure of a passage or vessel. This may be due to the intestine twisting (VOLVULUS), or herniation of the intestine. Strangulation of a blood vessel and/or airway affects the organs being supplied and if vital organs are affected, can prove fatal.

STRANGURY the desire to pass water, which can only be done in a few drops and with accompanying pain. It is symptomatic of an irritation of the base of the bladder by a stone, cancer at this site, or CYSTITIS or PROSTATITIS.

STRAPPING the application of layers of adhesive plaster to cover part of the body and maintain moderate pressure, so as to prevent too much movement and provide rest, as with fractured ribs.

STREPTOCOCCUS a genus of Gram-positive (see GRAM'S STAIN) spherical bacteria that form chains. Many species are responsible for a variety of infections including scarlet fever, ENDOCARDITIS and pneumonia.

STRESS FRACTURE a fracture created by making excessive demands on the body, as commonly happens in sport. Treatment involves rest and analgesics for the pain.

STRICTURE a narrowing of a passage in the body, e.g. the URETHRA, OESOPHAGUS, or URETER. It may result from inflammation, a spasm, growth of a tumour or pressure from surrounding organs. In many cases it is due to ulceration and contraction of the subsequent scar tissue. With a urethral stricture, it becomes increasingly difficult to pass urine.

STRIDOR the noise created on breathing in when there is a narrowing of the upper airway, especially the LARYNX.

STROKE (or **APOPLEXY**) the physical effects, involving some form of paralysis, that result from an interruption to the brain's blood supply. The effect in the brain is secondary and the cause lies in the heart or blood vessels and may be a THROMBOSIS, EMBOLUS, or HAEMORRHAGE. The severity of a stroke varies greatly from a temporary weakness in a limb, or tingling, to paralysis, coma and death.

ST VITUS' DANCE the former name for Sydenham's CHOREA.

STYE a bacterial infection and inflammation of a gland at the base of an eyelash, resulting in a pus-filled cyst.

SUBARACHNOID HAEMORRHAGE bleeding into the SUBARACHNOID SPACE due often to a ruptured cerebral ANEURYSM. Initial symptoms are a severe headache, stiff neck, followed by vomiting, drowsiness and there may be a brief period of unconsciousness after the event. Brain damage is possible but severe haemorrhages may result in death.

SUBARACHNOID SPACE the space between the arachnoid and pia mater MENINGES covering the brain and spinal cord. It contains cerebrospinal fluid and blood vessels.

SUBCUTANEOUS general term meaning beneath the skin.

SUBDURAL term meaning below the dura mater, and referring to the space between this and the arachnoid MENINGES around the brain.

SUBPHRENIC ABSCESS an abscess occurring beneath the diaphragm and commonly on the right side. It may be due to infection after an operation or perforation of an organ, e.g. a peptic ulcer. Surgery is usually necessary although antibiotics may be effective.

SUDDEN INFANT DEATH SYNDROME (*or* COT DEATH) the sudden death of a baby, often occurring overnight, from unknown causes. A significant proportion (c. 20% in U.K.) of infant deaths occur this way. Although the cause is unknown numerous suggestions have been put forward from viral infection and allergic reaction to poor breathing control that be particularly susceptible to mild infections. Research continues.

SULPHONAMIDE one of a group of drugs containing the chemical group - SO_2NH_2. These drugs do not kill bacteria, but prevent bacterial growth and are thus very useful in controlling infections. Some side effects may occur but in general these are outweighed by the benefits.

SUNBURN skin damage caused by exposure to the ultra-violet rays in sunlight. This may vary from a reddening of the skin and itching to formation of blisters which can cause shock if a large area is affected. Fair-skinned people are more susceptible than others and it is advisable to take sun in gradual stages.

SUNSTROKE *see* HEATSTROKE.

SUPINE the position in which someone is lying on their back, face upwards.

SUPPOSITORY medication prepared in a form which enables it to be inserted into the rectum (or vagina). It may be a lubricant, drugs for treatment in the area of the rectum or anus, or for absorption. The suppository has to be inserted beyond the sphincter muscle to ensure retention.

SUPPURATION pus formation, whether on the surface (ulceration) or more deep seated (as with an ABSCESS).

SURGEON a qualified practitioner specializing in surgery.

SURGERY the branch of medicine that through operation treats disease and injuries or deformities.

SUSCEPTIBILITY when there is a lack of resistance to disease, due either to poor general health, or a deficiency in defence mechanism because of another condition, e.g. AIDS. Susceptibility can be decreased by vaccination, etc.

SUTURE the means whereby a wound or incision is closed in surgery, using threads of silk or catgut. There are several types of suture to deal with diverse situations.

Also, a type of joint across which there is no movement, e.g. as in the skull, where there are several sutures.

SWAB a general term applied to a pad of material used in various ways. It can be used to clean wounds, apply medication, remove blood during operations, and obtain samples from infected areas, e.g. throat, for further examination.

SWEAT *see* PERSPIRATION.

SWEAT GLANDS the glands in the EPIDERMIS of SKIN that project into the dermis and are under the control of the sympathetic nervous system (*see also*

PERSPIRATION). The glands occur over most of the body but are especially abundant on the forehead, palms of the hands and soles of the feet and under the arms.

SYMPATHETIC the term for a symptom or disease that occurs as a result of disease elsewhere in the body, e.g. injury of one eye and a related inflammation in the other due to them being connected by the lymphatics.

SYMPATHETIC NERVOUS SYSTEM with the parasympathetic nervous system (and acting in opposition to it), this makes up the AUTONOMIC NERVOUS SYSTEM. NORADRENALINE and ADRENALINE are the main NEUROTRANSMITTERS released by its nerve endings. Its functions include raising the heart beat rate, constricting blood vessels and inhibiting secretion of saliva.

SYMPTOM any evidence of a disease or disorder.

SYNAPSE the junction between two nerve cells, at which there is a minute gap. A nerve impulse bridges the gap via a NEUROTRANSMITTER (see also ACETYLCHOLINE). The chemical diffuses across the gap that connects the axon of one nerve cell to the dendrites of the next. Some brain cells have many thousand synapses.

SYNCOPE (fainting) a temporary loss of consciousness due to a fall in blood pressure and reduced supply of blood to the brain. It may occur after standing for a long time (particularly in hot weather), after shock or injury. Typical signs before an attack are sweating and light-headedness.

SYNDACTYLY a fusion of fingers or toes which is a CONGENITAL effect. It may affect two or more fingers through webbing, or result in complete fusion of all digits.

SYNDROME a number of symptoms and signs that together constitute a particular condition.

SYNOVIAL FLUID see SYNOVIAL MEMBRANE.

SYNOVIAL MEMBRANE (or **SYNOVIUM**) the inner membrane of a capsule that encloses a joint that moves freely. It secretes into the joint a thick lubricating fluid (synovial fluid) which may build up after injury to cause pain.

SYNOVITIS inflammation of the SYNOVIAL MEMBRANE that lines a joint capsule. The result is swelling with pain. It is associated with rheumatic disease, injury or infection (e.g. chronic tuberculosis). The treatment depends upon the cause of the condition and often a sample of the synovial fluid is taken for examination.

SYPHILIS an infectious, sexually-transmitted disease, caused by the bacterium *Treponema pallidum* which shows symptoms in three stages. Bacteria enter the body through mucous membranes during sexual intercourse and an ulcer appears in the first instance. Within a short time the LYMPH NODES locally and then all over the body enlarge and harden and this lasts several weeks. Secondary symptoms appear about two months after infection and include fever, pains, enlarged lymph nodes and a faint rash which is usually noticed on the chest. The bacterium is found in enormous numbers in the primary sores and any skin lesions of the secondary stage. The final stage may not appear until many months or years after infection and comprises the formation of numerous tumour-like masses throughout the body (in skin, muscle, bone, brain, spinal cord and other organs such as the liver, stomach. etc.).. This stage can cause serious damage to the heart, brain or spinal cod resulting in blindness, TABES DORSALIS, and mental disability. CONGENITAL syphilis is much rarer than the former, *acquired*, type. It is contracted by a developing foetus from the mother, across the placenta and symptoms show a few weeks after birth. Treatment of syphilis is with penicillin, but it should be administered early in the development of the disease.

SYRINGE an instrument used for injecting fluids into the body or the removal of body fluids for examination. In such cases, it comprises a hollow needle connected to a piston within a tube. Larger metal syringes are used to wash the outer ear and remove wax.

SYRUP a mixture of sugar, water and drug, used for the easy administration of medications which may taste unpleasant. It also provides a means of delivering drugs which would otherwise deteriorate when exposed to air.

SYSTEMIC general term referring to the body as a whole.

SYSTOLE the contraction of the heart that alternates with the resting phase (diastole). It usually refers to ventricular systole which at 0.3 seconds is three times longer than atrial systole.

SYSTOLIC PRESSURE see BLOOD PRESSURE.

TABES DORSALIS medically known as LOCOMOTOR ATAXIA, this is a complication of syphilis occurring 5 to 20 years after the initial infection. It affects the sensory nerves especially of the trunk and legs causing stabbing pains and unsteadiness in walking. There is often loss of bladder control and disturbance of vision if the optic nerves are involved. Treatment is by means of penicillin and the condition may be associated with *taboparesis* which is also called *general paralysis of the insane*.

TACHYCARDIA increased rate of heart beat which may be caused naturally as with exercise or be symptomatic of disease.

TALUS the ankle bone which articulates with the lower leg bones (TIBIA and FIBULA) above and also with the heel bone (*calcaneus*) below (see TARSUS).

TAMOXIFEN a drug used in the treatment of certain breast cancers.

TAMPON a plug of compressed gauze or cotton wool inserted into a wound or cavity to absorb fluid or blood.

TARGET CELL an abnormal form of ERYTHROCYTE (red blood cell) which is large and has a ringed appearance when stained and viewed microscopically, resembling a target. These cells are present in several kinds of anaemia including those due to iron-deficiency. They are also found when there is liver disease, a small SPLEEN, haemoglobin abnormalities (haemoglobinopathies) and THALASSAEMIA.

TARSUS a part of the foot in the region of the instep consisting of seven bones, chiefly the TALUS and the *calcaneus* (heel bone) and also the cuboid, navicular and three cuneiform bones.

TASTE the perception of flavour which is brought about by chemoreceptors (the TASTE BUDS) situated on the TONGUE. There are four main categories of taste: salt, sour, sweet and bitter.

TASTE BUDS the sensory receptors responsible for the perception of taste, located in the grooves around the papillae of the TONGUE, in the epiglottis, parts of the PHARYNX and soft palate. The taste buds are stimulated by the presence of dissolved food in the saliva and messages are sent via nerves to the brain where the information is interpreted and perceived.

TAXIS the returning to their normal position of displaced organs, parts of organs or bones by manipulation (see HERNIA).

TEETH see TOOTH.

TEMPERATURE (of the body) the normal body temperature is around 37°C (98.4°F) but it varies considerably both between individuals and in one person throughout the day. In addition, temperature differences occur between various areas of the body being lower in the skin than internally.

TEMPLE the side of the head above the level of the eye and the ear.

TEMPORAL relating or referring to the temple, e.g. *temporal artery*.

TEMPORAL LOBE one of the main areas of the CEREBRAL CORTEX in each of the CEREBRAL HEMISPHERES of the brain, occurring in the TEMPORAL region of the skull. A cleft known as the *lateral sulcus* separates it from the frontal lobe.

TEMPORAL LOBE EPILEPSY EPILEPSY which is centred within the temporal lobe caused by disease within the cortex. It is characterized by hallucinations involving the senses of taste, smell, hearing and sight and memory disturbances. During an attack, the person usually remains conscious but not fully and normally aware, and afterwards may not have any memory of what has occurred.

TENDINITIS inflammation of a tendon which often results from excessive or unaccustomed exercise but may also result from infection. Treatment involves rest, possibly splinting of an affected joint and corticosteroid injections, and the taking of ANALGESIC drugs.

TENDON a tough and inelastic white cord composed of bundles of COLLAGEN fibres which attaches a muscle to a bone. A tendon concentrates the pull of the muscle onto one point on the bone and the length and thickness varies considerably. The fibres of a tendon pass into, and become continuous with, those of the bone it serves. Many tendons are enclosed in tendon sheaths lined with SYNOVIAL MEMBRANE containing synovial fluid which reduces friction and enables easy movement to occur.

TENNIS ELBOW a form of TENDINITIS affecting the tendon at the outer part of the elbow which becomes inflamed and painful. It is caused by hard and excessive use of the arm and the treatment involves rest and corticosteroid injections.

TERATOGEN a substance or disease or any other factor which causes the production of abnormalities in a foetus. The drugs in this category include thalidomide and alcohol. German

measles and cytomegalovirus are among the infections.

TERATOGENESIS the processes which result in the development of physical abnormalities in a foetus.

TERATOMA a tumour that is composed of unusual tissues not normally found at that site and derived from partially developed embryological cells. Teratomas are most common in the ovary and testicle (particularly if latter undescended).

TESTICLE (TESTIS) one of the pair of male sex organs which are situated within the SCROTUM and which produce spermatozoa and secrete the hormone TESTOSTERONE. The testicles develop within the abdomen of the foetus but descend around the time of birth into the scrotum. Each testicle has an outer double membrane layer known as the *tunica vaginalis*. The tunica vaginalis contains an inner fibrous layer called the *tunica albuginea* which protects the testicle. The bulk of the testicle consists of numerous fine, convoluted tubules called seminiferous tubules which are lined with cells that produce the spermatozoa. In addition, other cells known as *sertoli cells*, occur which provide support and possibly nourishment for the developing spermatozoa. The tubules are supported by connective tissue containing nerves and blood vessels and also the *cells of Leydig* which are responsible for hormone production. The tubules connect with another highly folded tube called the *epididymis* which is about 7m long and connects with the VAS DEFERENS which leads to the URETHRA. The spermatozoa are passed by passive movement along the epididymis, completing their development as they go and are stored in the lower part until ejaculation.

TESTIS *see* TESTICLE.

TESTOSTERONE the male sex hormone secreted by the TESTES (*see also* ANDROGEN).

TETANUS a very serious and sometimes fatal infectious disease, the non-medical name for which is *lockjaw*.

It is caused by the bacterium *Clostridium tetani*, spores of which enter through a wound. Rapid multiplication of the bacteria produces a toxin which affects the nerves resulting in rigidity and spasm of muscles. Often there is high fever and the spasms cause extreme agony.
If respiratory muscles are involved death may occur by asphyxia. Effective antitoxin is available, although its effects are not permanent and it needs to be regularly maintained. Antibiotics such as penicillin are also effective against the bacteria.

TETANY an abnormal condition due to calcium metabolism disorder which may occur with a deficiency of vitamin D, hypoparathyroidism or ALKALOSIS. It results in convulsions, cramps and muscle twitching, particularly in the face, feet and hands.

THALAMUS one of a pair of masses of grey matter located within each side of the forebrain. Each is a centre for co-ordinating and relaying sensory information concerned with all the senses apart from that of smell.

THALASSAEMIA also known as *Cooley's anaemia*, this is an inherited form of ANAEMIA in which there is an abnormality in the HAEMOGLOBIN.
There is a continuation in the production of foetal haemoglobin and two forms of the disorder are recognized, T. major in which the disorder is inherited from both parents (HOMOZYGOUS) and T. minor. The *minor* form is usually symptomless but the *major* type causes, in addition to the severe anaemia, bone marrow abnormalities and enlargement of the spleen. Treatment is by means of repeated blood transfusions. The disease is widespread throughout the Mediterranean, Asia and Africa.

THALIDOMIDE a TERATOGENIC drug which was formerly prescribed for treatment of MORNING SICKNESS in pregnancy. It was withdrawn when it was discovered that it caused developmental damage to the foetus, particularly malformation of limbs.

THERAPEUTICS the area of medicine concerned with the various methods of healing and treatment.

THERAPY the treatment of disease.

THERMOGRAPHY a method of recording the heat produced by different areas of the body using photographic film sensitive to infrared radiation. Areas with good blood circulation produce more heat and this can occur abnormally if a tumour is present. The record thus obtained is a *thermogram* and this is one of the techniques used to detect breast tumours (*mammothermography*).

THIAMINE *see* VITAMIN B.

THIERSCH'S GRAFT a type of skin graft in which thin strips of skin, involving the epidermis and the upper layer of the dermis, are taken from one part of the body and placed on the wound which requires to be healed.

THIGH the part of the leg above the knee.

THORACOCENTESIS also known as *pleuracentesis*. The withdrawal, by means of a hollow needle inserted through the chest wall, of fluid from the pleural cavity.

THORAX the chest.

THROMBIN an enzyme derived from prothrombin, its inactive precursor, which is formed and is active during the final stages of blood clotting (*see* COAGULATION).

THROMBOCYTOPENIA a reduction in the number of PLATELETS in the blood associated most commonly with tumours (whether benign or malignant) or the reaction of the immune system to drugs. It is a common cause of bleeding disorders.

THROMBOEMBOLISM the situation in which a blood clot (THROMBUS) forms in one part of the circulation, usually a vein in the leg (phlebothrombosis), and a portion breaks off and becomes lodged elsewhere causing a total blockage (EMBOLISM). The embolism often involves the pulmonary artery or one of its branches and this is known as PULMONARY EMBOLISM.

THROMBOLYSIS the dissolving of

blood clots by enzyme activity. Natural enzymes produced within the body have this effect but drug treatment, especially involving streptokinase, may be used to break up clots following PULMONARY EMBOLISM, CORONARY THROMBOSIS and PHLEBOTHROMBOSIS.

THROMBOPHLEBITIS inflammation of the wall of a vein along with clot formation in the affected section of the vessel.

This is a complication of pregnancy and may be dangerous, involving a deep vein thrombosis which can result in PULMONARY EMBOLISM. The condition known as WHITE LEG, (plegmasia alba dolens) is thrombophlebitis especially of the femoral vein which can occur after childbirth.

THROMBOSIS the process of clotting within a blood vessel producing a THROMBUS. It may occur within an artery or vein, often one which is diseased or damaged, and can be very serious or even fatal, e.g. STROKE, CORONARY THROMBOSIS.

THROMBUS a blood clot within a vessel which partially or totally obstructs the circulation.

TROPHOBLASTIC relating to the tissue forming the wall of the BLASTO-CYST, the outer of which forms the outer layer of the placenta. Also used therefore to categorise related diseases e.g. cancer of the uterus, trophoblastic cancer.

THRUSH an infection caused by the fungus *Candida albicans* which affects the mucous membranes of the mouth and vagina producing white patches. It is a popular name given to a group of infections known as *candidiasis*.

THYMUS a gland, divided into two lobes, which is present in the neck and which forms a vital part of the immune system. It is especially large in children and important in the development of the immune response and the production of lymphoid tissue. After puberty, the thymus gradually begins to shrink. Bone marrow cells, known as *stem cells*, undergo maturation within the thymus

and one group, the *T. lymphocytes*, are dependent upon the gland. These are very important cells in the body which produce ANTIBODIES.

THYROIDECTOMY surgical removal of the thyroid gland.

THYROID GLAND a bilobed endocrine gland situated at the base and front of the neck. It is enclosed by fibrous tissue and well-supplied with blood, and internally consists of numerous vesicles containing a jelly-like colloidal substance. These vesicles produce thyroid hormone, which is rich in iodine, under the control of *thyroid stimulating hormone* (THYROTROPHIN STIMULATING HORMONE) released from the PITUITARY GLAND. Two hormones are produced by the gland, thyroxine and triiodothyronine, which are essential for the regulation of metabolism and growth. *See also* CRETINISM, MYXOEDEMA and HYPERTHYROIDISM.

THYROTOXIC ADENOMA a form of THYROTOXICOSIS or GRAVES' DISEASE.

THYROTOXICOSIS *see* GRAVES' DISEASE.

THYROTROPHIN RELEASING HORMONE a hormone produced and released from the HYPOTHALAMUS which acts on the anterior lobe of the PITUITARY GLAND which then releases THYROTROPHIN STIMULATING HORMONE (*see* THYROID).

THYROTROPHIN STIMULATING HORMONE a hormone produced and released by the anterior pituitary gland which stimulates the THYROID GLAND to produce its hormones (*see* THYROID).

THYROXINE an important hormone produced by the thyroid gland and used medically to treat conditions resulting from underactivity of this gland, e.g. CRETINISM and MYXOEDEMA.

TIBIA the larger of the two bones in the lower leg known as the shin bone articulating above with the FEMUR and with the TALUS of the ankle below.

TINNITUS any ringing or buzzing sound in the ear which does not have a real external cause. Many disorders of the ear can cause this, for example, hardened wax, Ménière's disease, drugs including aspirin and quinine, and damage to the auditory nerve. In many cases no underlying cause is found. Tinnitus cannot usually be suppressed altogether although certain drugs can help to dampen its effects.

TOLERANCE the adaptation of the body to a particular drug or substance so that over a period of time, there is a reduction in the response to a particular dose. Usually a larger dose must now be given to produce the same effect as before.

TOMOGRAPHY a particular technique using X-rays or ultrasound so that structures at a given depth are brought into sharp focus while those at other levels are deliberately blurred. In this way, pictures of *slices* of the body are obtained at different levels to build up a three-dimensional image. The image obtained is called a *tomogram*.

TONGUE the muscular and highly mobile organ attached to the floor of the mouth, the three main functions of which are manipulation of food during chewing prior to swallowing, taste and production of speech. The three areas of the tongue are the tip, body and root and it is covered with a mucous membrane which unites with that of the mouth and pharynx.

The tongue is anchored at the root by various muscles which attach it to the back of the mouth. In addition, the undersurface of the tongue is attached in the midline to the floor of the mouth by a fold of mucous membrane called the *frenulum lingae*. If this is attached too far forward to restrict the movement at the tip it causes the condition known as *tongue tie*.

The tongue has a furred appearance because its surface is covered with minute projections called papillae, of which there are three different kinds, filiform, fungiform and circumvallate. There are grooves surrounding the papillae in which the TASTE BUDS occur.

The tongue is well supplied with blood and receives branches from five different nerves on each side.

TONSILLECTOMY surgical removal of the TONSILS.

TONSILLITIS inflammation of the tonsils caused by bacterial or viral infection. The symptoms include a severe sore throat causing painful swallowing, accompanied by fever and earache, especially in children. The tonsils are swollen and white in appearance due to infected material exuded from them and glands in the neck are enlarged. Treatment is by means of antibiotics, especially penicillin and erythromycin, along with analgesics for pain relief.

TONSILS usually refers to the two small masses of lymphoid tissue situated on either side at the back of the mouth (the *palatine tonsils*). However, another pair occur below the tongue which are the *lingual tonsils* while the ADENOIDS are the PHARYNGEAL TONSILS. All are part of the body's protective mechanism against infection.

TOOTH a hard structure used for biting and chewing. Each tooth consists of a *root* embedded in a socket within the jawbone to which it is attached by the fibrous *periodontal membrane*. The projecting part of the tooth is called the *crown* which is covered with a hard resistant layer of *enamel*, (composed primarily of calcium phosphate and calcium carbonate). The root is covered with a thin hard layer of cementum. Most of the interior of the tooth consists of *dentine*, a hard ivory-like substance which surrounds the inner core or pulp. The pulp contains blood vessels and nerve fibres and is connected with the dentine by means of fine cellular processes. There are four different types of teeth, canine, incisor, premolar and molar.

TORPOR a state of physical and mental sluggishness which accompanies various mental disorders, some kinds of poisoning and may be present in elderly people with arterial disease.

TORSION twisting, often referring to an abnormal state of the whole or part of an organ which impairs the nerve and blood supply. Examples are a torsion of a loop of bowel or of the spermatic cord of the testicle. Surgery is usually required to correct a torsion.

TOUCH the sense which is conferred by specialized sensory receptors present in the skin (and also in muscles and other areas of the body), which enable sensations of pain, temperature, pressure and touch to be perceived. The sense organs involved are specially adapted to respond to particular sensations conveying their messages to the brain along different nerve pathways.

TOURNIQUET a device used to arrest bleeding, usually from an artery in a limb, which may be a length of bandage, rubber tube or cord tied tightly round generally as an emergency measure. Direct pressure on a wound is now considered to be preferable as a first aid measure, because a tourniquet can deprive all the tissues of oxygen by arresting the circulation, and there is a risk of damage and of gangrene.

TOXAEMIA blood poisoning resulting from the toxins produced by rapidly multiplying bacteria at a localized site of infection such as an abscess. Symptoms are varied including fever, vomiting and diarrhoea and a general feeling of being unwell. The source of the infection has to be treated with antibiotic drugs. Toxaemia of pregnancy involves two relatively rare conditions known as ECLAMPSIA and PRE-ECLAMPSIA.

TOXICOLOGY the scientific study of poisons and their effects.

TOXIC SHOCK SYNDROME a state of acute shock due to SEPTICAEMIA and caused by toxins produced by *staphylococcal* bacteria. The symptoms include high fever, skin rash and diarrhoea and can prove rapidly fatal if not adequately treated with antibiotics,

especially PENICILLIN and *cephalosporin*, along with fluid and salt replacement. The syndrome is associated with the use of tampons by women during menstruation. It is thought that young women or girls whose immune system is not fully developed may be at greater risk, particularly if a tampon is left in place too long. However, the syndrome can also occur in other people and is in all cases rare.

TOXIN a poison produced by bacteria and by many species of plant and also present in snake venom. In the body, a toxin acts as an ANTIGEN and provokes the production of special antibodies called antitoxins. The antitoxins produced may be used in IMMUNIZATION to protect against the disease as with tetanus and diphtheria. An *endotoxin* is contained within the bacterial cell and only released when the organism dies and decays. Endotoxins do not provoke antitoxin production (*see* TOXOID).

TOXOCARIASIS a disease caused by the larvae of roundworms which normally infect the domestic dog (*Toxicara canis*) and cat (*Toxicara cati*), but can be passed to man by swallowing material contaminated with eggs in infected faeces.

Those most at risk are children, especially at a young age when hands may become infected while playing. Once swallowed, the larvae which hatch from the eggs travel around the body in the circulation and can cause considerable damage to, for example, the lungs and liver. Also, the larvae may lodge in the retina of the eye causing inflammation and the production of abnormal granulated tissue called granuloma. Symptoms of the infection include muscular pain, fever, skin rash, respiratory problems, vomiting and convulsions. Treatment is with drugs, such as diethylcarbamazine and thiabendazole.

TOXOID a preparation of TOXIN which has been treated with chemicals so that it cannot cause disease but is able to provoke the production of antitoxin. This is the basis of VACCINES against diphtheria and tetanus.

TOXOPLASMOSIS an infectious disease caused by a protozoan organism known as *Toxoplasma*. The infection is either transmitted by eating undercooked meat or through direct contact with contaminated soil or especially with infected cats. This form of the infection is mild and causes few ill effects. However, a much more serious form of the disease can be passed from a mother infected during pregnancy to her unborn baby. The newborn infant may suffer from HYDROCEPHALUS, mental retardation, blindness or may even be stillborn. Treatment is by means of sulphonamide drugs and pyrimethamine.

TRACER a substance which is marked so that when it is introduced into the body its progress can be followed e.g. radioactive tracers used in the detection of brain tumours and thyroid disease.

TRACHEA the windpipe which is the part of the air passage that is situated between the LARYNX and the bronchi.

TRACHEITIS inflammation of the trachea, often accompanying a viral infection of the upper respiratory tract. The symptoms include a persistent painful cough and sore chest and it often accompanies BRONCHITIS and also DIPHTHERIA.

TRACHEOSTOMY (or TRACHEOT-OMY) a surgical procedure in which a hole is made in the trachea to allow direct access of air to the lower respiratory passages. This may be performed in an emergency if there is an obstruction in breathing. However, usually this operation is carried out in hospital, especially on patients in intensive therapy who require long-term artificial ventilation. This is to avoid the damage to the trachea which is caused by the long-term use of an endotracheal breathing tube (inserted through the nose or mouth) which would normally be used first.

Tracheostomy is also used in cases of diphtheria, where the obstruction is a large tumour or where there is nerve damage. Once the opening has been made a double tube is inserted and held in place by tapes around the neck. The inner tube can be freely withdrawn and replaced and needs to be kept scrupulously clean and free from any obstruction.

TRACTION the use of weights and pulleys to apply a pulling force on a broken bone, to ensure that it is kept correctly aligned while healing takes place.

TRANCE a sleep-like state in which a person ceases to react normally to the environment and loses the power of voluntary movement, but remains aware. It can be induced by HYPNOSIS, meditation, hysteria, CATATONIA and drug abuse.

TRANQUILLIZER a drug that has a soothing and calming effect, relieving stress and anxiety. Minor tranquilizers such as diazepam and chlordiazepoxide are widely used to relieve these symptoms which may arise from a variety of causes. There is a danger of dependence with long-term use. Major tranquillizers e.g. chlorpromazine and haloperidol are used to treat severe mental illnesses such as SCHIZOPHRENIA.

TRANSFUSION *see* BLOOD TRANSFUSION.

TRANSPLANTATION the transfer of an organ or tissue from one person to another (*called an allotransplant*) or within the body of an individual (*autotransplant*). It overwhelmingly refers to skin and bone GRAFTING. The person from whom the organ is obtained is known as the *donor* and the one who receives it is known as the *recipient*. Organ transplants involving the kidney, heart, bone marrow, cornea, lungs and liver have all become more common. Success varies but is improving in all areas especially with the advent of *immunosuppressive* drugs to prevent organ rejection by the recipient's immune system. *See also* IMMUNOSUPPRESSION and GRAFT.

TRAUMA an event which causes physical damage such as a fracture or an emotional shock brought about by a harmful and upsetting circumstance.

TREMOR involuntary movements which may involve the whole of a muscle or only part of it and produce fine trembling or more pronounced shaking. Tremors are classified according to the type of movement produced and are a symptom of many diseases including CHOREA, MULTIPLE SCLEROSIS and PARKINSONISM.

TRENCH FEVER an infectious disease caused by *Rickettsia quintana* which was epidemic among troops in the First World War and still occurs in Mexico. It is transmitted to man by the body louse and causes fever, rash, leg aches and general weakness.

TRICEPS a three-headed muscle present in the upper arm which extends the forearm.

TRICHOMONIASIS two types of infection caused by a protozoan organism which either attacks the digestive system causing DYSENTERY (*Trichomonas hominis*), or causes vaginal inflammation and discharge (*Trichomonas vaginalis*). In the latter case the infection can be transmitted to a male sexual partner. The drug metronidazole is highly effective.

TRICHORRHOEA the medical name for the falling out of hair which may be due to disease such as typhoid fever or scarlet fever or have no apparent cause.

TRICUSPID VALVE a valve with three flaps or cusps that controls the passage of blood from the right ATRIUM to the right VENTRICLE of the heart and normally prevents backflow (*see* HEART).

TRIGEMINAL NERVE the fifth and largest of the cranial nerves which has three divisions, the *mandibular, maxillary* and *ophthalmic* nerves. The ophthalmic and maxillary nerves are sensory nerves and the mandibular has both sensory and motor functions. Hence the trigeminal nerve is involved in the relaying and perception of sensations (temperature, touch, pain, etc.) from the whole of the face and mouth and also in controlling the muscles involved in chewing.

TRIGEMINAL NEURALGIA also known as Tic Doulourex. This is a severe form of NEURALGIA which can affect all the divisions of the trigeminal nerve. It affects women more commonly than men, especially those over the age of 50. It causes severe pain of a burning or cutting nature which can be constant or spasmodic and may be provoked by simple actions such as eating or by heat or cold. The skin of the face may be inflamed and the eye red and watery and the neuralgia is usually confined to one side. The condition is debilitating in that the pain is so intense and interferes with sleeping and eating but the drug carbamazepine is proving to be highly beneficial.

TRIGLYCERIDES fats consisting of three fatty acid molecules combined with glycerol which are the form in which the body stores fat. Triglycerides are derived from the digestion of fats in food.

TROPHIC a term referring to nutrition, e.g. trophic fracture which occurs when the bone is weakened due to poor nourishment in the person concerned.

TRUSS a device consisting of a pad attached to a belt with spring straps to maintain its position, which is worn under clothing to support a HERNIA.

TRYPANOSOMIASIS *see* SLEEPING SICKNESS.

TRYPSIN an important enzyme involved in the digestion of proteins. Its inactive precursor, trypsinogen, is secreted by the PANCREAS and converted to trypsin in the DUODENUM by the action of another enzyme called enteropeptidase.

TUBERCLE either a small rounded knob on a bone e.g. on the ribs or a minute nodular tissue mass (lesion) which is characteristic of TUBERCULOSIS.

TUBERCULOSIS a group of infections caused by the bacillus (bacterium) *Mycobacterium tuberculosis* of which pulmonary tuberculosis of the lungs (consumption or phthisis) is the best known form. The pulmonary disease is acquired through inhalation of air containing the organism from an infected person, or dust laden with bacteria.

People infected in this way can show no symptoms but still be carriers. In the lungs, the infection causes formation of a *primary tubercle* which spreads to lymph nodes to form the *primary complex*.

The disease may wax and wane for years as the body's natural immune system acts against the infection. If the infection is severe, symptoms include fever, wasting, night sweats and the coughing up of blood. The bacteria may enter the blood stream and spread throughout the body setting up numerous tubercles in other tissues (*miliary tuberculosis*).

The organism may also be acquired by eating contaminated food, especially milk, in which case the production of a primary complex in abdominal lymph nodes can lead to PERITONITIS. Rarely, the infection is acquired via a cut from contact with an infected person or animal.

Tuberculosis affects people throughout the world (about 6000 new cases each year in England and Wales). Many people acquire the infection and recover without suspecting its presence and the disease is curable with antibiotics, e.g. streptomycin. In addition, BCG VACCINATION as a preventive measure is given to children in the UK, in addition to X-ray screening to detect carriers.

TUMOUR any abnormal swelling occurring in any part of the body consisting of an unusual growth of tissue and which may be malignant or benign. Tumours tend to be classified according to the tissue of which they are composed, e.g. FIBROMA (mainly fibrous tissue) and

MYOMA (largely muscle fibres).

TURGOR a state of being distended, engorged or swollen.

TURNER'S SYNDROME a genetic disorder affecting females in which there is only one X chromosome instead of the usual two. Hence those affected have 45 instead of 46 chromosomes, are infertile (as the ovaries are absent), menstruation is absent and breasts and body hair do not develop. Those affected are short, may have webbing of the neck and other developmental defects. The heart may be affected and there can be deafness and intellectual impairment. In a less severe form of the disorder, the second X chromosome is present but abnormal, lacking in normal genetic material.

TYMPANIC MEMBRANE the eardrum which separates the middle and outer ears and which vibrates in response to sound waves transmitting the vibrations to one of the ear ossicles (the *malleus*). See EAR.

TYPHOID FEVER a severe infectious disease of the digestive system which is caused by the bacterium *Salmonella typhi* and causes symptoms including a rise in temperature, a rash on the abdomen and chest, headache and nosebleeds.

The temperature rise occurs in a characteristic fashion known as a *step-ladder temperature*. In severe cases there may be ulceration of the intestinal wall leading to PERITONITIS if an ulcer bursts, or haemorrhage from the bowels and inflammation of the lungs, SPLEEN and bones. In these cases the disease can prove to be fatal.

The infection is acquired through ingesting contaminated food or water hence preventive measures involving high standards of hygiene and sanitation are important. Drug treatment is by means of antibiotics such as chloramphenicol and ampicillin. Inoculation with TAB vaccine confers temporary immunity.

TYPHUS FEVER *see* RICKETTSIA.

ULCER a break on the skin surface or on the MUCOUS MEMBRANE lining within the body cavities that may be inflamed and fails to heal. Ulcers of the skin include BEDSORES and varicose ulcers (which are caused by defective circulation). For ulcers of the alimentary tract, see DUODENAL ULCER, GASTRIC ULCER and PEPTIC ULCER.

ULNA one of the two bones making up the forearm. It is the inner and longer of the two bones (the other being the radius). It articulates with the radius at both ends and additionally with the humerus above, and indirectly with the wrist below.

ULTRASOUND (*or* **ULTRASONIC WAVES**) high frequency sound waves (above 20 kHz), beyond the range of the human ear. Ultrasound is used to examine the body's organs, ducts, etc. in addition to assessing the progress of a developing foetus. The patient is not submitted to harmful radiation as with other techniques and no contrast medium is required. It can be used to examine the liver, kidney, bladder, pancreas, ovaries and is used in diagnosing brain tumours. The vibrations of the sound waves can be used in other ways, e.g. breaking up kidney stones.

UMBILICAL CORD the cord connecting the foetus to the placenta, containing two arteries and one vein. It is approximately 60cm long and after birth it is severed and the stump shrivels to leave a scar, the navel or *umbilicus*.

UMBILICUS the navel (*see* UMBILICAL CORD).

UNCONSCIOUSNESS the state of being partially or totally unaware of the surroundings and lacking in response to stimuli. Sleep is a natural form of unconsciousness. Unnatural states of unconsciousness can be due to numerous causes including injuries to the brain resulting in compression or concussion, fainting due to insufficient blood supply to the brain, EPILEPSY, poisoning and various diseases, e.g. DIABETES MELLITUS.

UNDULANT FEVER *see* BRUCELLOSIS.

UNGUAL a term meaning relating to the fingernails or toenails.

UNGUENTUM the term in pharmacy for an ointment.

UNGUIS a fingernail or toenail.

URAEMIA the condition where there is excess UREA in the blood due to kidney disease or failure. Waste products are usually excreted by the kidneys but accumulation in the blood leads to headaches, drowsiness and lethargy, nausea and vomiting and diarrhoea. Eventually, without treatment, death follows. Haemodialysis on a kidney machine may be necessary or even a renal transplant.

URATAEMIA the presence in the blood of urate compounds (*see* URIC ACID), associated with GOUT, when urates are deposited in the body.

UREA a metabolic byproduct of the chemical breakdown of protein and the form in which excess nitrogen is removed from the body, in urine. It is formed in the LIVER and taken in the blood to the KIDNEYS. The amount excreted daily is 30-35gm. Although urea is not poisonous in itself, an excess in the blood (URAEMIA) implies a defective kidney which will cause an excess of other waste products that may be poisonous.

UREAPLASMA microorganisms responsible for diseases such as PROSTATITIS, non-specific URETHRITIS and infertility and NEONATAL death. The latter can be associated with infection of the placenta by *Ureaplasma urealyticum*.

URETER the tubes joining the KIDNEYS to the bladder and through which urine passes. The muscular ureter walls contract to force urine into the bladder.

URETERECTOMY surgical excision of a URETER, usually with the removal of the associated kidney.

URETERITIS inflammation of the URETER which usually occurs with bladder inflammations.

URETEROENTEROSTOMY the creation by surgery of a link between the URETER and the bowel, thus bypassing the bladder. The join is made at the SIGMOID COLON and is made to pass a diseased bladder. The urine is then passed with the faeces, thus avoiding an external opening for collection of urine.

URETEROPLASTY reconstruction of a damaged or diseased ureter by surgery, using bowel or bladder tissue.

URETEROSCOPE an instrument introduced into a dilated URETER often to locate a stone or remove stone fragments created by ultrasonic destruction of a larger stone.

URETEROSTOMY the creation of an external opening to the URETER whereby the ureter is brought to the surface to permit drainage.

URETEROTOMY an incision into the URETER, commonly to remove a stone.

URETHRA the duct carrying urine from the bladder out of the body. It is about 3.5cm long in women and 20cm in men. The male urethra runs through the penis and also forms the ejaculatory duct.

URETHRITIS inflammation of the mucous lining of the urethra which may be associated with CYSTITIS, often being the cause of the latter. The commonest cause or urethritis is GONORRHOEA (*specific*). Alternatively, it may be due to infection with microorganisms (causing *non-specific* urethritis). The symptoms include pain on passing urine, a discharge, and possible inflammations in other organs such as the bladder and testicle. Sulphonamide and antibiotic drugs are effective, once the infecting organism is identified.

URIC ACID an organic acid that contains nitrogen and is the end-product of the metabolism of protein. It occurs in the urine but in small amounts (<1gm). It is formed in the liver and excreted by the kidneys but in excess, salts (urates) form and occur as stone in the urinary tract. Deposits of urates in joints is a feature of GOUT.

URINARY ORGANS the system responsible for the extraction of components from the blood to form urine, its storage and periodic discharge from the body. The organs are the kidneys, ureters, bladder and urethra (*see individual entries*).

URINARY TRACT the system of ducts that permit movement of urine out of the body from the kidneys, i.e. the URETERS, BLADDER and URETHRA.

URINATION (*or* **MICTURITION**) the discharge of urine from the body via the URETHRA. It is begun by a voluntary relaxation of the sphincter muscle below the bladder.

URINE the body's fluid waste excreted by the KIDNEYS. The waste products include UREA, URIC ACID and creatinine (produced by muscles) with salt, phosphates and sulphates and ammonia also present. In a solution with about 95-96% water, there may be 100 or more compounds but the vast majority occur only in trace amounts.
Many diseases alter the quantity and composition of urine and its analysis is standard procedure to assist diagnosis of diseases.

URINE RETENTION the condition when urine is produced by the kidneys but it is retained in the bladder. This may be due to an obstruction, or a weakness in the bladder (less common).
Enlargement of the PROSTATE GLAND is a common cause of blockage. It may also be caused by a STRICTURE due to injury scar or ulceration.

URINOGENITAL a collective descriptive term relating to all organs and tissues involved in excretion and reproduction, because they are closely linked anatomically and functionally.

UROLOGY the subdiscipline of

medicine dealing with diseases of the urinary tract, from the kidney to the urethra.

URTICARIA (*or* **NETTLE RASH**) an allergic reaction by an individual to some substance to which they are hypersensitive, in which the allergic response is manifested on the skin. Raised red patches develop which may last for hours or days. There is intense itching. The sensitivity may be to certain foods, e.g. shellfish, and the effect may occur anywhere on the body, but commonly erupts on the face and trunk. If it also affects the tongue or throat, there is danger of a blockage of the airway which would need urgent attention.

UTERINE relating to the UTERUS.

UTERUS (*or* **WOMB**) a vaguely pear-shaped organ within the cavity of the pelvis that is specialized for the growth and nourishment of a foetus. FALLOPIAN TUBES connect to the upper part and the lower part joins the VAGINA at the CERVIX. It has a plentiful blood supply with lymphatic vessels and nerves. During pregnancy it enlarges considerably and the SMOOTH MUSCLE walls thicken. Contractions of the muscular wall push the foetus out via the vagina at childbirth. If there is no pregnancy the lining undergoes periodic changes (MENSTRUATION).

UVEA the middle pigmented layer of the EYE consisting of the IRIS, choroid and ciliary body.

UVEITIS inflammation of any part of the UVEA. The iris and ciliary body are often both inflamed (*anterior uveitis*) producing a painful condition, unlike *posterior uveitis* (when the choroid is affected). The disease may follow from affected areas elsewhere in the eye. Symptoms may include blurred vision with discomfort or pain and diseases or conditions with which it is known to be linked are arthritis, tuberculosis, syphilis, viral and parasitic infections.

VACCINATION the production of immunity to a disease by inoculation with a VACCINE or a specially prepared material that stimulates the production of antibodies. It was used initially to refer only to cowpox virus (which also protected against SMALLPOX) but now is synonymous with inoculation, in immunizing against disease.

VACCINE a modified preparation of a BACTERIUM or VIRUS that is no longer dangerous but will stimulate development of antibodies and therefore confer immunity against actual infection with the disease. Other vaccines consist of specific toxins (e.g. tetanus), or dead bacteria (e.g. cholera and typhoid). Live but weakened organisms are used against smallpox and tuberculosis.

VAGINA the lower part of the female reproductive tract that leads from the uterus to the outside. It receives the erect penis during sexual intercourse, the semen being ejaculated into the upper part from where the sperms pass through the CERVIX and UTERUS to the FALLOPIAN TUBES. The vagina is essentially a muscular tube lined with mucous membrane.

VAGINISMUS a sudden and painful contraction of muscles surrounding the VAGINA in response to contact of the vagina or VULVA, e.g. an attempted intercourse. It may be due to a fear of intercourse or an inflammation.

VAGINITIS inflammation of the vagina due to infection or deficiency in diet, or hygiene. There may be itching, a discharge and pain on urination.

VAGOTOMY the cutting of fibres of the vagus nerve to the stomach. The operation can be performed to reduce the stomach's acid and pepsin secretion, in treatment of a PEPTIC ULCER.

VAGUS the tenth cranial nerve which comprises motor, sensory, vasodilator and secretory fibres. It supplies the muscles for swallowing and fibres go to the heart, throat, lungs and stomach and other organs in the abdomen. It also carries the taste sensation from the mouth.

VALVE a structure within an organ or vessel that restricts flow to one direction, whether the fluid be blood or lymph. The valves comprise cusps on the vessel wall. The cusp is like a membranous pocket that fills with blood should it flow back and the cusps distend and close the valve.

VALVULAR HEART DISEASE affects mainly the AORTIC and MITRAL VALVES which may narrow (STENOSIS) or weaken. Aortic valve disease is associated more with old age while mitral valve disease is rheumatic in origin.

VALVOTOMY an operation undertaken to open a stenosed heart valve and render it functional. A number of techniques are available including surgery, an inflating balloon or a dilating instrument.

VALVULITIS inflammation of a valve, particularly in the heart. It is commonly due to rheumatic fever.

VAPORIZER a device that produces a mist of liquid medication for inhalation. It is commonly used in the treatment of asthma.

VARICOSE VEINS veins that have become stretched, distended and twisted. The superficial veins in the legs are often affected although it may occur elsewhere. Causes include congenitally defective valves, obesity, pregnancy and thrombophlebitis (inflammation of the wall of a vein with secondary THROMBOSIS in the affected part of the vein). Elastic support is a common treatment although alternatives are SCLEROTHERAPY and PHLEBECTOMY.

VARIOLA a name for SMALLPOX.

VAS a vessel or duct, especially those carrying blood, lymph or spermatozoa.

VASCULAR relating to blood vessels; supplied with blood vessels.

VASCULITIS inflammation of the blood vessels that may cause damage to the linings and cause narrowing. It may result from several conditions including acute NEPHRITIS and SERUM SICKNESS.

VAS DEFERENS the tubes that join the testes to the ejaculatory duct via the PROSTATE GLAND. It carries spermatozoa to the URETHRA on ejaculation, aided by contraction of its muscular wall.

VASECTOMY the cutting of the VAS DEFERENS, which is performed on both ducts causing sterility, although the effect is not immediate.

VASOCONSTRICTION the narrowing of blood vessels with a consequent reduction in blood supply to that part of the body supplied. A variety of circumstances can cause vasoconstriction including cold and shock.

VASODILATION (VASODILATATION) the increase in diameter of blood vessels producing a lowering of blood pressure.

VASOPRESSIN (ANTIDIURETIC HORMONE) a PITUITARY GLAND hormone that constricts blood vessels and reduces urine secretion by increasing the quantity of water reabsorbed by the KIDNEY.

VASOVAGAL ATTACK fainting, precipitated by a slowing of the heart and a fall in blood pressure. This may be due to shock, severe pain, fear, etc. and is caused by excessive stimulation of the VAGUS nerve which participates in the control of breathing and the circulation.

VASOVASOSTOMY the reversal of VASECTOMY.

VECTOR commonly an insect that carries parasitic microorganisms between people, or from animals to people, e.g. mosquitoes carrying malaria.

VEIN one of the numerous blood vessels carrying deoxygenated blood to the right atrium of the heart (the one exception is the PULMONARY vein). Each vein has three tissue layers, similar to the layers of the heart. Veins are less elastic than arteries and collapse when cut. They also contain VALVES to prevent backflow.

VENA CAVA either of two major veins carrying blood from other veins to the right ATRIUM of the heart. The *inferior* vena cava takes blood from the body below the DIAPHRAGM and the *superior* vena cava takes blood from the head, neck, arms and thorax.

VENEREAL DISEASE (or SEXUALLY TRANSMITTED DISEASE) a disease transmitted by sexual intercourse. This includes AIDS, SYPHILIS, GONORRHOEA, non-specific URETHRITIS, etc.

VENOGRAPHY examination of veins using X-rays after injection of a radio-opaque substance. This enables leaks, blockages or other abnormalities to be identified.

VENOM the poisonous substance produced by snakes, scorpions, etc. which in humans may produce only localized pain and swelling, or in serious cases cause more general effects and even death.

VENTILATION the means whereby air passes into and out of the lungs, aided by movement of the diaphragm. *Artificial* ventilation is the usse of a machine (VENTILATOR) to regulate and perform a person's breathing. This may be during an operation. Also, damage to the relevant part of the brain, chest injury, lung disease or nerve and muscle disorders may all require the use of artificial ventilation.

VENTILATOR the machine used to provide an air supply to the lungs of patients who cannot breathe normally for themselves. Blood gases and other body functions can be monitored at the same time.

VENTOUSE (or VACUUM EXTRACTOR) a machine used in childbirth. It comprises a suction cup which is attached to the head of the foetus enabling it to be gently pulled out of the uterus. It is an alternative to the use of forceps.

VENTRICLE one of the two major chambers within the heart. They are thick-walled and muscular and form the main pumping chamber. The right ventricle receives blood from the right ATRIUM and venae cavae and its outflow is the pulmonary artery. The left ventricle takes blood from the pulmonary vein via the left atrium, and its outflow is the AORTA. Also cavities within the brain, filled with cerebrospinal fluid.

VENTRICULAR FIBRILLATION a rapid ARRHYTHMIA of the ventricle which is dangerous.

VERRUCA a term for WART.

VERRUCOSE covered with WARTS.

VERSION also known as *turning*, the procedure to move a foetus in the uterus to a more normal position, to make delivery easier.

VERTEBRA (plural VERTEBRAE) any of the bones making up the vertebral column. Each has a cavity (the vertebral canal or foramen) and various processes for attachment of muscles or articulation of adjacent vertebrae. The spinal cord passes through the vertebral canal (*see* SPINAL COLUMN).

VERTEBRAL COLUMN *see* SPINAL COLUMN.

VERTIGO a condition in which a person has a false sensation of imbalance and of the surroundings moving. It is commonly a sensation of spinning but may be as if the ground is tilting. The semicircular canals of the ear are fundamental in the maintenance of balance and vertigo is generally due to some problem with this mechanism or with the appropriate centres in the brain.

VESICULAR BREATHING soft, normal sounds of breathing heard in the lung by means of a stethoscope. The sounds change when the lungs are diseased and the different sounds help a doctor diagnose the disease.

VESSEL any tube that carries fluid, particularly blood or lymph.

VESTIGIAL the term applied to an organ that has progressively, over a long time, lost its function and structure to become rudimentary.

VILLUS (plural VILLI) *see* JEJUNUM.

VINCENT'S ANGINA a former name

for ulcerative GINGIVITIS and ulcerative inflammation of the throat, caused by bacteria.

VIRAL HAEMORRHAGIC FEVER a viral disease with a high mortality rate. After the incubation period there is headache, fever, severe internal bleeding, diarrhoea and vomiting. Death may follow, usually eight or nine days later. Serum taken from someone recovering from the disease is a useful source of antibodies.

VIRAL PNEUMONIA an acute lung infection caused by one of a number of viruses. The symptoms include fever, headache, muscle pains and a thick sputum associated with the cough. It often occurs after a viral infection and treatment, in the main, deals with the symptoms only.

VIROLOGY the study of viruses.

VIRULENCE the ability of a bacterium of virus to cause disease, measured by numbers of people infected, the speed with which it spreads through the body, etc.

VIRUS the smallest microbe that is completely parasitic, because it is only capable of replication within the cells of its host. Viruses infect animals, plants and microorganisms. Viruses are classified according to their nucleic acids and can contain double or single-stranded DNA or RNA. In an infection the virus binds to the host cells and then penetrates to release the viral DNA or RNA which controls the cell's metabolism to replicate itself and form new viruses. Viruses cause many diseases including influenza (single-stranded RNA), herpes (double-stranded DNA), AIDS (a RETROVIRUS, single-stranded RNA) and also mumps, chickenpox and polio.

VISCERA the term for organs within the body cavity, usually the abdominal cavity.

VISION the capacity for sight. Light enters the eye through the cornea and the aqueous humour. Next, it passes through the pupil, lens and vitreous humour to impinge upon the retina. There the ROD and CONE cells detect light and send impulses to the nerve fibres, impulses which are relayed to the visual cortex in the brain. Visual acuity is the sharpness of vision, dependent upon a healthy retina and accurate lens (*see* SNELLES CHART).

VITAL CAPACITY the largest volume of air that can be exhaled after breathing in deeply.

VITAMIN any of a group of organic compounds required in very small amounts in the diet to maintain good health. Deficiencies lead to specific diseases. Vitamins are divided into two groups: vitamins A, D, E and K are fat-soluble while C and B are water soluble.

VITAMIN A (*or* RETINOL) a fat-soluble vitamin that must be in the diet as it cannot be synthesized in the body. It occurs in dairy products, egg yolk and liver and is available as a precursor in green vegetables. It is essential for vision in dim light, growth and the maintenance of mucous tissue.

VITAMIN B any of a group of vitamins that although they are not related chemically, they are often found in the same types of food (*see following entries and* BIOTIN).

VITAMIN B1 (THIAMINE) a vitamin active in the form thiamine pyrophosphate, a deficiency of which leads to BERIBERI. Thiamine can be found in cereals, meat, beans, nuts and potatoes.

VITAMIN B2 (RIBOFLAVIN) a vitamin important in tissue respiration (enzyme reactions in cells) although a deficiency is not serious. Sources are milk, liver and eggs.

VITAMIN B3 (PANTOTHENIC ACID) a vitamin that occurs widely in foods and which is therefore unlikely to be lacking in the diet.

VITAMIN B6 (PYRIDOXINE) a vitamin found in many foods (liver, fish, yeast and cereals). It is important in the metabolism of several amino acids.

VITAMIN B12 (CYANOCOBALAMIN) an important vitamin, in the synthesis of nucleic acids, maintenace of MYELIN surrounding nerve fibres and in the production of red blood cells. It is found in fish, liver, eggs and dairy products. A deficiency produces anaemia and degeneration of the nervous system.

VITAMIN C (ASCORBIC ACID) a vitamin found in citrus fruits and vegetables. It is essential in maintaining cell walls and connective tissue and a deficiency leads to fragility of tendons, blood vessels and skin - all characteristic of the disease called scurvy. The presence of ascorbic acid is believed to assist the uptake of iron during digestion.

VITAMIN D this vitamin occurs as two steroid derivations: D_2 or calciferol in yeast and D_3 or cholecalciferol which is produced by the action of sunlight on the skin. The dietary source of vitamin D is fish liver oils, eggs and dairy products and it is vital in control of blood calcium levels. It prompts an increase in calcium takeup in the gut, increasing the supply for the production of bone. It also affects phosphorus uptake. A deficiency leads to RICKETS and OSTEOMALACIA.

VITAMIN E a group of compounds (tocopherols) thought to prevent damage to cell membranes. Vitamin E is found in cereal grains, green vegetables and eggs. A deficiency is unusual due to its widespread occurrence in foods.

VITAMIN H see BIOTIN.

VITAMIN K a vitamin that is essential for the clotting of blood as it is involved in the formation of prothrombin (the inactive precursor of THROMBIN) in the liver. The main food sources are spinach, leafy vegetables and liver but a deficiency rarely occurs because the vitamin is synthesized by bacteria in the large intestine.

VITREOUS HUMOUR the jelly-like substance occurring between the lens and the retina in the EYE.

VOCAL CORDS two membranes in the LARYNX that vibrate to produce sound when air is expelled over them. Tension in the cords is controlled by muscles and tendons, thus changing the sound generated.

VOLKMANN'S CONTRACTURE a condition often caused by pressure from

a cast or tight bandage on the arm. The result is persistent contraction (flexion) of forearm muscles and decreased blood supply to hand and arm. The muscles then swell and become fibrosed.

VOLUNTARY MUSCLE (or STRIATED MUSCLE) muscle that is under conscious control, e.g. those muscles operating the skeleton. It consists of bundles of elongated fibres surrounded by connective tissue. A tendon at the end of the muscle attaches it to the bone. Each muscle fibre comprises smaller fibres (myofibrils) with alternating dark and light bands (sarcomeres), which produce the striated appearance and provide the contractile function. A flexor (or agonist) muscle contracts, becoming shorter thus moving bones closer to each other. An extensor or antagonist muscle works in the opposite sense.

VOLVULUS a twisting of part of the bowels which usually results in some obstruction which may reduce the blood supply, ending in gangrene. It may right itself spontaneously or may be righted by manipulation. However, surgery is often necessary.

VOMITING (emesis) the reflex action whereby the stomach contents are expelled through the mouth, due to the contraction of the diaphragm and abdominal wall muscles. Vomiting is due to stimulus of the appropriate centre in the brain but the primary agent is usually a sensation from the stomach itself, e.g. a gastric disease, or some irritant. Other causes may be the action of drugs, some effect on the inner ear (e.g. travel sickness), migraines, etc.

VON RECKLINGHAUSEN'S DISEASE a congenital disorder, neuro-fibromatosis, in which soft tissue tumours form along nerves and beneath the skin. There are often other anomalies such as decalcification of bones, FIBROSIS of the lungs and formation of kidney stones.

VULVA the external female genitals comprising two pairs of fleshy folds surrounding the vaginal opening.

VULVECTOMY surgical removal of the VULVA, the extent of which depends upon where there is a malignant or non-malignant growth.

VULVITIS inflammation of the VULVA.

VULVOVAGINITIS inflammation of both the VULVA and VAGINA.

WARFARIN an anticoagulant given to reduce the risk of EMBOLISM. It may be administered orally or by injection and the significant side effect is bleeding, usually from the gums and other mucous membranes.

WART (VERRUCA) a solid, benign growth in the skin caused by a virus. They are infectious and spread rapidly in schools, etc. There are several types: *plantar*, on the foot; *juvenile* in children and *venereal*, on the genitals. Warts often disappear spontaneously, but can be dealt with in several ways, e.g. cryosurgery (freezing), laser treatment, and electrocautery (burning away with an electrically heated wire or needle).

WATER BED a bed with a water-containing mattress which readily accommodates a patient's posture. This is useful to avoid bedsores.

WATER ON THE BRAIN *see* HYDROCEPHALUS.

WEAL (or WHEAL) an area of the skin that is temporarily raised and coloured red, or pale with red margins. It may be due to an allergy (*see also* URTICARIA), nettle rash or a sharp blow, and in the former cases may be accompanied by itching.

WEBBED FINGERS *see* SYNDACTYLY.

WEBER'S TEST assessing a person's deafness using a tuning fork. The stem of a vibrating fork is placed on the forehead or maxillary incisors and if the hearing is normal, the sound is equal in both ears. It helps to diagnose whether hearing loss is due to a middle ear disorder or a neurosensory loss.

WEIL'S DISEASE *see* LEPTOSPIROSIS.

WEN *see* SEBACEOUS CYST.

WERTHHEIM'S HYSTERECTOMY a major form of hysterectomy undertaken to deal with uterine or ovarian cancer. It involves the removal of the uterus, ovaries, Fallopian tubes, upper part of the vagina and the surrounding lymph nodes.

WHEEZE the sound produced by the long drawn-out breathing associated with ASTHMA. It also occurs when bronchial tubes are narrowed, e.g. as in BRONCHITIS.

WHIPLASH INJURY damage caused by the sudden jerking backwards of the head and neck, as in a road accident. A severe whiplash can cause death, but injury is the usual outcome. The vertebrae, spinal cord, ligaments and nerves in the neck may all be damaged. Treatment usually involves wearing a special collar to immobilize the affected area.

WHIPPLE'S DISEASE a rare disease of the intestines resulting in malabsorption of food. Symptoms include anaemia, weight loss, arthritis, skin pigmentation, chest pain and a non-productive cough. It seems to be caused by microorganisms in the mucosa. It responds to extensive antibiotic treatment.

WHITE LEG *see* THROMBOPHLEBITIS.

WHITE MATTER nerve tissue in the CENTRAL NERVOUS SYSTEM, composed primarily of nerve fibres in light-coloured MYELIN sheaths. In the brain it occupies the central part of the cerebral cortex.

WHITLOW inflammation of tissues in the finger tip, and usually an abscess affecting the fat and fibrous tissues that comprise the pulp of the finger.

WHOOP the noisy and characteristic drawing in of breath following a coughing attack in WHOOPING COUGH.

WHOOPING COUGH (*pertussis*) an infectious disease caused by the bacterium *Bordetella pertussis*. The mucous membranes lining the air passages are affected and after a one to two week incubation period, fever, catarrh and a cough develop. The cough then becomes paroxysmal with a number of short coughs punctuated with the 'whooping' drawing in of breath. Nosebleeds and vomiting may follow a paroxysm. After about two weeks the symptoms abate but a cough may continue for some weeks. Whooping cough is not usually serious and immunization reduces the severity of an attack. However, a child may be susceptible to pneumonia and tuberculosis during the disease.

WILM'S TUMOUR a tumour of the kidney (nephroblastoma) in infancy. Early removal of the kidney with radiotherapy and chemotherapy confers a high survival rate.

WINDPIPE see TRACHEA.

WISDOM TOOTH the last (third) molar tooth on each side of either jaw. The teeth normally erupt last, around the age of 20 to 25 although some remain impacted in the jaw bone.

WITHDRAWAL SYMPTOMS a characteristic feature when someone stops using a drug upon which they have become dependent. The hard drugs such as heroin and cocaine induce dependence as does alcohol, nicotine and amphetamines. Symptoms include shivering, tremors, vomiting and sweating.

WOMB see UTERUS.

WOUND a sudden break in the body tissues and/or organs caused by an external agent. There are four types based upon the result of the injury: incisions, punctures, lacerations and contusions.

WRIST the joint between the hand and forearm. The wrist region comprises eight carpal bones and five metacarpal bones joined by strong ligaments. The wrist joint then articulates with the RADIUS and ULNA. The joint can move in all directions with little risk of dislocation.

WRITER'S CRAMP an involuntary contraction of the hand muscles when

writing, but not when using those muscles to undertake other functions. A similar condition may arise with musicians (guitarists and pianists), typists and computer operators.

WRYNECK (TORTICOLLIS) when the head is twisted to one side due to a scar contracting or, more commonly, to excessive muscle contraction.

XANTHELASMA yellow fatty deposits in the eyelids and skin around the eyes. It often occurs in elderly people, when it is insignificant, but a severe case may be due to a fat metabolism disorder.

XANTHOCHROMIA a yellow colouring, e.g. the skin in jaundice, or the cerebrospinal fluid when it contains haemoglobin breakdown products.

X CHROMOSOME the sex chromosome present in male and female although women have a pair, and men just one (with the Y CHROMOSOME). Certain disorders such as HAEMOPHILIA are carried as genes on the X chromosome.

XERODERMA a condition of the skin which manifests itself as a dryness and roughness with the formation of scales. It is a mild form of ICHTHYOSIS.

XIPHOID PROCESS (or **XIPHOID CARTILAGE**) the lowest part of the STERNUM. It is a flat cartilage that is progressively replaced by bone, a process completed sometime after middle age.

X-RAYS the part of the electromagnetic spectrum with waves of wavelength 10^{-12} to 10^{-9}m and frequencies of 10^{17} to 10^{21}Hz. They are produced when high velocity electrons strike a target. The rays penetrate solids to a depth that depends upon the density of the solid.

X-rays of certain wavelengths will penetrate flesh but not bone. They are therefore useful in therapy and diagnosis within medicine.

YAWNING a reflex action when the mouth is opened wide, air drawn into the lungs and slowly released. It is usually, though not exclusively, associated with tiredness or boredom.

YAWS an infectious disease of the tropics caused by a spirochaete (a type of bacterium) *Treponema pertenue*, usually in unhygienic conditions. The bacteria enter through abrasions and after about two weeks, during which time there is fever, pain and itching, small tumours appear each with a yellow crust of dried serum. These may eventually form deep ulcers. The final stages may not appear until after several years and include LESIONS of skin and bone. Fortunately, penicillin works dramatically and effectively in this disease.

Y CHROMOSOME the small chromosome that carries a dominant gene conferring maleness. Normal males have 22 matched chromosome pairs and one unmatched pair comprising one X and one Y chromosome.

During sexual reproduction the mother contributes an X chromosome, but the father contributes an X or Y chromosome, XX produces a female offspring, XY male.

YELLOW FEVER an infectious viral disease in tropical Africa and South America. Transmitted by mosquitoes, it causes tissue degeneration in the liver and kidneys. Symptoms include headache,

back pains, fever, vomiting, jaundice, etc., and an attack can prove fatal. Vaccination will prove effective and anyone recovering from an attack has immunity conferred.

ZIDOVUDINE an antiviral drug (trade name **RETROVIR**) that is used to treat AIDS. Although it slows the growth of the HIV virus, it does not effect a cure.

ZOLLINGER-ELLISON SYNDROME an uncommon disorder resulting in diarrhoea and multiple PEPTIC ULCERS. The cause is a pancreatic tumour or enlarged pancreas which in turn leads to high levels of the hormone gastrin which stimulates excess production of acidic gastric juice, causing the ulceration. Surgery is usually effective.

ZOONOSIS (*plural* **ZOONOSES**) an infectious animal disease that can be transmitted to man. Some of the 150 or so diseases are: anthrax, brucellosis, bovine tuberculosis, Rift Valley fever, rabies, leptospirosis and typhus (*see individual entries*).

ZOOPHOBIA an unnatural and strong fear of animals.

ZYGOMATIC ARCH the arch of bone of either side of the face, below the eyes.

ZYGOMATIC BONE a facial bone and one of a pair of bones that form the prominence of the cheeks.

ZYGOTE the cell produced by the fusion of male and female germ cells (GAMETES) during the early stage of fertilization, i.e. an ovum fertilized by a sperm. After passing down the FALLOPIAN TUBE, it implants in the uterus, forming the embryo.